HIV/AIDS
Global frontiers in prevention/intervention

"This impressive new volume examines HIV/AIDS from a historical, social, political, and biomedical perspective while traversing issues of culture, gender, and geography. Timely and comprehensive, this thought-provoking volume provides a detailed description of the context of HIV/AIDS and invigorates the reader to address this epidemic locally to globally for future generations."

Sally J. Stevens, Women's Studies, University of Arizona

"Bringing together leading experts in the social and behavioral sciences, global health and public policy as well as AIDS activists, this book provides a uniquely clear, balanced and highly readable introduction to HIV and AIDS. The outstanding range of articles—from thoughtful theoretical chapters and case studies on why and how global society has responded to the AIDS epidemic, to individual accounts of working with and living with HIV and AIDS—provides the reader with an excellent understanding of current policies, practices and emerging concerns. An excellent book for any course on AIDS, global health, or social medicine, this book should also be on the bookshelves of practitioners and advocates. It is an important contribution to the field."

Nora Ellen Groce, Yale School of Public Health

This economically and visually appealing reader showcases articles and essays specifically written for this volume, all within an interdisciplinary, global framework. The book includes some of the most well-known HIV researchers along with emerging voices and cutting-edge issues in HIV research, policymaking, and advocacy, and integrates viewpoints from public health, epidemiology, and social and behavioral sciences.

The goal is for this reader to be useful as a foundation text for various university classrooms and serve as a reference book for researchers and libraries.

Cynthia Pope is Associate Professor of Geography at Central Connecticut State University and Lecturer in Global Health at Yale University. Her work deals with the intersections of geopolitics, gender, and HIV risk in the developing world, particularly Latin America and the Caribbean.

Renée T. White is Professor of Sociology and co-director of Black Studies at Fairfield University. She is co-editor of the *Journal of HIV/AIDS Prevention in Children and Youth*. Her research focuses on health disparities, reproductive and AIDS-related social policy, urban inequalities, and social justice.

Robert Malow is Professor of Public Health at Florida International University and is associated editor of *AIDS Education and Prevention*. He has authored over 150 scientific publications and has led over a dozen National Institutes of Health-funded projects in the area of HIV and substance abuse.

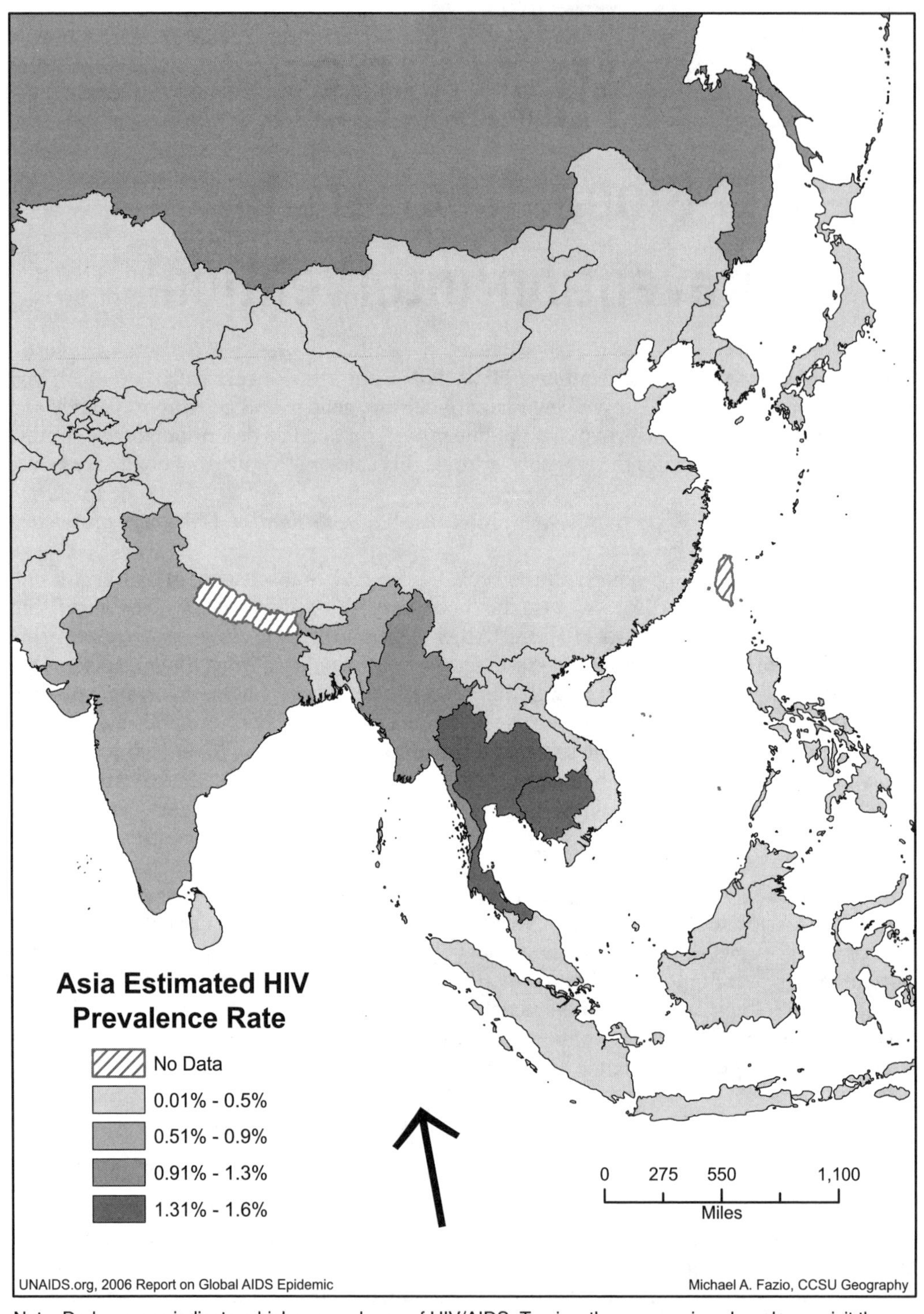

Note: Darker areas indicate a higher prevalence of HIV/AIDS. To view these maps in color, please visit the companion website for this volume at www.routledge.com/textbooks/9780415953832.

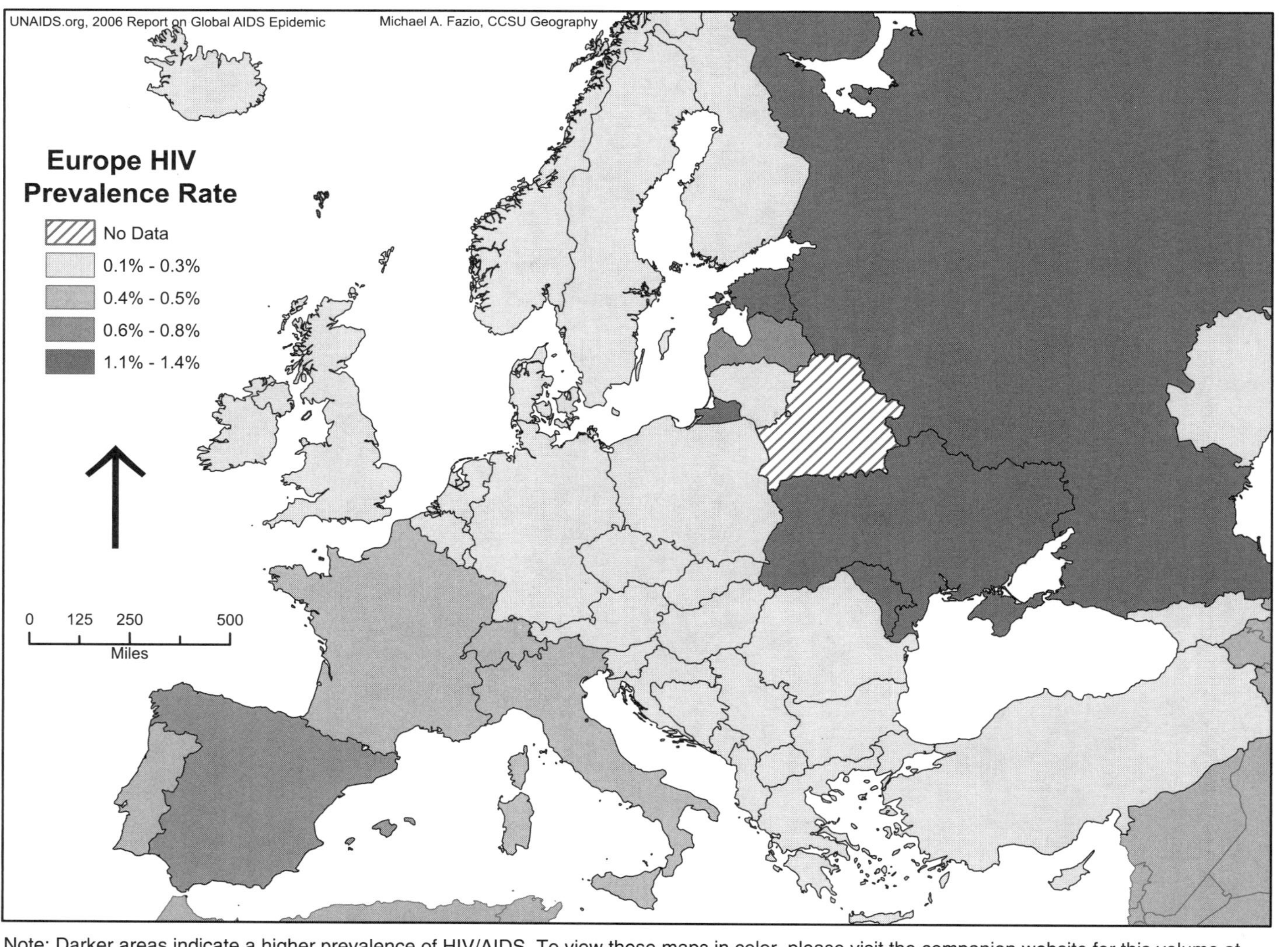

Note: Darker areas indicate a higher prevalence of HIV/AIDS. To view these maps in color, please visit the companion website for this volume at www.routledge.com/textbooks/9780415953832.

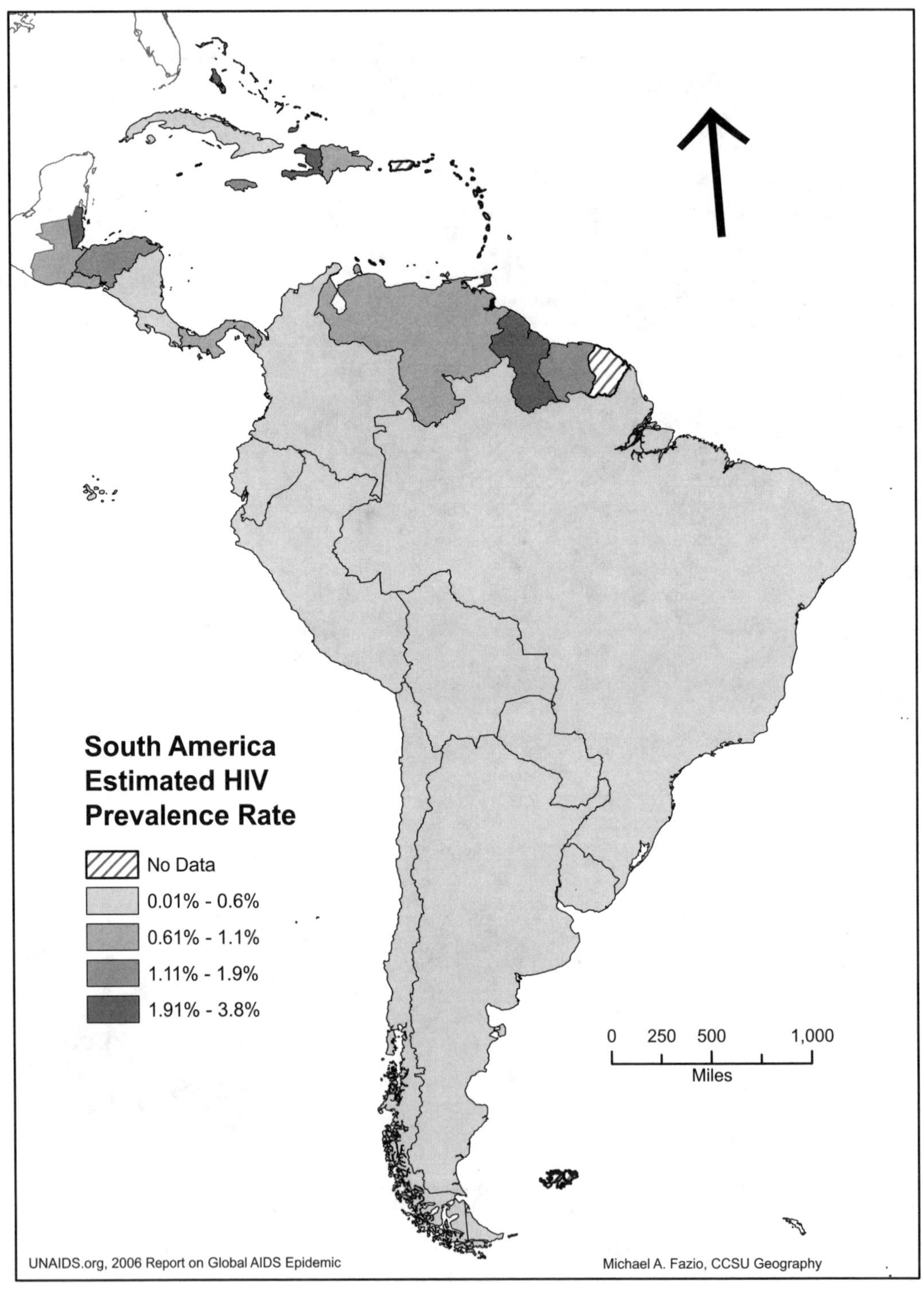

Note: Darker areas indicate a higher prevalence of HIV/AIDS. To view these maps in color, please visit the companion website for this volume at www.routledge.com/textbooks/9780415953832.

HIV/AIDS
Global frontiers in prevention/intervention

Edited by Cynthia Pope, Renée T. White, and Robert Malow

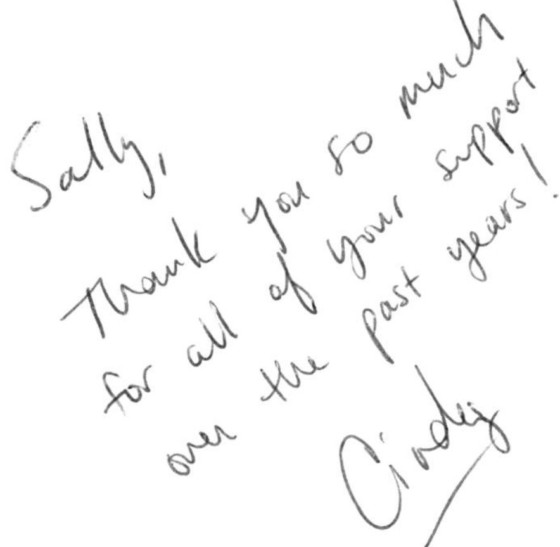

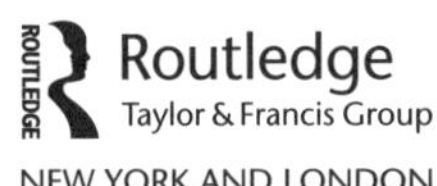

NEW YORK AND LONDON

First published 2009
by Routledge
270 Madison Ave, New York, NY 10016

Simultaneously published in the UK
by Routledge
2 Park Square, Milton Park, Abingdon, Oxon OX14 4RN

Routledge is an imprint of the Taylor & Francis Group, an informa business

Typeset in Sabon by RefineCatch Limited, Bungay, Suffolk
Printed and bound in the United States of America on acid-free paper by
Edwards Brothers, Inc

Library of Congress Cataloging-in-Publication Data
HIV/AIDS : stories of a global epidemic / edited by Cynthia Pope, Renée T. White, and Robert Malow.
p. ; cm.
Includes bibliographical references.
1. AIDS (Disease)—Cross-cultural studies. 2. HIV infections—Cross-cultural studies. I. Pope, Cynthia. II. White, Renée T. III. Malow, Robert.
[DNLM: 1. Acquired Immunodeficiency Syndrome. 2. HIV Infections. 3. Disease Outbreaks. 4. Health Planning. 5. Health Policy. 6. Risk Assessment. WC 503 H6729 2008]
RA643.8.H578 2008
362.196′9792—dc22
2007052736

ISBN10: 0–415–95382–0 (hbk)
ISBN10: 0–415–95383–9 (pbk)

ISBN13: 978–0–415–95382–5 (hbk)
ISBN13: 978–0–415–95383–2 (pbk)

CONTENTS

SECTION 5. POLICIES OF (IN)JUSTICE: STRUCTURAL RESPONSES TO HIV

SECTION 6. MEDIA AND HIV/AIDS

SECTION 7. VULNERABLE POPULATIONS: CONFLICT, NATURAL DISASTER, AND MIGRATION

ACKNOWLEDGMENTS

The authors would like to thank Joseph Parys, Brendan Kelly, Elaine Samsell, Heather Webb for her research assistance, cartographer Mike Fazio, and graduate assistant Bethany Dunbar. The cartogram on the cover was created by Dr Mark Newman, University of Michigan.

ILLUSTRATIONS

Maps

FOREWORD

Globalization, Vulnerability, and the Response to HIV and AIDS

In less than three decades, the global HIV epidemic has rapidly emerged to become one of the most complex problems facing the contemporary world. From initial reports of scattered cases among what were perceived to be relatively small and socially marginal groups such as gay men and injecting drug users, HIV and AIDS have rapidly evolved to be among the most important issues of public health globally. The epidemic has impacted severely upon social and economic development, and has more recently been identified as a growing threat to national and international security. From its devastating effects in specific societies (both north and south of the equator) to its perceived potential at a global level, in a remarkably short period of time HIV and AIDS have changed the way we think and the way we live in communities and countries around the world. This book is an attempt to analyze some of these changes—to explore the forces that have shaped the global epidemic, the communities that it has affected, the ways in which governments and institutions have responded, and the lessons that this experience might be able to teach us if only we were willing to learn.

One of the key insights that forms the basis for the selection of texts included in this volume is an understanding of the extent to which a range of structural inequalities intersect and combine to shape the character of HIV and AIDS everywhere, both North and South, in resource-rich and resource-poor countries. In all societies, regardless of their degree of development or prosperity, the HIV epidemic affects the most marginalized sectors of society, living in situations characterized by diverse forms of structural violence. It is in the spaces of poverty, racism, gender inequality and sexual oppression that vulnerability to HIV infection is greatest—in large part unencumbered by formal public health and education programs and barely impacted upon by the advances in treatment therapies and access that have taken place in recent years. It is from the growing polarization between the very rich and the very poor, from the exclusion of whole segments of society, together with the perverse integration of others (for example, in criminal economies or informal labor markets), and from increasing forms of social and economic inequality (that appear to be such an integral part of the processes of globalization based upon neoliberal economic policies), that the HIV epidemic has gained strength. Perhaps no other major global health problem so clearly has its origins in, and reflects, the unequal social, political, and economic architecture of the contemporary world system.

These are the kinds of issues that the analyses brought together in this volume seek to develop and extend—offering key insights into the broad range of structural factors that have shaped the epidemic and conditioned our responses to it. Now, more than ever, it is crucial that we work to analyze and understand these social, cultural, and economic processes. Clearly, research and analysis has a key role to play in seeking to build the intellectual bridges that will be necessary in order to understand the health consequences of the models of social and economic development that have been pursued globally in recent decades—and the ways in which these models have contributed to new forms of insecurity in the world we now live in. It is within this context that it is crucial to develop an understanding of the broader structural forces that have shaped HIV and AIDS as a kind of quintessential epidemic of a truly globalized world. The future of the global epidemic, and of the millions of lives affected by it, depends upon our ability to develop this understanding, and to build upon it in seeking to confront the challenges posed by HIV and AIDS for communities and societies around the world.

Beyond critique and careful analysis, however, it is essential to take action, bringing hope to those communities most affected by HIV and AIDS, and utilizing the insights and skills that have arisen in response to the epidemic. Nowhere is this more important than in relation to the greater involvement of people living with HIV in the national and international response. For if there is one thing that the epidemic has taught us, it is that the seeds to success have their origins in the actions of communities most affected. Only by working together and in partnership can advance take place. The texts included in this volume make a key contribution in this direction, opening up new insights and stimulating new debates that take crucial steps forward in responding to HIV and AIDS in the contemporary world.

Peter Aggleton
Institute of Education, University of London
Richard Parker
Mailman School of Public Health, Columbia University

December 2007

OVERVIEW

Global Convergences: Emerging Issues in HIV Risk, Prevention, and Treatment

Cynthia Pope, Renée T. White, and Robert Malow

The purpose of this reader is to present cutting-edge research and emerging issues in HIV research, advocacy, and policies at both the U.S. and international scales. Using primarily original manuscripts, the volume presents work from established scholars, international policymakers, activists, and people living with HIV. In this way, we hope to provide a fertile ground for discussing the emerging, and sometimes controversial, issues about HIV in the classroom setting. This book uses globalization and global processes as a lens to interpret the current underpinnings of HIV theory and vulnerability as well as the emerging debates and future issues. As the three editors of this volume represent different disciplinary approaches to the HIV/AIDS pandemic, they bring various perspectives to this collection, and indeed to the evolution of research, policymaking, and activism surrounding HIV globally.

A hitherto-unnamed cancer (Kaposi's syndrome) became the first alert to the epidemic over twenty-five years ago when it was detected in a small group of men who had sex with men in the western United States (Centers for Disease Control and Prevention 2006). It was soon thereafter that HIV was isolated and named in France, and then found in other parts of the world. Quickly, the "4-Hs" became designated HIV risk groups (hemophiliacs, homosexuals, heroin addicts, Haitians). However, after these original labels, the definition of HIV vulnerability shifted to behavior, and then once again more recently to encompass structure and ecology in terms of risky conditions. Now, with important work by Farmer (2005), Patton (2002), and others (D'Adesky 2004; Engel 2006), we see that behavior is couched in terms of social and built environments as well as structural forces that can contribute to risk (Frye et al. 2006).

As AIDS became truly global by the late 1980s, social scientists and critics responded to the various social movements to call attention to the fact that HIV was, more than anything else, a disease of marginalization (Kramer 1994). Even as new drugs were being developed in the late 1980s and early 1990s, the issue of access, and thus social and economic marginality, particularly in the United States, became pivotal. Eventually, protests in front of government buildings in the United States that opened up access to the first round of protease inhibitors (refer to Kaiser Family Foundation timeline on pages 551–62; ACT-UP 1990; Kramer 1994; Crimp 1988; Rimmerman 2007).

The expansion in research focus (from risky groups to risky environments) followed HIV's progression from a localized population-specific phenomenon to a global pandemic. Instead of men who have sex with men being the most vulnerable group, we now see that women have become increasingly more vulnerable for biological, social, and political reasons (Go et al. 2003; Gupta and Weiss this volume; Kelly et al. 2004; Kramer 1994; Taigy Thomas et al. this volume; Turmen 2003). The regional impact of HIV has shifted, as well. While sub-Saharan African countries continue to be hit hardest by this modern plague, India and China are emerging as areas of concern, particularly as more data has become available. Another emergent region is Central Asia and the former Soviet republics, as two authors in this volume describe (Hankivsky and Atlani-Duault). Thus, it is becoming impossible to pigeonhole risk groups or risky regions given the widespread diffusion of the virus.

Thus, an important framework in this book is the examination of HIV transmission and risk at various scales from the very local (such as the household) to the international (including international organizations, such as UNAIDS, the Global Fund, World Bank) (De Cock and Weiss 2006; Garrett and Rosenstein 2005). Another important aspect to highlight is the intersections of these chapters. While the sections were organized to maintain balance and present global impacts on the pandemic, the reader will notice that there are chapters that have some overlapping ideas. This is intended to show how different disciplines interpret various themes in HIV transmission, prevention, and treatment.

Having stated that marginality (economic, political, social, sexual orientation) is one of the primary reasons for HIV transmission, we must delve deeper into social structures to understand why women, who are certainly not a minority in the world, are most at risk to contract HIV in most societies. Indeed, women have traditionally played the role of villain in the spread of HIV, as they can be considered the "fifth H" in the "4-H" category of risk groups—hookers. Women in the early epidemic were relegated to the role of prostitutes (and later, more accurately, commercial sex workers) as "reservoirs of disease," waiting to infect unsuspecting males (Chan and Reidpath 2003; Gilman 1988; Sacks 1996). Later, this locus of blame expanded to include their reproductive role (mother-to-child transmission through childbirth and breastfeeding). As the virus has spread beyond social boundaries, though, women are becoming infected with greater frequency. It is not only women in these marginalized social settings, but also those who represent traditional gender norms (see Cheng this volume). By virtue of their roles, they often acquire the virus from their male partners' behaviors, whether sexual or otherwise.

In conjunction with marginalization, the second social epidemiological fact of the epidemic has become the growing shift from an acute to a chronic disease. Given that more people living with HIV/AIDS (PLWHA) are gaining access to increasingly improved antiretroviral medications, there is and will continue to be enhancement in longevity, health, and sexual desire in these infected individuals. This in turn will increase the likelihood of further viral spread and further psychosocial complexity to prevention. This is particularly true with around forty million people currently living with the virus. Given the genetic make-up of the virus and the facility with which it mutates, there is no evidence that a vaccine will become the panacea needed to save many people and several countries in the world (Cohen 2001). Indeed, the traditional issue of lack of access to heath care in the poorest countries will continue to affect lack of access to HIV medications as well (Gallo 2005, 2006).

We realize that HIV readers can become quickly out of date, because information surrounding the virus changes rapidly, HIV research has become more popular, and research funding has increased exponentially since the early days of the epidemic. Given the number of publications on HIV, as editors we understand that it is a daunting task for students or new researchers to even find a place to begin their work. We also acknowledge that there is no single reader that can accurately depict all facets of HIV. Taking these three concerns into account, we decided to focus on intersections of the social and behavioral sciences, emphasizing global contexts and concerns. While biological advancements are beginning to emerge because of the genomic revolution, significant translation into pharmacological remediation and clinical settings has not yet resulted, leaving the social and behavioral sciences as a core anchor for prevention research and for understanding the myriad complicated and overlapping concerns that individuals living with HIV deal with on a daily basis. Also, thematically, we decided on these sections as they are fertile ground for some of the most exciting research and activism currently taking place.

In Section 1, the authors present contemporary theories and case studies of harm reduction and HIV risk. While heroin addicts were accused as being one of the risk groups causing diffusion of HIV in the early 1980s, literature on this behavior has become more theoretical and multidisciplinary. Burris et al.'s framing essay contextualizes the section with a social ecological model that highlights the importance of structural interventions internationally. Duke et al. and Clair et al. provide case studies from emerging epidemics in China and Brazil, respectively. Brazil will continue to be a country of interest as the government has refused United States' economic aid for HIV programs due to several onerous provisions, including requiring a faith-based (Christian) model, promoting abstinence, and targeting sex workers (D'Adesky 2004). Comfort uses a social ecology approach to frame the issues of HIV in correctional institutions in the United States.

As part of Section 1, it must be mentioned that syringe exchange programs (SEPs) are increasingly important for harm reduction among injection drug users. SEPs can be conceptualized as the prototypical harm reduction intervention for injection drug users (Ksobiech and Malow 2005) and international evidence reviewed in Semaan, Des Jarlais, and Malow (2007) and Wodak and Cooney (2006) indicates strong support for this approach in reducing HIV and other sexually transmitted infections. Given that cost-effectiveness (such as societal savings for infections averted through SEP services) has been well documented (Ksobiech and Malow 2005), a crucial next step is to begin governmental funding of SEPs, and associated programs, to reduce harm to injection drug users (IDUs) personally and the community overall. This is now occurring in many locales (e.g., San Francisco, New York, Amsterdam, Rio de Janeiro). However, there has been considerable resistance to this effort at the federal level in the United States. Although certain locations have initiated programs, solutions to public and political concerns have not been adequately focused on by public health professionals and elected officials. Problem-solving models from other contentious public policy domains, such as natural resource management, need to be utilized in this effort, in order to shift the dialogue from conflict to negotiation. Public health models, such as Community Readiness, discussed in McCoy et al.'s chapter in this volume, could also be applied to this effort.

Section 2 focuses on gender, sexuality, and HIV risk globally. This theme has continued to evolve and influence research and policymaking since the 1980s. The chapters address women's vulnerabilities for HIV, as well as issues of masculinity and HIV transmission. The framing essay, by Gupta and Weiss, sets the context for preventing HIV in women who have sex with men and lays out a framework for addressing gender inequalities within the context of HIV prevention programming. Through the focus on HIV globally, the inherent or potential dangers of women's traditional roles have come to the forefront. Rosenberg and Malow, for example, highlight that biology, in addition to social structures, must be understood to properly flesh out arguments about, and programs on, women's vulnerability to HIV. Orchard et al. analyze the cultural systems of Karnataka and Rajasthan that produce sex work as a community-sanctioned occupation. Another articulation of sexuality, gender, and ethnicity is salient in Dilger's work in Tanzania. Both Hankivsky and Atlani-Duault highlight Central Asia, although with different foci. Hankivsky's case study addresses the growing needs of HIV positive women in Ukraine, while Atlani-Dualt uses a sociohistorical framework to analyze how Central Asian men who have sex with men have been targets of social and legal discrimination. However, paradoxically, the pandemic there has also provided an opportunity for self-identified homosexual men to fight for civil rights. Also focusing on men, Thomas et al. discuss the Philippines as an example of a country with limited resources which can serve as an example of how to maintain a low HIV rate.

Section 3 examines the intersections of biomedicine and more recent literature addressing the development, starting in 1996, of a new generation of HIV medication, protease inhibitors. Jones provides an overview of HIV antiretroviral drugs (ARVs) from AZT and HAART in the 1990s to more recent ARV medications. Sylla and Kaplan offer the possibility of Microbicides as another technological advance to decrease women's risk for HIV. Particularly important is the fact that women would be able to use Microbicides as an undetectable method to protect themselves from possible HIV and other sexually transmitted infections.

Durvasula et al. highlight some of the most cutting-edge interdisciplinary research in biology and behavioral sciences by showing that HIV decision-making can be impacted by the spread of the disease throughout the biological system, by a drug regimen, or co-infection with other diseases, such as tuberculosis. Simoni et al. provide an overview of drug regimen adherence issues worldwide, followed by Berkley-Patton et al., who offer a case study of success stories about ARV adherence.

Section 4 focuses on intervention and prevention programs from different cultural contexts around the world. The framing essay by DiClemente et al. highlights recent scholarship on an often-overlooked population—adolescents. The authors anchor HIV in terms of other sexually transmitted infections and the effect worldwide of these infections among adolescents. McCoy et al. examine the Community Readiness Model of HIV prevention as applied in the U.S. Virgin Islands, while Dévieux et al. examine sociocultural barriers to care among Haitians living with HIV, discussing not only prevention programs but also treatment protocols. Haiti is a particularly important country to examine because of its central role in the history and stigmatization of HIV. Ibembe also highlights an important and controversial program of the ABC HIV prevention strategy (Abstain, Be faithful, use Condoms), from his perspective as a Ugandan policymaker. Goggin et al. provide the first published data showing the importance of traditional health providers for the treatment of South Africans. The authors highlight that traditional and allopathic healers must work together in a complementary, rather than a contradictory, manner to improve HIV treatment adherence.

Section 5 deals implicitly with the idea of structural responses to HIV, which were highlighted in the first section of the introduction. This section shows that social, economic, political, and historical structures are at the heart of transmission, prevention, and treatment. In the framing essay, by White, Pope, and Malow, the interplay of economic policies and structural responses are examined in terms of how they contribute to a social justice framework. Craddock continues with a social justice paradigm by examining whether the patterns of this pandemic, as dictated by political, economic, and pharmaceutical structures, can be deemed genocidal in sub-Saharan Africa. Craddock uses the example of the TRIPS program, which requires all countries to buy HIV drugs from certain pharmaceutical companies by 2020. Bayer and Oppenheimer continue the section's themes, using ethnographic techniques to highlight the personal experiences of structural constraints of ARV therapies in South Africa, while Frasca examines the structures that have led to HIV transmission in Latin America. Unlike Africa, Latin America has received relatively little international media attention and global funding. One of the reasons is the relatively low rates of HIV compared with other affected regions, but Frasca argues that there are still communities with high rates of HIV that cannot go overlooked. Padamsee discusses the national policies of the United States and the United Kingdom, highlighting that different health care systems and cultural philosophies lead to the creation of different programs. Estrada and Estrada also utilize a structural framework, but in a unique context, the United States–Mexico border. As the longest border between an economically developing and developed country, this border is a focus of contested policy debate on immigration and related health and social policy concerns. The United States side receives federal funding for building more border walls and increasing the border patrol presence, but it receives very little funding for health care or other social services required by HIV-positive individuals living in the area.

Section 6 examines how the media portrays HIV/AIDS and the influence of media globally in prevention and treatment practices. Noar's framing essay traces the history of "old" and "new" media by examining mass communication campaigns and newer computer and internet-based interventions. Kylie Thomas views media in a different light by showing how photojournalist Gideon Mendel's photographs of people living with HIV/AIDS were a way to contest the South African government's portrayal of HIV/AIDS. Barker examines yet another route of communication, the soap opera, and its effects on individuals across the globe.

Finally, Cheng, in a very moving personal narrative, tells of becoming involved with the Cambodian media after she discovers she is infected with HIV.

Spiegel and Bennedsen's essay anchors section 7 on the relationship between vulnerable populations and geography, whether geography means living in environmentally susceptible areas (such as hurricane and earthquake zones) or living in or near war zones. Wagner et al. discuss the interrelated factors of Hurricane Katrina, post-traumatic stress disorder, and substance abuse on HIV risk. Kalipeni, Oppong, and Gosh focus on sub-Saharan geography to examine the interplay of history, political economy, and environment to contextualize HIV in the region. Westerhaus et al. research conflict zones in Africa and present evidence that individual behavior modification must be couched in culturally and historically specific terms. Repercussions of war not only lead to widespread rape of women (and thus an important transmission route to consider), but also hinders the development of a sound health care system and transportation routes. This section also addresses another influential geographic aspect—migration. This topic is addressed by McLean, who calls for more attention to adolescents and other groups in the Caribbean who are mobile and vulnerable to HIV.

As more individuals become infected with HIV, it is important to use their experiences to create effective prevention and treatment programs. The authors in Section 8 advocate integrating the experiences of people living with HIV/AIDS (PLWHA) into policymaking at local, national, and global levels. Faubion's framing essay captures the most recent publications contextualizing the various meanings that living with HIV has taken around the world, as well as the roles of stigma in susceptibility to HIV. Mary Fisher, a well-known artist and AIDS advocate, first came into the U.S. national spotlight as a keynote speaker during the Republican National Convention in 1992. Her work for this volume emphasizes the need for advocates and policymakers to work together to create innovative responses to the pandemic. Aspaas uses rural East African communities to show another facet of living with HIV, that of the caregivers. These caregivers illustrate the resilience of individuals in regions and communities with a high rate of HIV and how they have formed a safety net for orphans in lieu of state programs. Mayer shows that a connection between academia and advocacy is possible through his personal narrative of working in Ghana with patients who have HIV. The final chapter of the section, by Moore, also takes place in Africa. She presents results from a study exploring the meanings that seropositive parents and seronegative caregivers give to their experiences as a way of coping effectively with the physical and mental challenges of caregiving.

The final section, Section 9, deals explicitly with globalization, providing an anchor for this book. While from different disciplinary and geographic backgrounds, each author highlights the importance of dealing with local constraints and opportunities when addressing HIV. Friedman et al., for example, write in their framing essay about globalization and other large-scale social and economic processes affecting transmission. These processes include wars (addressed by others in Section 7), falling profit rates, sociopolitical transitions, and even global warming, among others. Myers and Kearns employ a health geography framework to explore the HIV-positive body as a site of struggle, leading to newer understandings of the role of globalization on conceptions of the body and its place (literal and metaphorical) in New Zealand society. Patton highlights a critical aspect of global policy, that of managing the different levels of HIV medications delivery in the World Health Organization's "3X5" Program. She highlights the challenges in reconciling different levels of frameworks (community through international) when translating biomedical science into public health policy. Sufian uses a regional approach to highlight an area that is often overlooked in HIV research and funding, the Middle East and North Africa. The little attention the region has received has focused recently on a case in which foreign doctors and nurses worked in a Libyan hospital where HIV was transmitted to children. The doctors and nurses were sentenced to death before an international negotiating team was able to get them extradited to their home countries. However, there is a dire need for more research in this region, particularly given the misconceptions about religion, gender, and cultural constructions of meanings about HIV. The final chapter in this book, by Nguyen represents one direction in which research on HIV at the global scale is heading. Nguyen highlights the different ways in which policy responses to HIV enhance and reproduce processes of globalization. Thus HIV is not only a product of global process, but also creates global linkages. Not only does globalization produce the circumstances for the transmission of HIV around the world, but HIV itself serves as a way to increase international interaction.

FUTURE RESEARCH DIRECTIONS INTO GLOBALIZATION AND HIV

Since globalization is a dynamic phenomenon, and the AIDS pandemic affects societies from the macro-structural to the individual levels, it would be impossible for this book to provide an exhaustive review of the emergent issues and hot spots of HIV incidence. For example, recent research about the MSM (men who have sex with men) community and re-emerging HIV is important to examine. There is evidence that the new generation of gay men, particularly in Western Europe and North America, feel removed from the virus and the political and social action of elders in their community (Fenton and Imrie 2005).

One of the newest, and most controversial, prevention methods to be espoused by the World Health Organization includes male circumcision. The controversy highlights an important issue in HIV research and prevention policies globally—a fissure between public health officials and those concerned with the implications of colonialism and imperialism on the male African body, a history that began with colonialism and may be perpetuated with this sort of policy (Aggleton 2007; Niang and Boiro 2007). One of the most neglected resources for the international community in addressing the meanings and safety of circumcision is in the public health and medical research in Israel, which not only has a long history with the procedure, but also a rare experience of diverse immigrant experiences, particularly from Africa (Schenker 2007; UNAIDS 2006; Weiss and Polonsky 2007). Interestingly, an emerging issue that has received very little attention to date is female circumcision, and the repercussions that using dirty razor blades or scissors may have on HIV transmission.

Another important development is the co-infection between tuberculosis, hepatitis, and HIV. Recent clinical research has begun to explore whether co-infection results in the emergence of a drug-resistant strain of HIV. There have been news reports of such a super-strain in New York City since 2005, but recent research indicates that, while virulent, it appears to be more difficult to transmit (Russell 2005).

We also would have liked to cover the newer faith-based approaches in more depth. The United States has launched a multi-year $15-billion HIV-reduction and prevention global initiative. This has the potential to make ARVs more accessible to people in the most affected regions of the world. However, there has been expressed concern that the donor's political and theological stances could impede the success of programs (Pope and White 2003).

REFERENCES AND FURTHER READING

ACT UP/New York Women and AIDS. *Women, AIDS, and Activism*, Boston: South End Press, 1990.

Aggleton, Peter. "'Just a Snip'?: A Social History of Male Circumcision." *Reproductive Health Matters* 15(29) (2007): 15–21.

Centers for Disease Control and Prevention. "25 Years of AIDS: Current and Former CDC HIV/AIDS Leaders to Discuss State of U.S. Epidemic Centers for Disease Control and Prevention." May 5, 2006. http://www.kaisernetwork.org/health_cast/uploaded_files/050506_kff_cdc_transcript.pdf

Chan, Kit Yee and Daniel D. Reidpath. "'Typhoid Mary' and 'HIV Jane': Responsibility, Agency and Disease Prevention." *Reproductive Health Matters* 11(22), 2003: 40–50.

Cohen, Jon. *Shots in the Dark: The Wayward Search for an AIDS Vaccine*. New York and London: W.W. Norton and Company, 2001.

Crimp, Douglas (ed.) *AIDS: Cultural Analysis Cultural Activism*, Cambridge, MA: MIT Press, 1988.

D'Adesky, A.-C. *Moving Mountains: The Race to Treat Global AIDS*. London and New York: Verso, 2004.

De Cock, K.M. and H.A. Weiss. "The Global Epidemiology of HIV/AIDS." *Tropical Medicine and International Health* 5(7) (2000): A3–A9.

Engel, Jonathan. *The Epidemic: A Global History of AIDS*. New York: Smithsonian Books, 2006.

Farmer, Paul. *Pathologies of Power: Health, Human Rights, and the New War on the Poor*. Berkeley and Los Angeles: University of California Press, 2005.

Fenton, K.A. and J. Imrie. "Increasing Rates of Sexually Transmitted Diseases in Homosexual Men in Western Europe and the United States: Why?" *Infectious Disease Clinics of North America* 19 (2005): 311–331.

Frye V, M.H. Latka, B. Koblin, P.N. Halkitis, S. Putnam, S. Galea, and D. Vlahov. "The Urban Environment and Sexual Risk Behavior Among Men Who Have Sex with Men." *Journal of Urban Health* 83(2) (2006): 308–324.

Gallo, R.C. "The End of the Beginning of the Drive to an HIV-Preventive Vaccine: a view from over 20 Years." *Lancet* 366 (2005): 1894–1898.

Gallo, R.C. "A Reflection on HIV/AIDS Research after 25 Years." *Retrovirology* 3(72) (2006). http://www.retrovirology.com/content/3/1/72

Garrett, L. and S. Rosenstein. "Missed Opportunities." *Harvard International Review*. 27(1) (2005): 64–69.

Gilman, S. *Disease and Representation: Images from Madness to AIDS*. Ithaca, NY: Cornell University Press, 1988.

Go, V.F., C.J. Sethulakshmi, M.E. Bentley, S. Sivaram, A.K. Srikrishnan, S. Solomon, and D.D. Celentano. "When HIV-Prevention Messages and Gender Norms Clash: The Impact of Domestic Violence on Women's HIV Risk in Slums of Chennai, India." *AIDS and Behavior* 7(3) (2003): 263–272.

Gruskin, S., L. Ferguson, and D. O. Bogecho. "Beyond the Numbers: Using Rights-Based Perspectives to Enhance Antiretroviral Treatment Scale-Up." *AIDS* 21(Suppl 5) (2007): S13–S19.

Hirsch, J, R.G. Parker, and P. Aggleton. "Social Aspects of Antiretroviral Therapy Scale-Up: Introduction and Overview." *AIDS*. 2(Suppl 5) (2007): S1–S4.

Hoffman, S., T. M. Exner, C.-S. Leu, A.A. Ehrhardt, and Z. Stein. "Female-Condom Use in a Gender-Specific Family Planning Clinic Trial." *American Journal of Public Health* 93(11) (2003): 1897–1903.

Kaiser Family Foundation. "HIV/AIDS Global Policy Fact Sheet." 2006. http://www.kff.org/hivaids/upload/3030-07.pdf

Kelly, J.A., A. Amirkhanian, E.K. Abakchieva, P. Csepe, D.W. Seal, R. Antonova, A. Mihaylov, and G. Gyukits. "Gender Roles and HIV Sexual Risk Vulnerability of Roma (Gypsies) Men and Women in Bulgaria and Hungary: An Ethnographic Study." *AIDS Care* 16(2) (2004): 231–246.

Kramer, L. *Reports from the Holocaust: The Story of an AIDS Activist*. New York: St. Martin's, 1994.

Ksobiech, K. and R. Malow. "Injection Drug Use, Poverty, and HIV among U.S. minorities: The necessity of targeted intervention approaches." *Newsletter of Addiction Division of the American Psychological Association* 12(2) (2005): 10–12.

Lichtenstein, B. "Stigma as a Barrier to Treatment of Sexually Transmitted Infection in the American Deep South: Issues of Race, Gender and Poverty." *Social Science and Medicine* 57(12) (2003): 2434–2445.

Nguyen, V.-K., C.Y. Ako, P. Niamba, A. Sylla, and I. Tiendrébéogo. "Adherence as therapeutic citizenship: impact of the history of access to antiretroviral drugs on adherence to treatment." *AIDS* 21(Suppl 5) (2007): S31–S35.

Niang, C.I. and H. Boiro. "You Can Also Cut My Finger!: Social Construction of Male Circumcision in West Africa, A Case Study of Senegal and Guinea-Bissau." *Reproductive Health Matters* 15(29) (2007): 22–32.

Patton, C. *Globalizing AIDS*. Minneapolis and London: University of Minnesota Press, 2002.

Pope, C. and R. White. "Keep Ideology Out of Fight against AIDS." *Hartford Courant*, Op-Ed article, February 24, 2003.

Pope, C. and R. White. "Global Impact: U.S. Sexual Health and Reproductive Policy." In *21st Century Sexualities*, ed. G. Herdt and C. Howe, New York: Routledge, 2007.

Rimmerman, C.A. "ACT UP." http://www.thebody.com/content/art14001.html. Accessed November 15, 2007.

Russell, S. "Conference Questions 'Super-Strain' of HIV Experts Unsure if N.Y. Case is Unique or a General Threat." *San Francisco Chronicle* A3, February 25, 2005.

Sacks, V. "Women and AIDS: An Analysis of Media Misrepresentations." *Social Science and Medicine* 42(1) (1996): 59–73.

Santana. "AIDS Prevention, Treatment and Care in Cuba." In *AIDS in Africa and the Caribbean*, ed. G.C. Bond, J. Kreniske, I. Susser, and J. Vincent, 65–84. Boulder, CO: Westview Press, 1997.

Schenker, I. "Managing Adult Male Circumcision for HIV/AIDS Prevention in Africa: A Model for International Health Workforce Collaboration in an Urgent Public Health Crisis." Presentation: American Public Health Association, Washington, DC, 2007.

Semaan, S., D.C. Des Jarlais, and R.M. Malow. "Sexually Transmitted Diseases among Illicit Drug Users in the United States: The Need for Interventions." In *Behavioral Interventions for Prevention and Control of Sexually Transmitted Diseases*, ed. S.O. Aral, J.M. Douglas Jr., 297–432. New York: Springer Science, 2007.

Shilts, R. *And the Band Played On: Politics, People, and the AIDS Epidemic*. New York: St. Martin's Press, 1987.

Steen, R. and G. Dallabetta. "Sexually Transmitted Infection Control with Sex Workers: Regular Screening and

Presumptive Treatment Augment Efforts to Reduce Risk and Vulnerability." *Reproductive Health Matters* 11(22) (2003): 74–90.

Treichler, P. "AIDS, Homophobia and Biomedical Discourse: An Epidemic of Signification." *Cultural Studies* 43 (1987): 31–70.

Turmen, T. "Gender and HIV/AIDS." *International Journal of Gynecology and Obstetrics* 82 (2003): 411–418.

UNAIDS. "Israel—HIV Education in a Multi-Cultural Society." 2006. http://www.unaids.org/en/PhotoGallery/2006/20060829-israel/20061011-israel01.asp. Accessed November 15, 2007.

Weiss, H. and J. Polonsky. *Male Circumcision: Global Trends and Determinants of Prevalence, Safety and Acceptability*. World Health Organization and UNAIDS, 2007. http://www.who.int/hiv/topics/malecircumcision/JC1320_MaleCircumcision_Final_UNAIDS.pdf

Wodak, A. and A. Cooney. "Do Needle Syringe Programs Reduce HIV Infection among Injecting Drug Users: A Comprehensive Review of the International Evidence." *Substance Use and Misuse*. 41(6–7) (2006): 777–813.

SECTION 1

Evolving Theories of Harm Reduction and HIV Risk

FRAMING ESSAY

Addressing the "Risk Environment" for Injection Drug Users

The Mysterious Case of the Missing Cop[1]

Scott Burris, Martin Donoghoe, Kim M. Blankenship, Susan Sherman, Jon S. Vernick, Patricia Case, Zita Lazzarini, and Steve Koester

ABSTRACT

Ecological models of the determinants of health and the consequent importance of structural interventions have been widely accepted, but operationalizing these models in research and practice has been challenging. This chapter reviews international evidence that laws and law enforcement practices influence IDU risk. It argues that more research is needed at four levels—laws; management of law enforcement agencies; knowledge, attitudes, beliefs and practices of front-line officers; and attitudes and experiences of IDUs—and that such research can be the basis of interventions within law enforcement to enhance IDU health.

OVERVIEW

In many places in the world, injection drug users (IDUs) are at a heightened risk of tuberculosis (TB), HIV, hepatitis C virus (HCV), hepatitis B virus (HBV), and other sexually transmitted infections, and face a significant risk of fatal overdose. Despite a growing awareness in public health of the need to address risk-determining factors in the social and physical environment, investigators seeking to unravel causes and cures for blood-borne disease among IDUs long turn to a set of usual suspects: individual risk factors and educational or behavioral interventions. While acknowledging the importance of a comprehensive approach to IDUs' health, including behavioral interventions and access to drug treatment, the available evidence points to a promising new target: the criminal justice system. From the laws on the books, through police practices on the streets, through the operation of courts, to the conditions of prisons and jail, the criminal justice system contributes significantly to the shape of everyday life among IDUs living at or beyond the margins of legality. In this chapter, we argue that greater attention to and work with law enforcement should be an important public health priority. After describing the ecological approach that comprises the framework of this chapter, we will review the evidence that law and law enforcement practices are influencing the spread of communicable disease among IDUs, and then discuss the implications of this for public health research and intervention.

AN ECOLOGICAL APPROACH TO PUBLIC HEALTH AND THE LAW

An enduring strain of thinking in epidemiology and public health ascribes to the social and physical environment a crucial role in determining a population's level and distribution of health (Berkman and Kawachi 2000; Krieger 2001; Link and Phelan 1995; Susser and Susser 1996a, 1996b). This ecological approach to health focuses on how social, political, and economic factors as well as characteristics of the physical environment interact with personal characteristics to determine health. Such an approach is at once "big," in that it identifies pervasive characteristics of social ordering (such as inequality (Kawachi 2000) and collective efficacy (Sampson and Morenoff 2000)) that are linked to distributions of health, and particular or contextual, in its attempt to understand how characteristics of the social and physical environment are operationalized or "reproduced" in daily life (Link and Phelan 2002; Marmot 2000).

To posit that health has determinants in the social and physical environment is to suggest that interventions can promote public health by changing the environment. Such ecologically oriented efforts are now frequently referred to as "structural interventions" (Blankenship et al. 2006) and have been defined as "interventions that work by altering the context within which health is produced and reproduced" (Blankenship et al. 2000). Law can be seen as an ecological cause of risk and a medium of structural intervention to reduce risk. As a causal factor, law contributes to the construction of ecological determinants, and also operates as a mechanism through which ecological characteristics operate to produce health outcomes. For example, the daily interactions of law enforcement agents and IDUs in particular places are a mechanism through which ecological conditions are transformed into risks and outcomes (Burris et al. 2002). Law is also a prime potential mode of structural intervention, for it sets broad and effective rules of behavior. Both new and well-established public health interventions rely on law as a means of structuring an environment in healthy ways. For example, a law requiring customers in brothels to use condoms changes the context in which sex workers and clients negotiate safe sex (Albert et al. 1995).

"Law" can be understood to include not only the rules as they are to be found "on the books" in statutes, regulations, and court decisions, but also in the institutions and practices through which these laws are implemented "on the streets" (Black 1976), and indeed in the understanding of the rules and the system in the minds of people in the population (Ewick and Silbey 1998). Law, then, consists of four distinct components, which are illustrated in the simple heuristic in Exhibit FE1.1. The "law on the books" includes the formal, written, legal rules—statutes, constitutions, and regulations—as well as court decisions interpreting the law. The boundaries of this formal body of law may vary somewhat from place to place (in China, for example, sociolegal scholars treat speeches and rules of the Communist Party as the equivalent of formal law), but by and large this domain is straightforward to delineate. In the context of criminal law, law on the books broadly defines the roster of criminal acts, and sets the mission and powers of law enforcement agencies.

Exhibit FE1.1 From drug policies to health outcomes of injection drug users

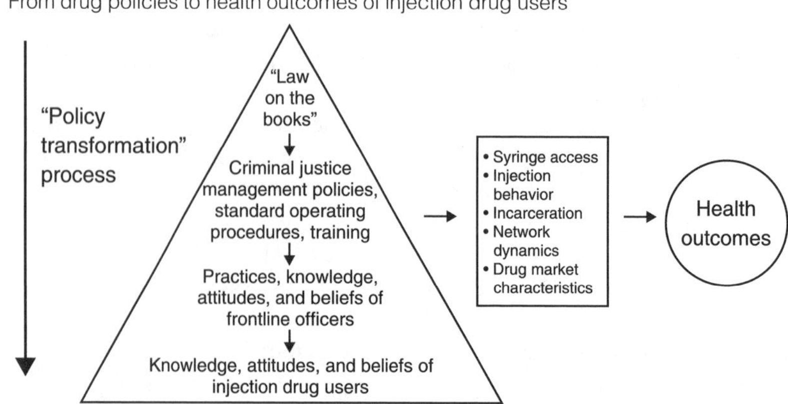

Law on the books is only part of the picture. Implementation research has long demonstrated that the actual application of law is subject to many institutional, individual and environmental factors, which form a gap between law as written and law as actually applied (Bardach 1977). So significant is the difference that the implementation of laws has been called a "policy transformation" process (Percy 1989). Policy implementation begins with the management tools of the implementing agencies—training, work rules, policies, and standard operating procedures—but extends through the practices, knowledge, attitudes, and beliefs of the line personnel who are expected to enforce the law. In Exhibit FE1.1, we also include the knowledge, attitudes, and beliefs of regulated parties, whose understanding of and reaction to the law and the way it is enforced influences its effectiveness.

In the remainder of this chapter, we apply this model to understand how law influences the health of IDUs. It is important to note that, in doing so, we are accepting as *given* a prohibitionist drug policy—i.e., the enforcement of criminal laws prohibiting drug use or possession. An ecological approach to the health of IDUs, and a structural approach to interventions, invites consideration of more upstream questions, such as ecological elements that may be influencing both what laws are enacted and how they are implemented. Why drug use is seen substantially as a matter for criminal control in the first place, and what forces shape attitudes towards drug use and drug users are complex questions. We will address them in a limited way at the end of this chapter, but the chapter proceeds on the premise that there are meaningful steps to be taken within the current approach to drug control that will alter the risk environment for IDUs.

HIV AND HEPATITIS RISK AMONG IDUS: REVIEWING THE EVIDENCE

There is considerable evidence that IDUs are at elevated risk of communicable disease, and in many places injection drug use contributes significantly to the spread of these diseases (UNAIDS and World Health Organization 2006). It is estimated that 22 percent of AIDS cases (Centers for Disease Control and Prevention 2005), at least 10 percent of HBV cases (Goldstein et al. 2002), and 68 percent of new HCV infections in the United States are injection-related (Alter 2002). The rates are higher in women and African-American men (Centers for Disease Control and Prevention 2005). Injection drug use is the main mode of HIV transmission in the countries of Eastern Europe and Central Asia, where approximately two-thirds of all reported HIV cases are among injecting drug users (European Centre for the Epidemiological Monitoring of AIDS 2006; UNAIDS and World Health Organization 2006); in several countries, IDUs contribute over 90 percent of reported HIV cases (Rhodes et al. 1999a). Injection drug use is the source of a significant proportion of recent HIV, HBV, and HCV outbreaks in India, Afghanistan, and Pakistan (Cohen 2004; Kuo et al. 2006; Rai et al. 2007; UNAIDS and World Health Organization 2006). In China and Southeast Asia, injection drug use is a major driver of the rapid spread of HIV and HCV (Shao 2006; UNAIDS and World Health Organization 2006; Zhang et al. 2002). By the early 1990s, HIV prevalence in Brazilian IDUs had reached 50–60 percent in Santos and 25 percent in Rio (Bastos et al. 2005), and, despite recent improvements, remains substantial (Bastos et al. 2005).

Individual Risk Behaviors and Related Interventions

Identified individual risk factors include "sharing" (serial reuse) of syringes, cotton filters, water (for dissolving drug powder), or "cookers" (bottle caps or similar vessels used to prepare an injectable solution); using a common syringe to divide a dose of drug solution among multiple users; not being in drug treatment; and injecting at "shooting galleries" where IDUs congregate to consume drugs and in other semi-public areas (such as rooftops, abandoned buildings, parked cars, and so on) (Celentano et al. 1991; Friedman et al. 1995;

Jose et al. 1993; Latkin et al. 1996; Needle et al. 1998). Intervention strategies targeted to these individual risk factors have depended heavily on education, outreach, counseling, and substance abuse treatment to modify individual behavior (Academy for Educational Development 2000; Coyle et al. 1998; McCoy et al. 1998).

Ecological Approaches to Risk and Structural Interventions

It has become evident that interventions targetting individual risk factors are insufficient. IDUs exist in complex "risk environments" (Rhodes 2002) in which behaviors are shaped by limited availability of resources (such as clean syringes, hygienic places to inject, or drug treatment), societal norms that stigmatize drug users, the structure of social networks (Galea and Vlahov 2002; Latkin et al. 2003; Sherman and Latkin 2002), low levels of social capital and social and economic power among drug users, and a legal and policy environment that focuses on social control and punishment of drug users. In this chapter, we focus on evidence that demonstrates that criminal law and associated law enforcement practices comprise significant ecological factors structuring risk and behavior among IDUs. Moreover, laws and legal practices are among the more readily identifiable and, in some settings, malleable ecological risk factors influencing IDUs.

Drug Law, Police Practice, and their Effects on IDU Risk and Attitudes

In the United States, where laws on the books commonly prohibit possession of drug paraphernalia, a substantial body of ethnographic and quantitative research indicates that fear of police involvement deters IDUs from carrying syringes and encourages hurried, unsterile injection (Bluthenthal et al. 1999a, 1999b; Bourgois 1998; Clatts et al. 1998; Cooper et al. 2005; Feldman and Biernacki 1988; Gleghorn et al. 1995; Grund et al. 1992; Koester 1994; Small et al. 2006; Waldorf et al. 1990; Zule 1992). In their report of needle use practices in Seattle, Washington, where needle purchase is legal, Calsyn and colleagues observed lower rates of needle sharing compared to regions where needle purchase and possession was illegal (Caslyn et al. 1991). Bluthenthal and colleagues found that IDUs concerned about arrest while carrying needles were over 1.5 times more likely to report sharing (Bluthenthal et al. 1999b). In a number of studies, IDUs who shared needles reported more arrests or other unpleasant encounters with the law (Metzger et al. 1991; Rhodes et al. 2004). Laws limiting access to syringes are significantly associated with high prices for syringes obtained from street sellers, which in turn limits the ability of IDUs to purchase sufficient syringes to use one new syringe for every injection (the public health ideal (Rich and Foisie 2000)). Two different analyses found that punitive drug policies predicted higher incidence and prevalence of HIV infection in U.S. metropolitan areas (Friedman et al. 2001a, 2006).

Police practices may be, to some extent, independent of the written law concerning syringe possession and drug use. Police generally have the discretion and the dexterity to deploy a wide variety of criminal and public order laws to accomplish their street control and public safety mission, and research indicates that they do so in the area of drug use (Cooper et al. 2004; Lovell 2002; Maher and Dixon 1999). In Russia, where syringe possession is not a crime, possessing a syringe marks an individual as an IDU and exposes him or her to punishment on other grounds. Police may confiscate syringes; they may arrest drug users and require them to be screened and, if positive, registered as habitual users at a government narcological institution or confined for treatment. Possession of even small amounts of drug can lead to charges, and the threat of any of these measures may be used to extort bribes (Bidordinova 2002). The impact is borne out by Grund's study, in which 40 percent of IDUs surveyed in five Russian cities said that they did not routinely carry injection equipment, in part to avoid attracting attention from the police (Grund 2001).

Such direct behavioral influence is not, however, the only way in which laws or law enforcement practices may influence HIV risk. A high prevalence of incarceration as a punishment for drug use can make prisons key sites for the transmission of HIV, TB, and other diseases, because of overcrowding, poor nutrition, limited access to health care, continued drug use and unsafe injecting practices, unprotected sex, and tattooing (Carbonara et al. 2005; Fullilove 2007; Galea and Vlahov 2002; Hammett et al. 2002; Okie 2007; Sarmati et al. 2007). TB outbreaks and HIV risk behavior and infection have been reported even in countries with substantial budgets to invest in hygienic prison conditions (Bergmire-Sweat et al. 1996; Centers for Disease Control and Prevention 2006; Rotily et al. 2001; Taylor et al. 1995; WHO Regional Office for Europe 2005). In Russia and Ukraine, significant outbreaks of HIV and multi-drug-resistant TB have been reported in prisons (Bobrik et al. 2005; Grange and Zumla 2002; Holden 1999; Stern 2001; Trebucq 1999), making imprisonment itself an important risk factor for disease. In a particularly dramatic example, 284 cases of HIV were discovered at a Lithuanian prison, a number that was greater than the total number of HIV infections previously recorded by national health authorities (UNAIDS and World Health Organization 2002).

Law enforcement practices are also of interest in the context of increasing attention to the important role of network dynamics in the spread of HIV among IDUs (Friedman and Aral 2001; Potterat et al. 1999). Networks of injectors who only share injection equipment with others in their network may in theory be retarding factors in the spread of HIV, even if other networks become saturated with the virus. However, high arrest and incarceration rates, or other police practices that influence injection partnering, could be actively causing the disruption of stable networks and the reconstitution of seromixed networks that facilitate HIV spread (Friedman et al. 2000; Rhodes et al. 2002). Differences in the intensity of police activity and the attendant disruption of networks could be a factor in substantial differences in HIV rates exhibited within and across nations with significant amounts of injection drug use (Singer 2004).

Drug laws and enforcement practices also may reshape drug markets and drug use patterns, exposing new populations to injecting drug use and consequently HIV and other blood-borne viruses. In the late 1980s in some countries of Southeast Asia, for example, vigorous enforcement of laws against the use of smokable opium led to increased injection of heroin (Costigan et al. 2003). Criminal laws and enforcement practices can also influence IDU risk by affecting the ability of public health agents to effectively deliver prevention services. In the U.S., law enforcement activity has been found to hamper both illegal and legal syringe exchange programs (SEPs). Studies have reported that arrests of staff or attendees have reduced SEP attendance, limited their expansion, and may have increased the length of time contaminated needles circulated on the streets (Bluthenthal 1997, 1998). In a California study, IDUs attending legal exchanges were actually 1.6 times more likely than those attending an illegal exchange to report citations or arrests for drug paraphernalia possession (Martinez et al. 2007).

Ethnographically, Maher and Dixon's (1999) study of the drug scene in Cabramatta (Sydney), Australia has documented the role of a climate of fear in promoting unhygienic use of the mouth or nose to store drug packets (increasing the risk of HBV or HCV transmission), a reluctance to carry injection equipment, and pressure to consume drugs less safely (Maher and Dixon 1999). A police crackdown was found to have similar results in the Melbourne area (Aitken et al. 2002), where another study observed IDUs consciously running a higher risk of fatal overdose by selecting injection sites that were secluded from police surveillance (Dovey et al. 2001). In the United States, shooting galleries, sites where large numbers of drug users congregate to inject drugs, are associated with very high HIV risks. IDU use of shooting galleries has been attributed in part to fear of arrest (Celentano et al. 1991; Miller et al. in press).

Summary

If it is recognized that the criminal justice system itself creates incentives for risky behavior, then these institutions are crucial to public health research and action. Interventions among and collaborations with law enforcement are also necessary as a practical matter to ensure that public health programs aimed at marginalized populations can be authorized and successfully implemented. In the remainder of this chapter, we examine some plausible directions for research and intervention to demonstrate that, even without answers to all of the methodological or practical questions about social epidemiology and structural interventions, there is ample opportunity for immediate work.

CONDUCTING RESEARCH ON LAW, LAW ENFORCEMENT, AND IDU HEALTH

Consistent with the diagram in Exhibit FE1.1, this work may focus on any one of four different dimensions of law. In this section, we discuss these in greater detail.

Law on the Books

Law on the books is the starting point for analysis of how laws and their implementation affect IDU health. In the U.S.A., state and national law is readily available to legal researchers, as it is in many wealthier countries with high-functioning legal systems. Many countries facing HIV are not so well off in terms of policy research capacity or infrastructure. In these countries identifying and then obtaining relevant law can be an onerous task, requiring considerable legal expertise (Butler 2005). There is also considerable room for more systematic research on how variations in law on the books are associated with the health risks and health behaviors of IDUs. For example, differences in state laws between the amount of crack and the amount of powder cocaine that will trigger sales or trafficking charges or mandatory minimums have been shown to be associated with higher rates of HIV/AIDS among African Americans (Blankenship et al. 2003), who can expect to spend significantly more time in prison than white Americans (Hogg et al. 2008).

In researching the impact of formal law on IDU health, it is also important to pay careful attention to the question of what law is "relevant" among the huge body of rules that obtain in a modern state. It may be that the vulnerability of drug users depends less in some places on criminal laws explicitly forbidding drug behavior and more on other laws that police deploy to accomplish their mission. For example, in Russia, police officers in at least some places use public intoxication or disorderly conduct charges to arrest IDUs (Rhodes et al. 2002). Also relevant may be laws that create long-term social or economic penalties for IDUs or their families, including exclusion from benefits programs, public housing or the franchise.

Management Policies, Procedures, and Training

The first important level of implementation is the embodiment of rules in the management tools of the agencies charged with enforcing the laws. "Drug czars," mayors, and police chiefs set a tone and often concrete priorities for the deployment of law enforcement resources. Police agencies issue directives to officers, create standard operating procedures, launch special initiatives of high-intensity policing, and train new staff (Fagan and Davies 2000). Public prosecutors devise guidelines on charging, and plea bargaining. Data on this level of policing are rather limited. Some management factors may be collectible in the form of written policies or manuals, but many will require interviews with cooperative managers to acquire.

Practices, Knowledge, and Attitudes of Street-Level Criminal Justice Personnel

In the area of policing, research has long shown that the implementation gap between "law on the books" and "law on the streets" exists not just between law on the books and management practices but also between management directives and street practice (Bayley and Bittner 1984). Discretion in the deployment of laws is both central and essential: central because the day-to-day work of the officer and its effect on the policed community are shaped by how he or she uses the power of the police; and essential because rigid enforcement of every law as much as possible as written would quickly paralyze the officer and the system (Holmberg 2000; Shearing and Ericson 1991).

In spite of the large body of work on police generally, and a growing interest in public health law, largely missing from current research is a focus on police and other criminal justice actors from a health perspective. Research cited here has shown how law and police work influences IDUs, but with a few exceptions its focus has been on the effect rather than the cause. Research has documented how IDUs respond to police, but as yet has not focused on the behavior of police towards IDUs or the factors that drive it. Key issues to explore include the knowledge, attitudes and beliefs of front-line staff and managers concerning drug use, HIV prevention and the impact of law enforcement on IDUs; the organizational structures and incentives that influence how drug laws are enforced; and how people within the system think it could or should be changed to bring about different practices with respect to IDUs (Beletsky et al. 2005; Rhodes et al. 2006). The same sorts of questions can and should be asked regarding prosecutors, probation and parole officers, prison officials, and judges. Rapid assessment and response methods appear to be particularly useful in identifying local law enforcement risk factors within a time frame that allows response to be timely enough to make a difference (Rhodes et al. 1999a, 1999b). But a greater scrutiny of law enforcement officials and the drivers of their behavior is an important way to begin to grapple with ecological approaches to intervention.

Attitudes, Knowledge, and Experiences of IDUs

The final important component of law is the way the IDU experiences the rules. For the people governed by law, "law" is less a matter of formal rules than of the street rules they actually experience in their day-to-day experiences with the enforcement system (Ewick and Silbey 1998). The studies described above demonstrate the value of ethnographic research in explaining how perceptions of the law and experiences with police and other system agents shape the behavior of injection drug users.

Efforts to determine relationships between laws on the books and health can be rendered much more powerful by data on the actual implementation practices of system actors and the responses of IDUs (Birkhead et al. 2002; Cotten-Oldenburg et al. 2001), as well as by more accessible data on key measures of system activity, such as crackdowns and drug paraphernalia arrests and convictions (Case 1998; Davis et al. 2005). Major "non-health" interventions, such as drug courts and supply-side drug control interventions, require more extensive and rigorous evaluation in terms of their effect on IDU risk and risk behavior (Kerr et al. 2005).

DEVELOPING INTERVENTIONS AIMED AT LAWS AND LAW ENFORCEMENT PRACTICES

Interventions that change law, policy, or the attitudes and practices of law enforcement agents are "structural" with respect to IDUs because they alter the risk environment with which IDUs have to cope. With a necessary qualification as to the need for further research and evaluation, it can be argued that plausible interventions are available at all four levels of the law in our schema—and beyond.

Changes in Law on the Books

Law on the books is an important structural factor for public health in part because it can usually be changed to some extent, on occasion substantially. Public health research and advocacy can be an important part of the process of guiding legal change in ways that promise to promote health. The formal law can also be changed by litigation, which in some countries affords a means through which advocates for marginalized people, or for public health generally, can have an effect even in the absence of the money or other resources necessary to effect legislative change. The leading recent examples of substantial formal policy change include elimination of criminal penalties for possession of small amounts of drug in Russia (Butler 2005), and adoption of needle exchange and methadone maintenance as important components of HIV prevention in China (Wu et al. 2007).

The list of legal changes that could predictably have an effect on IDU vulnerability to blood-borne disease includes deregulating the possession of syringes and needles (including the decriminalization of the possession of trace amounts of drug in the barrel of a used syringe so that IDUs can carry their used syringes to appropriate disposal sites without fear of arrest), legalizing methadone and other forms of opiate agonist therapy, and minimizing regulatory barriers to their use. In countries that rely on high levels of incarceration in dealing with drug users, efforts to reduce imprisonment and encourage diversion to treatment would be helpful. These include diversion programs, drug courts, and, in places like countries of the former Soviet Union, new rules for bail, probation, and parole.

Changing law is useful as a means to instigate management change, but it is neither sufficient nor essential to such change. It may be possible for there to be considerable cooperation at a management level in harm reduction efforts, even though the law on the books remains highly punitive. Thus in some communities in the U.S.A., syringe exchanges operate by local interpretation of laws that state-level officials may believe prohibit SEPs, or without claim to legality but with the tacit support of local law enforcement officials (Burris et al. 1996).

Management and Training Changes

Incorporating harm reduction and disease prevention into national drug strategies, as has happened in Australia and to a limited degree in Europe (Aitken et al. 2002; European Monitoring Center for Drugs and Drug Addiction 2002), is an important initial step in harmonizing health and law enforcement. The United Kingdom has adopted a policy of encouraging the identification and treatment of drug users at every stage of the criminal justice process (Kothari et al. 2002). Formal cooperative structures bringing together health, law enforcement, and other government managers is a promising way to begin to change priorities and cultures while exchanging useful information. Such structures have been developed in the U.K. and Australia (Midford et al. 2002), and may be created at the local or state level in the absence of a national plan. In some Australian and American states, for example, management policies have been implemented to discourage police from making arrests at drug overdose scenes, in order not to deter help-seeking behavior (Burris et al. 2001). In New York City, police managers issued orders against arresting people for syringe possession after the passage of legislation to encourage pharmacy sale of syringes to IDUs (Roe V. City of New York 2002).

Better management of courts, bail systems, and prisons can improve conditions even without fundamental changes in law. Drug courts and other alternatives to incarceration may be organized without changes in the overall legal framework. Condom, syringe, and bleach distribution within prisons, and better prison health care and health education may help reduce disease transmission within the system, and more effective management of health issues at release could potentially reduce the risk of overdose among newly freed prisoners (Binswanger et al. 2007). Also, making health a relevant outcome for assessing the performance of law enforcement managers could be a way to encourage more attention to these issues. Of course, both legal and policy changes must be supported by the commitment of resources.

Management structures that encourage interaction across government provide health and law enforcement managers an opportunity to educate each other informally, as can advocacy from outside government. The International Harm Reduction Development Program (IHRD) of the Open Society Institute has for several years organized study tours for police officers to visit sites where a public health or harm reduction approach is integrated into policing. Once management has accepted the importance of health concerns in policing, police training becomes a prime means of fostering attitudinal and behavior change within the organization.

Street Level Changes

Even if changes in law and management policies successfully addressed top-down factors that created tensions between law enforcement and health promotion, there would still be a need to deal with the bottom-up factors embodied in the knowledge, attitudes, and beliefs of the police officers, attorneys, probation officers, and others who apply the law day to day. Education and police reform are both part of this cultural change. In practice, most interventions among marginalized populations already entail negotiation with the local law enforcement agency and front-line staff, but these "educational" interventions are not documented and evaluated as such. Research on law enforcement workers is needed to formulate attitudinal interventions and incentives to take health into consideration in their interactions with marginalized populations.

Paradigm Changes in Drug and Security Policy

Proponents of the current approach to drug control may argue that public health and harm reduction approaches to drug use weaken the normative or deterrent power of drug control laws and will ultimately hurt more than they help as the overall rate of drug use increases in response. Those who favor drug legalization may find our ambitions too limited, or suggest that it is naive to imagine that policing practices can change significantly in the absence of more fundamental change in the laws the police are enforcing. It can be argued that ecological approaches that fall short of pursuing fundamental change in the deep social determinants they identify lack the courage of their convictions, and may in the end accomplish little more than shifting the blame for ill health from disadvantaged individuals to disadvantaged communities (Muntaner and Lynch 1999). From this view, perhaps only changes at the deepest level of social structure—in this case, changes that would transform the punitive approach to drugs and drug use, and deal with related matters of race and class—can properly be called "structural interventions."

That said, the agenda we propose here deploys tried and true tools of institutional change that are capable of producing meaningful improvements in the risk environment for IDUs (Burris and Strathdee 2006). Significant change can be catalyzed from within police organizations, through a process that changes the organizational mentality with respect to drug abuse. Public health movements have traditionally relied on data to awaken concern about social problems and channel that concern into advocacy for political and institutional change. Epidemiological data have facilitated the enhancement of syringe access for IDUs just as they have stricter control of smoking and drunken driving. "Harm reduction" as a grassroots social movement has achieved real success in the form of thousands of functioning programs around the world (Friedman et al. 2001b). Needle exchanges, safe-injecting rooms, overdose prevention campaigns, and drug treatment initiatives have helped demonstrate that the case for a public health approach to drug use is a strong one. The changes in U.S. drug control law catalyzed by public health and harm reduction arguments have been substantial even if not radical (Burris et al. 2003).

More broadly, a public health perspective might also loose the Gordian knot of drug policy by reframing the debate from one that contrasts prohibition with legalization to one that focuses on the nature of policing and its relationship to security. Looking beyond existing law enforcement approaches, a health perspective resonates with efforts within criminology and policing to promote innovation in the governance of security. Providing safe, well-ordered communities is an essential obligation of the state, but there may be better ways to do this. In particular places, or in relation to particular kinds of disorder, it may be possible to devise new security systems that draw upon different tools and ways of thinking, and free police resources to deal with matters to which coercive, retributive approaches are better suited.

CONCLUSION

Both law enforcement and public health are directed to the promotion of good health and good order in the community. We have argued that law enforcement agents are of substantial importance in the search for environmental determinants of IDU health. We have suggested a change in focus in research to address a need that has remained unmet for some years, not just with respect to IDUs but also commercial sex workers, illegal migrants, and other populations living at or beyond the margins of legality. The recognition of the importance of structural factors in health has thus far outstripped research and intervention premised on that ecological view of health. It is imperative that we deploy an ecological approach to studying law and law enforcement practices as contributing causes of HIV and targets of prevention intervention.

The significance of this change in focus is substantial. Rather than looking solely at the population at risk of HIV, such research would take seriously the notion of social causes of disease or risk environment by directing significant attention toward *other people and institutions* that structure disease risks among marginalized populations. A focus on law enforcement responds to these risk-structuring factors with a research aimed at producing structural interventions—that is, interventions that try to change the social-environmental risks, as well as continuing to help IDUs cope with aspects of their risk environment that may be immutable. Looking away from the population immediately at risk and in the direction of institutions whose behavior creates risk offers many new opportunities for prevention work.

NOTE

1. This article was originally published in volume 82 of the *Milbank Quarterly*. It is reprinted with permission, and has been updated to reflect studies published through July 2007.

REFERENCES AND FURTHER READING

Academy for Educational Development. 2000. "A Comprehensive Approach: Preventing Blood-Borne Infections Among Injection Drug Users." Washington, DC: Academy for Educational Development.

Aitken, Campbell, David Moore, Peter Higgs, Jenny Kelsall, and Michael Kerger. 2002. "The Impact of a Police Crackdown on a Street Drug Scene: Evidence from the Street." *International Journal of Drug Policy* 13: 189–98.

Albert, A. E., D. L. Warner, R. A. Hatcher, J. Trussell, and C. Bennett. 1995. "Condom Use Among Female Commercial Sex Workers in Nevada's Legal Brothels. [Comment]." *American Journal of Public Health* 85: 1514–20.

Alter, M. J. 2002. "Prevention of Spread of Hepatitis C." *Hepatology* 36: S93–S98.

Bardach, Eugene. 1977. *The Implementation Game: What Happens After a Bill Becomes Law*. Cambridge, MA: MIT Press.

Bastos, F. I., V. Bongertz, S. L. Teixeira, M. G. Morgado, and M. A. Hacker. 2005. "Is Human Immunodeficiency Virus/Acquired Immunodeficiency Syndrome Decreasing Among Brazilian Injection Drug Users? Recent Findings and How to Interpret Them." *Memorias do Instituto Oswaldo Cruz* 100: 91–6.

Bayley, D., and E. Bittner. 1984. "Learning the Skills of Policing." *Law and Contemporary Problems* 47: 35–59.

Beletsky, Leo, Grace Macalino, and Scott Burris. 2005. "Attitudes of Police Officers towards Syringe Access, Occupational Needle-Sticks, and Drug Use: A Qualitative Study of One City Police Department in the United States." *International Journal of Drug Policy* 16: 267–74.

Bergmire-Sweat, D., B. J. Barnett, S. L. Harris, J. P. Taylor, G. H. Mazurek, and V. Reddy. 1996. "Tuberculosis Outbreak in a Texas Prison, 1994." *Epidemiology and Infection* 117: 485–92.

Berkman, Lisa, and Ichiro Kawachi, eds. 2000. *Social Epidemiology*. New York: Oxford University Press.

Bidordinova, Asya. 2002. "Who Benefits from the War on Drugs in Russia." in *4th National Harm Reduction Conference*. Seattle, WA.

Binswanger, Ingrid A., Marc F. Stern, Richard A. Deyo, Patrick J. Heagerty, Allen Cheadle, Joann G. Elmore, and Thomas D. Koepsell. 2007. "Release from Prison—A High Risk of Death for Former Inmates." *New England Journal of Medicine* 356: 157–65.

Birkhead, G. S., S. J. Klein, A. R. Candelas, H. A. Plavin, and M. Narcisse-Pean. 2002. "New York State's Expanded Syringe Access Demonstration Program (ESAP): A Statewide Intervention to Prevent HIV/AIDS." Abstract # TuOrF1165. in *14th International AIDS Conference*. Barcelona, Spain.

Black, D. 1976. *The Behavior of Law*. New York: Academic Press.

Blankenship, K. M., Sarah Bray, and Michael Merson. 2000. "Structural Interventions in Public Health." *AIDS* 14 Supplement 1: S11–S21.

Blankenship, K. M., S. R. Friedman, S. Dworkin, and J. E. Mantell. 2006. "Structural Interventions: Concepts, Challenges and Opportunities for Research." *Journal of Urban Health*.

Blankenship, K. M., K. Mattocks, and M. Stolar. 2003. "Drug policy, incarceration and black-white disparities in HIV/AIDS." in *131st Annual Meeting of the American Public Health Association*. San Francisco, CA.

Bluthenthal, R. N. 1997. "Impact of Law Enforcement on Syringe Exchange Programs: A Look at Oakland and San Francisco." *Medical Anthropology* 18: 61–83.

Bluthenthal, R. N. 1998. "Syringe exchange as a social movement: a case study of harm reduction in Oakland, California." *Substance Use and Misuse* 33: 1147–71.

Bluthenthal, R.N., A. H. Kral, E. A. Erringer, and B. R. Edlin. 1999a. "Drug Paraphernalia Laws and Injection-Related Infectious Disease Risk Among Drug Injectors." *Journal of Drug Issues* 29: 1–16.

Bluthenthal, R. N., J. Lorvick, A. H. Kral, E. A. Erringer, and J. G. Kahn. 1999b. "Collateral Damage in the War on Drugs: HIV Risk Behaviors among Injection Drug Users." *International Journal of Drug Policy* 10: 25–38.

Bobrik, A., K. Danishevski, K. Erosina, and M. McKee. 2005. "Prison Health in Russia: The Larger Picture." *Journal of Public Health Policy* 26: 30–59.

Bourgois, P. 1998. "The Moral Economies of Homeless Heroin Addicts: Confronting Ethnography, HIV Risk, and Everyday Violence in San Francisco Shooting Encampments." *Substance Use and Misuse* 33: 2323–51.

Burris, S., B. Edlin, and J. Norland. 2001. "Legal Aspects of Providing Naloxone to Heroin Users in the United States." *International Journal of Drug Policy* 12: 237–48.

Burris, S., D. Finucane, H. Gallagher, and J. Grace. 1996. "The Legal Strategies Used in Operating Syringe Exchange Programs in the United States." *American Journal of Public Health* 86: 1161–6.

Burris, S., I. Kawachi, and A. Sarat. 2002. "Integrating Law and Social Epidemiology." *Journal of Law, Medicine and Ethics* 30: 510–21.

Burris, S., and S. Strathdee. 2006. "To Serve and Protect? Toward a Better Relationship Between Drug Control Policy and Public Health." *AIDS* 20: 117–18.

Burris, S., S. Strathdee, and J. Vernick. 2003. "Lethal Injections: The Law, Science and Politics of Syringe Access for Injection Drug Users." *University of San Francisco Law Review* 37: 813–83.

Butler, W. E. 2005. *Narcotics and HIV/AIDS in Russia: Harm Reduction Policies Under Russian Law*. London: Wildy, Simmonds and Hill Law Publishing.

Calsyn, D. A., A. J. Saxon, G. Freeman, and S. Whittaker. 1991. "Needle-Use Practices Among Intravenous Drug Users in an Area where needle purchase is legal." *AIDS* 5: 187–93.

Carbonara, S., S. Babudieri, B. Longo, G. Starnini, R. Monarca, B. Brunetti, M. Andreoni, G. Pastore, V. De Marco, G. Rezza, and Glip. 2005. "Correlates of Mycobacterium Tuberculosis Infection in a Prison Population." *European Respiratory Journal* 25: 1070–76.

Case, P. 1998. "Arrests and Incarceration of Injection Drug Users for Syringe Possession in Massachusetts: Implications for HIV Prevention." *Journal of Acquired Immune Deficiency Syndromes* 18 Supplement 1: S71–S75.

Celentano, D. D., D. Vlahov, S. Cohn, J. C. Anthony, L. Solomon, and K. E. Nelson. 1991. "Risk Factors for Shooting Gallery Use and Cessation among Intravenous Drug Users." *American Journal of Public Health* 81: 1291–5.

Centers for Disease Control and Prevention. 2005. "HIV/AIDS Surveillance Report, 2005." Atlanta: Department of Health and Human Services, Centers for Disease Control and Prevention.

Centers for Disease Control and, Prevention. 2006. "HIV Transmission among Male Inmates in a State Prison System—Georgia, 1992–2005." *MMWR—Morbidity and Mortality Weekly Report* 55: 421–6.

Clatts, M.C., J. L. Sotheran, P. A. Luciano, T. M. Gallo, and L. M. Kochems. 1998. "The Impact of Drug Paraphernalia Laws on HIV Risk among Persons who Inject Illegal Drugs: Implications for Public Policy." In *How to Legalize Drugs*, ed. J. M. Fish, 80–101. Northvale, NJ and London: Jason Aronson Inc.

Cohen, J. 2004. "HIV/AIDS in India. The Needle and the Damage Done." *Science* 304: 509–12.

Cooper, H., L. Moore, S. Gruskin, and N. Krieger. 2004. "Characterizing Perceived Police Violence: Implications for Public Health." *American Journal of Public Health* 94: 1109–18.

Cooper, H., L. Moore, S. Gruskin, and N. Krieger. 2005. "The Impact of a Police Drug Crackdown on Drug Injectors' Ability to Practice Harm Reduction: A Qualitative Study." *Social Science and Medicine* 61: 673–84.

Costigan, G., N. Crofts, and G. Reid. 2003. *The Manual for Reducing Drug Related Harm in Asia*. Melbourne: The Centre for Harm Reduction, MacFarlane Burnet Centre for Medical Research and Asian Harm Reduction Network.

Cotten-Oldenburg, N. U., P. Carr, J. M. DeBoer, E. K. Collison, and G. Novotny. 2001. "Impact of Pharmacy-Based Syringe Access on Injection Practices among Injecting Drug Users in Minnesota, 1998 to 1999." *Journal of Acquired Immune Deficiency Syndromes* 27: 183–92.

Coyle, S. L., R. H. Needle, and J. Normand. 1998. "Outreach-Based HIV Prevention for Injecting Drug Users: A Review of Published Outcome Data." *Public Health Reports* 113 Supplement 1: 19–30.

Davis, C., S. Burris, D. Metzger, J. Becher, and K. Lynch. 2005. "Effects of an Intensive Street-Level Police Intervention on Syringe Exchange Program Utilization: Philadelphia, Pennsylvania." *American Journal of Public Health* 95: 233–6.

Dovey, K., J. Fitzgerald, and Y. Choi. 2001. "Safety Becomes Danger: Dilemmas of Drug-Use in Public Space." *Health and Place* 7: 319–31.

European Centre for the Epidemiological Monitoring of AIDS. 2006. "HIV/AIDS Surveillance in Europe, End-Year Report 2005." Saint-Maurice: Institut de Veille Sanitaire.

European Monitoring Center for Drugs and Drug Addiction. 2002. "Strategies and Coordination in the Field of Drugs in the European Union: A Descriptive Review." Lisbon, Portugal.

Ewick, P., and S. Silbey. 1998. *The Common Place of Law: Stories from Everyday Life*. Chicago: University of Chicago Press.

Fagan, J., and G. Davies. 2000. "Street Stops and Broken Windows: *Terry*, Race, and Disorder in New York City." *Fordham Urban Law Journal* 28: 457–504.

Feldman, H. W., and P. Biernacki. 1988. "The Ethnography of Needle Sharing Among Intravenous Drug Users and Implications for Public Policies and Intervention Strategies." In *Needle Sharing Among Intravenous Drug Abusers: National and International Perspectives*, ed. R. J. Battjes and R. W. Pickens, 28–39. Rockville, MD: National Institute on Drug Abuse.

Friedman, S. R., and S. Aral. 2001. "Social Networks, Risk-Potential Networks, Health, and Disease." *Journal of Urban Health* 78: 411–18.

Friedman, S. R., H. L. Cooper, B. Tempalski, M. Keem, R. Friedman, P. L. Flom, and D. C. Des Jarlais. 2006. "Relationships of Deterrence and Law Enforcement to Drug-Related Harms among Drug Injectors in U.S. Metropolitan Areas." *AIDS* 20: 93–9.

Friedman, S. R., B. Jose, S. Deren, D. C. Des Jarlais, and A. Neaigus. 1995. "Risk Factors for Human Immunodeficiency Virus Seroconversion among Out-of-Treatment Drug Injectors in High and Low Seroprevalence Cities. The National AIDS Research Consortium." *American Journal of Epidemiology* 142: 864–74.

Friedman, S. R., B. J. Kottiri, A. Neaigus, R. Curtis, S. H. Vermund, and D. C. Des Jarlais. 2000. "Network-Related Mechanisms May Help Explain Long-Term HIV-1 Seroprevalence Levels that Remain High but Do Not Approach Population-Group Saturation." *American Journal of Epidemiology* 152: 913–22.

Friedman, S. R., T. Perlis, and D. C. Des Jarlais. 2001a. "Laws Prohibiting Over-the-Counter Syringe Sales to Injection Drug Users: Relations to Population Density, HIV Prevalence, and HIV Incidence." *American Journal of Public Health* 91: 791–3.

Friedman, S. R., M. Southwell, R. Bueno, D. Paone, J. Byrne, and N. Crofts. 2001b. "Harm Reduction—A Historical View from the Left." *International Journal of Drug Policy* 12: 3–14.

Fullilove, R. E. 2007. "Sociocultural Factors Influencing the Transmission of HIV/AIDS in the United States: AIDS and the Nation's Prisons." In *Comprehensive Textbook of AIDS Psychiatry*, ed. Mary Ann Cohen and Jack M. Gorman, 49–60. New York: Oxford University Press.

Galea, S., and D. Vlahov. 2002. "Social Determinants and the Health of Drug Users: Socioeconomic Status, Homelessness, and Incarceration." *Public Health Reports* 117: S135–S145.

Gleghorn, A. A., T. S. Jones, M. C. Doherty, D. D. Celentano, and D. Vlahov. 1995. "Acquisition and Use of Needles and Syringes by Injecting Drug Users in Baltimore, Maryland." *Journal of Acquired Immune Deficiency Syndromes* 10: 97–103.

Goldstein, S. T., M. J. Alter, I. T. Williams, L. A. Moyer, F. N. Judson, K. Mottram, M. Fleenor, P. L. Ryder, and

H. S. Margolis. 2002. "Incidence and Risk Factors for Acute Hepatitis B in the United States, 1982–1998: Implications for Vaccination Programs." *Journal of Infectious Diseases* 185: 713–19.

Grange, J. M., and A. Zumla. 2002. "The global emergency of tuberculosis: what is the cause?" *Journal of the Royal Society of Health* 122: 78–81.

Grund, J. P. C. 2001. "A Candle Lit from Both Ends: The Epidemic of HIV Infection in Central and Eastern Europe." In *HIV and AIDS: International Perspectives*, ed. K. McElrath, 41–67. Westport, CT: Greenwood Press.

Grund, J. P., L. S. Stern, C. D. Kaplan, N. F. Adriaans, and E. Drucker. 1992. "Drug Use Contexts and HIV-Consequences: The Effect of Drug Policy on Patterns of Everyday Drug Use in Rotterdam and the Bronx." *British Journal of Addiction* 87: 381–92.

Hammett, T. M., M. P. Harmon, and W. Rhodes. 2002. "The Burden of Infectious Disease Among Inmates of and Releasees From U.S. Correctional Facilities, 1997." *American Journal of Public Health* 92: 1789–94.

Hogg, R. S., E. F. Druyts, S. Burris, E. Drucker, and S. A Strathdee. 2008. "Years of Life Lost to Prison: Racial and Gender Gradients in the United States of America." *Harm Reduction Journal* 5: doi:10.1186/1477–7517–5–4.

Holden, C. 1999. "Stalking a Killer in Russia's Prisons." *Science* 286: 1670.

Holmberg, L. 2000. "Discretionary Leniency and Typological Guilt: Results from a Danish Study of Police Discretion." *Journal of Scandinavian Studies in Criminology and Crime Prevention* 1: 179–94.

Jose, B., S. R. Friedman, A. Neaigus, R. Curtis, J. P. Grund, M. F. Goldstein, T. P. Ward, and D. C. Des Jarlais. 1993. "Syringe-Mediated Drug-Sharing (Backloading): A New Risk Factor for HIV among Injecting Drug Users." *AIDS* 7: 1653–60.

Kawachi, I. 2000. "Income Inequality and Health." In *Social Epidemiology*, ed. I. Kawachi and L. Berkman, 76–94. New York: Oxford University Press.

Kerr, T., W. Small, and E. Wood. 2005. "The Public Health and Social Impacts of Drug Market Enforcement: A Review of the Evidence." *International Journal of Drug Policy* 16: 210–20.

Koester, S. 1994. "Copping, Running, and Paraphernalia Laws: Contextual and Needle Risk Behavior Among Injection Drug Users in Denver." *Human Organization* 53: 287–95.

Kothari, G., J. Marsden, and J. Strang. 2002. "Opportunities and Obstacles for Effective Treatment of Drug Misusers in the Criminal Justice System in England and Wales." *British Journal of Criminology* 42: 412–32.

Krieger, N. 2001. "Theories for Social Epidemiology in the 21st Century: An Ecosocial Perspective." *International Journal of Epidemiology* 30: 668–77.

Kuo, I., S. ul-Hasan, N. Galai, D. L. Thomas, T. Zafar, M. A. Ahmed, and S. A. Strathdee. 2006. "High HCV Seroprevalence and HIV Drug Use Risk Behaviors among Injection Drug Users in Pakistan." *Harm Reduction Journal* 3: 26–35.

Latkin, C. A., V. Forman, A. Knowlton, and S. Sherman. 2003. "Norms, Social Networks, and HIV-Related Risk Behaviors among Urban Disadvantaged Drug Users." *Social Science and Medicine* 56: 465–76.

Latkin, C., W. Mandell, D. Vlahov, M. Oziemkowska, and D. Celentano. 1996. "People and Places: Behavioral Settings and Personal Network Characteristics as Correlates of Needle Sharing." *Journal of Acquired Immune Deficiency Syndromes and Human Retrovirology* 13: 273–80.

Link, B. G., and Jo Phelan. 1995. "Social Conditions as Fundamental Causes of Disease." *Journal of Health and Social Behavior* Supplement: 80–94.

Link, B. G., and J. C. Phelan. 2002. "McKeown and the Idea that Social Conditions are Fundamental Causes of Disease." *American Journal of Public Health* 92: 730–32.

Lovell, A. M. 2002. "Risking Risk: The Influence of Types of Capital and Social Networks on the Injection Practices of Drug Users." *Social Science and Medicine* 55: 803–21.

Maher, L., and D. Dixon. 1999. "Policing and Public Health: Law Enforcement and Harm Minimisation in a Street-Level Drug Market." *British Journal of Criminology* 39: 488–511.

Marmot, M. 2000. "Multilevel Approaches to Understanding Social Determinants." In *Social Epidemiology*, ed. L. and I. Kawachi, 349–67. New York: Oxford University Press.

Martinez, A. N., R. N. Bluthenthal, J. Lorvick, R. Anderson, N. Flynn, and A. H. Kral. 2007. "The Impact of Legalizing Syringe Exchange Programs on Arrests among Injection Drug Users in California." *Journal of Urban Health* 84: 423–35.

McCoy, C. B., L. R. Metsch, D. D. Chitwood, P. Shapshak, and S. T. Comerford. 1998. "Parenteral Transmission of HIV among Injection Drug Users: Assessing the Frequency of Multiperson Use of Needles, Syringes, Cookers, Cotton, and Water." *Journal of Acquired Immune Deficiency Syndromes and Human Retrovirology* 18 (Supplement 1): S25–S29.

Metzger, D., G. Woody, D. De Philippis, A. T. McLellan, C. P. O'Brien, and J. J. Platt. 1991. "Risk Factors for Needle Sharing among Methadone-Treated Patients." *American Journal of Psychiatry* 148: 636–40.

Midford, R., J. Acres, S. Lenton, W. Loxley, and K. Boots. 2002. "Cops, Drugs and the Community: Establishing Consultative Harm Reduction Structures in two Western Australian Locations." *International Journal of Drug Policy* 13: 181–8.

Miller, C. L., M. Firestone, R. Ramos, S. Burris, M. E. Ramos, P. Case, K. C. Brouwer, M. A. Fraga, and S. A. Strathdee. In press. "Injecting Drug Users' Experiences of Policing Practices in Two Mexican–U.S. Border Cities: Public Health Perspectives." *International Journal of Drug Policy*.

Muntaner, C., and J. Lynch. 1999. "Income Inequality, Social Cohesion, and Class Relations: A Critique of Wilkinson's Neo-Durkheimian Research Program." *International Journal of Health Services* 29: 59–81.

Needle, R. H., S. Coyle, H. Cesari, R. Trotter, M. Clatts, S. Koester, L. Price, E. McLellan, A. Finlinson, R. N. Bluthenthal, T. Pierce, J. Johnson, T. S. Jones, and M. Williams. 1998. "HIV Risk Behaviors Associated with the Injection Process: Multiperson Use of Drug Injection Equipment and Paraphernalia in Injection Drug User Networks." *Substance Use and Misuse* 33: 2403–23.

Okie, S. 2007. "Sex, Drugs, Prisons, and HIV." *New England Journal of Medicine* 356: 105–108.

Percy, S. L. 1989. *Disability, Civil Rights, and Public Policy: The Politics of Implementation*. Tuscaloosa, AL: University of Alabama Press.

Potterat, J. J., R. B. Rothenberg, and S. Q. Muth. 1999. "Network Structural Dynamics and Infectious Disease Propagation." *International Journal of STD and AIDS* 10: 182–5.

Rai, M. A., H. J. Warraich, S. H. Ali, and V. R. Nerurkar. 2007. "HIV/AIDS in Pakistan: The Battle Begins." *Retrovirology* 4: 22.

"Roe v. City of New York." 232 *F.Supp*.2d 240 (S.D. N.Y. 2002).

Rhodes, T. 2002. "The 'Risk Environment': A Framework for Understanding and Reducing Drug-Related Harm." *International Journal of Drug Policy* 13: 85–94.

Rhodes, T., A. Ball, G. V. Stimson, Y. Kobyshcha, C. Fitch, V. Pokrovsky, M. Bezruchenko-Novachuk, D. Burrows, A. Renton, and L. Andrushchak. 1999a. "HIV Infection Associated with Drug Injecting in the Newly Independent States, Eastern Europe: The Social and Economic Context of Epidemics." *Addiction* 94: 1323–36.

Rhodes, T., A. Judd, L. Mikhailova, A. Sarang, M. Khutorskoy, L. Platt, C. M. Lowndes, and A. Renton. 2004. "Injecting Equipment Sharing among Injecting Drug Users in Togliatti City, Russian Federation: Maximizing the Protective Effects of Syringe Distribution." *Journal of Acquired Immune Deficiency Syndromes: JAIDS* 35: 293–300.

Rhodes, T., L. Mikhailova, A. Sarang, A. Rylkov, C. Lowndes, M. Khutorskoy, L. Platt, D. Burrows, C. Fitch, and A. Renton. 2002. "Situational Factors Influencing Drug Injecting, Risk Reduction and Syringe Exchange in Togliatti City, Russian Federation: A Qualitative Study of Micro Risk Environment." *Social Science and Medicine* 57: 39–54.

Rhodes, T., L. Platt, A. Sarang, A. Vlasov, L. Mikhailova, and G. Monaghan. 2006. "Street Policing, Injecting Drug Use and Harm Reduction in a Russian City: A Qualitative Study of Police Perspectives." *Journal of Urban Health* 83: 911–25.

Rhodes, T., G. V. Stimson, C. Fitch, A. Ball, and A. Renton. 1999b. "Rapid Assessment, Injecting Drug Use, and Public Health." *Lancet* 354: 65–8.

Rich, J. D., and C.K. Foisie. 2000. "High Street Prices of Syringes Correlate with Strict Syringe Possession Laws." *American Journal of Drug and Alcohol Abuse* 26: 481–7.

Rotily, M., C. Weilandt, S. M. Bird, K. Kall, H. J. Van Haastrecht, E. Iandolo, and S. Rousseau. 2001. "Surveillance of HIV Infection and Related Risk Behaviour in European Prisons. A Multicentre Pilot Study." *European Journal of Public Health* 11: 243–50.

Sampson, R., and J. Morenoff. 2000. "Public Health and Safety in Context: Lessons from Community-Level Theory on Social Capital." In *Promoting Health: Intervention Strategies from Social and Behavioral Research*, ed. Brian Smedley and S. Leonard Syme, 366–89. Washington DC: National Academy Press.

Sarmati, L., S. Babudieri, B. Longo, G. Starnini, S. Carbonara, R. Monarca, A. R. Buonomini, L. Dori, G. Rezza, M. Andreoni, and Penitenziari Gruppo di Lavoro Infettivologi. 2007. "Human Herpesvirus 8 and Human Herpesvirus 2 Infections in Prison Population. *Journal of Medical Virology* 79: 167–73.

Shao, Y. 2006. "AIDS Epidemic at Age 25 and Control Efforts in China." *Retrovirology* 3: 87.

Shearing, C., and R. Ericson. 1991. "Culture as Figurative Action." *British Journal of Sociology* 42: 482–506.

Sherman, S. G., and C. A. Latkin. 2002. "Drug Users' Involvement in the Drug Economy: Implications for Harm Reduction and HIV Prevention Programs." *Journal of Urban Health* 79: 266–77.

Singer, M. 2004. "Why is it Easier to Get Drugs than Drug Treatment?" In *Unhealthy Health Policy: A Critical Anthropological Examination*, ed. A. Castro and M. Singer. Walnut Creek, CA: Altamira Press.

Small, W., T. Kerr, J. Charette, M. T. Schechter, and P. M. Spittal. 2006. "Impacts of Intensified Police Activity on Injection Drug Users: Evidence from an Ethnographic Investigation." *International Journal of Drug Policy* 17: 85.

Stern, V. 2001. "Problems in Prisons Worldwide, with a Particular Focus on Russia." *Annals of the New York Academy of Sciences* 953: 113–19.

Susser, M., and E. Susser. 1996a. "Choosing a Future for Epidemiology: I. Eras and Paradigms." *American Journal of Public Health* 86: 668–73.

Susser, M., and E. Susser. 1996b. "Choosing a Future for Epidemiology: II. From Black Box to Chinese Boxes and Eco-Epidemiology." *American Journal of Public Health* 86: 674–7.

Taylor, A., D. Goldberg, J. Emslie, J. Wrench, L. Gruer, S. Cameron, J. Black, B. Davis, J. McGregor, and E. Follett. 1995. "Outbreak of HIV Infection in a Scottish Prison." *British Medical Journal* 310: 289–92.

Trebucq, A. 1999. "Tuberculosis in Prisons." *Lancet* 353: 2244–5.

UNAIDS, and World Health Organization. 2002. "AIDS Epidemic Update: 2002." Geneva: UNAIDS.

UNAIDS, and World Health Organization. 2006. "AIDS Epidemic Update: December 2006." Geneva: Joint United Nations Programme on HIV/AIDS.

Waldorf, D., C. Reinarman, and S. Murphy. 1990. "Needle Sharing, Shooting Galleries, and AIDS Risks among Intravenous Drug Users in San Francisco: Criminal Justice and Public Health Policy." *Criminal Justice Policy Review* 3: 321–43.

WHO Regional Office for Europe. 2005. "Status Paper on Prisons, Drugs and Harm Reduction." De Leeuwenhorst, Netherlands: WHO Regional Office for Europe.

Wu, Z., S. G. Sullivan, Y. Wang, M. J. Rotheram-Borus, and R. Detels. 2007. "Evolution of China's Response to HIV/AIDS." *Lancet* 369: 679–90.

Zhang, C. Y., R. G. Yang, X. S. Xia, S. Y. Qin, J. P. Dai, Z. B. Zhang, Z. Z. Peng, T. Wei, H. Liu, D. C. Pu, J. H. Luo, T. Takebe, and K. L. Ben. 2002. "High Prevalence of HIV-1 and Hepatitis C Virus Coinfection among Injection Drug Users in the Southeastern Region of Yunnan, China." *Journal of Acquired Immune Deficiency Syndromes* 29: 191–6.

Zule, W. 1992. "Risk and Reciprocity: HIV and the Injection Drug User." *Journal of Psychoactive Drugs* 24: 242–9.

Shooting gallery

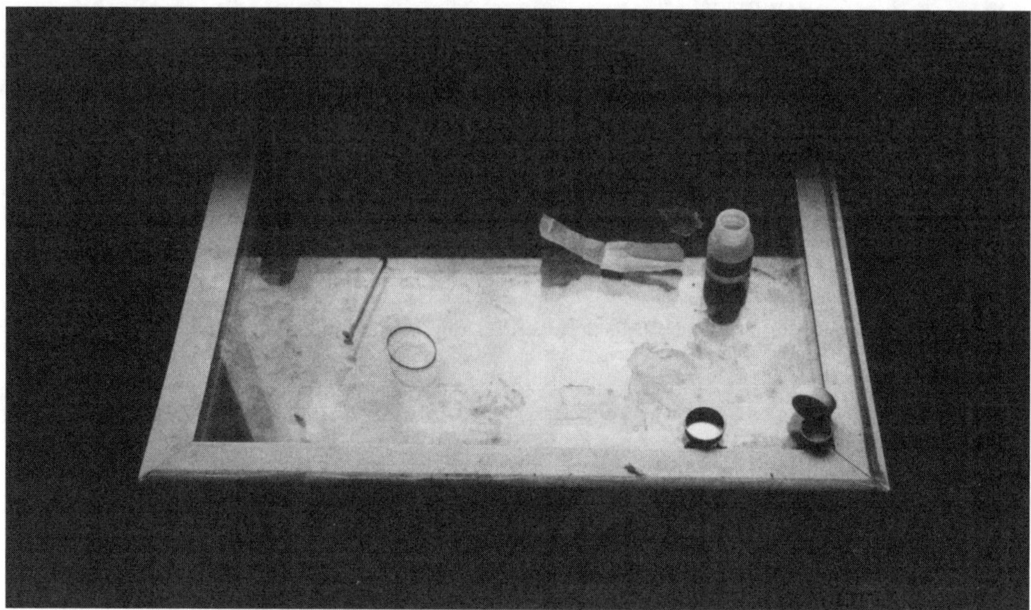

Source: Photo courtesy of Delia Easton

CHAPTER 1

Inside and Out

Incarceration, HIV/AIDS, and Public Health in the United States

Megan Comfort

ABSTRACT

This chapter discusses the particular hazards of carceral environments regarding HIV transmission and treatment and how the prevalence of HIV/AIDS in jails and prisons affects public health on a scale far exceeding the 2.18 million individuals residing behind bars. Jail detainees and prisoners in the United States are known to have levels of HIV prevalence and confirmed AIDS cases that are substantially higher than those of the general population. Of particular concern is the vulnerability to HIV infection experienced by people involved in intimate relationships with former inmates.

During the last thirty years, the United States has been engaged in a continuous and now-infamous rise in incarceration that is unprecedented in the nation's history. From the 1920s to the mid-1970s, the national incarceration rate hovered around a stable mean of 110 inmates per 100,000 residents (Tonry 2001: 8). However, as of mid-year 2005 the U.S. incarceration rate reached 738 inmates per 100,000 residents, bringing the carceral population to an all-time high of 2,186,230 bodies behind bars (Harrison and Beck 2006).[1] Today the United States is a penal outlier among its "peer" nations, which—despite significant rises in their own incarceration rates—confine their residents at levels similar to those of America before 1980: 65 inmates per 100,000 residents in Norway, 88 in France, 97 in Germany and Italy, 116 in Canada, 127 in the Netherlands, and 145 in England and Wales (International Centre for Prison Studies 2005).

Beyond the debate over whether being the number one incarcerator in the developed world has had any beneficial impact on social order and crime reduction (see Tonry 1995; Tonry 1999; Zimring, Hawkins, and Kamin 2001; Clear 2002; Rose and Clear 2003), social scientists are just beginning to map out the consequences of large-scale confinement on family relations, employment and housing stability, civic participation, and other areas of socioeconomic concern (Mauer and Chesney-Lind 2002; Travis and Waul 2003; Pattillo, Weiman, and Western 2004). In recent years, public health researchers have raised their own alarm, noting that jail detainees and prisoners in the United States are known to have levels of HIV prevalence and confirmed AIDS cases that are substantially higher than those of the general population (Hammett, Harmon, and Rhodes 2002).[2] Inmates also have rates of hepatitis and sexually transmitted diseases that are notably higher than those of the general population (Hammett 1998; Rohde 2001; Solomon et al. 2004). According to *The Health Status of Soon-to-Be-Released Inmates*, a report by the National Commission on Correctional Health Care (2002), 1.3 million people released from American prisons and jails in 2002 were estimated to be infected with the hepatitis C virus (HCV), 137,000 with human immunodeficiency virus (HIV), and 12,000 with active tuberculosis (TB) (not including the 566,000 people with latent TB). These figures represent 29 percent, 13–17 percent, and 35 percent respectively of the total number of Americans living with these infections.

This chapter discusses the particular hazards of carceral environments regarding HIV transmission and treatment and how the prevalence of HIV/AIDS in jails and prisons affects public health on a scale far exceeding the 2.18 million individuals residing behind bars. First, though, it is imperative to specify the demographic profile of the nation's inmates in order to clarify who is bearing the impact of the dramatic rise of incarceration rates in the United States and who is, in turn, most vulnerable to HIV infection and illness in connection with punitive confinement. Incarceration policies linked to the War on Drugs have wrought specific devastation on African Americans, and in particularly on young African-American men (Tonry 1995; Miller 1996; Mauer 1999; Western 2006): 93 percent of state prisoners and 87 percent of jail inmates are male (Harrison and Beck 2006). African-American men, who constitute 12 percent of American males, represent 43 percent of male prisoners and 39 percent of jail inmates (U.S. Census Bureau 2005; Harrison and Beck 2006). Among all men aged 25 to 29, 12.6 percent of African Americans were behind bars in 2004, compared to 3.7 percent of Hispanics and 1.7 percent of whites (Harrison and Beck 2006). Even more strikingly, sociologists Becky Pettit and Bruce Western (2004) have determined that nearly 60 percent of African-American male high-school dropouts born between 1965 and 1969 had been to prison at least once by 1999. Although women constitute a much smaller percentage of the overall carceral population, in recent years the annual growth rate of the number of incarcerated women has exceeded that for men, with African-American and Hispanic women being the fastest-growing incarcerated populations (Harrison and Beck 2006).

The majority of incarcerated people are taken from and subsequently returned to concentrated inner-city areas, which are predominantly low-income neighborhoods of color (Clear 2002; Braman 2004; Lynch and Sabol 2004). One study identified the phenomenon of "million-dollar blocks" in which more than one million dollars annually is spent to incarcerate and return residents to city blocks in neighborhoods with high incarceration rates (Cadora, Swartz, and Gordon 2003). Researchers studying such a neighborhood found that 64.5 percent of denizens either had themselves been incarcerated or knew someone who had been incarcerated (Rose and Clear 2004). It is therefore evident that any socioeconomic or health outcome related to incarceration will disproportionately affect young African-American men, African-American and Hispanic women, and the neighborhoods to which they return upon their release from jail or prison. Indeed, recent studies have linked racial disparities in incarceration to health disparities, including disparities in HIV/AIDS (Freudenberg 2002; Blankenship et al. 2005; Golembeski and Fullilove 2005; Iguchi et al. 2005; Johnson and Raphael 2005).

HIV TRANSMISSION AND TREATMENT BEHIND BARS

In 2003 the prevalence of confirmed AIDS cases among the nation's prisoners was nearly 3.5 times that in the general population (0.5 percent vs. 0.15 percent) and 2 percent of state prisoners were known to be HIV positive (Maruschak 2005).[3] Interviews conducted in 2002 determined that nearly two-thirds of jail inmates had ever tested for HIV, and 2.5 percent of inmates who had tested after admission to jail were HIV positive (Maruschak 2004). The majority of inmates are male, with women constituting 7 percent of prisoners and 13 percent of jail detainees (Harrison and Beck 2006), but the prevalence of HIV infection is notably higher among female inmates: in 2002, 1.2 percent of male jail inmates and 2.3 percent of female jail inmates were known to be HIV positive (Maruschak 2004) and in 2003, 1.9 percent of male state prisoners and 2.8 percent of female state prisoners were known to be HIV positive (Maruschak 2005). Over 10 percent of female prisoners were known to be HIV positive in two states, New York (14.6 percent) and Maryland (11.1 percent), whereas only one state reported over 5 percent of its male population being HIV positive (New York, 7.3 percent) (Maruschak 2005). High HIV prevalence among women may be attributable to higher proportions of women inmates having histories of injection drug use, sexual relationships with injection drug users, histories of sexual abuse, or involvement in sex work (Hammett and Drachman-Jones 2006; Braithwaite, Treadwell, and Arriola 2005). Transgender people, who are particularly vulnerable to HIV infection both when incarcerated and when not in correctional custody due to social marginalization, sex work, hormonal injections, and sexual victimization (Bockting, Robinson, and Rosser 1998; Clements-Nolle et al. 2001; Kenagy 2002), are not accounted for in official statistics on HIV in correctional institutions.

Since HIV-testing policies in correctional facilities vary by jurisdiction and not all inmates are required to test for HIV, the actual percentage of HIV-positive inmates is likely to be higher than reported in the official statistics (Lanier and Paoline 2005). Mirroring the overall organization of U.S. correctional institutions, testing policies for HIV are determined at the city or county level (for jails) or the state or federal level (for prisons). Jails have high population turnover rates and therefore tend not to emphasize HIV testing, since individuals may not be around long enough to receive a test result or to embark upon a course of treatment. Currently about one-third of state prisons implement mandatory HIV testing for all prisoners at intake while the rest have voluntary testing only (Hammett 2006). National statistics on the total number of inmates offered HIV testing and the number who refuse testing are not available. In New York state, where the Department of Health estimates the number of HIV-infected inmates using blinded seroprevalence studies, prisoners with HIV/AIDS constituted 7.6 percent of the total prison population in 2003 (Maruschak 2005). In 2003 the New York, Florida, and Texas state prison systems housed 48 percent of all known HIV-positive prisoners (Maruschak 2005).

Due to the absence of systematic testing policies in U.S. correctional facilities, it is presently impossible to determine how many HIV-positive inmates were infected prior to their arrest and incarceration and how many became infected during their time of confinement. While recent research indicates that a significant number of people are already HIV positive at the time of their admission to jail or prison (Macalino et al. 2004; Taussig et al. 2006; Hammett 2006), the lack of availability of condoms, sterile injecting equipment, and other materials needed for safer behaviors in correctional facilities suggests that these institutions are high-risk environments for HIV transmission (Kane and Mason 2001) and HIV seroconversion during incarceration has been demonstrated (Horsburgh et al. 1990). Inmates are vulnerable to HIV infection during imprisonment due to injection drug use, consensual sexual activity, sexual violence, and tattooing (Rothenberg 1983; Slater 1986; Doll 1988; Kantor 1990; Loimer and Werner 1992; Braithwaite, Hammett, and Mayberry 1996; Dolan 1997; Kane and Mason 2001; Lanier and Paoline 2005). The correctional environment both increases the likelihood that people will engage in risky behaviors they avoid in the community and escalates the risk associated with these behaviors. A prime example is consensual sex among men (Nacci and Kane 1983; Solursh, Solursh, and Meyer 1993; Wohl et al. 2000). Although this subject is difficult to systematically document due to stigma, reports from inmates indicate that voluntary male-to-male penetrative sex is common in correctional facilities, often among men who identify as heterosexual and only have female partners when not incarcerated (Stephens, Cozza, and Braithwaite 1999; Lichtenstein 2000; Koscheski et al. 2002; Taussig et al. 2006). Since state laws explicitly prohibit the distribution of condoms in prisons in nearly every state (Polonsky et al. 1994; LRP Publications 2005) and the distribution of condoms in jails is the exception rather than the rule, the vast majority of inmates do not have the option to choose protected sex.

In addition, sexual violence and rape are ritualized elements of prison culture and may be perpetrated against people who are not targets of such violence when outside of prison walls (Rideau and Wikberg 1992; Kupers 1999; Sabo, Kupers, and London 2001). The national organization Stop Prisoner Rape estimates that one in five male inmates is a victim of sexual violence while incarcerated (Stop Prison Rape 2003), and the first ever survey of administrative records on sexual violence in adult and juvenile facilities found that males comprised 90 percent of victims and perpetrators of inmate-on-inmate nonconsensual sex acts (Beck and Hughes 2005). Women and transgender inmates have been found to be at risk of sexual assault by, or coercive sexual relationships with, male correctional officers (Members of the ACE Program of the Bedford Hills Correctional Facility 1998; LeBlanc 2003). Sexual abuse of women also has been noted to occur at the hands of correctional staff during routine medical examinations (Braithwaite, Treadwell, and Arriola 2005).

Many studies have documented considerable levels of risky drug injection among inmates (Toepell 1992; ECAP 1994; Braithwaite, Hammett, and Mayberry 1996; Dufour et al. 1996; Luekefeld et al. 1999). Although needle exchange programs have been successfully implemented in some European prisons (Dolan, Rutter, and Wodak 2003), no American jurisdiction allows syringe distribution or exchange. This policy means that inmates who inject drugs typically reuse and share smuggled or makeshift syringes (Muller et al. 1995; Darke, Kaye, and Finlay-Jones 1998). Likewise, despite the cultural importance and centrality of tattooing in prison and jail gang culture (Phillips 2001), standard policies prohibit this activity behind bars and therefore inmates reuse and share "homemade" tattoo needles (Demello 1993; Doll 1988). Notably, the significant health risks posed by in-prison tattooing prompted the Correctional Service of Canada to undertake a pilot program of supervised tattoo parlors in six prisons in 2005 (Krauss 2005).

As with testing, the treatment of HIV-positive inmates again depends on the city, county, or state in which they are incarcerated. Some correctional systems operate segregated housing units for seropositive inmates, while others send seriously ill convicts to a designated medical facility but keep healthier HIV-positive people in the "general population," that is, in the regular housing units. Depending on the facility, seropositive inmates sometimes reside in "chronic-care" housing units where they live alongside people suffering from diabetes, asthma, and other treatable health problems. In any case, the rigorous protection of the confidentiality of medical information that is considered paramount for most Americans does not exist for inmates who test positive or voluntarily disclose their positive status while behind bars. Standing in line daily for medication, requesting to see the designated HIV doctor, or having a correctional officer discuss information gleaned through a monitored phone call or letter quickly spreads talk of one's serostatus throughout the carceral microcosm—and possibly beyond, if any fellow inmates or officers know one's family or associates in the outside world (Murphy 2004). Not surprisingly, in facilities where testing is not mandatory some people (particularly those serving shorter sentences) forego testing or conceal their already-known positive status while incarcerated in order to preserve their medical privacy (McTighe 2005).

Physicians and nurses working behind bars find their efforts to provide care complicated by prison-specific impediments such as mandatory racial segregation (which can prevent inmates of different races/ethnicities from being in the infirmary simultaneously, ostensibly to avoid gang violence), lack of equipment and supplies, high costs for security when transporting inmates to and from outside hospitals, and severe understaffing (ratios of one doctor to a thousand or more inmates are not uncommon) (Sterngold 2005). Furthermore, serious errors, neglect, and incompetence can impede diagnosis and treatment for HIV-positive inmates since doctors and other medical personnel who have been sanctioned for poor standards of practice and who have had their general licenses revoked are allowed to continue to work in correctional facilities (Pollack, Khoshnood, and Altice 1999; Hylton 2003). Inmates who require medication for HIV may receive outdated treatments that are modified according to correctional policies; for instance, requiring inmates to "prove compliance" on single-drug regimens before being allowed to receive more advanced multidrug therapies. Medications also may be improperly administered, as in the case of a Florida prisoner who was routinely given his pills with meals, despite the interdiction on eating two hours before and one hour after taking his HIV medication (Cusac 2000). Recent lawsuits filed by or on behalf of ill inmates are bringing questions of state liability for medical malpractice and neglect to the fore: in 2005, federal judge Thelton Henderson cited "horrifying" and "abysmal" conditions in his decision to place California's prison health care system under receivership (Bee 2005; Sterngold 2005). A suit in Alabama brought forward by HIV-positive inmates forced the state's Department of Corrections to change its medical provider and the settlement required regular inspections of medical, housing, and nutritional conditions by an independent consultant and the hiring of a full-time nurse to coordinate HIV services (Jafari 2004).

Importantly, the health care someone receives in a correctional facility may be better than that which he or she can scrounge together when *not* behind bars (Conklin, Lincoln, and Tuthill 2000). The U.S. Census Bureau reports that in a nation lacking a system of universal coverage for its citizens, 44 million people found themselves uninsured in 2003. Ironically, inmates are the only group entitled by the Eighth Amendment of the U.S. Constitution to the right to medical care—for as long as they remain within correctional walls (McDonald 1999: 430). No wonder, then, that "the sad truth is that some individuals deliberately return to incarceration because they feel that they can obtain better care there than in the community" (Hammett 2000: 4). This paradox has resulted in the nation's detention centers and cellblocks becoming central hubs of primary-care opportunities for the poor, and the ramifications of this organization of the health care system are forcibly felt in the low-income and working-class neighborhoods to which millions of inmates return each year (Hammett 2001).

FROM INSIDE TO OUTSIDE

When considering HIV/AIDS and incarceration, one must remember that the majority of inmates are released back into society at some point. On any given day in the United States there are 2.18 million people behind bars, but 15 million people cycle through the criminal justice system each year (Bureau of Justice Statistics 2003; Harrison and Beck 2006). Public health researchers are beginning to examine the impact of this exodus on the neighborhoods to which inmates return (Travis 2000; Hammett 2000; National Commission on Correctional Health Care 2002). Of particular concern is the vulnerability to HIV infection experienced by people involved in intimate relationships with former inmates. Low-income women and women of color—that is, the women most likely to experience the incarceration of their sexual partners—are disproportionately affected by HIV/AIDS (Zierler and Krieger 1997; Dawson 2005; Whitmore et al. 2005). African Americans and Hispanics accounted for 83 percent of AIDS diagnoses among women reported in 2003 (Centers for Disease Control and Prevention 2004), and HIV was the leading cause of death for African-American women aged 25 to 34 in 2001 (NCHS 2003). Increasingly, researchers are asserting that "the higher incarceration rates among black males . . . explain a substantial share of the racial disparity in AIDS infection between black women and women of other racial and ethnic groups" (Johnson and Raphael 2005).

As explained above, given current HIV-testing policies, it is difficult to ascertain whether the high prevalence of HIV in correctional institutions is directly related to people becoming infected while they are behind bars, or whether jails and prisons are simply concentrated environments of people who were vulnerable to HIV infection "on the outside." However, when considering the health of women who are intimately involved with ex-inmates, the impact of a man's incarceration on relationship dynamics factors into women's HIV risk. For example, open communication about sex and HIV exposure is associated with higher levels of condom use and lower levels of unprotected sex (Ahlemeyer and Ludwig 1997; Van Campenhoudt and Cohen 1997; Bruhin 2003; Klein, Elifson, and Sterk 2004). Correctional rules and a lack of privacy can impede a couple's willingness or ability to address sexual health issues when communicating with each other during the incarceration period. Phone calls placed by inmates are typically monitored (as stated at the beginning of the call by a recording) and letters delivered to or sent by inmates are opened and read (Fishman 1988; Girshick 1996; Hairston 1998, 1999; Braman 2004). There are two primary types of visits held in most correctional facilities: "non-contact visits" (conducted over telephones or speaker systems with a Plexiglas separation barrier) and "contact visits" (held in cafeteria-style rooms) (Fishman 1990; Girshick 1996; Comfort 2003; Nurse 2002). The booths in which non-contact visits are held typically are not enclosed and correctional officers and other visitors are easily able to overhear anything that is said. Contact visits are held in large public spaces with other visitors and inmates, and the visiting rooms often become crowded, preventing private conversations. In addition, strict regulation of physical contact between inmates and visitors disrupt women's feelings of closeness to their partner and dissuade them from discussing personal topics such as HIV testing or condom use during their visits (Comfort et al. 2005).

Communication difficulties do not immediately abate when a man is released from jail or prison. Stress over finding employment, contributing to the household, and avoiding trouble can cause men to withdraw emotionally and become depressed (Hagan and Coleman 2001; Travis and Waul 2003; Braman 2004). As a result, difficult issues such as sexual health and HIV risk that were not discussed during the incarceration period are left unaddressed post-release. In the meantime, since correctional facilities generally provide regular meals, sheltered housing, and some degree of health care, people enduring poverty, homelessness, and other hardships in the "outside world" may consider jails or prisons to be relatively *healthy* environments, especially when they see their partner return to the streets well-rested, sufficiently nourished, and "buffed up" from long hours of exercise (Bourgois 1995: 109). Indeed, the wives and girlfriends of ex-inmates often do not perceive carceral settings to be particularly risky in terms of acquiring illness and therefore do not avoid unprotected sex with someone who has recently rejoined society (Comfort et al. 2000; Grinstead et al. 2005).

Surveillance by probation or parole agents further hampers couples' communication. When inmates are released before the end of their sentence, they are required to serve out the remainder of that sentence under the supervision of a probation or parole agent. During this time, people must meet a variety of requirements; for example, parolees in California are not allowed to carry weapons or to travel more than fifty miles from their residence, and they must submit to their person, residence, or vehicle being searched at any time by police or parole agents (Petersilia 1999). Failure to meet any parole condition is considered a "violation" and can result in an immediate return to prison. People may feel that the encroachment on their and their partner's privacy in the form of surveillance and searches inhibits the feelings of relaxation and intimacy needed to discuss sensitive issues like HIV risk (Comfort et al. 2005). The possibility that a man might be abruptly reincarcerated discourages couples who desire pregnancy from waiting six months to confirm a negative HIV test before having unprotected sex, as is generally recommended by HIV prevention practitioners.

Couples' relationships often span multiple periods of incarceration, with men serving several months in jail or years in prison, then spending a few weeks or months living with their female partners, then going back to jail or prison for another sentence, only to return to the female partner once again (Braman 2004; Nurse 2004). Unprotected sexual intercourse has emotional and practical importance within a larger context of romantic connectedness and societal reintegration for couples coping with these cycles of freedom and confinement (Comfort 2002; Comfort et al. 2005). Women experience a range of strong emotions, including stress, loss, ambivalence, and relief, about their romantic relationships during men's prison sentences (Fishman 1990; Comfort 2008). Romantic scripts advising women to "stand by your man" when he is incarcerated can deepen women's commitments to their relationships when their partner is detained (McDermott and King 1992). Drawing on narratives of rehabilitation and personal transformation, inmates may consider the incarceration period as a time of atonement for and rectification of past mistakes. The ensuing apologies and promises of forgiveness intensify feelings of closeness and intimacy because the couple has "been through a lot together," which in turn causes women to place a high value on expressions of trust and commitment like unprotected intercourse and conceiving children (Comfort 2007). In the framework of these demonstrations of attachment, the suggestion by either partner of using condoms upon an inmate's release can be seen as disrespectful to the relationship or as negating a new level of commitment, trust, and intimacy (Sobo 1995; Stevens 1995).

In addition, one's own incarceration and the incarceration of one's partner have been repeatedly associated with greater prevalence of concurrent sexual partnerships (Gorbach et al. 2002; Manhart et al. 2002; Adimora et al. 2003a, 2003b; Johnson and Raphael 2005; Thomas and Sampson 2005). Sexual contact is typically forbidden during the incarceration period. Although some state prisons permit conjugal visits, eligibility requirements (including the necessity of the couple being legally married and the man having a low security status) and logistics result in only a tiny fraction of prisoners being able to participate. The prohibition of intimacy for extended periods of time leads to sexual frustration (Comfort et al. 2005), which may lead to sexual relations outside of the primary partnership. Similarly, the disruption of continuity in a primary relationship (Johnson and Raphael 2005; Stephenson et al. 2006), the desire to "make up for lost time" (Seal et al. 2003), or for men the need to reassert a diminished sense of masculinity (Sabo, Kupers, and London 2001), can also lead to concurrent partnerships upon release from prison.

Finally, structural issues such as lack of work opportunity, lack of child-care, uncertain or inadequate housing and other repercussions of racism, poverty, and sexism increase the vulnerability of women with incarcerated partners to HIV infection. These problems translate into HIV risk through lack of health care, illegal or hazardous work, violence, domestic abuse, and exposure to street drug and sex trade cultures. The incarceration of a partner may aggravate preexisting risk factors in women's lives or push women into risk behaviors they had previously managed to avoid, particularly if the man acted as a protector, advocate, or financial provider in the relationship prior to his arrest. Furthermore, a partner's imprisonment can cause or heighten women's feelings of loneliness, depression, anxiety, and powerlessness (Girshick 1996), emotions that may weaken women's bonds to societal support structures and precipitate "entrapment" in situations of severely limited options (for example, early pregnancy, abusive partnerships) that also increase risk of HIV transmission (Richie 1996). A partner's imprisonment may incur a drop in women's income due to the loss of contributions he previously made to the household (including child-care, food, or gifts) as well as the considerable financial cost of prison visiting and phone calls (Grinstead et al. 2001). As a result, some women may engage in sex work to combat financial problems during a partner's prison term, while others become involved with secondary or multiple partners during a primary partner's incarceration in order to obtain financial, physical, or practical support.

Although the above discussion only addresses female partners of male prisoners, it is obvious that the health repercussions of incarceration do not stop at the jail or prison gate, nor are they limited to the person who was incarcerated. More research is required to document, and more interventions are needed to ameliorate, the health risks posed to immediate family members, sexual partners, needle-sharing partners, and other residents of neighborhoods to which men and women return after periods of incarceration.

CONCLUSION

The Constitutional mandate to provide health care to inmates presents a propitious occasion for the advancement of public health, as nurses and physicians can provide infectious-disease prevention information, treatment counseling, substance-abuse rehabilitation, and basic care to people who otherwise have scant chances of receiving non-urgent medical attention (Freudenberg 2001; Hammett 2006). Working with jail and prison administrators to develop protocols for protecting confidentiality and the right to refuse compulsory testing, ensuring proper laboratory analysis, and mandating care that meets basic professional standards must be intrinsic to this effort, both from the ethical standpoint of the humane treatment of a powerless population and from the pragmatic perspective of the state's liability for those in its charge. Peer education and counseling programs for inmates have been found to be effective in correctional settings and should be a focus of further development and implementation (Grinstead et al. 1999; Collica 2002). Parallel measures to reduce the risks of disease transmission behind bars by implementing condom distribution (as has recently been proposed in the California and New York state assemblies) and needle exchange for drug or tattoo use (following the highly successful examples in Switzerland, Germany, and Spain (Dolan, Rutter, and Wodak 2003)) are similarly important. Looking beyond this country's borders, particularly to Canada and Europe, one finds models of effective HIV-prevention and treatment strategies that could be adopted to ameliorate the public health threat posed by the current policies of the United States' correctional institutions (Gatherer, Moller, and Hayton 2005). Underlying each of these efforts must be forceful advocacy for a continuum of care beyond the carceral border, the amelioration of discrepancies in access to health services, movement toward a decrease in the national incarceration rate to ensure that the poor are not reliant on punitive institutions to provide HIV/AIDS diagnosis and treatment, and public health in low-income communities not being perpetually at the mercy of correctional institutions and policies (Rich et al. 2001; Richie, Freudenberg, and Page 2001; Freudenberg et al. 2005).

NOTES

1. This figure includes people confined in jails (operated on a local level by cities or counties and holding new arrestees awaiting trial, plus convicts sentenced to under one year of detention), state prisons (run by each state's Department of Corrections and containing felons serving over one year as well as parole violators), and federal prisons (controlled by the Federal Bureau of Prisons and inhabited by offenders convicted of federal crimes).
2. In this chapter, I use the term "inmate" to refer to people incarcerated in any correctional facility, while "prisoner" refers only to those held in state or federal prisons and "detainee" indicates someone in a city or county jail.
3. The figures in this chapter are the most recent available at the time of this writing. Readers are encouraged to consult the Bureau of Justice Statistics website (www.ojp.usdoj.gov/bjs) for the most up-to-date reports.

REFERENCES AND FURTHER READING

Adimora, Adaora A., Victor J. Schoenbach, Francis E. A. Martinson, Kathryn H. Donaldson, Tonya R. Stancil, and Robert E. Fullilove. 2003a. "Concurrent Partnerships among Rural African Americans with Recently Reported Heterosexually Transmitted HIV Infection." *Journal of Acquired Immune Deficiency Syndromes* 34: 423–429.

——. 2003b. "Concurrent Sexual Partnerships among African Americans in the Rural South." *AIDS Education and Prevention* 14: 155–160.

Ahlemeyer, H. W., and D. Ludwig. 1997. "Norms of Communication and Communication as a Norm in the Intimate Social System" in *Sexual Interactions and HIV Risk*, ed. L. Van Campenhoudt, M. Cohen, G. Guizzardi, and D. Hausser, 22–43. Bristol, PA: Taylor and Francis.

Beck, Allen J., and Timothy A. Hughes. 2005. "Sexual Violence Reported by Correctional Authorities, 2004." Washington DC: Bureau of Justice Statistics.

Bee, Claire Cooper. 2005. "Prison Health Care Seized Citing Some 'Outright Depravity,' U.S. Judge Will Pick Overseer." *Sacramento Bee*. July 1, A1.

Blankenship, K. M., A. B. Smoyer, S. J. Bray, and K. Mattocks. 2005. "Black–White Disparities in Hiv/Aids: The Role of Drug Policy and the Corrections System." *Journal of Health Care for the Poor and Underserved* 16 (Supplement B) (November 2005): 140–146.

Bockting, W. O., B. E. Robinson, and B. R. Rosser. 1998. "Transgender HIV Prevention: A Qualitative Needs Assessment." *AIDS Care* 10: 505–525.

Bourgois, Philippe. 1995. *In Search of Respect: Selling Crack in El Barrio*. Cambridge: Cambridge University Press.

Braithwaite, R., T. Hammett, and R. Mayberry. 1996. *Prisons and AIDS: A Public Health Challenge*. San Francisco: Jossey-Bass.

Braithwaite, Ronald L., Henrie M. Treadwell, and Kimberly R. J. Arriola. 2005. "Health Disparities and Incarcerated Women: A Population Ignored." *American Journal of Public Health* 95: 1679–1681.

Braman, Donald. 2004. *Doing Time on the Outside: Incarceration and Family Life in Urban America*. Ann Arbor: University of Michigan Press.

Bruhin, E. 2003. "Power, Communication and Condom Use: Patterns of HIV-Relevant Sexual Risk-Management in Heterosexual Relationships." *AIDS Care* 15: 389–401.

Bureau of Justice Statistics. 2003. "Sourcebook of Criminal Justice Statistics." Washington DC: U.S. Department of Justice.

Cadora, Eric, Charles Swartz, and Mannix Gordon. 2003. "Criminal Justice and Health and Human Services: An Exploration of Overlapping Needs, Resources, and Interests in Brooklyn Neighborhoods." In *Prisoners Once Removed: The Impact of Incarceration and Reentry on Children, Families, and Communities*, ed. Jeremy Travis and Michelle Waul, 285–311. Washington DC: Urban Institute Press.

Centers for Disease Control and Prevention. 2004. "HIV/AIDS Surveillance Report 2003." Atlanta: U.S. Department of Health and Human Services, CDC.

Clear, Todd R. 2002. "The Problem with 'Addition by Subtraction:' The Prison-Crime Relationship in Low-Income Communities" in *Invisible Punishment: The Collateral Consequences of Mass Imprisonment*, ed. Marc Mauer and Meda Chesney-Lind, 181–193. New York: New Press.

Clements-Nolle, K., R. Marx, R. Guzman, and M. Katz. 2001. "HIV Prevalence, Risk Behaviors, Health Care Use, and Mental Health Status of Transgender Persons: Implications for Public Health Intervention." *American Journal of Public Health* 91: 915–921.

Collica, Kimberly. 2002. "Levels of Knowledge and Risk Perceptions About HIV/AIDS among Female Inmates in New York State: Can Prison-Based HIV Programs Set the Stage for Behavior Change?" *Prison Journal* 82: 101–124.

Comfort, Megan. 2002. "'Papa's House:' The Prison as Domestic and Social Satellite." *Ethnography* 3: 467–499.

——. 2003. "In the Tube at San Quentin: The 'Secondary Prisonization' of Women Visiting Inmates." *Journal of Contemporary Ethnography* 32: 77–107.

——. 2007. "'It's a Lot of Good Men Behind Walls!': Mass Incarceration and the Transformation of Romance in the United States." *Actes de la recherche en sciences sociales*.

——. 2008. *Doing Time Together: Forging Love and Family in the Shadow of the Prison*. University of Chicago Press.

Comfort, Megan, Olga Grinstead, Bonnie Faigeles, and Barry Zack. 2000. "Reducing HIV Risk among Women Visiting Their Incarcerated Male Partners." *Criminal Justice and Behavior* 27: 57–71.

Comfort, Megan, Olga Grinstead, Kathleen McCartney, Philippe Bourgois, and Kelly Knight. 2005. "'You Can't Do Nothing in This Damn Place!' Sex and Intimacy among Couples with an Incarcerated Male Partner." *Journal of Sex Research* (Special Issue on Sexuality and Place) 42: 3–12.

Conklin, Thomas J., Thomas Lincoln, and Robert W. Tuthill. 2000. "Self-Reported Health and Prior Health Behaviors of Newly Admitted Correctional Inmates." *American Journal of Public Health* 90: 1939–1941.

Cusac, Anne-Marie. 2000. "'The Judge Gave Me Ten Years. He Didn't Sentence Me to Death.' Inmates with HIV Deprived of Proper Care." *The Progressive* July, http://www.progressive.org/amc0700.htm.

Darke, S., S. Kaye, and R. Finlay-Jones. 1998. "Drug Use and Injection Risk-Taking among Prison Methadone Maintenance Patients." *Addiction* 93: 1169–1175.

Dawson, George. 2005. "HIV Disease and Black Women." *Journal of the National Medical Association* 97: 1449–1450.

Demello, Margo. 1993. "The Convict Body: Tattooing among Male American Prisoners." *Anthropology Today* 9: 10–13.

Dolan, K. 1997. "AIDS, Drugs, and Risk Behaviour in Prison: State of the Art." *International Journal of Drug Policy* 8: 5–17.

Dolan, K., S. Rutter, and A. D. Wodak. 2003. "Prison-Based Syringe Exchange Programmes: A Review of International Research and Development." *Addiction* 98: 153–158.

Doll, D. C. 1988. "Tattooing in Prison and HIV Infection." *Lancet* 2: 66.

Dufour, A., M. Alary, C. Poulin, F. Allard, L. Noel, G. Trottier, D. Lepne, and C. Hankins. 1996. "Prevalence and Risk Behaviours for HIV Infection among Inmates of a Provincial Prison in Quebec City." *Aids* 10: 1009–1015.

ECAP (Expert Committee on AIDS and Prison). 1994. "HIV/AIDS in Prisons: Summary Report and Recommendations of the Expert Committee on AIDS and Prisons." Ministry of Supply and Services Canada catalogue no. JS82-68/1-1994E. Ottawa, Canada: Correctional Service of Canada.

Fishman, Laura T. 1988. "Prisoners and Their Wives: Marital and Domestic Effects of Telephone Contacts and Home Visits." *International Journal of Offender Therapy and Comparative Criminology* 32: 55–66.

——. 1990. *Women at the Wall: A Study of Prisoners' Wives Doing Time on the Outside*. Albany: State University of New York Press.

Freudenberg, Nicholas. 2001. "Jails, Prisons, and the Health of Urban Populations: A Review of the Impact of the Correctional System on Community Health." *Journal of Urban Health* 78: 214–235.

——.2002. "Adverse Effects of U.S. Jail and Prison Policies on the Health and Well-Being of Women of Color." *American Journal of Public Health* 92: 1895–1899.

Freudenberg, Nicholas, Jessie Daniels, Martha Crum, Tiffany Perkins, and Beth E. Richie. 2005. "Coming Home from Jail: The Social and Health Consequences of Community Reentry for Women, Male Adolescents, and Their Families and Communities." *American Journal of Public Health* 95: 1725–1736.

Gatherer, Alex, Lars Moller, and Paul Hayton. 2005. "The World Health Organization European Health in Prisons Project after 10 Years: Persistent Barriers and Achievements." *American Journal of Public Health* 95: 1696–1700.

Girshick, Lori B. 1996. *Soledad Women: Wives of Prisoners Speak Out*. Westport, CT: Praeger Publishers.

Golembeski, Cynthia, and Robert E. Fullilove. 2005. "Criminal (In)Justice in the City and Its Associated Health Consequences." *American Journal of Public Health* 95: 1701–1706.

Gorbach, P. M., B. P. Stoner, So Aral, et al. 2002. " 'It Takes a Village:' Understanding Concurrent Sexual Partnerships in Seattle, Washington." *Sexually Transmitted Diseases* 29: 453–462.

Grinstead, Olga, Bonnie Faigeles, Carrie Bancroft, and Barry Zack. 2001. "The Financial Cost of Maintaining Relationships with Incarcerated African American Men: A Survey of Women Prison Visitors." *Journal of African-American Men* 6: 59–70.

Grinstead, O., B. Faigeles, M. Comfort, D. Seal, J. Nealey-Moore, L. Belcher, and K. Morrow. 2005. "HIV, STD, and Hepatitis Risk to Primary Female Partners of Men Being Released from Prison." *Women and Health* 41: 63–80.

Grinstead, Olga, Barry Zack, Bonnie Faigeles, Nina Grossman, and Leroy Blea. 1999. "Reducing Postrelease HIV Risk among Male Prison Inmates: A Peer-Led Intervention." *Criminal Justice and Behavior* 26: 468–480.

Hagan, John, and Juleigh Petty Coleman. 2001. "Returning Captives of the American War on Drugs: Issues of Community and Family Reentry." *Crime and Delinquency* 47: 352–367.

Hairston, Creasie Finney. 1998. "The Forgotten Parent: Understanding the Forces That Influence Incarcerated Fathers' Relationships with Their Children." *Child Welfare* 77: 617–639.

——. 1999. "Kinship Care When Parents Are Incarcerated." In *Kinship Care: Improving Practice through Research*, ed. James P. Gleeson and Creasie Finney Hairston, 189–211. Washington DC: CWLA Press.

Hammett, Theodore M. 1998. "Research in Brief: Public Health/Corrections Collaborations: Prevention and Treatment of HIV/AIDS, STDs, and TB." Washington DC: National Institute of Justice, Center for Disease Control and Prevention.

——. 2000. "Health-Related Issues in Prisoner Reentry to the Community." Reentry Roundtable. Washington DC: The Urban Institute, Justice Policy Center, October 12–13.

——. 2001. "Making the Case for Health Interventions in Correctional Facilities." *Journal of Urban Health* 78: 236–240.

—— 2006. "HIV/AIDS and Other Infectious Diseases among Correctional Inmates: Transmission, Burden, and Appropriate Response" *American Journal of Public Health* 96: 13–17.

Hammett, Theodore M., and Abigail Drachman-Jones. 2006. "HIV/AIDS, Sexually Transmitted Diseases, and Incarceration among Women: National and Southern Perspectives." *Sexually Transmitted Diseases* 33: S17–S22.

Hammett, Theodore M., Mary Patricia Harmon, and William Rhodes. 2002. "The Burden of Infectious Disease among Inmates of and Releasees from Correctional Facilities, 1997." *American Journal of Public Health* 92: 1789–1794.

Harrison, Paige M., and Allen Beck. 2006. "Prison and Jail Inmates at Midyear 2005." Washington DC: Bureau of Justice Statistics, U.S. Department of Justice.

Horsburgh, C. R. Jr. J. Q. Jarvis, T. MacArther, and et al. 1990. "Seroconversion to Human Immunodeficiency Virus in Prison Inmates." *American Journal of Public Health* 80: 209–210.

Hylton, Wil S. 2003. "Sick on the Inside: Correctional HMOs and the Coming Prison Plague." *Harper's Magazine*, August: 43–54.

Iguchi, M. Y., J. Bell, R. N. Ramchand, and T. Fain. 2005. "How Criminal Justice Racial Disparities May Translate into Health Disparities." *Journal of Health Care for the Poor and Underserved* (Supplement B) (November)16: 48–56.

International Centre for Prison Studies. 2005. "World Prison Brief." London: King's College, University of London. http://www.kcl.ac.uk/depsta/rel/icps/worldbrief/world_brief.html

Jafari, Samira. 2004. "Settlement Requires Prison to Revise Care for HIV Inmates." Montgomery, AL: Associated Press, May 26.

Johnson, Rucker C., and Steven Raphael. 2005. "The Effects of Male Incarceration Dynamics on AIDS Infection Rates among African-American Women and Men." Unpublished manuscript.

Kane, Stephanie, and Theresa Mason. 2001. "AIDS and Criminal Justice." *Annual Review of Anthropology* 30: 457–479.

Kantor, E. 1990. "AIDS and HIV Infection in Prisoners: Epidemiology." In *The AIDS Knowledge Base*, ed. P. T. Cohen, M. A. Sande, and P. A. Volberding, 1–4. San Francisco: Medical Publishing Group, Section 1.1.8.

Kenagy, G. P. 2002. "HIV among Transgendered People." *AIDS Care* 14: 127–134.

Klein, Hugh, Kirk W. Elifson, and Claire E. Sterk. 2004.

"Partner Communication and HIV Risk Behaviors among 'At Risk' Women." *Soz.-Präventivmed* 49: 363–374.

Koscheski, Mary, Christopher Hensley, Jeremy Wright, and Richard Tewksbury. 2002. "Consensual Sexual Behavior." In *Prison Sex: Practice and Policy*, ed. Christopher Hensley, 111–131. Boulder: Lynne Rienner Publishers, Inc.

Krauss, Clifford. 2005. "A Prison Makes the Illicit and Dangerous Legal and Safe." *New York Times*, November 24, p. 4.

Kupers, Terry. 1999. *Prison Madness: The Mental Health Crisis Behind Bars and What We Must Do about It.* San Francisco: Jossey-Bass Publishers.

Lanier, Mark M., and Eugene A. Paoline III. 2005. "Expressed Needs and Behavioral Risk Factors of HIV-Positive Inmates." *International Journal of Offender Therapy and Comparative Criminology* 49: 561–573.

LeBlanc, Adrian Nicole. 2003. *Random Family: Love, Drugs, Trouble, and Coming of Age in the Bronx.* New York: Scribner.

Lichtenstein, Bronwen. 2000. "Secret Encounters: Black Men, Bisexuality, and AIDS in Alabama." *Medical Anthropology Quarterly* 14: 374–393.

Loimer, N., and E. Werner. 1992. "Tattooing and High Risk Behavior among Drug Addicts." *Medicine and Law* 11: 164–174.

LRP Publications. 2005. "California Chamber Approves Measure to Give Inmates Condoms: Cost of AIDS Care Weighs Heavy on Decision." *Corrections Professional* 10.

Luekefeld, C., T. K. Logan, D. Farabee, D. Watson, H. Spalding, and R. Purvis. 1999. "Drug Dependency and HIV Testing among State Prisoners." *Population Research and Policy Review* 18: 55–69.

Lynch, James P., and William J. Sabol. 2004. "Effects of Incarceration on Informal Social Control in Communities." In *Imprisoning America: The Social Effects of Mass Incarceration*, ed. Mary Pattillo, David Weiman, and Bruce Western, 135–164. New York: Russell Sage Foundation.

Macalino, Grace, D. Vlahov, S. Sanford-Colby, et al. 2004. "Prevalence and Incidence of HIV, Hepatitis B Virus, and Hepatitis C Virus Infections among Males in Rhode Island Prisons." *American Journal of Public Health* 94: 1218–1223.

Manhart, Lisa E., Sevgi O. Aral, King K. Holmes, and Betsy Foxman. 2002. "Sex Partner Concurrency: Measurement, Prevalence, and Correlates among Urban 18–39-Year-Olds." *Sexually Transmitted Diseases* 29: 133–143.

Maruschak, Laura. 2004. "HIV in Prisons and Jails, 2002." Washington DC: Bureau of Justice Statistics.

—— 2005. "HIV in Prisons, 2003." Washington DC: Bureau of Justice Statistics.

Mauer, Marc. 1999. *Race to Incarcerate*. New York: New Press.

Mauer, Marc, and Meda Chesney-Lind (eds.). 2002. *Invisible Punishment: The Collateral Consequences of Mass Imprisonment.* New York: The New Press.

McDermott, Kathleen, and Roy D. King. 1992. "Prison Rule 102: 'Stand by Your Man.' the Impact of Penal Policy on the Families of Prisoners." In *Prisoners' Children: What Are the Issues?*, ed. Roger Shaw, 50–73. London: Routledge.

McDonald, Douglas C. 1999. "Medical Care in Prisons." In *Prisons*, ed. Michael Tonry and Joan Petersilia, 427–478. Chicago: University of Chicago Press.

McTighe, Laura. 2005. "Prison Health Crisis—What You Can Do." *The Body* www.thebody.com.

Members of the ACE Program of the Bedford Hills Correctional Facility. 1998. *Breaking the Walls of Silence: Aids and Women in a New York State Maximum-Security Prison.* Woodstock and New York: The Overlook Press.

Miller, Jerome G. 1996. *Search and Destroy: African-American Males in the Criminal Justice System.* New York: Cambridge University Press.

Muller, R., K. Stark, I. Guggenmoos-Holzmann, D. Wirth, and U. Bienzle. 1995. "Imprisonment: A Risk Factor for HIV Infection Counteracting Education and Prevention Programmes for Intravenous Drug Users." *AIDS* 9: 183–190.

Murphy, Tim. 2004. "Getting out Alive." *POZ* (April): 34–41.

Nacci, Peter L., and Thomas R. Kane. 1983. "The Incidence of Sex and Sexual Aggression in Federal Prisons." *Federal Probation* 47: 31–36.

National Commission on Correctional Health Care. 2002. *The Health Status of Soon-to-Be-Released Inmates: A Report to Congress.* Volume 1. Chicago.

NCHS. 2003. "National Vital Statistics Report." Pp. 52(9).

Nurse, Anne M. 2002. *Fatherhood Arrested: Parenting from within the Juvenile Justice System.* Nashville, TN: Vanderbilt University Press.

——. 2004. "Returning to Strangers: Newly Paroled Young Fathers and Their Children." In *Imprisoning America: The Social Effects of Mass Incarceration*, ed. Mary Pattillo, David Weiman, and Bruce Western, 76–96. New York: The Russell Sage Foundation.

Pattillo, Mary, David Weiman, and Bruce Western (eds.). 2004. *Imprisoning America: The Social Effects of Mass Incarceration.* New York: Russell Sage Foundation.

Petersilia, Joan. 1999. "Parole and Prisoner Reentry in the United States." In *Prisons*, ed. Michael Tonry and Joan Petersilia, 479–529. Chicago: University of Chicago Press 479–529.

Pettit, Becky, and Bruce Western. 2004. "Mass Imprisonment and the Life Course: Race and Class Inequality in U.S. Incarceration." *American Sociological Review* 69: 151–169.

Phillips, Susan A. 2001. "Gallo's Body: Decoration and Damnation in the Life of a Chicano Gang Member." *Ethnography* 2: 357–388.

Pollack, Harole, Kaveh Khoshnood, and Frederick Altice. 1999. "Health Care Delivery Strategies for Criminal Offenders." *Journal of Health Care Finance* 26: 63–77.

Polonsky, S., S. Kerr, B. Harris, and J. Gaiter. 1994. "HIV Prevention in Prisons and Jails: Obstacles and

Opportunities." *Public Health Reports* 109: 615–626.

Rich, Josiah D., Leah Holmes, Christopher Salas, Grace Macalino, Deborah Davis, James Ryczek, and Timothy Flanigan. 2001. "Successful Linkage of Medical Care and Community Services for HIV-Positive Offenders Being Released from Prison." *Journal of Urban Health* 78: 279–289.

Richie, Beth E. 1996. *Compelled to Crime: The Gender Entrapment of Battered Black Women*. New York: Routledge.

Richie, Beth E., Nicholas Freudenberg, and Joanne Page. 2001. "Reintegrating Women Leaving Jail into Urban Communities: A Description of a Model Program." *Journal of Urban Health* 78: 290–303.

Rideau, Wilbert, and Ron Wikberg. 1992. *Life Sentences: Rage and Survival Behind Bars*. New York: Times Books.

Rohde, David. 2001. "A Health Danger from a Needle Becomes a Scourge Behind Bars." *New York Times*, August 6.

Rose, Dina R., and Todd R. Clear. 2003. "Incarceration, Reentry, and Social Capital: Social Networks in the Balance." In *Prisoners Once Removed: The Impact of Incarceration and Reentry on Children, Families, and Communities*, ed. Jeremy Travis and Michelle Waul, 313–341. Washington DC: The Urban Institute Press.

——. 2004. "Who Doesn't Know Someone in Jail? The Impact of Exposure to Prison on Attitudes Toward Formal and Informal Controls." *Prison Journal* 84: 228–247.

Rothenberg, David. 1983. "Sexual Behavior in an Abnormal Setting." *Corrective and Social Psychiatry and Journal of Behavior Technology, Methods and Therapy* 29: 78–81.

Sabo, Don, Terry A. Kupers, and Willie London (eds.). 2001. *Prison Masculinities*. Philadelphia: Temple University Press.

Seal, David Wyatt, Andrew D. Margolis, Jim Sosman, Deborah Kacanek, Diane Binson, and The Project START Study Group. 2003. "HIV and STD Risk Behavior among 18- to 25-Year-Old Men Released from U.S. Prisons: Provider Perspectives." *AIDS and Behavior* 7: 131–141.

Slater, R. G. 1986. "Psychiatric Intervention in an Atmosphere of Terror." *American Journal of Forensic Psychiatry* 7: 5–12.

Sobo, E. J. 1995. *Choosing Unsafe Sex: Aids-Risk Denial among Disadvantaged Women*. Philadelphia: University of Pennsylvania Press.

Solomon, Liza, Colin Flynn, Kelly Muck, and John Vertefeuille. 2004. "Prevalence of HIV, Syphilis, Hepatitis B, and Hepatitis C among Entrants to Maryland Correctional Facilities." *Journal of Urban Health* 81: 25–37.

Solursh, Lionel P., Diane S. Solursh, and Charles A. Meyer. 1993. "Is There Sex after the Prison Door Slams Shut?" *Medicine and Law* 12: 439–443.

Stephens, T., S. Cozza, and R. Braithwaite. 1999. "Transsexual Orientation in HIV Risk Behaviors in an Adult Male Prison." *International Journal of STD and AIDS* 10: 28–31.

Stephenson, B. L., D. A. Wohl, R. McKaig, et al. 2006. "Sexual Behaviors of HIV-Seropositive Men and Women Following Release from Prison." *International Journal of STD and AIDS* 17: 103–108.

Sterngold, James. 2005. "Overhaul of Prison Health System Delayed." *San Francisco Chronicle*, November 3, B1.

Stevens, Patricia E. 1995. "Impact of HIV/AIDS on Women in the United States: Challenges of Primary and Secondary Prevention. *Health Care of Women International* 16: 577–595.

Stop Prison Rape. 2003. "Prison Rape Elimination Act Becomes Federal Law." Press release, September 4.

Taussig, J., R. L. Shouse, M. LaMarre, L. Fitzpatrick, P. McElroy, C. B. Borkowf, R. MacGowan, A. D. Margolis, D. Stratford, E. McLellan-Lemal, K. Robbins, W. Heneine, A. Greenberg, P. Sullivan, Z. Henderson, and K. Jafa. 2006. "HIV Transmission among Male Inmates in a State Prison System: Georgia 1992–2005." *Morbidity and Mortality Weekly Report*, Centers for Disease Control 55: 421–426.

Thomas, J. C., and L. A. Sampson. 2005. "High Rates of Incarceration as a Social Force Associated with Community Rates of Sexually Transmitted Infection." *Journal of Infectious Diseases* 191: S55–S60.

Toepell, A. R. 1992. "Prisoners and AIDS: AIDS Education Needs Assessment." Toronto, Canada: John Howard Society of Metropolitan Toronto.

Tonry, Michael. 1995. *Malign Neglect: Race, Crime, and Punishment in America*. New York: Oxford University Press.

——. 1999. "Why Are U.S. Incarceration Rates So High?" *Crime and Delinquency* 45: 419–437.

——. 2001. "Punishment Policies and Patterns in Western Countries" in *Sentencing and Sanctions in Western Countries*, ed. Michael Tonry and Richard S. Frase, 3–28. New York: Oxford University Press.

Travis, Jeremy. 2000. "But They All Come Back: Rethinking Prisoner Reentry." U.S. Department of Justice, National Institute of Justice.

Travis, Jeremy, and Michelle Waul (eds.). 2003. *Prisoners Once Removed: The Impact of Incarceration and Reentry on Children, Families, and Communities*. Washington DC: Urban Institute Press.

U.S. Census Bureau. 2005. "We the People: Black Population in the United States." Washington DC.

Van Campenhoudt, L., and M. Cohen. 1997. "Interaction and Risk-Related Behaviour: Theoretical and Heuristic Landmarks." In *Sexual Interactions and HIV Risk*, ed. L. Van Campenhoudt, M. Cohen, G. Guizzardi, and D. Hausser, 59–74. Bristol, PA: Taylor and Francis.

Western, Bruce. 2006. *Punishment and Inequality in America*. New York: Russell Sage Foundation.

Whitmore, S. K., et al. 2005. "Epidemiology of HIV/AIDS among Non-Hispanic Black Women in the United States." *Journal of the National Medical Association* 97: S19–S24.

Wohl, A. R., D. Johnson, W. Jordan, S. Lu, G. Beall, J.

Currier, and P. R. Kerndt. 2000. "High Risk Behaviors During Incarceration in African-American Men Treated for HIV at Three Los Angeles Public Medical Centers." *Journal of Acquired Immune Deficiency Syndromes* 24: 386–392.

Zierler, Sally, and Nancy Krieger. 1997. "Reframing Women's Risk: Social Inequalities and HIV Infection." *Public Health* 18: 401–436.

Zimring, Franklin E., Gordon Hawkins, and Sam Kamin. 2001. *Punishment and Democracy: Three Strikes and You're out in California*. New York: Oxford University Press.

CHAPTER 2

Drug Use, Syringe Sharing, and HIV Risk in the People's Republic of China

Michael Duke, JiangHong Li, and Merrill Singer

ABSTRACT

In the People's Republic of China (PRC), the State's response toward the emerging HIV epidemic has changed dramatically over time, from a denial that the disease existed within its borders to grudging acceptance to an aggressive, comprehensive prevention campaign that includes harm reduction approaches. Although the majority of AIDS cases stem from unhygienic commercial blood and plasma donation schemes that flourished during the early to mid-1990s, the majority of reported infections derive from drug-related syringe sharing. Set against a backdrop of changing governmental response to the epidemic, this chapter presents the unique features and contexts of syringe sharing in Guangdong province, as well as recommendations for intervention strategies.

OVERVIEW

In the People's Republic of China (PRC), the State's response toward the emerging HIV epidemic has changed dramatically over time, from a denial that the disease existed within its borders to grudging acceptance to an aggressive, comprehensive prevention campaign that includes harm reduction approaches. Although a large number of AIDS cases stem from unhygienic commercial blood and plasma collection schemes that flourished before the mid-1990s, the majority of reported infections derive from drug-related syringe sharing. While there is a significant body of literature from Western societies indicating that injection drug users (IDUs) share syringes for practical (Page, et al. 1990; Koester 1994; Siegal, et al. 1994; Carlson, et al. 1996; Singer 1997) and social reasons (Price 1988; Des Jarlais and Friedman 1990; Friedman, et al. 1992; Zapka, et al. 1993; Friedman, et al. 1997; Neaigus, et al. 1994; Latkin 1995; Longshore and Anglin 1995; Neaigus, et al. 1996; Suh, et al. 1997; Li, et al. 2003), the causes and characteristics of syringe sharing in China remain poorly understood (Duke and Li 2006; Li, et al. 2003). Set against a backdrop of changing governmental response to the epidemic, this chapter presents the results of a pilot study of syringe sharing in a mid-sized city in Guangdong Province, in the south of China. In particular, we will discuss the unique features and contexts of syringe sharing in China.

HIV IN THE PEOPLE'S REPUBLIC OF CHINA: AN OVERVIEW

It is estimated that the People's Republic of China has over 800,000 HIV cases (China Ministry of Health 2003). Although the government has stated its commitment to keep HIV cases at under 1.5 million (AFP 2005), this number may reach between 10 and 25 million by 2010 (China Ministry of Health and the UN Theme Group on HIV/AIDS in

China 2002). The rapidly accelerating rate of HIV infection spreading across China, and the potential for infections to reach epidemic proportions in the near future and to potentially derail the PRC's otherwise dramatic economic growth, has spurred the government to take dramatic action in recent years. This proactive response differs markedly from earlier government approaches.

Although the PRC experienced its first documented case of AIDS in 1985, initial response to the epidemic consisted of either denial of the disease's existence or an understating of the severity of the epidemic on the part of government officials. This dismissive approach was due in part to the belief that HIV was a foreign disease (Bureau of Hygiene and Tropical Diseases 1987). As a consequence, early public health responses to the disease were limited, and were directed largely at foreign residents and visitors rather than Chinese nationals. For example, in 1986, mandatory HIV testing for foreign students was initiated. A year later, the PRC's Vice Minister of Public Health warned women to avoid sexual relations with foreigners in order to prevent the spread of AIDS among the national population (China Ministry of Health and UN Theme Group on HIV/AIDS in China 1997). Driving the focus on outsiders over Chinese nationals was the underlying assumption that China was free of the alleged moral failings of Western society that were seen as responsible for the spread of the epidemic: drug abuse, sexual relationships between men, prostitution. Indeed, by the end of the 1980s, AIDS came to be known as *aizibing*, the "loving capitalism disease" (Bureau of Hygiene and Tropical Diseases 1990; Kanabus 2005).

More importantly, the initial denial of the scope of the epidemic within the country's borders is related to the political fallout surrounding the proliferation of poorly regulated plasma collection centers that sprang up in rural areas during the early to mid-1990s. Because of concerns about the safety of foreign blood supplies, the Chinese government banned the importation of blood products. A number of commercial blood collecting companies filled this void (China Ministry of Health and UN Theme Group on HIV/AIDS in China 1997). Most of these firms established collection centers in rural areas, both because of the vast number of impoverished peasants willing to sell whole blood or plasma and because it allowed these often illegal operations to avoid government oversight (UNAIDS 2002). Collection practices at these facilities were often highly unsanitary. Syringes typically were reused and the equipment not properly sanitized. Furthermore, the blood of multiple donors was mixed together as part of the plasma extraction process, and the resulting stew would be reinjected back into the blood sellers after the plasma was extracted. Rural areas within the central Henan Province were hit especially hard by this mode of transmission, with some regions reporting higher than 40 percent HIV prevalence (State Council AIDS Working Committee Office and UN Theme Group on HIV/AIDS in China 2004).

As it became clear that HIV rates were increasing throughout the country, the routes of transmission growing more diverse, and the epidemic spreading to the general population, the disease became harder for the government to downplay. Overlaying all of these factors was the presence of an enormous "floating population" of peasants seeking to escape rural poverty by relocating to urban centers (UNAIDS 2002). Although the presence of a vast mobile, expendable, proletarianized labor force was proving to be an important component of the PRC's economic growth, this population also posed particular challenges, given the strong association of migrant groups and the spread of HIV.

By the turn of the century, international and public health officials recognized the potential for HIV to grow into an epidemic of catastrophic proportions. The failure of China's initial attempt to apply for Global AIDS funding, coupled with intensive international criticism about the State's inefficient response to the epidemic, caused Beijing to begin reassessing its response to the epidemic. More significantly, the government's largely successful experience in controlling the initial wave of the Severe Acute Respiratory Syndrome (SARS) epidemic has helped lead to a change in its response to HIV/AIDS. The SARS epidemic provided the government with a sobering assessment of what could happen to China's economy and the country's overall standing in the world should a more devastating epidemic like HIV/AIDS fail to receive adequate attention: loss of productivity, risk of jeopardizing international investment, and a challenge to the PRC's meticulously cultivated image as a global leader and economic superpower (Einhorn 2004; Kleinman and Watson 2006).

In recent years, the PRC has been aggressive in pursuing multiple prevention strategies, including greater oversight over the nation's blood supply (China Daily 2004, 2005) and media campaigns to promote safe sex and reduce AIDS stigma (UNAIDS 2004: 10–12). For example, in November 2004, President Hu Jintao made a highly publicized visit to an AIDS ward in a Beijing hospital, and the widely circulated images of him shaking hands with two patients was meant to dispel the still commonly held belief that HIV could be spread through casual contact. In addition, the government has pursued a variety of interventions that target particular risk groups, including sex workers, truck drivers and other transportation workers, and intravenous drug users (State Council HIV/AIDS Working Committee Office and UN Theme Group on HIV/AIDS in China 2004). As of the date of this writing, most of these interventions remain at the pilot stage, or have been initiated by provincial governments, such as Yunnan Province's ambitious "Six Frontage" Program, which seeks to promote condom use, syringe exchange, methadone maintenance, and AIDS care support centers (UNAIDS 2002: 12–13). However, HIV prevention programs are not yet disseminated into all affected regions, and HIV-related stigma remains a significant barrier at the local level (AFP 2005). For example, the two AIDS patients who shook hands with President Hu subsequently became ostracized in their village in Shanxi Province because their HIV status was made public (Reuters 2005). Nonetheless, the ruling party has made dramatic changes in its approach to HIV/AIDS, from denial of its existence within its borders and stigmatizing of most of the groups at high risk, to a multi-tiered effort and an increasing acceptance of harm-reduction approaches to prevention.

HIV AND INTRAVENOUS DRUG USE

In the PRC, there is significant variation in HIV sero-prevalence not only between the nation's thirty-one provinces, but within them as well. In addition, prevalence rates for the most highly at-risk groups vary significantly from region to region (State Council HIV/AIDS Working Committee Office and UN Theme Group on HIV/AIDS in China 2004). Overall, the highest number of existing AIDS cases is due to unhygienic commercial blood and plasma collection. However, most of these infections occurred between 1992 and 1996, and related deaths may have reached their peak among this group (State Council HIV/AIDS Working Committee Office and UN Theme Group on HIV/AIDS in China 2004). Currently, injection drug use is the most frequent mode of new transmission (41 percent) among all reported HIV/AIDS cases (State Council HIV/AIDS Working Committee Office and UN Theme Group on HIV/AIDS in China 2004). The national HIV/AIDS sentinel surveillance indicates, furthermore, that the sharing of drug injection equipment is widespread in China, and that HIV infection is diffusing rapidly among IDUs.

Since HIV spread from Yunnan to other provinces in 1994 (China Ministry of Health 1997), a process that was fueled largely by injection drug use, the HIV/AIDS epidemic in China has rapidly accelerated. The number of Chinese drug users is constantly increasing. By 1995, all thirty-one provinces, including the major cities and autonomous regions in China, reported drug use problems. The epidemic among IDUs began in rural areas and then spread to urban areas, from ethnic minority communities (such as southern Yunnan, Xinjiang, and Liangshan in Sichuan Province) to mixed Han and ethnic minority communities (i.e., Xichang in Sichuan), and further to Han communities (i.e., Zigong in Sichuan, and most areas in Guangdong). The HIV epidemic among IDUs has spread along the major drug trafficking routes, from

Yunnan to Guangxi, Xinjiang, Sichuan, Guangdong, and other provinces (Wang 1998; Wu, Rou, and Cui 2004).

While sharing of drug injection equipment is widespread in China, existing data indicate variable sharing rates (25 percent to 100 percent) across different regions (China Ministry of Health 1999; China Ministry of Health and the UN Theme group on HIV/AIDS in China 2002). In many regions, increasing numbers of drug users are becoming injectors, and increasing proportions of injectors are sharing needles (China Ministry of Health 2001). Three interlocked changes —rising rates of injecting drug use, increasing rates of injection equipment sharing, and increasing rates of HIV infection among IDUs—place China on the cusp of a potentially explosive drug-related HIV epidemic (State Council AIDS Working Committee Office and UN Theme Group on HIV/AIDS in China 2004). In addition, the increasing rate of heterosexual transmission, changes in sexual social norms, large-scale migration, and low levels of risk awareness among ordinary people suggest the potential for extensive secondary HIV spread from IDUs to the general population (State Council HIV/AIDS Working Committee Office and UN Theme Group on HIV/AIDS in China 2004). Nevertheless, there has been a general lack of knowledge on drug use process, particularly in terms of the cultural, social, structural, and epidemiological factors associated with the sharing of drug injection equipment in China.

SYRINGE SHARING IN GUANGDONG PROVINCE

In order to understand the sociocultural beliefs, meanings, and understandings that underlie injection equipment sharing among IDUs, the authors initiated a pilot study[1] in collaboration with the China Centers for Disease Control and Prevention (CDC) in a mid-sized city in Guangdong Province in 2002 and 2003. The initial findings are discussed below.

Guangdong Province is located along the South China Sea in southeastern China. Situated in close proximity to both Hong Kong and Macao, and dominated by a major shipping port in the provincial capital of Guangzhou, Guangdong has a long history as a hub of shipping and trade, as well as serving as a gateway to the outside world. The province, for example, was a major staging area for the Opium Wars launched by Great Britain against China during the nineteenth century in order to pressure the Chinese to purchase opium from the British. In more recent times, Guangdong is thought to be part of a major smuggling corridor for Ecstasy, methamphetamine, and other drugs, and a destination for heroin from Yunnan Province (Brzezinski 2002). Guangdong is one of five provinces with a major HIV epidemic among injection drug users, and injection drug use related infections account for about 90 percent of all cases locally (Cheng, et al. 2004; Fang, et al. 2004; Fu, et al. 2004; Guangdong Health Bureau 2004; Peng, et al. 2006; Xu 2005).

Covering 9,450 square kilometers and containing a population of four million, Jiayuan (a pseudonym) is considered a mid-sized city by PRC standards. The administrative center for five county-level cities within Guangdong, Jiayuan is in many respects a prosperous and modern metropolis. Despite this, the Jiayuan Prefecture, along with four additional city/prefectures, are responsible for 61 percent of all reported HIV/AIDS cases in the province (Xu 2005).

METHODS

The project integrated quantitative survey and qualitative in-depth interviewing. Both components took place at mandatory treatment centers in the prefecture. Treatment centers house people who are charged with drug-related crimes. These sites were selected because the feasibility of reaching active drug users in the community was unknown at that time. The research team utilized an established protocol to ensure that participant confidentiality was maintained and that project data should not end up in the hands of treatment center officials (who are physicians but also police officials) or other authorities.

To recruit the survey sample, research team members from the Jiayuan CDC regularly contacted the two collaborating drug detoxification centers in Jiayuan City to identify times when they would have an adequate number of potential participants who: 1) had injected drugs within thirty days before entering the treatment center; and 2) would be discharged within two weeks. At appropriate times, the provincial and city offices of CDC assembled a group of interviewers from a pool of researchers who had undergone extensive training led by the authors, to visit the treatment centers and to conduct survey interviews. The final survey sample consisted of 199 former IDUs between 18 and 46 years of age. The one-on-one survey interview included questions about: 1) syringe availability, including acquisition, source, price, convenience of source location, problems encountered in acquisition, stability of syringe supply, and related issues; 2) drug use patterns (quantity, frequency, drugs use duration, location of use; 3) syringe- and other equipment-sharing behaviors; 4) socioeconomic status; 5) emotional state, including depression; 6) perceived peer risks and risk norms; 7) drug network characteristics, including network member characteristics and network structural features; 8) social support (emotional, social, material); 9) HIV/AIDS risk behaviors, knowledge, and attitudes; and 10) post-treatment life plans.

From the main survey sample, we purposively selected fifty-three IDUs who were talkative, able to clearly articulate their views, and were willing to describe the behaviors and attitudes of interest to the project. During the in-depth interview, subsample participants were asked about their: 1) drug injection initiation; 2) drug use patterns, including both injecting with and in the presence of others; 3) acquisition of drugs and syringes; 4) decision-making and circumstances regarding sharing of drug and injection equipment; and 5) knowledge of needle sharing and associated behaviors as transmission routes for HIV and other blood-borne diseases.

DEMOGRAPHICS

The main sample was 83.6 percent male and 16.4 percent female with a mean and median age of 29 years. The ethnic distribution of the participants was 96.5 percent Han (the predominant ethnic group in China) and 3.5 percent others (including Zhuang, Miao, and Tujia). Most participants in our sample were from Guangdong Province (78.4 percent) and Jiayuan City (60.3 percent). The majority (86.9 percent) had nine years or fewer of formal school education. Notably, almost half (42.7 percent) were unemployed at the time they entered the treatment center, while another 21.6 percent had only a temporary job during the thirty days prior to entering the center.

DRUG USE AND ACQUISITION

Drug use patterns were generally comparable to IDUs in Western countries, with some unique features. Heroin was the most popular injected drug, and was used by 95 percent of our participants. A notable percentage of our participants, however, reported also using prescription drugs such as diazepam (21.6 percent) and triazolam (10.6 percent). These medications were sometimes mixed with heroin, but were also used as a substitute when heroin was unavailable. Some respondents noted that prescription medications had distinct advantages over heroin in that they were relatively easy to obtain and would not result in arrest for drug possession if the user was stopped by the police.

In-depth interview data showed that some drug users did not work because of their addiction and therefore had to engage in gambling and theft or other crimes to get money for drugs. Because of the unreliability of these revenue-generating activities and the need to apply available funds to drug purchases, participants did not always have the money to purchase a new syringe.

Another unique feature among the sample was the ways in which drugs were purchased and divided. Among habitual drug-using cohorts in the United States, these activities are frequently a source of conflict due to the anxiety of not receiving one's "fair share" of the drug (Singer 2006). In contrast, Jiayuan IDUs tended to treat members of their drug-using network differently than they did others who were outside the group. Among IDUs with a network relationship based on *guānxì* (reciprocity and mutual obligation) participants reported feeling obliged to pool money together to buy drugs in order to: 1) reduce the total cost for each network member, and; 2) to insure that those who did not have enough money on a given day could nonetheless use drugs. Expressing concern about whether or not everyone's contribution matched the amount of drugs he or she received was considered inappropriate. As one participant said: "We are very close, so we do not *feng* [divide something evenly]. Whoever has money takes it out to use first. When we finished it, when there are no more drugs left, we see how much money all of us have, pool it together, and see how much we can get. You don't need to *feng* drugs."

SYRINGE ACQUISITION

At the time of the study, Jiayuan did not have a syringe exchange or distribution program in place. Thus, most of our participants (86.9 percent) reported pharmacies as their primary syringe sources. Syringes could be purchased in the province for about one yuan each (about 12 cents, U.S.) from pharmacies without a prescription. A walking survey conducted at the beginning of the study found that there were numerous small pharmacies and convenience stores selling syringes without the required government license, in addition to licensed pharmacies. The number and location of pharmacies and other stores selling syringes appeared to make it relatively easy for IDUs to buy guaranteed sterile syringes. Indeed, 86.9 percent of participants reported pharmacies as their primary syringe source. Our in-depth interview data showed that government anti-drug campaigns or other types of governmental license checking could cause significant decreases in syringe selling at these businesses. Concerns about police interference and low night-time pharmacy accessibility were two other main barriers for sterile syringe access identified by the research. Unlike the U.S.A. (Stopka, et al. 2003), pharmacists' attitudes toward their drug-using customers did not appear to be a barrier to IDUs' access to sterile syringes, since respondents did not feel that they were discriminated against in these locales.

SYRINGE AND PARAPHERNALIA SHARING AND HIV RISK

The median number of injections per day among participant was 2.67. This figure fits within the lower range of injection frequency among U.S. drug-using populations studied by the authors (Singer, et al. 1998). Nearly 45 percent of participants reported that they would discard a syringe only once the needle point had become dull; that is, at the point at which it would become painful to puncture a vein and put the user at risk for causing vein damage. Jiayuan IDUs most often injected in the place where they currently lived (83.0 percent), while 12 percent of participants reported public places as the locale used most often for injection.

Notably, compared with our research data of U.S. drug users, Jiayuan IDUs were more likely to share drugs, syringes and other injection equipment with others. In the thirty days prior to entering the detoxification center, for example, 30.1 percent of respondents used other people's syringes, compared to 17 percent in a comparative sample of U.S. drug users (Singer, et al. 1992). Also, 33.8 percent of Guangdong IDUs injected drugs that were squirted from another syringe and 36.2 percent used drugs that were mixed, measured, or divided within a syringe that belonged to someone else. Other indirect and potentially risky sharing of syringes or injection paraphernalia (i.e., rinse water; cookers or filters; and drugs that were contaminated by others' syringes) was also common (23.2 percent, 24 percent, and 24.4 percent, respectively). Notably, 41.7 percent of participants reported at least one of these risk behaviors.

The most commonly cited reasons for reusing a syringe that was already owned was that it was convenient to do so (61.5 percent) and that the needle was still usable (39.2 percent). In terms of syringe sharing, participants' most commonly stated explanation was that they were suffering from drug withdrawals and did not have their own needle (68.9 percent) or that using another's syringe was more convenient (41.7 percent).

Among the 112 IDUs (57.4 percent of the sample) who had sex during the one-month period prior to entering treatment, only 25 percent reported always using a condom with casual sex partners. In fact, 63.6 percent reported that they never used condoms with their casual partners. Additionally, 6.3 percent of the survey participants reported that they sold sex for money; 32.1 percent indicated that they paid for sex; and 27.0 percent said that they had sex with other IDUs or someone suspected to be an IDU prior to entering treatment. The mean and median number of sex partners for members of the sample during the month before entering treatment were 1.7 and 1.0 respectively (SD=1.55). Survey findings on HIV risk behaviors and syringe sharing are summarized in Exhibits 2.1 and 2.2.

Other behaviors found to be associated with syringe sharing include the number of injections carried out per day, the frequency of injecting in the same location as other injectors, and positive results in the Peer Risk Behavior and Depression Scales. These findings are summarized in Exhibit 2.3.

EPIDEMIOLOGICAL AND CULTURAL ASPECTS OF SYRINGE SHARING

The message that sharing syringes can transmit HIV had circulated widely among the drug-using community in Guangdong. This was reflected in the initial reluctance of interview participants to admit that they had engaged in such activities. Many participants reported that they did not share syringes with others at the beginning of the in-depth interview. As the interview proceeded, however, they frequently would admit that they sometimes resorted to using another's equipment when they desperately needed to inject but did not have their own syringe with them, a pattern that is also typical among U.S. IDUs. Syringe sharing was particularly common at night, when most pharmacies were closed. Very often, the need to get high prevented

Exhibit 2.1 HIV risk behaviors of Jiayuan IDUs during last thirty days of drug use (N = 199)

	%
Used other people's syringes	30.1
Injected drugs that were squirted from another syringe	33.8
Indirect syringe or paraphernalia (cookers, filters, rinse water)	41.7
Always using a condom with casual sex partners	25.0
Never use condoms with casual sex partners	63.6
Sold sex for money	6.3
Paid for sex	32.1
Sex with other IDUs	27.0

Exhibit 2.2 Reasons for using others' syringes (N = 60)

I was sick and did not have a needle on me	68.9%
Convenient, didn't have to go buy one	41.7%
The needle was from my boyfriend/girlfriend	5.0%
I had the needle cleaned	11.5%
It was at night and I did not want to go out to get one	11.7%
There is no reason not to use others' needle	15.0%
Other	11.7%

Exhibit 2.3 Factors associated with drug or injection paraphernalia sharing

	Direct sharing of syringes	*Indirect sharing of syringe or injection equipment*
Number of injections per day	Pearson r = .254, p = .030	Pearson r = .294, p = .000
Frequency injecting with others	Pearson r = .230, p = .001	Pearson r = .220, p = .002
Peer Risk Behavior	Pearson r = .394, p = .000	Pearson r = .255, p = .009
Depression Scale (Lin 1989)	Pearson r = .229, p = .001	Pearson r = .116, p = .019

Note: No associations were found between the above variables and direct or indirect syringe sharing: age, sex, education level, income, AIDS Risk Behavior Knowledge (Kelly et al. 1989), and Individualism and Collectivism (Triandis 1995).

participants from focusing on other concerns, including the desire to stay healthy.

Our in-depth interview data suggest that Jiayuan IDUs' sharing behaviors (including direct and indirect sharing of injection equipment) were associated with the lack of availability of sterile syringes at the precise time of the injection act, as well as the lack of money to purchase a syringe when it was needed. In addition, respondents sometimes based their decision to share on inadequate HIV risk knowledge, such as the commonly held view that injection-related HIV risk was limited to the direct sharing of needles, and that the HIV virus would die a few seconds after leaving the body. Awareness of indirect sharing risks was limited.

The size of the syringe used by participants also appears to be a factor in sharing behaviors. While the most common syringe gauge of IDUs in the United States is between 0.5 cc and 1 cc with a needle length of between ½ and 5/8 inch, the most widespread syringe available in Jiayuan is 3 cc with a 9/10 inch needle. The barrel of these large syringes is thus of sufficient size to facilitate the mixing of drugs with water, and the needle is long enough to draw a portion of the resulting solution from the back of another's syringe. Participants characterized this strategy for dividing drugs, known in the United States as backloading, as particularly common. Indirect syringe sharing of this type is particularly risky if a previous user of the syringe is HIV positive, since trace amounts of blood containing the HIV virus may be present in the syringe barrel.

Lastly, respondents reported sharing syringes in order to maintain harmonious interpersonal relationships within their immediate drug-using network.

As in the general Chinese population, maintaining group harmony and integrity appears to be more important to a Chinese IDU than insisting on distributive equity. As noted above, among U.S. drug users, arguments over getting a fair portion when drugs are divided are quite common and can be intense—even among family members, intimate partners, and other close associates—and syringes without clearly identified calibration markers can therefore be useless (Weeks, et al. 1996).

However, a commonly accepted view among Jiayuan drug users is that "friends should help each other out." It is furthermore expected that "whoever has money pays for the group's drugs," and "the one who has more money contributes more, the one who has less contributes less." The most commonly expressed benefits of pooling money for drug purchases are that the one who has little or no money can still get the amount of drug he or she needs, and that pooling funds helps to lower the cost per individual over time. Expressing concern about fairness would disturb the *guānxì* relationship among network members and be considered socially inappropriate and insulting. If someone feels they are being called on too frequently to contribute more than their share for the drugs consumed among network members, participants reported they would not express their dissatisfaction. Instead, they might find an excuse to inject alone rather than hurt each other's *miànzi* (prestige or reputation) and *guānxì* by refusing to share. When someone is craving drugs, or has no syringes or other injection equipment, others are expected "to do this person a *rénqíng*"; that is, engage in reciprocity by offering drugs or a syringe to that person. The recipient is then expected to behave similarly at some point in the future and return the *rénqíng*. For example, our in-depth interviews show that Jiayuan drug users often maintain relationships by visiting each other and sharing drugs in the host's residence. The host is expected to offer his or her syringes (new or used) to those who did not bring their own syringes, which is often the case.

CONCLUSIONS

As the People's Republic of China's HIV epidemic is driven currently by injection drug use, it is critically important to understand the cultural, social, structural, and epidemiological dimensions of syringe-sharing behaviors in that country. The study outlined here offers a tantalizing glimpse into the ways in which these behaviors are manifested. However, further research is needed to determine the degree to which these results can be generalized in such a geographically vast and culturally diverse nation. A particularly fruitful area of investigation is the cultural dimension of relationship maintenance, including the nature of drug use networks, the various social exchange rules that inform interpersonal relations, and the motivations and decision-making patterns related to relationship maintenance and drug or injection equipment sharing. If, for example, there are significant cultural pressures placed on drug users to share their injection equipment despite their health concerns, this would pose significant challenges to any social marketing campaign designed to reduce direct and indirect syringe sharing. Fortunately, the government's growing willingness to treat HIV risk as a public health problem requiring multiple approaches, rather than approaching the epidemic in strictly moralistic or punitive terms, may help to lead the PRC away from the turmoil that would result should HIV rates spin out of control.

NOTE

1. Funding was provided by a grant from the National Institute on Drug Abuse (#R03 DA14705; PI: Jianghong Li).

REFERENCES AND FURTHER READING

AFP (Agence France Presse). "China Marks World AIDS Day, but Faces Uphill Battle Against Spread," *AFP (Agence France Presse)*. December 1, 2005.

Brzezinski, Matthew. "Re-Engineering the Drug Business." *New York Times Magazine*, June 23, 2002, 24–29, 46–55.

Bureau of Hygiene and Tropical Diseases. *AIDS Newsletter* (1987): news item 531.

Bureau of Hygiene and Tropical Diseases. *AIDS Newsletter* (1990): news item 213.

Carlson, Robert G., et al. "Attitudes Toward Needle Sharing Among Injection Drug Users: Combining Qualitative and Quantitative Research Methods." *Human Organization* 55(4) (1996): 361–369.

Cheng, Yu, et al. "Community Outreach: A Case Study among Guangzhou Injection Drug users." *Journal of Guangxi University for Nationalities* 26(4) (2004): 83–87.

China Daily "Suppliers of Blood Under Investigation." July 30, 2004.

China Daily "China Closes Blood Agencies to Curb AIDS." March 28, 2005.

China Ministry of Health, National Center for AIDS Prevention and Control. Beijing. *National HIV/AIDS Surveillance Report 1996*. 1997.

China Ministry of Health. "Current Status of HIV in China." Beijing, December 1999.

China Ministry of Health. *China Annual STI and HIV/AIDS Sentinel Surveillance Report. (1989–2000)*. Beijing 2001.

China Ministry of Health. News Conference. September 2003.

China Ministry of Health and the UN Theme Group on HIV/AIDS in China. "China Responds to AIDS." November 1997.

China Ministry of Health and the UN Theme Group on HIV/AIDS in China. *HIV/AIDS: China's Titanic Peril: 2001 Update of the AIDS Situation and Needs Assessment Report*. Beijing, UNAIDS, June 2002.

Des Jarlais, Donald C., and Samuel R. Friedman. "Shooting Galleries and AIDS: Infection Probabilities and 'Tough' Policies." *American Journal of Public Health* 80(2) (1990): 142–144.

Duke, Michael, and JiangHong Li. "Medical Anthropology in the U.S.A. and China in the Context of the AIDS Syndemic." *Journal of Guangxi University for Nationalities* 28(3) (2006): 9–13.

Einhorn, Bruce. "AIDS: China Opens it Eyes." *Business Week Online*, July 19, 2004.

Fang, Yang, et al. "Qualitative Study on Drug Use and Syringe Sharing among IDUs in Guangdong." *Southern China Journal of Preventive Medicine*. 30(6) (December 2004): 1–4.

Friedman, Samuel R., et al. "Social Intervention Against AIDS Among Injection Drug Users." *British Journal of Addiction* 87 (1992): 393–404.

Friedman, Samuel R., et al. "Network and Sociohistorical Approaches to the HIV Epidemic among Drug Injectors." In *The impact of AIDS: Psychological and social aspects of HIV infection*. ed. L. Sherr, J. Catalan, and B. Hedge, 89–113. Switzerland: Harwood Academic Publishers, 1997.

Fu, Xiaobing, et al. "2004 Epidemiological Survey of Poly-Drug Abuse among Injection Drug Users in Guangdong Province." *South China Journal of Preventive Medicine* 30(6) (December 2004): 8–11.

Guangdong Health Bureau. *Guangdong Province HIV Updates*, 2004.

Kanabus, Annabel. *HIV and AIDS in China* [online]. Horsham, West Sussex, UK: Avert. org, 2005. http://www.avert.org/aidschina.htm. Cited December 31, 2005.

Kelly, Jeffrey A., et al. "An Objective Test of AIDS Risk Behavior Knowledge: Scale development, Validation and Norms." *Journal of Behavior Therapy and Experimental Psychiatry*. 20 (1989): 227–234.

Kleinman, Arthur, and James L. Watson, eds. *SARS in China: Prelude to Pandemic?* Stanford, CA: Stanford University Press, 2006.

Koester, Stephen K. "The context of Risk: Ethnographic Contributions to the Study of Drug Use and HIV." *NIDA Research Monograph* 143 (1994): 202–217.

Latkin, Carl A. "A Personal Network Approach to AIDS Prevention: An Experimental Peer Group Intervention for Street-Injecting Drug Users: The SAFE Study." *NIDA Research Monograph 151* (1995): 181–195.

Li, JiangHong, et al. "Revealing Drug Users' Injection Practice and HIV Risks in Guangdong, China." Paper presented at AIDS Science Day, Yale University, New Haven, CT, April 2003.

Lin, N. "Measuring Depressive Symptomatology in China." Journal of Nervous and Mental Disease 177 (1989): 121–131.

Longshore, Douglas, and M. Douglas Anglin. "Intentions to Share Injection Paraphernalia: An Empirical Test of the AIDS Risk Reduction Model Among Injection Drug Users." *International Journal of the Addictions* 30(3) (1995): 305–321.

Neaigus, A., et al. "The Relevance of Drug Injectors' Social and Risk Networks for Understanding and Preventing HIV Infection." *Social Science and Medicine* 38(1) (1994): 67–78.

Neaigus, Alan, et al. "High-Risk Personal Networks and Syringe Sharing as Risk Factors for HIV Infection Among New Drug Injectors." *Journal of Acquired Immune Deficiency Syndrome and Human Retrovirology* 11(5) (1996): 499–509.

Page, J. Bryan, et al. "Intravenous Drug Use and HIV Infection in Miami." *Medical Anthropology Quarterly* 4(1) (1990): 56–71.

Peng Lin, et al. "Characteristics of Drug Use and Sexual Behaviors among Injection Drug Users in Guangdong Province." *Chinese Journal Of AIDS and STD* 12(2) (2006): 117–120.

Price, Rumi Kato, "Kicking the Habit: A Social Network Approach to Recovery from Opiate Addiction." Ph.D. Dissertation, Department of Sociology. Berkeley, CA, University of California at Berkeley, 1988.

Reuters. "Hu Handshakes Mean Mockery for China AIDS Victims." December 14, 2005.

Siegal, Harvey A., et al. "Injection Drug Users' Needle-Cleaning Practices." Letter to the editor. *American Journal of Public Health* 84(9) (1994): 1523–1524.

Singer, Merrill. "Needle Exchange and AIDS Prevention: Controversies, Policies and Research." *Medical Anthropology* 18(1) (1997): 1–12.

Singer, Merrill. *The Face of Social Suffering: The Life History of a Street Drug Addict*. Long Grove, IL: Waveland Press, 2006.

Singer, Merrill, et al. "AIDS and the IV Drug User: The Local Context in Prevention Efforts." *Medical Anthropology* 14 (1992): 285–306.

Singer, Merrill, et al. "Variation in Drug Injection Frequency Among Out-of-Treatment Drug Users: A National Study." *American Journal of Drug and Alcohol Abuse* 24(2) (1998): 321–341.

State Council HIV/AIDS Working Committee Office and UN Theme Group on HIV/AIDS in China. "A Joint Assessment of HIV/AIDS Prevention. Treatment and care in China," 2004.

Stopka, Thomas, et al. "Pharmacy Access to Over-the-Counter (OTC) Syringes in Connecticut: Implications for HIV and Hepatitis Prevention among Injection Drug Users." *AIDS and Public Policy Journal* 17(4) (2003): 115–126.

Suh, Tongwoo, et al. "Social Network Characteristics and Injecting HIV-Risk Behaviors Among Street Injection Drug Users." *Drug and Alcohol Dependence* 47(2) (1997): 137–143.

Triandis, Harry C. *Individualism and Collectivism*. Boulder, CO: Westview Press, 1995.

UNAIDS. *HIV/AIDS: China's Titanic Peril*, 2002.

Wang Zhe. "Current Epidemics of STDs and HIV/AIDS and Control Strategies and Programs in China." *Chinese Journal of Prevention and Control of STD and AIDS*. Supplement (1998): 1–4.

Weeks, Margaret, et al. "Community-Based AIDS Prevention: Preliminary Outcomes of a Program for African American and Latino Injection Drug Users." *Journal of Drug Issues* 26(3) (1996): 561–590.

Wu Zunyou, Keming Rou, and Haixia Cui. "The HIV/AIDS Epidemic in China: History, Current Strategies and Future Challenges." *AIDS Education and Prevention* 16, Supplement A (2004): 7–17.

Xu, Ruiheng. "Er Zhi Ai Zi Bing Liu Xing, Jia Kuai Shi Shi Jian Shao Wei Hai Ce Lue" ("Controlling the HIV Epidemic by Accelerating the Implementation of Harm Reduction Strategies"), Centers for Disease Control, Guangdong, China, November 30, 2005 (cited 15 December 2005). http://www.cdcp.org.cn/expert/aids3.pdf.

Zapka, Jane G., et al. "Social Network, Support and Influence: Relationships with drug-use and Protective AIDS Behavior." *AIDS Education and Prevention* 5, No. 4 (1993): 352–366.

CHAPTER 3

The Role of Drug Users in the Brazilian HIV/AIDS Epidemic

Patterns, Perceptions, and Prevention

Scott Clair, Merrill Singer, Francisco I. Bastos, Monica Malta, Claudia Santelices, and Neilane Bertoni

ABSTRACT

According to a report issued by the Brazilian Ministry of Health in 2001, the official estimated number of adults living with HIV/AIDS in 2000 was about half of what was predicted. This difference is attributable in large part to a comprehensive set of prevention and care initiatives. However, the majority of health professionals working in testing facilities do not receive proper training to provide culturally sensitive counseling and testing for drug-using populations. This is especially problematic because a substantial proportion of HIV/AIDS cases in Brazil have been attributed to drug use. This chapter examines the drug-use behaviors of street drug users in Brazil and assesses the feasibility of oral HIV tests now that Brazil has approved rapid oral testing for HIV.

Extrapolating from existing trends, in 1992 the Brazilian Ministry of Health (2001a) estimated that over a million adults in the country would be living with HIV/AIDS by the year 2000. Instead, according to a report issued by the Ministry in 2001, the official estimated number of adults living with HIV/AIDS in 2000 was about half of what was predicted. Based on various analyses, Brazilian and international experts are unanimous in concluding that the substantial difference between actual and estimated numbers of people living with HIV/AIDS (PLWHA) in Brazil is attributable in large part to a comprehensive set of prevention and care initiatives implemented by the Brazilian National STD/AIDS Program, state and municipal health secretariats, and nongovernmental organizations (NGOs) (Brazilian Ministry of Health 2000a, 2001a). While this is a significant achievement, especially in light of the continued global spread of the AIDS pandemic, to fully assess the effectiveness of AIDS prevention in Brazil it is necessary to identify who actually did become infected and the patterning of disease spread in a time of enhanced prevention efforts.

In the early 1980s, the HIV epidemic in Brazil, like many other developed Western countries, was largely restricted to people living in major urban centers, men who have sex with men (MSM), and people who received blood transfusions. In the mid-1980s, the epidemic began to spread to midsize cities and markedly increased among vulnerable groups, such as injection drug users (IDUs). In a third and ongoing phase, HIV has been spreading in smaller municipalities and among heterosexuals (Lowndes, et al. 2000; Szwarcwald, et al. 2000). Fortunately, scenarios that forecast a massive epidemic among heterosexuals throughout Brazil have not materialized to date. The Joint United Nations Program on HIV/AIDS (UNAIDS) estimates the current overall HIV prevalence in Brazil as 0.57

percent. HIV prevalence rates among specific subgroups are considerably higher—particularly among IDUs from Southern Brazil and female sex workers from the lower social strata. A 1998 study conducted among female sex workers in São Paulo, for example, documented 18 percent HIV prevalence rates (UNAIDS 2000).

While the overall prevalence of HIV has been declining in recent years throughout the country, prevalence continues to rise among poor women, IDUs, and the sexual partners of IDUs in specific geographic areas, such as the south of Brazil (Brazilian Ministry of Health 2001a; Hacker, et al. 2006; Szwarcwald, et al. 2001; UNAIDS 2000). These trends affirm the importance of better understanding of HIV/AIDS risk and prevention among drug users in Brazil, which is the focus of this chapter. Specifically, the chapter examines the role of drug users in the Brazilian epidemic, the current state of prevention and treatment initiatives targeted to this population, and the nature of HIV testing available to drug users, especially oral HIV testing, and presents suggestive findings from a National Institute on Drug Abuse (NIDA)-funded multimethod study of mismessaging in oral HIV testing among drug users in Rio de Janeiro that have direct implications for HIV prevention in Brazil.

HIV/AIDS AMONG DRUG USERS IN BRAZIL

Since the mid-1980s, an increasing proportion of HIV/AIDS cases in Brazil have been attributed to injection drug use. In the south and southeast metropolitan areas, in particular, IDUs and their sexual partners have played a pivotal role in local HIV/AIDS dynamics (Bastos et al. 1999; Bastos et al. 2002). IDUs constituted about 4 percent of HIV/AIDS cases in the early 1980s, but they now account for about 25 percent of new cases. HIV sero-prevalence rates among IDUs vary widely across cities in Brazil, ranging from a low of about 10 percent to as high as 70 percent in some metropolitan areas (Bastos, et al. 2002).

A unique characteristic of the drug scene in Brazil is that the major drug of abuse is cocaine. Due to the specific patterns of cocaine consumption—namely, constant and repetitive use in a single day—active cocaine users frequently engage in risk behaviors to maintain their established patterns of recurrent consumption (Inciardi and Surratt 2001; Latkin, et al. 2001). Additionally, many cocaine users are engaged in commercial sex, participate in dealing small amounts of illicit drugs, and are homeless or living in shelters. There is also a clear relationship between illicit drug use and HIV sexual risk in Brazil. Studies conducted with men who have sex with men and commercial sex workers found that illicit drug use (both injectors and non-injectors) was related to an increased likelihood of being HIV positive and engaging in higher levels of HIV sexual risk (Souza, et al. 2002; Szwarcwald, et al. 1998).

NEED FOR HIV TESTING

Brazil was the first middle-income country with a sizable epidemic to provide free, universal access to antiretroviral (ARV) therapy for the treatment of HIV/AIDS, followed by Argentina, and more recently by Botswana and Thailand. Universal access to ARV therapy was established by Brazilian Federal Law No. 9.313, implemented on November 13, 1996. This law states: "HIV-infected people and/or people living with AIDS are entitled to receive, at no cost, all medicines necessary for their treatment, from the National Health System" (Brazilian Ministry of Health 2000b). At present, more than 180,000 persons receive ARV therapy in Brazil. There are approximately 620,000 PLWHA currently in Brazil. This proportion of approximately 29 percent of PLWHA under ARV treatment corresponds to the number of persons who have been identified as needing such treatment by the Brazilian National Health System.

Treatment of drug users presents considerable challenges anywhere, but in developing countries there are additional problems due to scarce resources and poor infrastructure. Despite taking important steps to address the HIV/AIDS epidemic in Brazil, health professionals still lack adequate training regarding drug users and HIV; treatment facilities targeted to this population are relatively scarce; and the health infrastructure overall is inadequate in light of the significant health disparities that prevail in the country (Goldstein 2003). Therefore, some studies have concluded that HIV testing targeted to drug users is needed (Ferreira, et al. 2006). PLWHA who are also substance dependent in studies outside of Brazil have been found to usually face several barriers in accessing HIV testing, treatment and care; they generally receive poor HIV voluntary counseling and testing (VCT) and limited psychosocial support; and they are the recipients of suboptimal clinical follow-up (Barcellos, et al. 2003; Knowlton, et al. 2001; Malta, et al. 2003).

Despite substantial improvements in access to VCT generally in Brazil, many persons are still not being diagnosed until the later stages of HIV infection. Late diagnoses make the clinical care of HIV/AIDS more complicated and costly. To address this issue, the Brazilian Ministry of Health (BMH) has intensified the development of a comprehensive network of free and anonymous VCT units throughout the country. Currently, there are around 400 free public HIV testing units across Brazil (Brazilian Ministry of Health 2007). However, the vast majority of health professionals working in those facilities do not receive proper training to provide culturally sensitive counseling and testing for drug-using populations. In light of international studies that have documented that vulnerable populations, such as IDUs and poor women, have lower rates of early diagnosis and hence of initial and continued access to ARV therapy (Zorrilla 2000), there is a need for specialized intervention that is culturally and socially appropriate for and acceptable to these populations. Knowledge in this area in Brazil is limited, as are resources assigned to fill this gap in prevention services.

ORAL HIV TESTING

Oral HIV testing methods, which are now widely available internationally, have produced several tangible benefits over other methods of testing. These include lower personnel costs, increased portability of the test, less reluctance to provide oral specimens as opposed to blood draws (in that a notable number of street drug users feel uncomfortable with serum testing), the ability to test individuals with collapsed or hard-to-locate veins, and the removal of the possibility of needle-stick injuries to staff (Gallo, et al. 1997). Perhaps most importantly, early reports suggest that these methods have resulted in more people getting tested for HIV (Bureau of HIV/AIDS Early Intervention Section 1999). These advances in HIV testing have not resulted in a decrease in test accuracy, as shown in two large empirical studies conducted with the OraSure (Epitope, Beaverton, OR) oral HIV testing method (Gallo, et al. 1997; Soto-Ramirez, et al. 1992). In light of the importance of drug use in the spread of HIV/AIDS in Brazil, all of these findings suggest the value of implementing oral HIV testing targeted to Brazilian drug users.

Despite these benefits, there is the possibility of unintended consequences resulting from oral HIV testing. One such possible unintended effect is leading participants to believe, or perpetuating their existing belief, in the transmission of HIV through saliva (e.g., through kissing or sharing a drinking utensil). *Past research has found that the belief in the possible transmission of HIV through saliva is fairly widespread in some populations.* Research among Latinos in the U.S.A., for example, has found that they have lower AIDS knowledge scores than other ethnic groups (Nyamathi, et al. 2000; Scott, et al. 1998, Singer, et al. 1990).

Little, if any, research has been conducted on the potential effects of oral HIV testing on AIDS knowledge. Recent research by our research team, however, suggests that those tested with oral methods are more likely subsequently to believe that HIV can be transmitted through saliva (Clair, et al. 2003). In this study, we compared street-recruited drug users who had received oral HIV testing at baseline with those that had not on three different interview items that assessed HIV Saliva Risk Behavior Knowledge both at their baseline assessment and at a follow-up assessment approximately four months later. Participants who received HIV testing had higher scores on each of the three items at baseline compared to those who did not test. However, at Time 2 the accuracy of those who tested decreased and the accuracy of participants who did not test increased, such that at Time 2 those who did not test had higher scores on each of the three items. Examining the means over time for the two groups, we found that those who did not test were more accurate over time in their assessment of oral HIV risk and those who did test were less accurate over time.

While there are several benefits of oral HIV testing methods, this study suggests that there may also be important drawbacks to using these methods. Specifically, it appears that over time those persons who received oral HIV testing were more likely to believe in the possible transmission of HIV through saliva. The current study will help assess the generalizability of these findings to other social contexts and different populations of drug users.

IMPLICATIONS OF LOWER HIV KNOWLEDGE

There are real and tangible implications to increasing and/or perpetuating the belief in the transmission of HIV through saliva. Specifically: 1) those with lower AIDS knowledge scores are less likely to reduce their risky HIV behaviors, get tested for HIV or return for their test results; and 2) those who believe that HIV can be transmitted through saliva and casual contact in general are more likely to have prejudicial attitudes towards PLWHAs.

HIV knowledge is part of the foundation guiding most effective interventions (Dudley, et al. 2002; Laub, et al. 1999). Although some research among drug users has shown a direct link between AIDS knowledge and risk behavior, the consensus is that AIDS knowledge is a necessary but not a sufficient condition for reducing HIV risk behavior (Lewis, et al. 1997). Furthermore, successful prevention programs must include an HIV knowledge component, because knowing how HIV is transmitted is the first step in risk behavior reduction (Cerwonka, et al. 2000). Moreover, as Ingham (1995: 44) observed, mistaken beliefs about routes of HIV transmission can "engender a feeling of helplessness such that no changes are made." Recent research on the role of emotions in decision-making suggests that negative affect, such as the fear of contracting HIV, can result in an inability to generate alternative solutions, thus putting the individual more at risk (Dudley, et al. 2002). Lower HIV knowledge has also been linked to lower rates of HIV testing and participants being less likely to return for HIV test results (Nyamathi, et al. 2000; Simon, et al. 1996). Accurate HIV knowledge, in short, is essential for HIV prevention and risk reduction to be successful. In a country like Brazil, where drug users constitute a high and growing portion of infected individuals, accurate HIV knowledge in this population has national implications for halting the AIDS epidemic.

Moreover, 25 percent of those who believed HIV could be spread by sharing a drink, coughing, and sneezing showed stigmatized attitudes towards PLWHAs compared to 14 percent of those who stated that HIV could not be transmitted in these ways (Centers for Disease Control and Prevention 2000). Lew-Ting and Hsu (2002) similarly found that more accurate knowledge leads to less prejudicial attitudes. Specifically, they found that the instrument items "shaking hands" and "sharing of utensils" were the most predictive of prejudicial attitudes among those who thought you could get HIV in these ways. Ingham (1995) cautioned such beliefs could lead to fear and discrimination, which could potentially further stigmatize people living with HIV/AIDS. The in-depth interviews with our participants substantiate these concerns and show that these errant beliefs carry very significant and real consequences for the people affected by them in their own lives. In that experiencing HIV stigmatization creates burdens for sufferers that are equal to or even greater than infection itself, minimizing misinformation about HIV transmission is critically important.

METHODS

The goals of our project were to enhance our understanding of oral HIV testing among street drug users by implementing oral testing in a new setting, to increase the HIV testing capacity in Brazil by assessing the feasibility of oral testing, and to pilot-test a replicable approach for use in the U.S.A. and elsewhere through an enhanced counseling and testing protocol designed to minimize potential unintended consequences. The study employed a survey assessment, focus group interviewing, and in-depth interviewing with active drug users. Data for the current chapter come from the survey assessment and qualitative in-depth interviews, so we will focus our description on those.

Recruitment of Study Participants

Participants for all components of this study were recruited through street outreach by a trained team of community outreach workers. Outreach workers, primarily former drug users who lived in major slum areas, commonly referred to as favelas in Brazil, or other disenfranchised communities of Rio de Janeiro, recruited participants from local street drug scenes in these locations. Participants also were recruited at an assessment center for drug users sponsored by the Rio de Janeiro State Council for Drug Abuse.

Survey Assessment

The survey was administered at two time points, first at baseline and then at the four-month follow-up. The survey included several different measures including social and environmental factors, psychosocial factors, health outcomes, and HIV Transmission Knowledge.

In-Depth Interview

This component of the study involved the recruitment of a nested subsample of thirty-four active drug users from the larger survey sample for in-depth interviewing. The specific questions for the in-depth interview component of interest to the current chapter included: 1) participants' experiences with HIV testing, including experiences with the oral test; 2) their understanding of differences between the HIV oral and blood tests and the comparative acceptability of these two forms of testing among drug users; and 3) the participants' reactions about which type of HIV testing they thought would be more accepted in the general population and among drug users. Participants were paid R$24 (approximately $12) for each interview. Interviews were conducted in Portuguese and translated into English for analysis.

THE INTERVENTION

One goal of the project was to test an intervention designed to reduce the likelihood that individuals who undergo HIV testing with an oral test would be more likely to believe that HIV can be orally transmitted. The intervention we designed consisted of a pile-sort that was administered to participants after they had completed the survey. Participants in the experimental group were shown a set of thirteen picture cards that represented direct or indirect human interaction (e.g., two people kissing, one person handing another a glass, one person handing another a syringe). Participants were asked to sort the cards into two piles: interactions that are known to transmit HIV and those that have not been found to be routes of routine HIV transmission. If participants placed cards in the incorrect pile, the intervention staff discussed the item more fully with the participant and asked him or her if they still felt these cards belonged in the pile. Interviewers were trained to be able to fully and carefully explain the nature of HIV risk, and took as much time as necessary to assist the participants in understanding the explanation that was provided.

RESULTS

Sample Demographics

Two hundred and ninety five individuals participated in the survey component and, of

Exhibit 3.1 Demographic characteristics of survey and in-depth interview participants

	Survey	
	N	*%*
Gender		
Male	227	76.9
Female	68	23.1
Years of education		
<8 years	116	39.3
8 years (full basic education)	51	17.3
9–11 years	98	33.2
>11 years	30	10.2
Marital status		
Single	167	56.8
Married/living together	90	30.6
Separated	27	9.2
Divorced	7	2.4
Widowed	3	1.0
Income last month		
None	59	20.2
Less than R$300	91	31.2
R$300–R$599	93	31.8
R$600–R$1199	33	11.3
R$1200–R$1799	13	4.5
More than R$2400	1	0.3
Don't know/not sure	2	0.7

these, thirty-four individuals received in-depth interviews. Exhibit 3.1 displays the demographics for the survey sample. As reflected in the table, our participants were primarily male, with limited education, single, and relatively poor.

Drug Use

With a significant proportion of the HIV cases in Brazil occurring among drug users, it is important to understand more fully the drug use behaviors of this population. Exhibit 3.2 provides a summary of the survey participants' drug use. There are several results worth noting in this table. First, with regards to "harder" drug use (other than alcohol and marijuana), the sample reported a very high rate of cocaine use and very little heroin or speedball. This was expected given the availability of cocaine in Rio compared to heroin. Similarly, there was very little drug injection occurring in Rio, and most of the injection drug use in Brazil is located in the southeastern portion of the country. There were two additional findings worth noting. The first is the high rate of inhalant use in the population, with over 60 percent reporting ever using inhalants. More generally, the sample of drug users from Rio report currently using a much more extensive variety of drugs compared to U.S. samples, including over 20 percent (64/295) of the sample that report using inhalants in the past thirty days.

HIV Testing

One of the goals of the current project was to determine the feasibility of conducting oral HIV testing in Brazil in the hopes of expanding the number of HIV testing options available. Of the survey participants only 41 percent reported that they had previously received an HIV test. Of these, 86 percent returned to get their test results, 46 percent said they received pretest counseling, and 31 percent received posttest counseling, suggesting that there is room for improvement.

Exhibit 3.2 Reported drug use of survey and in-depth interview participants

	Survey	
	N	%
Ever used		
Alcohol	287	97.6
Marijuana/ Hashish	270	91.5
Crack	57	19.3
Cocaine (sniffed)	199	67.5
Cocaine (injected)	23	7.8
Heroin (sniffed)	15	5.1
Heroin (injected)	6	2.0
Speedball (heroin and cocaine)	8	2.7
Meth/amphetamines	33	11.2
Steroids (non-Rx)	31	10.5
Ecstasy (MDMA)	47	15.9
Inhalants	181	61.4
LSD	22	7.5
Barbituates (non-Rx)	35	11.9
Benzodiazepines (non-Rx)	25	8.5
Used in last thirty days (among those who have already used)		
Alcohol	257	92.3
Marijuana/hashish	210	78.7
Crack	29	50.9
Cocaine (sniffed)	143	72.2
Cocaine (injected)	9	42.9
Heroin (sniffed)	6	40.0
Heroin (injected)	4	66.6
Speedball (heroin and cocaine)	4	50.0
Meth/amphetamines	6	20.0
Steroids (non-Rx)	5	16.7
Ecstasy (MDMA)	20	43.5
Inhalants	64	37.6
LSD	8	36.4
Barbituates (non-Rx)	14	42.4
Benzodiazepines (non-Rx)	11	45.8

The responses to the in-depth interviews gave us more detailed information regarding the participants' positive reactions towards the oral test. As one participant noted:

> It's something new, brand new, I didn't know about this. It was very new, interesting, very practical and fast. This should be open to the public, so people would have more chances and would be easier [to get tested]. Sometimes people are concerned about going to a place to get tested, are afraid "I might do it later, everything is alright" . . . oral test would succeed, I think. (Participant #6)

This was particularly true when they explicitly compared it to a traditional blood draw test:

> . . . it's a bit strange, you put a "lollipop" in your mouth (laugh), sorry . . . I thought, well, it's new, maybe it can help people. I thought it's a bit strange, but it's cool. Strange because I was making fun . . . but it's OK . . . Blood test hurts, the needle hurts. I don't like needles, I suffer a lot the day I tested my blood, . . . I hoped it would not hurt and then I suffered a lot. I prefer the lollipop test, better than take out blood. (Participant #7)
>
> The oral test is rapid . . . there are lots of people who are afraid of donating blood, to take blood . . . the oral test is more practical. People won't be afraid of the stick [the antibody collector], just two minutes . . . and you put that stick inside the cup . . . There are some people who are afraid of blood tests, afraid of seeing blood, people who faint. The oral test no, it's more practical, you know. (Participant #5)

CONCLUSION

Brazil is an excellent example of how HIV rates have been reduced as a result of sound public health policies, but even in Brazil there is room for improvement. One noticeable gap is the continued higher HIV prevalence rates among drug users and the relative lack of services including HIV testing targeted to this population. The current chapter describes a project that is looking to expand the possible testing options available in the hopes of increasing the number of individuals that decide to get tested while seeking to limit any potential unintended consequences associated with oral testing by implementing a brief intervention. Concerning the project as a whole, there have been several successes so far. First, the project has been able to access the target population and in fact exceeded the original target recruitment number. The findings to date show that the population of drug users in Rio have a number of differences from participants in our previous studies of drug users in the northeastern U.S.A., including primary use of non-injection power cocaine and regular inhalant use. Concerning the HIV tests specifically, all of the survey participants were open to receiving the oral HIV test and in-depth interview responses suggest that they felt that the oral test would be more successful than a standard blood draw, demonstrating that implementing oral HIV testing is feasible and has a high rate of acceptability among street drug users. Once the data collection has been completed, we will know more about whether or not the brief intervention has been successful in preventing increased belief in the transmission of HIV through saliva as a result of receiving an oral HIV test; if so, then a specific plan of wider implementation in Brazil can be examined.

REFERENCES AND FURTHER READING

Barcellos, N.T., Fuchs, S.C., and Fuchs, F.D. (2003). Prevalence of and risk factors for HIV infection in individuals testing for HIV at counseling centers in Brazil. *Sex Transm Dis* 30(2): 166–173.

Bastos F.I., Pina M.F., and Szwarcwald C.L. (2002). The social geography of HIV/AIDS among injection drug users in Brazil. *International Journal of Drug Policy* 13: 163–169.

Bastos F.I., Strathdee S.A., and Derrico M. (1999). Drug use and the spread of HIV/AIDS in South America and the Caribbean. *Drug Education Prevention and Policy* 6: 29–50.

Brazilian Ministry of Health (2000a). *Brazilian Legislation on STD and AIDS* (BMH, Brasilia, 2000) (in Portuguese).

Brazilian Ministry of Health (2000b). *The Brazilian Response to HIV/AIDS—Best Practices.*

Brazilian Ministry of Health (2001a). *Implementation and Monitoring Report—AIDS II—December 1988–May 2001.* World Bank Loan BIRD 4392/BR (in Portuguese).

Brazilian Ministry of Health (2001b). *Epidemiological Bulletin* 13(3), October–December 2000 (in Portuguese).

Brazilian Ministry of Health (2007). *Network of Public VCT, Treatment and Care Facilities for People Living with HIV/AIDS* (in Portuguese). Available at www.aids.gov.br.

Bureau of HIV/AIDS Early Intervention Section (1999). *OraSure Uncovers Higher Seroprevalence in Some Florida Counties. Data at a Glance July, 1999.* Talahassee: Florida Department of Health.

Centers for Disease Control and Prevention (2000). HIV-related knowledge and stigma—United States—2000. *Morbidity and Mortality Weekly Report* 49: 1062–1064.

Cerwonka, E.R., Isbell, T.R., and Hansen, C.E. (2000). Psychosocial factors as predictors of unsafe sexual practices among young adults. *AIDS Education and Prevention* 12(2): 141–153.

Clair, S. Singer, M., Huertas, E., and Weeks, M. (2003). Unintended Consequences of Using an Oral HIV Test on HIV Knowledge. *AIDS Care* 15(4): 575–580.

Dudley, C., O'Sullivan, L.F., Moreau, D. (2002). Does familiarity breed complacency? HIV knowledge, personal contact, and sexual risk behavior of psychiatrically referred Latino adolescent girls. *Hispanic Journal of Behavioral Sciences* 24(3): 353–368.

Ferreira, A.D., Caiaffa, W.T., Bastos, F.I., Mingoti, S.A. and Projeto AjUDE-Brasil II (2006). Injecting drug users who are (un)aware of their HIV serostatus: findings from the multi-center study AjUDE-Brasil II. *Cad Saude Publica* 22(4): 815–826.

Gallo, D., George, J. R., Fitchen, J. H., Goldstein, A. S., and Hindahl, M. S., for the OraSure HIV clinical Trials Group (1997). Evaluation of a System Using Oral Mucosal Transudate for HIV-1 Antibody Screening and Confirmatory Testing. *JAMA* 227(3): 254–258.

Goldstein, D. (2003). *Laughter Out of Place: Race, Class, Violence, and Sexuality in a Rio Shantytown.* Berkeley: University of California Press.

Hacker, M.A., Leite, I.C., Renton, A., Torres, T.G., Gracie, R., and Bastos, F.I. (2006). Reconstructing the AIDS epidemic among injection drug users in Brazil. *Cad Saude Publica* 22(4): 751–60.

Inciardi J.A., and Surratt H.L. (2001). Drug use, street crime, and sex-trading among cocaine-dependent women: implications for public health and criminal justice policy. *Journal of Psychoactive Drugs* 33(4): 379–389.

Ingham, R. (1995). In *Sexual behavior and AIDS in the developing world*, ed. J. Cleland and B. Ferry, 43–74. London: University of Florida Press.

Knowlton A.R., Hoover D.R., and Chung S.E. (2001). Access to medical care and service utilization among injection drug users with HIV/AIDS. *Drug and Alcohol Dependence* 64(1): 55–62.

Latkin C.A., Knowlton A.R., and Sherman S. (2001). Routes of drug administration, differential affiliation, and lifestyle stability among cocaine and opiate users: implications to HIV prevention. *Journal of Substance Abuse* 13(1–2): 89–102.

Laub, C., Somera, D.M., Gowen, L.K., and Diaz, R. (1999). Targeting risky gender ideologies: Constructing a community-driven, theory-based HIV prevention intervention for youth. *Health Education and Behavior* 26: 185–199.

Lew-Ting, C.Y., and Hsu, M.L. (2002). Pattern of responses to HIV transmission questions: rethinking HIV knowledge and its relevance to AIDS prejudice. *AIDS Care* 14(4): 549–557.

Lewis, J.E., Malow, R.M., and Ireland, S.J. (1997). HIV/AIDS risk in heterosexual college students: A review of a decade of literature. *Journal of American College Health* 45: 147–158.

Lowndes, C.M., Bastos, F.I., Giffin, K., Reis, A.C.G.V., d'Orsi, E., and Alary, M. (2000). Differential trends in mortality from AIDS in men and women in Brazil, 1984–1995. *AIDS* 14: 1269–1273.

Malta, M., Carneiro-da-Cunha, C., Kerrigan, D., Strathdee, S.A., Monteiro, M., and Bastos, F.I. (2003). Case management of human immunodeficiency virus-infected injection drug users: a case study in Rio de Janeiro, Brazil. *Clin Infect Dis.* 37 (Supplement 5): S386–S391.

Nyamathi, A.M., Stein, J.A., and Swanson, J.M. (2000). Personal, cognitive, behavioral, and demographic predictors of HIV testing and STDs in homeless women. *Journal of Behavioral Medicine* 23(2): 123–147.

Scott, S.A., Jorgensen, C.M., and Suarez, L. (1998). Concerns and dilemmas of Latinos AIDS information seekers: Spanish speaking callers to the CDC National AIDS Hotline. *Health Education and Behavior* 25(4): 501–516.

Simon, P.A., Weber, M., Ford, W.L., Cheng, F., and Kerndt, P.R. (1996). Reasons for HIV antibody test refusal in a heterosexual sexually transmitted disease clinic population. *AIDS* (10): 1549–1553.

Singer, M., Flores, C., Davison, L., Burke, G., Castillo, Z., Scanlon, K., and Rivera, M. (1990). SIDA: The Sociocultural and Socioeconomic Context of AIDS among Latinos. *Medical Anthropology Quarterly* 4: 72–114.

Soto-Ramirez, L.E., Hernandez-Gomez, L., Sifuentes-Osornio, J., Barriga-Angulo, G., Duarte de Lima, D., Lopez-Portillo, M., and Ruiz-Palcios, G.M. (1992). Detection of Specific Antibodies in Gingival Crevicular Transudate by Enzyme-Linked Immunosorbent Assay for Diagnosis of Human Immunodeficiency Virus Type 1 Infection. *Journal of Clinical Microbiology*, 30 (11): 2780–2783.

Souza, C., Diaz, T., Sutmoller, F., and Bastos, F.I. (2002). The association of socioeconomic status and use of crack/cocaine with unprotected anal sex in a cohort of men who have sex with men in Rio de Janeiro, Brazil. *Journal of Acquired Immune Deficiency Syndromes*, 29(1): 95–100.

Szwarcwald, C.L., Bastos, F.I., Barcellos, C., Esteves, M.A., and Castilho, E.A. (2001). Spatial-temporal modeling: dynamics of the AIDS epidemic in the municipality of Rio de Janeiro, Brazil, 1988–1996 (in Portuguese). *Cadernos de Saúde Pública* 17: 1123–1140.

Szwarcwald, C.L., Bastos, F.I., Esteves, M.A.P. and Andrade, C.L.T. (2000). The spread of the AIDS epidemic in Brazil from 1987 to 1996: a spatial analysis (in Portuguese). *Cadernos de Saúde Pública 16 (Supplement 1)*: 7–19.

Szwarcwald, C., Bastos, F.I., Gravato, N., Lacerda, R., Chequer, P.N. and Castillo, E.A. (1998). The relationship of illicit drug consumption to HIV-infection among commercial sex workers (CSWs) in the city of Santos, Sao Paulo, Brazil. *International Journal of Drug Policy* 9(6): 427–436.

UNAIDS (2000). *Report on the Global HIV/AIDS Epidemic*. UNAIDS, Geneva.

Zorrilla, C. (2000). Antiretroviral Combination Therapy in HIV-1 Infected Women and Men: Are Their Responses Different? *International Journal of Fertility and Menopausal Studies* 45(2): 195–199.

SECTION 2

Gender, Sexuality, and HIV Risk

FRAMING ESSAY

Gender and HIV

Reflecting Back, Moving Forward

Geeta Rao Gupta and Ellen Weiss

Since the beginning of the AIDS epidemic, the disease has resulted in a staggering 25 million deaths. Over the years the epidemic has achieved for women in death what they had lacked in life—equality with men. In 1985 only about a third of those infected worldwide were female, whereas ten years later nearly half of the 39.5 million adults infected with HIV globally were women. But in sub-Saharan Africa, for every ten adult men infected with the virus, there are an estimated fourteen adult women also infected. And young women between the ages of 15 to 24 are the most vulnerable—approximately three young women are infected for every two young men (UNAIDS 2006; UNAIDS/WHO 2006).

As cases of HIV rose among women, so has our understanding of the reasons behind the statistics. Women's greater biological susceptibility to infection offered some explanation (Nicolosi et al. 1994). But findings from social science research in the late 1980s and early 1990s highlighted a variety of social, cultural, and economic factors that make it difficult for adolescent and adult women to adopt HIV prevention behaviors, namely abstinence, monogamy, and condom use, or ensure that the latter two are practiced by their partners (Worth 1989; Ulin 1992; Schoepf 1993; Gupta and Weiss 1993). For example, many women are economically dependent on men and this dependency can impede their ability to negotiate protection and to leave a relationship that they perceive to be risky (de Bruyn 1992, Heise and Elias 1995; Mane, Gupta, and Weiss 1994).

Such information about the reality of women's lives contributed to a paradigm shift in the HIV/AIDS discourse from individual risk to societal vulnerability (Whelan 1999). In the early years of the epidemic, individual-level behavioral models such as the Health Belief Model (Becker 1974) and the Theory of Reasoned Action (Ajzen and Fishbein 1980) were used to inform the design of HIV prevention interventions. These theories hypothesized that men and women were able to act on their choices after they acquired adequate knowledge, awareness, and skills (Exner et al. 2003). But the limitations of these theories to take into account the context in which sexual behavior takes place limited their usefulness, particularly when addressing the broader social forces that influence the lives of women and girls. Hence, researchers and policymakers began to highlight societal vulnerability, which results from the confluence of socioeconomic, cultural, and political factors that contribute to individual risk by significantly limiting individuals' choices and options for HIV prevention (Whelan 1999; Dworkin and Ehrhardt 2007).

One of the most important contextual variables to be identified that influences both women's and men's societal vulnerability to HIV is gender (Exner et al. 2003). Gender refers to the widely shared expectations and norms within a society about appropriate male and female behavior, roles and responsibilities, and the ways in which women and men interact with each other (Gupta 2001). Since gender is socially constructed, it is affected by a variety of other variables such as poverty, age, marital status, and occupational status (Theobald, Tolhurst, and Squire 2006). Gender is also a culture-specific construct—there are significant differences in what women and men can or cannot do in one culture as compared to another.

While that difference is more pronounced in some cultures, there is almost always a distinct difference between women's and men's roles, obligations and privileges, particularly in terms of access to productive resources, and decision-making authority. In most societies gender norms dictate that men are responsible for the productive activities outside the home while women are expected to be responsible for reproductive and productive activities within the home (Gupta 2001). And we know from over twenty-five years of research on women's roles in development that women have less access over and control of productive resources than men, as evidenced through persistent gender gaps in education, employment, income, ownership of land and housing, and access to credit (UN Millennium Project 2005).

Predictably, the inequality that characterizes the social and economic spheres of society, in which women have less access to productive resources than men, is often mirrored in sexual interactions, creating an unequal balance of power in sexual relations. As a result, many women have less control than men over when, where, why, with whom, and how sex takes place. This inequality in sexual decision-making is perpetuated by gender norms of femininity and masculinity that curtail women's sexual autonomy and expand men's sexual privilege, place greater emphasis on male pleasure over female pleasure, and cast women in the role of passive recipient rather than active actor. The complex interplay of social and economic gender differences and inequalities, combined with the unequal balance of power in sexual relations that favors men, significantly increases both women's *and* men's vulnerability to HIV (Gupta 2001; Dworkin and Ehrhardt 2007).

Gender is not synonymous with women. It is instead about the ways in which women and men relate to each other, about both women and men reinforcing traditional gender roles and enforcing sanctions against those who do not comply, and about men and women falling prey to gendered norms of sexual behavior that in this epidemic are harmful for all. Such an understanding of gender, even while acknowledging that gender inequality puts women at a significant disadvantage, requires that HIV interventions address both women's and men's needs and constraints in order to create interpersonal relationships and societal structures that support HIV prevention for all (Gupta 2001).

The focus of this chapter is on what can be done from a gender perspective to address the heterosexual transmission of HIV. The chapter begins by reviewing the ways in which gender inequalities contribute to women and men's vulnerability to HIV. The next section discusses key principles for creating an enabling context to foster HIV prevention among women and men, and lays out a framework for addressing gender inequalities within the context of HIV prevention programming. Drawing on research findings and program experiences, this section also highlights interventions that illustrate the different components of the framework. The chapter concludes by discussing some of the current debates related to HIV prevention and why a gender perspective is critical if the field is to move forward.

GENDER INEQUALITIES AND VULNERABILITY TO HIV

In many societies, norms of femininity and masculinity are quite distinct and may contribute to women's and men's vulnerability to HIV infection. For example, constructions of ideal feminine attributes and roles frequently emphasize sexual ignorance, virginity, and motherhood (Carovano 1992; Whelan 1999). This culture of silence and stigma that surrounds women and girls being informed about sexual matters can negatively impact their access to information and services. For example, a study in southeast Nigeria found that norms against pre-marital sex by single women limited their access to contraceptive information and methods (Ozumba, Obi, and Ijioma 2005). Such gender norms may also affect women's access to information about HIV prevention. Demographic and health survey data from six African countries show that women tend to have less HIV prevention knowledge than men (Glick and Sahn 2005). Moreover, data from 35 of 48 countries in sub-Saharan Africa reveal that, on average, young men were 20 percent more likely to know how to prevent the sexual transmission of HIV than young women (UNAIDS/WHO 2005).

Norms of masculinity that define men as being more knowledgeable and experienced about sex, for example, put men, particularly young men, at risk of infection because these norms discourage them from seeking information or admitting their lack of knowledge about sex or protection. Such norms also pressure men into experimenting with sex in unsafe ways, and at a young age, to prove their manhood (Whelan 1999; World Health Organization 1999). Gender norms in many societies also reinforce the belief that variety in sexual partners is essential to men's nature as men and that men must seek multiple partners for sexual release. Such beliefs make following prevention messages that call for fidelity in partnerships or a reduction in the number of partners a significant challenge (Mane, Gupta, and Weiss 1994; Heise and Elias 1995; Rivers and Aggleton 2001; Barker 2000). In creating a case for the need to understand the role of men's vulnerabilities in fueling the AIDS epidemic, Mane and Aggleton (2001) point out that "cultural and societal expectations and norms create an environment where risk is acceptable, even encouraged, for 'real' men."

Overall, support for such types of masculine ideologies begins in childhood as boys are taught to imitate male family members (World Health Organization 2007). Recent research has shown a strong association between risk-taking behavior and agreement with norms of masculinity that are detrimental to women and men. For example, findings from a study among young men in Brazil showed that support for inequitable gender norms was significantly associated with reported sexually transmitted infections (STI) symptoms, lack of contraceptive use, and both physical and sexual violence against a current or most recent partner (Pulerwitz et al. 2006). A study among sexually active men, aged 18–35 years, attending an urban community health center in Boston found that men who supported more traditional gender role ideologies within such domains as male toughness, anti-femininity, and male hypersexuality were significantly more likely to report unprotected vaginal sex in the past three months and intimate partner violence perpetration in the last year (Santana et al. 2006).

Violence is the most extreme form of gender inequality and is the direct result of gender norms that make male violence against women a socially acceptable way to control an intimate partner. Violence contributes directly and indirectly to women's vulnerability to HIV (Maman et al. 2000). Individuals who have been sexually abused are at immediate risk of HIV infection, but they are also more likely to engage in unprotected sex, have multiple partners, and trade sex for money or drugs (Heise, Ellsberg, and Gottemoeller 1999). Data from a Tanzanian study suggest that, for some women, the experience of partner violence could be a strong predictor of HIV. Maman and colleagues (2002) found that among women who sought services at a voluntary counseling and testing (VCT) center, those who were HIV positive were 2.6 times more likely to have experienced violence in an intimate relationship than those who were HIV negative. A similar association was found among women attending antenatal care centers in South Africa. After controlling for age, current relationship status, and women's risk behavior, intimate partner violence was significantly associated with HIV sero-positivity (Dunkle et al. 2004a).

Another source of inequality that is associated with HIV vulnerability is education. Gender gaps in education, which favor boys in most regions of the world and persist at both the primary and secondary school level, can increase women and girls' vulnerability. A recent review of the literature showed that there is a strong negative correlation between the number of years of schooling and HIV prevalence, particularly in countries with a high prevalence of HIV (Hargreaves and Boler 2006). The persistent gender gaps in secondary education, in particular, are of grave concern because the analysis also showed a stronger association of completion of secondary education with lower HIV risk, more condom use, and fewer sexual partners, as compared to primary education. In addition, the review showed that females who received more education were more likely to start having sex at a later age.

And finally, women's economic vulnerability and their dependency on men for economic security puts them at a clear disadvantage in terms of negotiating condom use or fidelity with a non-monogamous partner. It also makes it less likely that they will leave a relationship that they perceive to be risky because they lack bargaining power and fear abandonment and destitution (Worth 1989; Heise and Elias 1995; Weiss and Gupta 1998). Poverty and a lack of economic alternatives have repeatedly been identified as the reasons that many adult women and children become sex workers. In conditions of extreme poverty, many women and girls fall into sex work either because they are sold or trafficked into the sex industry or feel that they have no other option to economically sustain themselves and their children (Wojcicki 2002; Dunkle et al. 2004b; Harcourt and Donovan 2005).

Women's lack of access to and control over economic assets, such as land and housing, also makes them particularly vulnerable and can fuel a vicious intergenerational cycle of disease and death. Increasing women's economic security through ownership of and control over land and housing is an HIV prevention and control strategy because it protects women from complete economic devastation when husbands or fathers fall sick and die of AIDS. Without a guarantee of property and inheritance rights, the woman left behind is at risk of losing her home, inheritance, and possessions, either because the law of her land does not give her the right to own or inherit land or housing, or because of "property grabbing" by relatives and community members, with no accessible legal recourse to regain ownership of that property. Thrust into these difficult economic situations, women and girls may be forced into risky and unsafe sexual behaviors just to meet their own and their children's or siblings' basic needs for food, shelter, and clothing, or may fall prey to sexual predators, thereby perpetuating a vicious cycle of HIV infection, disease, and death (Strickland 2004).

It has also been known anecdotally for many years that control over land and housing can give women greater bargaining power within households, which may translate into greater leverage to negotiate HIV prevention behaviors, though this relationship is yet to be tested. Control over land and housing in some circumstances, however, may protect women against the risk of domestic violence, thereby indirectly reducing vulnerability to HIV. Research in Kerala, India, found that 49 percent of women with no property reported physical violence compared to only 7 percent of women who owned property (Panda 2002).

Yet, there are many countries in which women still do not have the right to own or inherit land and property—and even where such laws exist, most land and property is owned by men because of the poor enforcement of the laws or because of a conflict between statutory laws and customary laws.

CREATING AN ENABLING CONTEXT

A gendered response to the epidemic acknowledges that individual decision-making occurs within a gendered context. Thus to facilitate HIV prevention it is important to create an enabling environment for women and men that involves altering the ways in which HIV-related services are provided and programs are run to make them more gender sensitive; it requires putting in place community processes and programs to bring about normative changes in the definitions of masculinity and femininity; and, finally, it requires the creation of a policy and legislative context and effective enforcement mechanisms that promote gender equality and the empowerment of women.

Principles Underlying a Gender-Based Response

There are two principles that must guide the implementation of a gender-based response:

Women's and men's vulnerabilities vary and are context-specific

Women's and men's needs, constraints, and particular vulnerabilities are differentiated based on age, marital status, sexuality, socioeconomic status, ethnicity, race, place of residence, and many other variables. It is well-known, for example, that gender inequalities are much greater among the poor than the non-poor and that particular gender inequalities, such as in education or economic opportunity, are greater in some regions than others (UN Millennium Project 2005). The important first step in designing a gender-based response to contain the epidemic, as is true for any public health response, is to find out what is true for the majority of the population. This can be done through a context-specific gender analysis that maps the particular gender inequalities and sources of vulnerability that affect women and girls as well as men and boys (World Health Organization Department of Gender and Women's Health 2003; Warren 2007). The analysis must also be informed by the stage of the epidemic and its particular epidemiological context in order to determine which women and men, and which of their particular vulnerabilities, receive priority attention.

Effective HIV prevention requires services and community mobilization

The second principle, which is true for all HIV prevention programs but much more so for ones that seek to alter behavior by changing gender norms, is that creating an enabling context requires two simultaneous responses: first, basic HIV/AIDS interventions and services that are facility or community based; and second, actions that catalyze community-driven responses. The first is key to providing information, services, and technologies (e.g., male and female condoms), and for building skills. The second is instrumental in building social capital, developing local leadership, and mobilizing the community to take action, which may include grassroots educational campaigns or advocating for changes in broader laws and policies. For the best results in implementing a gender-responsive AIDS program, both of these sets of responses—AIDS services and community mobilization—must occur concurrently.

A Framework for a Gender-Based Response

The framework described below distinguishes between four levels of strategies that fall on a continuum of increasing degrees of responsiveness to gender inequality: do no harm, address gender differences, trigger transformation in gender roles and relationships; and empower women and girls. All four can be undertaken within AIDS programming, as traditionally defined, but the success of the fourth strategy, empower women, requires broader economic and social development actions.

Do no harm

To effectively address the intersection between HIV/ AIDS, gender, and sexuality requires at a minimum that interventions do not reinforce damaging gender and sexual stereotypes. Some efforts have fostered a predatory, irresponsible image of male sexuality and portrayed women as powerless victims or as repositories of infection. Posters in which a sex worker is portrayed as a skeleton, bringing the risk of death to potential clients, is an example of the latter which may do little other than stigmatize sex workers, thereby increasing their vulnerability to infection and violence.

Another example is programs that provide adolescents with "abstinence-only" prevention education that withholds any information on other methods of protection. These, too, can do damage—first, by denying that for many reasons (e.g., coercion, economic need, love) sexual activity is a reality in the lives of many female and male youths (Weiss, Whelan, and Gupta 2000) and males (Niang et al. 2003; World Health Organization 2007); and second, by presuming that the provision of comprehensive sexuality education will increase sexual activity when research evidence has proved otherwise (Kirby, Laris, and Rolleri 2005; Grunseit et al. 1997).

Address gender differences

A step up from merely doing no harm is to address the differential needs and constraints of individuals based on their gender. Providing a woman with a female condom or a microbicide is an example of such programming. It recognizes that the male condom is a male-controlled technology and that women need alternatives that they can initiate or control (Heise and Elias 1995; Mantell et al. 2006). Efforts to alter the timing of the provision of a service to better match women's daily schedules or provide services through a community outreach program in order to reduce the time and monetary impediments to women's use of services are examples of such an approach. Another is to integrate STI treatment and HIV prevention services with family planning services to help women access such services without social censure. Fleischman (2006) cites many positive program examples to make a powerful push for integrating reproductive health and HIV/AIDS programs, arguing that it makes practical sense to do so for reproductive age women, for whom both sets of services are critical.

Taegmeyer et al. (2006) describe a process of gender analysis undertaken at HIV VCT sites in Kenya to make services more responsive to the needs of women and men. They found that women were less likely to access VCT and, among those women who did access services, they were less likely than male clients to take home condoms. Married women in particular noted that they lacked power to negotiate protection and that they were vulnerable to marital rape. Using the findings, some VCT sites began demonstrating and offering female condoms, and established links with new comprehensive post-rape care services.

While such gender-responsive programming responds to felt needs and improves women's access to information, technologies, and services, by itself it does little to change fundamental social and economic inequalities or the larger contextual issues that lie at the root of women's vulnerability to HIV.

Trigger transformation in gender roles and relationships

These approaches aim to catalyze transformation in gender roles and create more gender-equitable relationships by building on what Barker calls "performances of resistance" by women and men to traditional views of manhood and womanhood. For example, in his work with young men whom he found to be more gender equitable, Barker found that such men had a high degree of self-reflection, acknowledged some benefits of gender equity, and had others around them who also questioned harmful gender norms and practices. This has several program implications, namely the need to engage participants in small group settings to share information, develop skills, and reflect critically about the costs of traditional gender ideologies; to create social support and safe spaces for this exploration; and to use participatory processes to trigger changes in values, attitudes, and behaviors (Barker 2000).

We highlight three examples of transformative interventions and the results from research to evaluate them. These programs use a wide range of activities—games, role-plays, and group discussions—to facilitate an examination of gender and sexuality and their impacts on relationships and HIV prevention. They are Program H, developed in Brazil for young men (Promundo 2004); Stepping Stones, developed in Uganda for men and women (Welbourn 1995) and recently adapted for use with young women and men in South Africa; and SISTA, an intervention for African-American women (DiClemente and Wingwood 1995).

Program H (which stands for *homen*, or "men" in Portuguese) draws upon an ecological model to address key gender-related issues at multiple levels, from the individual to the greater society. Program H focuses on helping young men question harmful norms related to masculinity and reflect on the costs of subscribing to these norms and the advantages of more gender-equitable views and behaviors. The version of Program H that was recently evaluated in Brazil contained two components: a curriculum and video for use with small groups of men; and a lifestyle social marketing campaign that emphasized how "cool" and "hip" it was to be a more "gender-equitable" man (Pulerwitz et al. 2006).

A quasi-experimental study to evaluate Program H found that support for inequitable gender norms decreased among young men who participated in the program, whereas there was no change in the control group. In addition, increases in condom use at last sex with primary partners and decreases in reported STI symptoms tended to be greater over time among young men who participated in group sessions and were exposed to a social marketing campaign that championed gender-equitable men, compared to young men who just participated in the group sessions or were in the control group (Pulerwitz et al. 2006). A program similar to Program H that was piloted in India was found also to reduce support for inequitable gender norms and decrease harassment of girls and women (Verma et al. 2006). The results suggest that the pilot was successful in reaching and engaging young men to critically discuss gender dynamics and health risk, and in shifting key gender-related attitudes.

In South Africa, the Stepping Stones program has been evaluated through a randomized control trial. Stepping Stones aims to foster gender-equitable relationships by increasing knowledge of sexual health, awareness of the risks and consequences of risk taking, and self-reflection on sexual behavior; and by strengthening communication and conflict resolution skills. The South African study collected data from 1400 young women and young men from 35 villages who participated in 17 group sessions over a period of 3–12 weeks and a similar number of youths from 35 control villages at baseline and at 12 and 24 months follow-up (Jewkes et al. 2006, 2007). The quantitative findings suggest that the program had a positive impact on male behaviors—reducing their number of partners, increasing correct condom use at last sex, and decreasing the perpetration of more than one episode of physical or sexual intimate partner violence. The qualitative data revealed increased sexual communication with partners, family, and community members; greater support for condom use; reduced support for violence against women; and greater use of conflict resolution skills among men. There were fewer improvements observed among young women who participated in the program, including around condom use, likely because they were in relationships with an unequal power balance (the intervention recruited individuals and not couples). However, women, as with men, reported improved communication and greater awareness that violence against women was wrong (Jewkes et al. 2007).

Although young women did not appear to benefit as much from the South Africa Stepping Stones trial, there are other examples of participatory group programs that have had a stronger impact on women, thus highlighting the benefits of this approach. One such program is SISTA, which is based on the Theory of Gender and Power (Wingwood and DiClemente 2000). DiClemente and Wingwood (1995) found that African-American women who participated in SISTA demonstrated an increase in consistent condom use, greater sexual self-control, greater sexual assertiveness, and increased support for safer sex norms at three-month follow-up compared to a control group. Among the program's core elements were small group sessions, utilization of cultural and gender-appropriate materials that foster pride and enhance self-worth, and discussion of cultural and gendered triggers that make it challenging for women to negotiate safer sex. Adapted versions of the intervention have been developed for African-American female adolescents (SiHLE) and HIV-positive women (WiLLOW), and have been found to be effective in randomized control trials (Wingwood and DiClemente 2006).

Empowering approaches

These strategies aim to complement transformative approaches by addressing the broader risk environment that constrains women's behaviors and choices and often go beyond the purview of traditional HIV programming. While transformative approaches are important for triggering changes in gender roles and interpersonal gender dynamics among women and men, empowering approaches are critical to reinforcing women's ability to protect themselves and to take charge of their own lives. In a recent review of the empirical and theoretical literature on women's empowerment, Malhotra and Schuler (2005) argue that "empowerment" is a process that engages women as active agents in the use of a range of resources, which brings about positive changes in women's environment, from one that undermines women's wellbeing to one that promotes it. Resources that are key for bringing about women's empowerment are information and education, economic opportunities and assets, decision-making opportunities, and security. Women's access to these resources can be increased through policies and programs that foster women's participation and decision-making.

Two programs highlighted below—the IMAGE Project and the Sonagachi Project—illustrate the feasibility and relevance of empowering women by addressing important contextual barriers to HIV prevention, namely partner violence, limited social capital, and economic vulnerability. Both programs focused on HIV prevention as a goal while providing women with needed resources through an empowering process, and showed measurable results in terms of their vulnerability to HIV.

The IMAGE (Intervention with Microfinance for AIDS and Gender Equity) Project highlights the importance for women of combining interventions that address individual and contextual barriers to behavior change with actions to stimulate community responses that foster an enabling environment. One component of the project involved providing micro-loans to women, which have been shown by previous research to contribute to increasing women's economic status and empowerment (Hashemi et al. 1996; Cheston and Kuhn 2002; Mayoux 2000). The other component was a ten-part gender and HIV training program called "Sisters for Life," which was integrated into fortnightly loan repayment meetings over a six-month period. More importantly, the IMAGE Project mobilized microfinance participants, who tended to be older women in the community, to be agents of change in their households and communities (RADAR 2002; Kim et al. 2007).

Using a randomized cluster design, the researchers found that, after two years, those in the intervention group compared to the control group (matched for age and poverty status) experienced greater improvements in assets, expenditures, and membership in informal savings groups. The intervention group also demonstrated improvements in empowerment indicators, such as challenging established gender roles and communication with household members about sexual matters, and in social capital measures, including participation in social groups and collective action. Indeed, as proof of increased empowerment and greater social capital, IMAGE participants organized over sixty community events (e.g., workshops, marches, and meetings with leadership structures) that addressed HIV, violence, rape, and abuse, and which engaged traditional leaders, police, school principals, and soccer clubs. The study also found that, among participants, the risk of physical and/or sexual intimate partner violence in the past year was reduced by 55 percent, from 11 percent to 6 percent. Among comparison group respondents the rate actually increased from 9 percent to 12 percent (Pronyk et al. 2006).

Qualitative data suggest that the intervention and the social mobilization that occurred enabled women to challenge the acceptability of such violence, to expect and receive better treatment from partners, and to leave abusive relationships (IMAGE Project 2006). The researchers concluded: "given the linkages between violence and HIV, existing development initiatives, such as microfinance, may provide an important entry point for addressing HIV in areas where poverty and gender inequalities continue to confound prevention efforts" (Kim et al. 2006).

A second example of an empowering program is the Sonagachi Project. It began by providing standard HIV services—behavior change communication, condom distribution, and STI management—to women who were sex workers. Over time, project leaders and participants recognized that sex workers' exclusion from access to material resources, civic participation, and decision-making contributed to a lack of power in their sexual relationships and their lives in general. This led the project to implement a wider variety of activities in order to develop a sense of community among sex workers, decrease their perceived powerlessness and insecurity, increase their access and control over material resources, increase their social participation, facilitate the social acceptance of sex workers, and stimulate community activism. Specifically, as the project evolved, literacy classes, a loan service, and a trade union were organized. (Jana et al. 2004).

As a result of the interventions and community responses, there was a significantly greater increase in condom use among sex workers living in the Sonagachi area compared to sex workers in the control sites (Basu et al. 2004). The Sonagachi Project highlights the importance of combining core prevention services that are of high quality with community processes that foster community ownership. It is only when the two are combined that changes in the normative context can occur.

CONCLUSION

This chapter has aimed to show that there is adequate conceptual clarity, programmatic experience, and empirical findings to justify increased resources on HIV prevention interventions that address gender differences, trigger transformation in gender roles and relationships, and that empower women. The examples highlighted in this chapter—together with blueprints that describe what programs and polices should be developed and how they should be carried out for reducing key barriers to prevention for women, including gender-based violence (Division for the Advancement of Women 2005; World Health Organization 2005), property and inheritance rights (Dohrn 2006; World Bank 2005), and economic empowerment (UN Millennium Project 2005)—point the way forward.

It is also clear that a gender lens is critical when dealing with a number of key programmatic and policy issues that have emerged in the past few years. For example, several randomized controlled trials in sub-Saharan Africa have shown that male circumcision reduces men's risk of acquiring HIV infection (Auvert et al. 2005; Bailey et al. 2007). While circumcision can address men's needs for a prevention technology, interventions that promote and offer services must take care that they do not harm both men and women by implicitly implying that the method is foolproof or that female circumcision can also be a positive practice.

Another example is the role of marriage as a risk factor for HIV acquisition. Some researchers have argued that marriage places women at a particular disadvantage for becoming infected with HIV (Clark 2004; Clark, Bruce, and Dude 2006). A study conducted in four African cities found that married young women were more likely to be HIV positive than similarly aged sexually active, unmarried women. In one of the cities, Kisumu, Kenya, a third of the married females in the study were infected with HIV compared to only 22 percent of their unmarried counterparts. Findings suggest that, because the women's husbands were considerably older and that intercourse tended to be unprotected and more frequent in marriage, these factors were more important in determining sero-positivity than the existence of multi-partnerships that characterize some unmarried girls' relationships (Clark 2004).

However, an analysis conducted by Mishra (2007) draws attention to the fact that, in a considerable proportion of discordant couples in eleven sub-Saharan countries, it is the female partners who are infected with HIV and a likely source of transmission to their male partners within marriage. Possible explanations are that extra-marital and pre-marital sex are more common among women than is generally reported. Regardless of the timing of women's infections, a gender approach is still warranted to understand the reasons for engaging in pre-marital or extra-marital sex (e.g., pleasure, economic gain, forced sex, loneliness), and to develop interventions at the individual, couple, and societal levels that respond to these factors.

REFERENCES AND FURTHER READING

Ajzen, I. and Fishbein, M. (1980). *Understanding Attitudes and Predicting Sexual Behavior*. Englewood Cliffs, NJ: Prentice Hall.

Auvert, B., Taljaard, D., Lagarde, E., Sobngwi-Tambekou, J., Sitta, R. and Puren, A. (2005). Randomized, controlled intervention trial of male circumcision of reduction of HIV infection risk: The ANRS 1265 trial. *PLOS Medicine*, Nov 2 (11), e298.

Bailey, R., Moses, S., Parker, C., Agot, K., Maclean, I., Krieger, J., Williams, C., Campbell, R. and Ndinya-Achola, J. (2007). Male circumcision for HIV prevention in young men in Kisumu, Kenya: A randomized controlled trial. *The Lancet*, 369 (9562), 643–656.

Barker, G. (2000). Gender equitable boys in a gender inequitable world: Reflections from qualitative research. *Sexual and Relationship Therapy*, 15 (6), 263–282.

Basu, I., Jana, S., Rotheram-Borus, M.J., Swendeman, D., Lee, S., Newman, P., and Weiss, R. (2004). HIV prevention among sex workers in India. *Journal of Acquired Immune Deficiency Syndrome*, 36 (3), 845–852.

Becker, M. (ed.) (1974). *The Health Belief Model and Personal Health Behavior*. Thorofare, NJ: Slack.

Carovano, K. (1992). More than mothers and whores: Redefining the AIDS prevention needs of women. *International Journal of Health Services*, 21, 131–142.

Clark, S. (2004). Early marriage and HIV risks in sub-Saharan Africa. *Studies in Family Planning*, 35 (3), 149–160.

Clark, S., Bruce, J. and Dude, A. (2006). Protecting young women from HIV/AIDS: The case against child and adolescent marriage. *International Family Planning Perspectives*, 32 (2), 79–88.

Cheston, S. and Kuhn, L. (2002). Empowering women through microfinance. In S.D. Harris (ed.), *Pathways out of Poverty: Innovations in Microfinance for the Poorest Families* (pp. 167–228). Bloomfield, CT: Kumarian Press.

de Bruyn, M. (1992). Women and AIDS in developing countries. *Social Science and Medicine*, 34(3), 249–262.

DiClemente, R.J. and Wingwood, G.M. (1995). A randomized controlled trial of an HIV sexual risk-reduction intervention for young African-American women. *JAMA*, 274 (16), 1271–1276.

Division for the Advancement of Women (2005). *Good Practices in Combating and Eliminating Violence Against Women*. Report of the Expert Group Meeting. Vienna, Austria.

Dohrn, S. (2006). *Governing Land: Reflections from IFPRI Research*. Washington DC: International Food Policy Research Institute.

Dunkle, K.L., Jewkes, R.K., Brown, H.C., Gray, G.E., McIntryre, J.A. and Harlow, S.D. (2004a). Gender-based violence, relationship power, and risk of HIV infection in women attending antenatal clinics in South Africa. *The Lancet*, 363 (9419), 1415–1421.

Dunkle, K.L., Jewkes, R.K., Brown, H.C., Gray, G.E., McIntryre, J.A. and Harlow, S.D. (2004b). Transactional sex among women in Soweto, South Africa: Prevalence, risk factors and association with HIV infection. *Social Science and Medicine*, 59 (8), 1581–1592.

Dworkin, S.L. and Ehrardt, A.A. (2007), Going beyond "ABC" to include "GEM:" Critical reflections on progress in the HIV/AIDS epidemic. *American Journal of Public Health*, 97 (1), 13–18.

Exner, T., Hoffman, S., Dworkin, S. and Erhardt, A.A. (2003). Beyond the male condom: The evolution of gender-specific HIV interventions for women. *Annual Review Sex Research*, 14, 114–136.

Fleischman, J. (2006). *Integrating Reproductive Health and HIV/AIDS Program: Strategic Opportunities for PEPFAR. A Report of the CSIS Task Force on HIV/AIDS*. Washington DC: Center for Strategic International Studies.

Glick, P. and Sahn, D.E. (2005). *Changes in HIV/AIDS Knowledge and Testing Behavior in Africa: How Much and for Whom?*. Cornell Food and Nutrition Policy Program Working Paper no. 173. Available at SSRN: http://ssrn.com/abstract=643161.

Grunseit, A., Kippax, S., Aggleton, P., Baldo, M. and Slutkin, G. (1997). Sexuality education and young people's sexual behavior: a review of studies. *Journal of Adolescent Research*, 12 (4), 421–453.

Gupta, G. Rao (2001). Gender, sexuality and HIV/AIDS: the what, the why, and the how. *SIECUS Report*. 29, 6–12.

Gupta, G. Rao and Weiss, E. (1993). Women's lives and sex: Implications for AIDS prevention. *Culture, Medicine and Psychiatry*, 17 (4), 399–412.

Harcourt, C. and Donovan, B. (2005). The many faces of sex work. *Sexually Transmitted Infections*, 81, 201–206.

Hashemi, S.M., Schulet, S.R. and Riley, A.P. (1996). Rural credit programs and women's empowerment in Bangladesh. *World Development*, 24 (4), 635–653.

Heise, L. and Elias, C. (1995). Transforming AIDS prevention to meet women's needs: A focus on developing countries. *Social Science and Medicine*, 40 (7), 933–943.

Heise, L., Ellsberg, M. and Gottemoeller, M. (1999). Ending violence against women. Baltimore, MD: Johns Hopkins University School of Public Health, Population Information Program. *Population Reports*, 27 (4), 1–20, 25–38.

Hargreaves, J. and Boler, T. (2006). *Girl Power: The Impact of Girls' Education on HIV and Sexual Behavior*. ActionAid International.

IMAGE Project (2006). *Using Microfinance to Empower Women and Address Poverty, Gender-based Violence and*

HIV. South Africa: Small Enterprise Foundation (SEF) and Rural AIDS and Development Action Research (RADAR).

Jana, S., Basu, I., Rotheram-Borus, M.J. and Newman, P. (2004). The Sonagachi Project: A sustainable community intervention project. *AIDS Education and Prevention*, 16 (5), 405–414.

Jewkes, R., Levin, J., Kristin, D., Jama, N., Khuzwayo, N., Koss, M., Nduna, M., Puren, A. and Duvvury, N. (2006). Results of the cluster RCT of the HIV behavioral intervention Stepping Stones. Poster presentation at the 16th International AIDS Conference, Toronto.

Jewkes, R. Nduma, M., Levin, J., Jama, N., Dunkle, K., Wood, K., Koss, M., Puren, A. and Duvvury, N. (2007). *Evaluation of Stepping Stones: A Gender Transformative HIV Prevention Intervention*. Policy Brief March 2007. Pretoria: Medical Research Council.

Kim, J., Watts, C., Hargreaves, J.R., Linda, M., Porter, J., Phetla, G., Ndhlovu, L., Busza, J. and Pronyk, P. (2006). Women's economic empowerment can reduce gender-based violence: Results from the IMAGE study, a cluster randomized trial in South Africa. Poster presentation at the 16th International AIDS Conference, Toronto.

Kim, J.C., Watts, C., Hargreaves, J.R., Ndhlovu, L., Pheta, G., Morison, L., Busza, J., Porter, J.D.H. and Pronyk, P. (2007). Understanding the impact of a microfinance-based intervention on women's empowerment and the reduction of intimate partner violence in South Africa. *American Journal of Public Health*, 97 (10), 1794–1802.

Kirby, D., Laris, B.A. and Rolleri, L. (2005). *Impact of Sex and HIV Education Programs on Sexual Behaviors of Youth in Developing and Developed Countries*. Youth Research Working Paper No. 2. Research Triangle Park, NC: Family Health International.

Malhotra, A. and Schuler, S.R. (2005). Women's empowerment as a variable in international development. In D. Narayan (ed.), *Measuring Empowerment: Cross-Disciplinary Perspectives*. Washington DC: The World Bank.

Maman, S., Campbell, J., Sweat, M.D. and Gielen, A.C. (2000). The intersections of HIV and violence: directions for future research and interventions. *Social Science and Medicine*, 50 (4), 459–478.

Maman, S., Mbwambo, J., Hogan, N.M., Kilonzo, G.P., Campbell, J.C., Weiss, E. and Sweat, M. (2002). HIV-positive women report more lifetime partner violence: Findings from a voluntary counseling and testing clinic in Dar es Salaam, Tanzania. *American Journal of Public Health*, 92, 1331–1337.

Mane, P. and Aggleton, P. (2001). Gender and HIV/AIDS: What do men have to do with it? *Current Sociology*, 49 (6), 23–37.

Mane, P., Gupta, G. Rao and Weiss, E. (1994). Effective communication between partners: AIDS and risk reduction for women. *AIDS*, 8 (1), S325–S331.

Mantell, J. E., Dworkin, S.L., Exner, T.M., Hoffman, S., Smit, J.A. and Susser, I. (2006). The promises and limitations of female-initiated methods of HIV/STI protection. *Social Science and Medicine*, 63 (8), 1998–2009.

Mayoux, L. (2000). *Micro-Finance and the Empowerment of Women*. Geneva: ILO.

Mishra, V. (2007). Why do so many HIV discordant couples in sub-Saharan Africa have female partners infected, not male partners? Paper presented at the HIV/AIDS Implementers' Meeting, Kigali, Rwanda, June 18, 2007.

Niang, C.I., Tapsoba, P., Weiss, E., Diagne, M., Niang, Y., Moreau, A.M., Gomis, D., SidbÉ Wade, A., Seck, K. and Castle, C. (2003). "It's raining stones": stigma, violence and HIV vulnerability among men who have sex with men in Dakar, Senegal. *Culture, Health and Sexuality*, 5 (6), 499–512.

Nicolosi, A., Correa Leite, M.L., Musicco, M., Arici, C., Gavazzeni, G. and Lazzarin, A. (1994). The efficiency of male-to-female and female-to-male sexual transmission of the Human Immunodeficiency Virus: A Study of 730 stable couples. *Epidemiology*, 5 (6), 570–575.

Ozumba, B.C., Obi, S.N. and Ijioma, N.N. (2005). Knowledge, attitude and practice of modern contraception among single women in a rural and urban community in Southeast Nigeria. *Journal of Obstetrics and Gynecology*, 25 (3), 292–295.

Panda, P. (2002). *Rights-Based Strategies in the Prevention of Domestic Violence*. Working Paper 344. Washington DC: International Center for Research on Women.

Promundo (2004). *Program H Manual Series*. Rio de Janeiro, Brazil: Promundo http://www.promundo.org.br/396?locale=en_US.

Pronyk, P.M., Hargreaves, J.R, Kim, J.C., Morison, L., Phetla, G., Watts, C., Busza, J. and Porter, J.D.H. (2006). Effect of a structural intervention for the prevention of intimate-partner violence and HIV in rural South Africa: A cluster randomized trial. *Lancet*, 368, 1973–1983.

Pulerwitz, J., Barker, G., Segundo, M. and Nascimento, M. (2006). *Promoting More Gender-Equitable Norms and Behaviors among Young Men as an HIV/AIDS Prevention Strategy*. Horizons Final Report. Washington DC: Population Council.

RADAR (2002). *Social Interventions for HIV/AIDS: Intervention with Microfinance for AIDS and Gender Equity*. IMAGE study intervention monograph no. 2. Rural AIDS and Development Action Research Programme. South Africa: School of Public Health, University of the Witwatersrand.

Rivers, K. and Aggleton, P. (2001). *Men and the HIV Epidemic*. New York: UNDP HIV and Development Programme.

Santana, M.C., Raj, A., Decker, M.R., La Marche, A. and Silverman, J.G. (2006). Masculine gender roles associated with increased sexual risk and intimate partner violence perpetration among young adult men. *Journal of Urban Health*, 83 (4), 575–585.

Schoepf, B. (1993). AIDS action-research with women in Kinshasa, Zaire. *Social Science and Medicine*, 37(11), 1401–1413.

Strickland, R. (2004). *To Have and to Hold: Women's Property and Inheritance Rights in the Context of HIV/AIDS in Sub-Saharan Africa*. Washington DC: International Center for Research on Women.

Taegmeyer, M., Kilonzo, N., Mung'ala, L., Morgan, G. and Theobald, S. (2006). Using gender analysis to build voluntary counseling and testing responses in Kenya. *Transactions of the Royal Society of Tropical Medicine and Hygiene*, 100, 305–311.

Theobald, S., Tolhurst, R. and Squire, S.B. (2006). Gender, equity: New approaches for effective management of communicable diseases. *Transactions of the Royal Society of Tropical Medicine and Hygiene*, 100, 299–304.

Ulin, P.R. (1992). African women and AIDS: Negotiating behavioral change. *Social Science and Medicine*, 34, 63–73.

UN Millennium Project (2005). *Taking Action: Achieving Gender Equality and Empowering Women*. Report of the Task Force on Education and Gender Equality. London: Earthscan.

UNAIDS (2006). Report on the Global AIDS Epidemic. May 2006. Geneva.

UNAIDS/WHO AIDS Epidemic Update (2005). Geneva http://www.unaids.org/epi/2005/doc/report_pdf.asp.

UNAIDS/WHO AIDS Epidemic Update (2006). Geneva. http://www.unaids.org/en/HIV_data/epi2006.

Verma, R. K., Pulerwitz, J., Mahendra, V., Khandekar, S., Barker, G., Fulpagare, P. and Singh, S.K. 2006. Challenging and changing gender attitudes among young men in Mumbai, India. *Reproductive Health Matters*, 14 (28): 135–143.

Warren, H. (2007). Using gender analysis frameworks: Theoretical and practical reflections. *Gender and Development*, 15(2), 187–198.

Weiss, E. amd Gupta, G. Rao (1998). *Bridging the Gap: Addressing Gender and Sexuality in HIV Prevention*. Washington DC: International Center for Research on Women.

Weiss, E., Whelan, D. and Gupta, G. Rao (2000). Gender, sexuality, and HIV making a difference in the lives of young women in developing countries. *Sexual and Relationship Therapy*, 15(3), 233–245.

Welbourn, A. (1995). *Stepping Stones: A Training Manual for Sexual and Reproductive Health Communication and Relationship Skills*. Strategies for Hope Training series No. 1. London: Actionaid.

Whelan, D. (1999). *Gender and HIV/AIDS: Taking Stock of Research and Programs*. Geneva: UNAIDS.

Wingwood, G. and DiClemente, R.J. (2000). Application of the theory of gender and power to examine HIV-related exposures, risk factors, and effective interventions for women. *Health Education and Behavior*, 27(5), 539–565.

Wingwood, G. and DiClemente, R.J. (2006). Enhancing adoption of evidence-based HIV interventions: Promotion of a suite of HIV prevention interventions for African American women. *AIDS Education and Prevention*, 18, Supplement A, 161–170.

Wojcicki, J.M. (2002). She drank his money: Survival sex and the problem of violence in taverns in Guateng Province, South Africa. *Medical Anthropology Quarterly*, 16(3), 267–293.

Wood, K., Bakam, K., Jewkes, R., Duvvury, N. and Skweyiya, Y. (2006). It has brought quietness in our relationship: young South Africans' experiences of the HIV behavioral intervention Stepping Stones. Poster presentation at the 16th International AIDS Conference, Toronto.

World Bank (2005). *Gender Issues and Best Practices in Land Administration Projects. A Synthesis Report*. Washington DC: The World Bank.

World Health Organization (1999). What about Boys? A Literature Review on the health and development of Adolescent Boys. Geneva: WHO Department of Child and Adolescent Health and Development.

World Health Organization (2005). *AIDS Epidemic Update 2005*. http://data.unaids.org/publications/IRC-pub06/epi_update2005_en.pdf.

World Health Organization (2007). *Engaging Men and Boys in Changing Gender-Based Inequity in Health: Evidence from Programme Interventions*. Geneva: WHO.

World Health Organization Department of Gender and Women's Health (2003). *Mainstreaming Gender in Health: A WHO Manual for Health Managers*. Geneva: World Health Organization.

Worth, D. (1989). Sexual decision-making and AIDS: Why condom promotion among vulnerable women is likely to fail. *Studies in Family Planning* 20, 297–307.

CHAPTER 4

The Hard Science of Hard Risks in Women's HIV Prevention

Making Biology Part of the Context

Rhonda Rosenberg and Robert Malow

ABSTRACT

The HIV epidemic in female populations, especially in resource-rich countries like the United States, has exposed the complex nature of risk and disease like few others. Prevention efforts have further advanced the contextual science of applied research in psychology, and the social and behavioral sciences. This chapter examines this history and then highlights major contributions from these sciences. It then discusses the neglected aspect of women's biology, its role in HIV behavioral interventions, and the challenges to researchers that are posed by the genomic era.

STUDY TARGET AND CONTEXT

Imagine a population in which the majority live below the poverty line and over one third operate on a level of human capital that does not include a high-school education. Unexceptional events in their lives include having no safe place to live, being physically attacked or raped, having no money for necessities, personal loss through death or break-up, and having children taken away. Up to 20 percent of this population report three or more of these during the past year (Moore et al. 1999). More than 60 percent have CES-D scores (Center for Epidemiologic Studies Depression Scale) indicating significant depression. Being married or monogamous may be their greatest risk factor.

This population is female and lives in the United States. It constitutes the HERS study cohort, the CDC/National Institute of Allergy and Infectious Disease's HIV Epidemiology Research Study, which prospectively followed both HIV-infected and at-risk women from four urban centers in the United States (Baltimore, The Bronx, Detroit, and Providence). Most were either black or Hispanic. Although to be eligible for this study women had to report drug or sexual risk, these cohort demographics nonetheless reflect national patterns for women at risk or infected with HIV: they are American women living in a developing country context.

ECONOMICS

Amartya Sen, a Nobel Laureate economist, once pressed this characterization in a keynote address before the World Health Assembly in Geneva (Sen 1999a). In illustrating the phenomenon of "Third World" deprivation for certain groups in wealthy countries, he pointed to mortality patterns among African-American women, whose chances of survival to older ages were no better than the Chinese and, in fact, were worse than that experienced in Kerala, a country-sized state in India. Kerala could do so much better even though per capita income was drastically lower than in the U.S.A., because of two factors according to Sen—investment in poverty removal and public health care.

In inter-country comparisons, the traditionally tight and predictive relationship between GNP per capita and life expectancy nearly disappears once these two expenditure categories are included (Sen 1999b), suggesting a pivotal role in biological health. This is not an undisputed issue, however. Public investment itself depends upon GNP. Such disputes reflect paradigmatic differences over the contributions of biomedicine and public health, markets versus more organic categories such as social capital, and whether the HIV epidemic is predominantly a structural, psychosocial, or biological problem. The ironic twist is that the sociocultural and psychological context of women's risk is demanding a return to biology, or rather a forward march to the new biology—that of neurogenetics and other related areas made possible by genomics. In mapping the human genome and thus beginning to see ourselves as a species, we may finally be able to do that and more for women and the concrete hardness of the risks for which they must have real strategies.

PUBLIC HEALTH

It is a fundamental principle of public health that the possibility of a "cure" has more to do with the hardness of life than with the grace of biomedical intervention. Even when it is a matter of a vaccine or a drug, the hardness of people's lives may prevent access to the intervention or interfere with making use of it. The history of tuberculosis should have made this clear. Yet it was the advent of AIDS that crystallized this public health principle as no other infectious disease had in human history.

Adequate nutrition, clean water, a sense of individual agency, and freedom from violence and social disarray are some of the touchstones of historical declines in infectious disease incidence and mortality. This history has been translated into social determinants research by epidemiologists and into development studies by economists. However, it has taken astronomical disease rates, principally in sub-Saharan Africa, along with drastic shifts in disease burden among different groups in the U.S. population, to clarify HIV/AIDS as something more than a problem of individual risk.

MINORITY U.S. WOMEN AND HIV/AIDS

Disproportionate rates among U.S. minorities have led researchers to look at health disparities and the need for tailored interventions. However, even this redefinition has proven inadequate to the most startling shift in the population patterns of the epidemic: the acceleration of HIV risk among women, particularly minority women (Gerberding 2004). In this, the U.S.A. has converged with Africa.

The distinguished public health scientist Tony McMichael (2001) has summed up the dynamic of the AIDS epidemic in the twenty-first century:

> Diseases such as tuberculosis, leprosy, cholera, typhoid and diphtheria are preeminently diseases of poverty. As happened historically with tuberculosis, HIV infection seems now to be entrenching itself among the world's poor and disempowered, especially in sub-Saharan Africa and South Asia. Much of the spread of HIV has been along international "fault lines," tracking the inequality and vulnerability which accompany migrant labour, educational deprivation and sexual commerce.

The gains in HIV/AIDS risk reduction among U.S. women have been meager compared to the escalating trajectory of the epidemic, which has exposed a new stratification into risk cultures in our society (minority, ethnic/immigrant culture, inner-city, drug culture). It is increasingly evident that interventions remain insufficiently focused on the *hardness* of women's risks, specifically the life situation and disparities in norms and institutional structures that even American women must navigate. Typically, this is manifested in recurrent interruptions in protective sexual behavior in the face of financial, physical, or emotional threat. Health is frequently neglected and services underutilized. A history of victimization and stigma is common.

The perpetual state of coping observed in the most vulnerable female groups can easily appear amorphous and unsolvable. Individual efforts to reduce HIV risk are often trumped by problems related to finances, housing, child care, transportation, looking for or holding down multiple low-skilled jobs, barriers to medical care, maintaining intimate relationships, and personal/neighborhood substance abuse and crime (Barthwell 1993; Kalichman et al. 1995; Kalichman, Hunter, and Kelly 1992; Wingood and DiClemente 1998).

Transactional sex is a known risk factor for women in a fight for survival in the developing world, but it is also an experience shared by women in the United States who live in a similar context, especially those with substance abuse problems (Logan, Cole, and Leukefeld 2002). McGowan et al. (2004) have identified it as a major barrier to HIV prevention with high-risk seropositive women. In their interviews with women receiving antiretroviral therapy, 41 percent stated that they continued to have unprotected sex, and the significant contributing factor was trading sex for drugs or money. Recent research indicates, however, that even in this HIV preventionists must take a tailored approach. Other factors besides deprivation may trigger transactional sex, requiring different intervention components for different subgroups of women (Maganja et al. 2007).

Let us be very specific about some of the ways in which poverty and its consequences synergize HIV risk. Women who are addicted often exchange sex for the drugs they need. Women without housing often give sex to men who offer them a safe place to spend a night. Women in violent relationships fear requesting that their partners use condoms because of the threat of partner retaliation for perceived infidelity. Women who cannot pay rent are often forced to give their landlords sex to avoid being expelled from their homes. Women lacking job skills have sex with their superiors to avoid being fired. Women who are incarcerated are subjected to forced sex and the use of unclean needles (O'Leary 2001; O'Leary and Jemmott 1995; O'Leary and Martins 2000).

PRINCIPLES FROM HIV/AIDS SOCIOBEHAVIORAL RESEARCH

HIV/AIDS sociobehavioral research has produced several organizing principles to avoid policy malaise in addressing women and HIV:

1. HIV prevention with persistently high-risk groups should be treated as a syndemic rather than merely an epidemic. A syndemic is the co-occurrence of epidemics in a population and describes the synergistic phenomenon that links poverty, limited free agency, and HIV/AIDS. An empirical syndemic model goes the extra step needed in developing an evidence-based science that can be funded to fight such a problem. This is why the recent research by Stall et al. (2003) is so significant. They were able to statistically demonstrate a linked set of four psychosocial health problems, which were each individually excessive in their study population and additively increased the risk of HIV: polydrug use, depression, childhood sexual abuse, and partner violence. Their study population was urban MSM (men who have sex with men) from four major U.S. cities. Similar survey research is needed for high-risk female populations. A tutorial to this approach can be found on the Centers for Disease Control and Prevention (CDC) website: www.cdc.gov/syndemics/index.htm.
2. Tailored intervention design means documenting the "hardness of risk" for vulnerable female groups. Hardness of risk can be defined as what makes potential exposure to HIV so difficult to avoid and bear or a therapeutic regimen so prohibitive once infected. The importance of this research is that it moves the prevention community beyond the measurement of individual risk and into intervention models that can encompass the context and heterogeneity of women. Foremost, it has had the effect of guiding intervention research toward those studies that can identify factors that mediate and moderate intervention effects. Such

research values the incorporation of social and contextual factors. Green and Glasgow (2006) have stressed the strategic use of mediating/moderating analyses in adapting interventions and overcoming ecological barriers to reducing risk. The cumulation of research on the hardness of risk has allowed increasingly precise statements about such influences, as illustrated in the review by McNair and Prather (2004) on the social and contextual risks of African-American women. However, as they noted, HIV/AIDS intervention design specifically tied to these factors has lagged behind in prevention with women.

3. The couple and the group are the new targets of intervention. Women's experience with HIV/AIDS has sharpened attention on the most basic of facts: Transmission risk is negotiated in couples or dyads and inside of groups. Even when it may be prohibitive to involve the sexual partner in an intervention protocol, this relationship as well as other types of relationships must be brought to the foreground in prevention efforts if outcomes are to be meaningful.
4. Empowerment needs to be tailored, too. Participatory designs have opened a promising avenue for HIV prevention with women, through peer support, family communication, and sociopolitical activation. Holtgrave and Crosby (2003) have identified an AIDS-related social capital effect by replicating the approach used by Harvard's Kawachi, in which state-level surveillance data are used with Putnam's social capital indicators of trust, density of organized groups, and participation (see Holtgrave and Crosby 2003, for their review of this approach). Yet a social capital approach to group influence is rare in HIV prevention, and we still do not have a knowledge base for deciding when an empowerment intervention is appropriate and for whom.

   There are indications that the impact of empowerment approaches may be a function of gender, and that women may gain more if interventions can also build a perceived sense of community (Peterson et al. 2005). Women may be particularly sensitive to interventions that foster a group experience, such that even participation in a research study can influence risk behavior. Dworkin et al. (2006) conducted a posttrial evaluation of the successful gender-specific intervention called Project FIO (the Future Is Ours), and found that gains in a sense of empowerment were reported by women across all three arms of the randomized trial, including the assessment-only control group. Women especially responded to opportunities to share their experience with family, peers, and the wider community. Referrals to services and social support were important not only to participants in the most intensive experimental group, but also to those in the control group, suggesting that brief HIV interventions can have real impact on accessing services even outside of case management approaches.
5. HIV prevention research has documented that mental health is critical to protective behavior and medication adherence (Prince et al. 2007). Moreover, therapy matters, even in the most environmentally deprived and disorganized communities. A poignant illustration is a randomized controlled trial of group psychotherapy for HIV-linked depression conducted in Uganda (Bolton et al. 2003). The research team led by Paul Bolton had already determined the significance of depression in Ugandan areas hardest hit by the epidemic. The intervention trial demonstrated that group psychotherapeutic approaches can be adapted with efficacy in a developing country context. Signs of positive impact on relational health between marital/sexual partners and on the social and financial empowerment of women were identified as areas for further research. This study was also reported by Marc Lacey in the *New York Times* on January 15, 2004.

MISSING VARIABLES

Castro and Farmer (2005) have emphasized that tying HIV prevention to poverty and health disparities is not enough and can result in approaches that caricature the target population as hollow victims. Their major point is that populations will respond and change behavior when health care infrastructures and interventions are available that work, and they present evidence from interventions in Haiti as illustration. In addition, Menon-Johansson (2005) has shown that HIV prevalence is higher in countries with poor governance. The U.N. Commission on HIV/AIDS and Governance in Africa is indicative of the growing importance of institutional design in fostering sustained outcomes from HIV interventions (see www.uneca.org/CHGA/about.htm). This effort and others, which tie governance and infrastructure to women's empowerment, have been fostered by the current U.S. Global AIDS Program.

But it is the World Bank that has been initially able to spotlight the need for empowering women in HIV prevention efforts. In this instance, an economic model has brought attention to individual and group capacity in adopting protective behavior. HIV behavioral interventions have typically neglected issues of human and social capital. Human capital is the education and training that the individual can summon in making use of HIV prevention programs; social capital is the collective values that social groupings can bring to bear, such as connectedness, trust, and associational ethics or habits (see Ziersch et al. 2005).

One initial step that can be taken in HIV behavioral prevention in this regard, however, is known as "linking." This involves incorporating linkage mechanisms within or in tandem with proven behavioral interventions that will go beyond information and referral and actually train and direct women to establish linkages with health services and social support. Such an approach offers a first step in building individual health capital—one dimension of human capital (Grossman 1972; Becker 2007)—and also affects health sector social capital in a given community, by increasing connective or service network capacity, at least in one problem area (see Hendryx and Ahern 2000; Rosenheck et al. 2001; Scott and Hofmeyer 2007). Although not targeted to women, a good example of this approach is ARTAS, the Antiretroviral Treatment Access Study (Gardner et al. 2005; see http://ssrg.med.miami.edu/x27.xml). In our own work, we have incorporated a linking skills-building strategy in a prevention intervention design for pregnant women in substance abuse treatment and are currently testing it in a randomized trial (Malow, PI "Multi-Level HIV Prevention for Pregnant Drug Abusers," NIDA R01 DA021521, 09/30/06–05/31/11).

Recent research from the New York City Health Department may indicate how essential such linkage mechanisms may be. Statistics reported in the *New York Times* by Marc Santora (2006) reveal that ethnic minorities, particularly Black women, in Central Harlem are more likely to die of AIDS than are people living in Chelsea, which actually has the highest rate of new cases. Financial obstacles to antiretroviral treatment are noted as very minimal in the city. The difference is being attributed to variations in help-seeking between ethnic minorities and the large gay white male population in Chelsea. Stigma in ethnic minority communities and heterosexual partnerships is evidently proving harder to negotiate.

The hardest hit are Blacks—male and female—not only in New York City but across the country. The February 10, 2006 *Morbidity and Mortality Weekly Report* (CDC 2006) is arresting in its portrayal of the pervasive disparity of experience with HIV/AIDS among Blacks in the United States. If preliminary suppositions from New York City are valid, what appears crucial to recognize is the important effect emotional life has on outcomes in this epidemic. Emotional life is at the core of an adequate response to stigma and undermining heterosexual partnerships. Interventions that do not take account of the affective dimensions of the factors that mediate and moderate outcomes—whether they pertain to individual, familial, cultural, or adverse socioeconomic issues—will be unable to sustain women through the inevitable losses and disappointments that accompany attempted adherence to the intervention.

Even now, the key outcome to be measured is still condom use, no matter how deep the poverty or health disparity. As attention is turned to macrocontextual issues, it is important to keep in mind that condom use to prevent HIV transmission is also about sexuality, intimacy, and loss. After nearly thirty years of the epidemic, the affective dimensions of both the macro- and the microcontext of condom use are still absent from most measurement methodologies of HIV/AIDS interventions. Even with cognitive–behavioral approaches and targeted psychological outcomes, the psychology of condom use, so to speak, is still waiting to be explored.

BIOLOGY

The most neglected variable in HIV prevention interventions, however, may be women's biology. In the first two decades of the epidemic, the predominant knowledge domain available to interventionists was social and behavioral science. Moreover, the most rigorous intervention studies, guided by testable theoretical models, time and again confirmed the importance of motivation, behavioral skills, and contextual factors, which frequently outweighed the contribution of HIV information in improving risk outcomes.

However, advancements in basic biological science are returning the HIV prevention community to two long-forgotten characteristics of transmission risk:

- individual variation in susceptibility—to both infection and risk behavior; and
- the unique biological vulnerability of the female genital tract.

Ames and McBride (2006) identify the first as the focus of one of the major tasks facing preventionists in the coming decades, which will involve the translation of genetics, neuroscience, and cognitive science into disease prevention. Advances in these areas, in large part driven by the genomic revolution, are expected to turn personalized medicine and individualized risk assessment from cliché and superficiality into realities with meaningful consequences. Already it is clear that there is a potentially malleable biological basis to how individuals respond to rewards (and losses), environmental cues, and novelty, which all may be important to HIV risk behavior and drug abuse.

The neuroscientist Nancy Andreasen (2001), a pioneer of neuroimaging applied to mental disorders, has emphasized the fundamental importance of integrating the principle of brain and gene plasticity into our models of intervention. This will mean considering the neurochemical messages as well as the social messages that may encumber vulnerable women in trying to utilize prevention interventions. This in turn means integrating new modes of assessment—neuroimaging and genetic markers—into our methods of observation and intervention. Research on neurochemical messaging or neurotransmitter systems, such as the serotonin and dopamine systems, increasingly shows the importance of their consideration in the prevention of co-morbid psychological and substance misuse disorders (Bryant 2006; Volkow and Li 2005).

Cicchetti and Blender (2006) have explained how neurobiological data can be studied as variables that may moderate intervention effects, and have suggested that it will also be possible to monitor "the extent to which neural plasticity may be promoted" by a given intervention. Hutchison et al. (2004) have elaborated on the logic of incorporating genetic markers in psychosocial studies related to substance abuse prevention, which may have far-reaching implications for HIV prevention with high-risk groups facing multiple psychosocial problems.

It is these methodologies that will be of increasing interest and necessity to HIV preventionists in future behavioral intervention trials. They are associated with the new field of neurogenetics and allow investigators to identify the molecular pathways through which genes act, opening the possibility for remedial intervention and deeper understanding of the mechanism of action in interventions. The National Institute of Neurological Disorders and Stroke (NINDS) has created a webpage devoted to this emerging area of study: http://www.ninds.nih.gov/funding/areas/neurogenetics/index.htm). The newly elected president of the American Public Health Association, Deborah Klein Walker (2007), has called for public health professionals to integrate genomics into their research and practice. This stems from her work on the Institute of Medicine's Committee on Genomics and the Public's Health in the Twenty-First Century (see workshop summary, http://www.nap.edu/openbook.php?isbn=0309096073). While genetics dealt primarily with single diseases governed by single genes, genomics is concerned with the more complex disorders that are actually more common in human populations, which may be shaped by many genes in interaction with the environment and behavior—exactly the kind of disease risk presented by HIV and related risk behaviors. One of the next frontiers for biological and sociobehavioral scientists will be behavioral phenotyping (outward manifestation). An initial step in this effort may be to begin incorporating neuropsychological and molecular-genetic data as moderators in HIV behavioral intervention trials. This is the strategy chosen by us in a newly funded study examining neurobehavioral factors in a randomized trial of an adaptation of Holistic Health Recovery Program (HHRP) for HIV-positive male and female substance abusers (PI, Malow, "Intervening with HIV+Alcohol Abusers: Influence of Neuro-Behavioral Factors," R01AA017405).

Hirbod and Broliden (2007) have expressed the importance of the second characteristic listed above like no others in the recent literature: "[t]he main biological factor contributing to female vulnerability to heterosexual transmission of HIV-1 is the substantial mucosal exposure of the female genital tract to seminal fluids." They go on to discuss how advances in immunologic and genetic science are rapidly improving our ability to interrupt this predisposing factor. Yet, how many women (or men) come away from current interventions really knowing what constitutes their main biological risk? While there have been Institute of Medicine reports reviewing how certain knowledge bases are being translated into HIV prevention science, there are none that have studied if or how well these biological advancements are being communicated to study participants, particularly when the information is gender-specific.

Boerma and Weir (2005) have offered what they call the Proximate-determinants framework as a means for refocusing attention on the biological mechanisms that contribute to transmission risk: "the rate of contact between susceptible and infected persons, the efficiency of transmission during exposure between susceptible and infected partners, and the duration of infectivity." In turn, efficiency of transmission depends on the degree of pathogenic virulence, pathogenic concentration in bodily fluids, and individual biologic susceptibility. The question their work raises is whether these pathways should be included in the information component of interventions for women. Although women may know more about their behavioral risk because of current risk reduction efforts, there has been no evaluation of whether they know anything about their specific biologic risk consistent with the advancement in our knowledge of HIV, such as the effect of ulcerative STDs on infectiousness and susceptibility during HIV exposure.

CONCLUSION

The available evidence indicates that the success of future interventions for women will depend on a goodness of fit in which empowerment may be central. Yet, until HIV preventionists fully integrate how they themselves have been empowered by the mapping of the human genome, this goodness of fit will remain mostly a problem of adapting interventions to fit the sociocultural needs of women and controlling group susceptibility rather than addressing individual variations. As already noted in reference to Castro and Farmer (2005), this is a necessary but not sufficient condition for intervening in the twenty-first century. Their fundamental message is that women can respond to facts on the ground and in their bodies. How many women know that HIV is a species and interacts with their bodies like an organism in an ecosystem, which means that it is capable of evolving, mutating, and becoming resistant to medications? If asked, would most just say that HIV is a germ? If so, they are only being empowered to face the nineteenth century. Even in highly undermined societies like Haiti, researchers have discovered the continuing and statistically significant importance of HIV knowledge to empowering women to negotiate sexual risk (Kershaw et al. 2006). The next frontier for women's HIV prevention is biology and governance—a *bio-psychosocial-democratic* model of intervention.

ACKNOWLEDGMENT

This research was supported, in part, by a grant from the National Institute on Drug Abuse (R03-DA 21982; PI, Malow) and the National Institute on Alcohol Abuse and Alcoholism (R01AA017405; PI, Malow).

REFERENCES AND FURTHER READING

Ames, S., and McBride, C. "Translating genetics, cognitive science, and other basic science research findings into applications for prevention." *Evaluation & the Health Professions* 29 (2006): 277–301.

Andreasen, N.C. *Brave New Brain: Conquering Mental Illness in the Era of the Genome*. New York: Oxford University Press, 2001.

Barthwell, A. "African American women and drug-related HIV infection and AIDS." *Center for Substance Abuse Prevention Monograph* 13 (1993): 113–129.

Becker, G.S. "Health as human capital: a synthesis and extensions." *Oxford Economic Papers* 59(3) (2007): 379–410.

Boerma, J., and Weir, S. "Integrating demographic and epidemiological approaches to research on HIV/AIDS: the proximate-determinants framework." *Journal of Infectious Diseases* 191 (2005): S61–S67.

Bolton, P., Bass, J., Neugebauer, R., Verdeli, H., Clougherty, K.F., Wickramaratne, P., Speelman, L., Ndogoni, L., and Weissman, M. "Group interpersonal psychotherapy for depression in rural Uganda: a randomized controlled trial." *Journal of the American Medical Association* 289 (2003): 3117–3124.

Bryant, K.J. "Expanding research on the role of alcohol consumption and related risks in the prevention and treatment of HIV/AIDS." *Substance Use and Misuse* 41 (2006): 1465–1507.

Castro, A., and Farmer, P. "Understanding and addressing AIDS-related stigma: from anthropological theory to clinical practice in Haiti." *American Journal of Public Health* 95 (2005): 53–59.

Centers for Disease Control and Prevention. "Racial and ethnic disparities in diagnoses of HIV/AIDS in 33 states: 2001–2004." *Morbidity and Mortality Weekly Report* 55(5) (2006, February 10): 121–125. Also available on-line at www.cdc.gov/mmwr/preview/mmwrhtml/mm5505a1.htm?s_cid=mm5505a1_e.

Cicchetti, D., and Blender, J. "A Multiple-Levels-of-Analysis Perspective on Resilience Implications for the Developing Brain, Neural Plasticity and Preventive Interventions." *Annals of the New York Academy of Sciences* 1094 (2006): 248–258.

Dworkin, S.L., Exner, T., Melendez, R., Hoffman, S., and Ehrhardt, A.A. "Revisiting 'success': posttrial analysis of a gender-specific HIV/STD prevention intervention." *AIDS and Behavior* 10(1) (2006): 41–51.

Gardner, L.I., Metsch, L.R., Anderson-Mahoney, P., Loughlin, A.M., del Rio, C., Strathdee, S., Sansom, S.L., Siegal, H.A., Greenberg, A.E., and Holmberg, S.D. Antiretroviral Treatment and Access Study Group. "Efficacy of a brief case management intervention to link recently diagnosed HIV-infected persons to care." *AIDS* 19 (2005): 423–431.

Gerberding, J.L. "Women and infectious diseases." *Emerging Infectious Diseases* 10 (2004): 1965–1967.

Green, L.W., and Glasgow, R.E. "Evaluating the relevance, generalization, and applicability of research." *Evaluation & the Health Professions* 29(1) (2006): 126–153.

Grossman, M. "On the concept of health capital and the demand for health." *Journal of Political Economy* 80(2) (1972): 223–255.

Hendryx, M.S., and Ahern, M.M. "Access to mental health services and health sector social capital." *American Journal of Community Psychology* 28(2) (2000): 149–173.

Hirbod, T., and Broliden, K. "Mucosal immune responses in the genital tract of HIV-1-exposed uninfected women." *Journal of Internal Medicine* 262 (2007): 44–58.

Holtgrave, D.R., and Crosby, R.A. "Social capital, poverty, and income inequality as predictors of gonorrhea, syphilis, chlamydia and AIDS case rates in the United States." *Sexually Transmitted Infection* 79 (2003): 62–64.

Hutchison, K.E., Stallings, M., McGeary, J.M., and Bryan, A. "Population stratification in the case-control design: fatal threat or red herring?" *Psychological Bulletin* 130 (2004): 66–79.

Kalichman, S.C., Adair, V., Somlai, A.M., and Weir, S.S. "The perceived social context of AIDS: study of innercity sexually transmitted disease clinic patients." *AIDS Education and Prevention* 7 (1995): 298–307.

Kalichman, S.C., Hunter, T.L., and Kelly, J.A. "Perceptions of AIDS susceptibility among minority and non-minority women at risk for HIV infection." *Journal of Consulting and Clinical Psychology* 60 (1992): 725–732.

Kershaw, T.S., Small, M., Joseph, G.,Theodore, M., Bateau, R., and Frederic, R. "The influence of power on HIV risk among pregnant women in rural Haiti." *AIDS and Behavior* 10(3) (2006): 309–318.

Logan, T., Cole, J., and Leukefeld, C. "Women, sex, and HIV: social and contextual factors, meta-analysis of published interventions, and implications for practice and research." *Psychological Bulletin* 128 (2002): 851–885.

McGowan, J.P., Shah, S.S., Ganea, C.E., Blum, S., Ernst, J.A., Irwin, K.L., Olivo, N., and Weidle, P.J. "Risk behavior for transmission of human immunodeficiency virus (HIV) among HIV-seropositive individuals in an urban setting." *Clinical Infectious Diseases* 38 (2004): 122–127.

McMichael, T. *Human Frontiers, Environments and Disease*. New York: Cambridge University Press, 2001.

McNair, L.D. and Prather, C.M. "African American women and AIDS: factors influencing risk and reaction to HIV disease." *Journal of Black Psychology* 30 (2004): 106–123.

Maganja, R.K., Maman, S., Groues, A., and Mbwambo, J.K. "Skinning the goat and pulling the load: transactional sex among youth in Dar es Salaam, Tanzania." *AIDS Care* 19(8) (2007): 974–981.

Menon-Johansson, A.S. "Good governance and good health: the role of societal structures in the human immunodeficiency virus pandemic." *BMC International Health and Human Rights* 5(1) (2005): 4. http://www.biomedcentral.com/content/pdf/1472-698x-5-4.pdf.

Moore, J., Schuman, P., Schoenbaum, E., Boland, B., Solomon, L., and Smith, D. "Severe adverse life events and depressive symptoms among women with or at risk for HIV infection in four cities in the United States of America." *AIDS* 13 (1999): 2459–2468.

O'Leary, A. "Substance use and HIV: disentangling the nexus of risk." *Journal of Substance Abuse* 13 (2001): 1–3.

O'Leary, A., and Jemmott, L. *Women at Risk: Issues in the Primary Prevention of AIDS*. New York: Plenum Press, 1995.

O'Leary, A., and Martins, P. "Structural and policy factors affecting women's HIV risk: a lifecourse example." *AIDS* 14(Supplement) (2000): S68–S72.

Peterson, N.A., Lowe, J.B., Aquilino, M.L., and Schneider, J.E. "Linking social cohesion and gender to intrapersonal and interactional empowerment: support and new implications for theory." *Journal of Community Psychology* 33(2) (2005): 233–244.

Prince, M., Patel,V., Saxena, S., Maj, M., Maselko, J., Phillips, M.R., and Rahman, A. "No health without mental health." *Lancet* 370 (2007): 859–877.

Rosenheck, R., Morrisssey, J., Lam, J., Calloway, M., Stolar, M., Johnsen, M., Randolph, F., Blasinsky, M., and Goldman, H. "Service delivery and community: social capital, service systems integration, and outcomes among homeless persons with severe mental illness." *Health Services Research* 36(4) (2001): 691–710.

Santora, M. "Report highlights AIDS risk to black men and women." *New York Times*, (February 4, 2006). Retrieved February 5, 2006 from the New York Times Company website: www.nytimes.com/2006/02/04/nyregion/04aids.html.

Scott, C. and Hofmeyer, A. "Networks and social capital: a relational approach to primary healthcare reform." *Health Research Policy and Systems* 5(1) (2007): 1–27. Open access BioMed Central.

Sen, A. "Health in Development." Keynote address to the 52nd World Health Assembly, Geneva, May 18, 1999. *Bulletin of the World Health Organization* 77 (1999a).

Sen, A. "Economics and Health." *The Lancet* (354) (December 1999b, Suppl.): SIV 20.

Stall, R., Mills, T.C., Williamson, J., Hart, T., Greenwood, G., Paul, J., Pollack, L., Binson, D., Osmond, D., and Catania, J.A. "Association of co-occurring psychosocial health problems and increased vulnerability to HIV/AIDS among urban men who have sex with men." *American Journal of Public Health* 93 (2003): 939–942.

Volkow, N.D., and Li, T.K. "Drugs and alcohol: treating and preventing abuse, addiction and their medical consequences." *Pharmacology and Therapeutics* 108 (2005): 3–17.

Walker, D.K. "Public health must embrace informatics, genomics fields." *Nation's Health* (October 2007).

Wingood, G.M., and DiClemente, R.J. "The influence of psychosocial factors, alcohol, drug use on African-American women's high-risk sexual behavior." *American Journal of Preventive Medicine* 15 (1998): 54–59.

Ziersch, A.M., Baum, F.E., MacDougall, C., and Putland, C. "Neighborhood life and social capital: the implications for health." *Social Science and Medicine* 60 (2005): 71–86.

CHAPTER 5

HIV/AIDS Prevention Programming with "Traditional" Sex Workers in Rural India

Challenges for the Empowerment Approach in Community-Sanctioned Sex Work Environments

Treena Orchard, John D. O'Neil, James Blanchard, Aine Costigan, and Stephen Moses

ABSTRACT

This chapter addresses HIV/AIDS prevention programs with sex workers in Devadasi *communities in Karnataka and* Nat *communities in Rajasthan, India. Both sets of communities sanction the socialization and initiation of adolescent girls into sex work and the economies of the communities are to a large extent dependent on sex work. Developing and implementing prevention initiatives in traditional female sex work communities requires an understanding of the social and economic structures in the community that determine sex work patterns. Program implementation must be monitored closely to ensure project activities are consistent with shifting power relationships in these communities, and supportive of empowerment strategies for the sex workers themselves.*

OVERVIEW

This chapter provides a descriptive overview and analysis of two projects designed to prevent HIV infection in traditional sex work communities in the Indian states of Rajasthan and Karnataka. These projects were implemented by the India–Canada Collaborative HIV/AIDS Project (ICHAP), funded by the Canadian International Development Agency from 2001 to 2006. Traditional sex work occurs in communities with cultural, religious, and caste-based traditions that sanction sex work as a legitimate economic strategy for the survival of the community.[1] This type of female sex work differs from the majority of sex work in India, where women usually enter the occupation from many sectors of society, often as a result of traumatic social circumstances such as spousal abuse and abandonment, extreme poverty, drug abuse, and/or exploitation by criminal elements (Chattopadhyay and McKaig 2004: 162; Sleightholme and Sinha 1996: 4). In these latter circumstances, sex workers usually do not maintain connections with their families of origin, and are not members of a cultural community that exists independent of their occupation. In situations of traditional sex work, community sanctions, practices, and expectations can have a significant impact on the implementation of programs designed to protect or improve the health of sex workers. Discerning the community response and impact in this setting is particularly challenging given the paucity of studies on rural sex work in India generally and rural traditional sex work specifically.

HIV/AIDS prevention programs with traditional sex workers are able to achieve better results when they are well informed by a critical evidence base. A primary objective of

ICHAP has been to build an applied research focus into all program activities, and to ensure that project implementation is constantly adjusted as new information about the target community and project activities becomes available. This process has involved a rapid ethnographic assessment, situation assessment and mapping, behavioral surveys, and ongoing monitoring and evaluation. However, the present material focuses on program implementation, beginning with an overview of HIV/AIDS in India and the sociocultural context of the traditional sex work communities in which these projects were based. This is followed by information on the different stages through which the demonstration projects were developed. The conclusion features a comparative analysis of lessons learned from the projects and a series of recommendations for implementing HIV/AIDS prevention and care programs in traditional sex work communities in India and elsewhere.

HIV/AIDS IN INDIA

Globally, India has recently surpassed South Africa in terms of the overall number of people living with HIV/AIDS (UNAIDS 2006). UNAIDS estimates that the number of Indians living with HIV/AIDS increased from 5.3 million in 2003 to 5.7 million in 2005. By the end of July 2005, the total number of AIDS cases reported in India was 111,608, of whom 32,567 were women (NACO 2005). These data also indicated that 37 percent of reported AIDS cases were diagnosed among people under 30, and that 86 percent of these cases occurred via sexual transmission. While the disease was first detected among sex workers (Amin 2004: 6), there is evidence to demonstrate that the epidemic has crossed over into "mainstream" populations. Indeed the situation in India is characterized by multiple epidemics, and in some places they occur within the same state. The epidemics vary, from states with mainly heterosexual transmission of HIV, to some states where injecting drug use is the main route of HIV transmission (AVERT 2006).

It is difficult to calculate the contribution of commercial sex to the evolution of the disease, but mathematical modeling suggests that prevention interventions directed at female sex work alone could end the HIV epidemic (Nagelkerke, Jha, and de Vlas 2002). Certain groups of high-risk men, such as migrant workers, truck drivers, and men who have sex with men, have also been identified as important to HIV transmission dynamics (Mane and Aggleton 2001; Rao et al. 1994). It has been demonstrated that the epidemic disproportionately affects those of lower socioeconomic status, and most female sex workers in India are women from poor, socially disadvantaged backgrounds (Bhave et al. 1995: S24; Brahme et al. 2006: 108). There is also evidence that HIV infection is well established in rural populations, particularly in the southern states of Maharashtra, Andhra Pradesh, Tamil Nadu, and Karnataka. A substantial proportion of sex workers come from communities where the practice is embedded within their socioeconomic, religious, and cultural history. For example, approximately 26 percent of female sex workers in Karnataka entered sex work through the *Devadasi* tradition (Blanchard et al. 2005: S141).

SOCIOCULTURAL CONTEXT OF TRADITIONAL SEX WORK IN RAJASTHAN: THE *NAT* COMMUNITY

Mapping exercises in Rajasthan have shown that a high proportion of women and girls in prostitution are from traditional sex work communities. Traditionally, members of the *Nat* community entertained feudal rulers and the masses through acrobatics, rope dance, and traditional plays. Among certain groups of powerful men, *Nat* women were kept as mistresses. With the decline of the *Rajput* ruling houses, the *Nats* have lost their patrons and many women from these communities have been initiated into sex work. Sex work or *dhandha*[2] is currently the primary occupation of *Nat* women for family survival. There is no prohibition of commercial sex by females and the caste Panchayat (political authority) has sanctioned this practice (Swarankar 1999a).

Parents, retired sex workers (*patelans*), and other community members often join forces when deciding on the fate of girl children and whether or not they will take up *dhandha* as a profession (Swarankar 1999a, 1999b). Once the decision is made and the girl is informed that her future is in *dhandha*, a *patelan* guides the socialization process by bringing her into closer contact with other sex workers and with clients. After attaining menarche a girl is ready for the *nath utrai* (sex initiation) ceremony. During this ceremony, the girl is dressed like a high-caste Hindu bride and a first client is selected based on the price he is willing to pay for the pleasure/honor of deflowering the girl. The ceremony reaps a considerable amount of money, ranging from INR 5,000/- 10,000/- (U.S.$ 200) in the villages to as high as INR 50,000/-100,000/- (U.S.$ 2,000) if the client is very wealthy or if the initiation takes place in urban centers (Swarankar 2001). Out of the total amount received, half is usually given to the parents of the girl and the remaining amount is utilized for a feast for family and other community members.

After the *nath utrai* and the community feast, a girl is socially permitted to pursue *dhandha* openly in the community. These activities are not only sanctioned by the community, they are under the control of the *Nat* caste Panchayat and enforced through the office of the *patelan* (Swarankar 1999a). The *patelan* charges a fixed commission from sex workers under her tutelage, irrespective of the amount received from a client. The *patelan* may also enter into a contract with the girl's parents, where she will ensure that a portion of the girl's fees is paid to the parents over a period of time.

Nat women who are sex workers cannot marry, but they may be allowed to keep a male partner referred to as "*ghar janwai*" (temporary husband). These individuals have usually been long-term clients of the sex worker and they have developed an emotional bond with the woman (Swarankar 2001). Children are often born from these unions and the *ghar janwai* may stay at a woman's house and assume economic responsibility for the family. Sex workers are supposed to abandon *dhandha* after developing a relationship with a *ghar janwai*, but many sex workers continue to practice *dhandha* when their partners are absent.

ICHAP IN RAJASTHAN

In the context of HIV in India, Rajasthan has been recategorized from a relatively low-risk state to one that is considered highly vulnerable, and there are many compelling reasons to prioritize HIV/AIDS initiatives in this state. Rajasthan is one of the largest and poorest states in India, has an estimated population of 56.47 million (2001 Census), a high degree of in-and-out migration, a large volume of daily intra-inter-state trucks on the move, a thriving tourist industry, and a considerable amount of rural, traditional caste-based sex work.

While the organization of traditional sex work within *Nat* communities has changed with modernization, the communities' economic dependence upon the women and girls' earnings ensures that this form of sex work persists in many communities throughout the region. Although it is widespread in Rajasthan, the caste-based stigma associated with sex work makes these women and other members of their community quite difficult to reach. This stigma and discrimination, combined with negative experiences with previous social/development projects, has bred significant mistrust among the community leaders and the women. This was an important factor to consider as a potential impediment to the project's development, but also as a more general comment on how threatening HIV prevention programs may appear for such communities which are almost entirely dependent upon sex work for their survival.

THE DESIGN PHASE OF THE *SAKSHAM* PROJECT (2001–JULY 2003)

As mentioned, few program models exist to address the complexities of HIV prevention in the context of rural, traditional caste-based sex work. However, the *Saksham* project, which in Hindi means "to enable/

empower," was implemented to help empower rural sex workers and to help reduce their risk and vulnerability to HIV/AIDS. The project areas are Alwar, Jaipur, and Tonk districts of eastern Rajasthan, which feature rural traditional female sex workers (RTFSW) from the *Nat*, *Kanjar*, and *Bediya* communities. Sex work in these districts has certain characteristics, which prompted a three-location design for *Saksham* at sex work places (along national and state highways), "habitats" (the women's home communities), and economic destinations like the large city of Mumbai.

In early 2001, ICHAP initiated preliminary ethnographic research with a non-governmental organization (NGO), the Hear Society, which was headed by a local social anthropologist with previous experience working in traditional sex work communities. One of the first studies examined the dynamics of the leadership within several RTFSW communities. Given the overarching political and social power of male community and caste leaders in these locales, the perception was that access to the women would depend upon the approval and involvement of these leaders. The study suggested that, although sex workers have interactions with leaders at the local level, their relationship with men at the higher levels is very limited. The women's role in decision-making is also quite small in scope, except in certain circumstances that directly pertain to their individual lives. Although most of the women were satisfied with their relationship with community leaders, 25 percent of participants reported a negative response to community leaders, an important indicator when trying to assess the "real" political power women are able to exercise.

OPERATIONALIZING THE COMMUNITY-BASED MODEL (JULY–DECEMBER 2003)

This phase of the project required initial outreach work with women in several traditional sex work communities and the implementation of a more formalized project design. A shift in the focus of the project activities also took place, and instead of concentrating on sex work places along the highways, smaller villages or "habitats" were included. Developing an approach to reach the RTFSWs who had migrated to Mumbai was also identified as a programmatic concern. The following schematic reflects the program design that emerged during the early part of this phase (Exhibit 5.1).

Exhibit 5.1 *Saksham* design framework

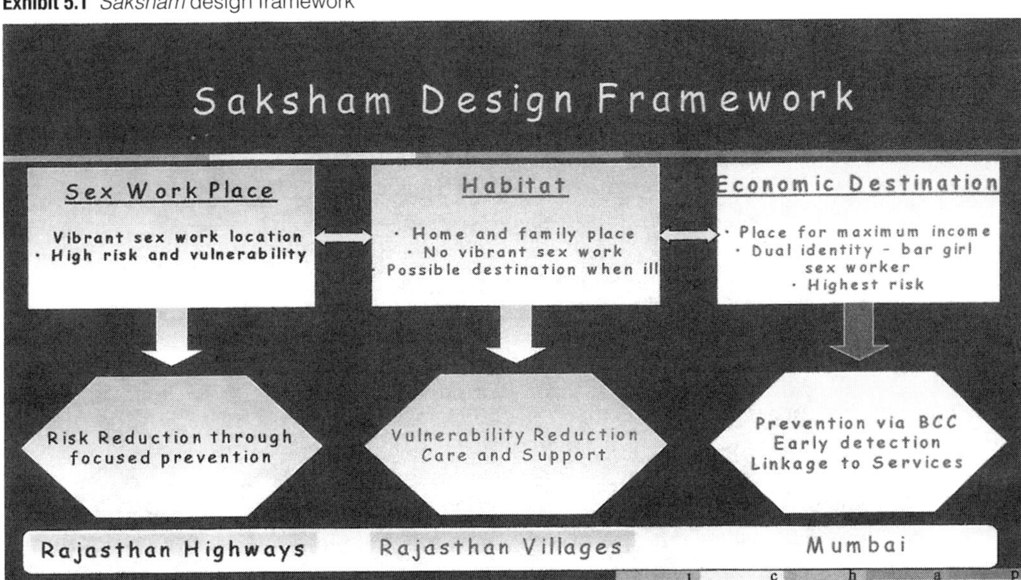

Source: ICHAP Annual Report

In July 2003, project activities were initiated in sex work places in Tonk and Jaipur. The teams consisted of two men from the *Nat* community and two young women from the general population, who were directed by local NGOs that were hired to help facilitate *Saksham*. They began visiting the women in these districts, but no specific mention was made initially of HIV/AIDS. Instead, the focus was on women's health issues. The main goal at this point was to gain the confidence and trust of the women, and the teams established good rapport with the sex workers, the madams, the community men, and the *Nat* leader. Over time, the sex workers became interested in the goals of the project, but continued to express concerns about whether the outreach workers had ulterior motives.[3]

The team continued with general outreach activities, mainly condom demonstrations and STI information sessions, and began to make plans for implementing the baseline behavioral survey. However, they encountered difficulties when trying to formalize the questions with stakeholders, primarily the *Nat* caste leaders. The survey had 150 questions and was based on one that had been administered to sex workers in the Karnataka project. After much discussion, the survey was reduced to 43 questions, with many questions related to the social and economic context of sex work eliminated. *Nat* caste leaders were strongly opposed to the collection of any data related to the "business" side of sex work.

The conduct of the *Nat* community men employed by the project was also becoming problematic. The NGOs were concerned because the men did not always follow the instructions of the NGO supervisors. The young women who were paired with them also experienced difficulties because the men resisted taking part in activities that involved issues of sexuality and the body, which are considered inappropriate topics to discuss with sex workers and women generally. For their part, the community men were equally unhappy with the attitude of the NGOs towards them.

This was a critical point in the project because it challenged our original assumption of the importance of working through community political structures and male leaders to access the women. The situation also drew attention to the limited participation of women in the development of the project. Although they were part of the power struggle, it did not stem from their direct resistance to the project or the wider political structures that dominated the project and the nature of their participation.

ADAPTING THE MODEL TO LOCAL CONDITIONS (JANUARY 2004–OCTOBER 2005)

To resolve this conflict the community men were removed from the NGO teams and placed under the jurisdiction of Akhil Rajasthan Nat Samaj Samiti (ARNSS), a community-based organization established for the *Nat* leaders. The baseline behavioral survey began in July of 2004 in sex work places and "habitats" outside the jurisdiction of ARNSS because the *Nat* leader and the community men were still uncomfortable with many of the questions relating to sexuality and financial concerns.

The first program implementation strategy adopted during this phase addressed both health and socioeconomic issues. ICHAP trained seven to ten doctors from the districts to which the women could be referred for both syndromic and presumptive treatment of sexually transmitted infections (STIs). STI kits were prepared[4] and the doctors used syndromic case management.

The strategy included the introduction of health camps, which provide information and health services to community members over the course of a three- to five-day period. This approach initially created problems because non-sex-working community members felt it was only geared toward sex workers. Given the low attendance of sex workers (10/170) the teams offered the camps to everyone, which helped establish rapport with the community at large. Referral slips were also introduced so that sex workers and clients or lovers could receive care. In addition, health diaries were developed so that

Exhibit 5.2 Total coverage under *Saksham*

Sample number	*District*	*Total number of sex workers*	*Total number of clients*	*Total number of adolescents*	*Other community members*	*Dhabhawalas, barbers, grocers*	*Total number*
1	Jaipur	532	1,432	173 girls 262 boys	727	66	3,192
2	Alwar	578	1,278	537 girls 757 boys	2,933	48	6,131
3	Tonk	557	1,394	337 girls 424 boys	1,810	75	4,597
Total	Three districts	1,667	4,104	1,047 girls 1,443 boys	5,470	189	13,920

women could monitor presumptive treatments, their health status, and condom use.

Outreach workers (ORWs) spent a considerable amount of time in the field, to gather as much information as possible and to demonstrate their commitment to the women. The ORWs' individual sessions with the women (five to ten per day) dealt primarily with HIV education, STIs, reproductive tract infections, general health, hygiene, and contraceptives. Projects were also organized for the retired sex workers as a way for them to earn small amounts of money, such as preparing the client STI kits and making greeting cards for various festivals.

Equally important was the team's participation in community celebrations with the women, including birthdays, marriages, and other important social ceremonies. In doing so they reassured the women that they were not only concerned about HIV/AIDS, but that they cared about them as people. Their social interactions with the women and community members were such that the team members were considered part of the sex workers' "extended family" (Exhibit 5.2).

IMPLEMENTING THE EMPOWERMENT MODEL (NOVEMBER 2005–MARCH 2006)

Central to making the transition from an outreach model to an empowerment paradigm is devolving the role of the NGOs and developing the capacity of the women. Particularly important to this process are the *sahcharis*, which in Hindi translates as "friends" and represents the peer-educator component. There are approximately 25 *sahcharis* per district, for a total of 75 in the three districts. Unlike madams, who often function as peer educators in other peer-education programs, these "friends" are sex workers who are about the same age as other working women. They meet monthly to deal with issues in the different sites, to meet with doctors and beauticians for information sessions, and to share their joys and sorrows with one another.

The women also attended a series of meetings with project coordinators and participants in an urban-based sex worker project in Ahmedabad, Gujurat, which is an instructive example of a project transferring its control to the sex workers. Following these meetings, several *sahcharis* indicated that they wanted to take greater responsibility for their project. With this in mind, the *Saksham* team took steps to help the women get their groups formally registered. As of January 2006, *Saksham Mahila Ekai* in Tonk and *Saksham Mahila Samiti* in Alwar have been registered. Jaipur is not registered yet because of the influence of the *Nat* leaders and the community men who work under their guidance, who are still resistant to certain issues pertaining to *Saksham*.

TRADITIONAL SEX WORK WITHIN KARNATAKA: THE *DEVADASIS*

Approximately 26 percent of female sex workers in Karnataka enter sex work through the *Devadasi* tradition (Blanchard et al. 2005: S141). The *Devadasi* ("female slave/servant of the God") system originated around the sixth century A.D., mainly in south India (Shankar 1990: 42). *Devadasis* were women dedicated through ritual marriage to different deities, after which they became the wives/servants of the Gods and performed various temple duties (Tarachand 1991). These duties included decorating shrines, dancing in important ceremonies, and delivering prayers and food to Gods (Kersenboom 1987; Orr 2000). The women also provided sexual services to male temple attendants, priests, and men who could be regarded as patrons or clients. As "wives" of deities, *Devadasis* were spared the stigmatized status of widowhood, and this was a primary reason for their auspiciousness within Indian society (Marglin 1985).

During social reforms of the nineteenth century, the colonial government introduced legislation that eroded the spiritual role and social position of *Devadasis* (Levine 2003). Campaigns to abolish the practice of dedicating women to temples in present-day Karnataka began around 1910 and spread to other parts of India. The 1982 Karnataka *Devadasi* (Prohibition of) Act, which was amended in 1984, is the most recent legislation designed to regulate the *Devadasi* system in the state (Jordan 1993: 272). This Act prohibits the dedication ceremony of young girls to the deity and criminalizes the activities of those involved in the process, including priests, parents, and agents.

Despite being illegal, the *Devadasi* system still exists in Karnataka and it provides a substantial portion of community income in many small towns and villages throughout northern areas of the state. Between the ages of 6 to 10, young girls are dedicated to a God or Goddess, and following menarche clients for the "first client ceremony," called *hennu madodu*, are sought. In addition to large fees (ranging from INR 1,500/- (U.S. $37) to INR 15,000/- (U.S. $373)), gifts of money, gold, sarees, and other forms of wealth (jewelry, bed sheets), are given to the girls' family. Since this initial wealth and a portion of the *Devadasi*'s future earnings go to the family, there is continued pressure in poor, low-caste families in rural areas to dedicate their daughters.

The advent of HIV/AIDS has engendered significant changes in the women and girls' lives, namely a drop in earnings due to lower client numbers and increased fears of infection. It has also altered components of the *Devadasi* system itself, as multiple first client ceremonies are now common,[5] dedications have been driven underground, and many older *Devadasis* want new dedications to cease. The Belgaum Integrated Rural Development Society (BIRDS), an NGO based in northern Karnataka, has been conducting HIV/AIDS education and prevention with *Devadasis* and other sex workers in the region since 1997. BIRDS has trained a group of AIDS counselors and outreach workers, who have been instrumental in developing and helping support *Devadasi*-run Collective organizations, called *sanghas*. The initial emphasis was on condom distribution and HIV/AIDS awareness; however, with their increased involvement in the ICHAP project, the *sanghas* have moved beyond condom distribution into areas that have programmatic implications, e.g., STI treatment and promotion of HIV voluntary counseling and testing (VCT). The women's participation in the project has also provided valuable experience as they work towards more empowering forms of social organization.

ICHAP IN KARNATAKA

Within India, Karnataka is regarded as one of the six "high-prevalence" states where the HIV/AIDS epidemic has become "generalized," with a sero-prevalence of more than 1 percent of the general population.[6] In 2003 it was estimated that there may be 500,000 HIV-positive persons in Karnataka alone, with the vast majority of cases (85–90 percent) resulting from sexual transmission (*Deccan Herald*, November 28, 2003). Sentinel surveillance in Karnataka has demonstrated that there is higher HIV prevalence in the northern districts and in districts surrounding the capital city of Bangalore, which indicates both a rural and urban distribution

(Karnataka State AIDS Prevention Society 2004).

In order to develop and pilot program models through demonstration projects, ICHAP designed and implemented the Bagalkot District Demonstration Projects (BDP), consisting of the Rural Demonstration Project (RDP) and a Sex Workers Demonstration Project (SWDP). The BDP develops and delivers HIV/AIDS prevention, care, and support services in rural and urban areas of Bagalkot district. The SWDP focuses these sets of interventions among female sex workers, primarily *Devadasis*. ICHAP has fostered a relationship with several *Devadasi* communities throughout northern Karnataka since 2001, when an ethnographic assessment of female sex workers was undertaken in the northern districts of Dharwad, Belgaum, Bijapur, and Bagalkot (see Blanchard et al. 2005; O'Neil et al. 2004).

IMPLEMENTATION PROCESS: THE INITIAL STAGE

The processes surrounding the implementation of the SWDP were profoundly affected by the larger sociopolitical structures within which the project took place, namely ICHAP's concerns regarding the women's control over the project, the influence of BIRDS, and the women's uncertainty about taking over the SWDP through their Collective, Chaitanya AIDS Prevention Mahila Sangha (CAPMS). CAPMS is a sex worker Collective that has been conducting HIV/AIDS education and prevention since 1999. It uses the peer-education model, and each woman is responsible for two *talukas* (subdistricts) and supervises a team of four to twelve peer educators, each of whom in turn works with ten to fifteen sex workers. The peer educators have a number of tasks, including condom distribution, conducting literacy classes, conducting awareness sessions, and making referrals to VCT and STI clinics.

Based on evidence from the ethnographic research that the project would be more effective and empowering if the women implemented it, ICHAP decided to fund the sex worker demonstration project directly through CAPMS. However, BIRDS wanted to retain some control over the direction of the project by continuing to advise the Collective. Supporting direct community participation, ICHAP asked the women to appoint an advisor, and after considerable discussions a new advisor was hired who had no affiliation with BIRDS or ICHAP. BIRDS and their counselors remained involved with the project though, as members of the Project, Steering Committee.

The project began with condom promotion as its primary activity, which the women were comfortable with, because it was a central exercise under BIRDS. It became apparent though that the project needed to expand its outreach because the Collective was limited to areas with a high volume of female sex workers and young girls were not being reached. However, because the Collective inherited its structure from BIRDS, the members were apprehensive about reorganizing their recruitment strategies. These underlying dilemmas were resolved when a mapping exercise was conducted to demonstrate the value of expanding their coverage. The women realized the importance of expansion and that it was only possible with additional peer educators.

Other problems arose when the project attempted to move beyond condom promotion to establish STI treatment services. The Collective was not willing to attend clinics manned by clinicians identified by the project, and so the project asked the Collective to help construct a preferred list of clinicians. The women complied, but the SWDP was not able to move forward with this initiative because the women eventually stopped accessing the preferred list. After much reflection and discussion, a functional literacy program and self-help groups were initiated, which were identified by *Devadasis* as desirable empowerment-oriented initiatives.

THE ISSUE OF EMBEDDING THE PROJECT

Shortly after this challenging first phase, the Rural Demonstration Project (RDP) assumed responsibilities for the SWDP. The sex work staff members expressed concern about embedding their SWDP within the larger RDP. The women were worried about data confidentiality and the difficulties associated with adapting their original organizational structure to a new model and unfamiliar leadership. They were also somewhat mistrustful of ICHAP and feared being dropped by project coordinators or being criticized if they made mistakes along the way.

However, CAPMS's fears of coordinating with the RDP diminished when the two teams began working together on several programmatic activities. The RDP also developed joint STI services with the Collective and began attending cluster meetings as one way to support the efforts put forth by CAPMS. The promotion of self-help groups began in the second and third year of the project. Doctors were identified for STI treatment and those preferred by CAPMS were also trained.

There were many important outcomes of embedding the SWDP within the RDP, including the teams' ability to combine and share resources, management responsibilities, and various capacity-building measures. The teams make each other accountable for project activities and evaluation, and the sex workers are also able to access more "mainstream" services that might otherwise not be available to them if they were being serviced by separate facilities. The mutual support that members of these two programs developed speaks volumes for overall project successes and of the value of integrating complementary programs.

STRATEGIES FOR REDUCING HIV-RELATED RISK AND VULNERABILITY

Five specific strategies were designed to help reduce risk and vulnerability to HIV infection: improving negotiation and decision-making skills for sex work encounters; ensuring access to condoms; working with clients of sex workers; providing training in safe sex, condom use, STI recognition and treatment; and reducing police violence and harassment.

Efforts towards reducing vulnerability were developed through seven separate strategies: providing economic alternatives to sex work; promoting legal reform of prostitution laws and the human rights of sex workers; educating clients and police against violence and harassment of sex workers; improving negotiation and decision-making skills for all non-sex work encounters; promoting the participation and decision-making of sex workers in sex work programs; providing care and support for sick and dying sex workers and their orphaned children; and providing literacy education to sex workers.

In December 2004, the SWDP began developing a more sophisticated outreach plan to reach greater numbers of sex workers and to get a sense of the women's different intervention needs based on client load. Villages having ten or more sex workers were identified, and formats developed to identify sex workers' client volume, based on weekly client numbers.[7] Peer educators identified sex workers with the help of relatives and friends and also educated family members and young girls about the effects of early sex work. Activities such as community meetings, home visits, folk shows, street plays, and sharing experiences of *Devadasi* women, served as a means to sensitize community leaders/members about the system. The folk media performances were perceived by the women as an especially empowering experience. During these events, some of the *Devadasis* spoke on stage, in front of male community leaders and others in attendance, which built their confidence and also helped establish CAPMS as a viable and important institution.

EMPOWERMENT EXAMPLES FROM THE PROJECT

Literacy Classes

To date, twelve literacy schools have been established, but they have achieved limited success. Although a number of women identified reading and writing as skills they would like to acquire, their support of the classes appears to be linked with wanting to adhere to suggestions made by ICHAP rather than being something the women view as useful to reducing their risk or vulnerability. The informal discussion aspect of the classes, which was intended to provide a forum for the women to talk about other issues in their lives, not just HIV prevention, was also unsuccessful because the classes were not of great interest to them.

Self-Help Groups

The SHGs were formed to promote savings among women, discuss micro-finance activities, and to promote a sense of social responsibility. The SWDP has facilitated seventeen such groups since 2003 and each has between twelve and twenty members. The SHG members consist of *Devadasi* women engaged in sex work, including the peer educators, and the peer coordinators. SHG members decide on their agenda, village or town problems, and loan activities, and discussions are held regarding the literacy school, training needs, and *Sangha* development plans. The SHG concept has potential and some groups have served as a forum for exchange of knowledge and skills. However, a practical and applicable skill base needs to be developed, with which to instruct the women about saving money and banking generally.

The Lovers' Workshop

In their relationships with lovers and regular partners, women's ability to enforce condom use is very limited. To address this, the SWDP introduced lovers' workshops, which are participatory gatherings that communicate facts about STI and HIV transmission, while emphasizing the importance of condom usage. Peer educators and a male office assistant were also trained to conduct outreach with lovers. The SWDP has conducted eight workshops with more than 350 lovers attending since January 2005. The workshops have developed the lovers' risk perception, and the men ask questions about the typology of sex work and the risks involved. Some of the lovers also became facilitators of project events. They have been mobilized for STI clinic attendance, have taken part in conducting meetings with lovers, and in some instances have even motivated sex workers for project activities. The project has observed that partner treatment and voluntary visits to voluntary counseling and testing centers (VCTCs) are on the rise. HIV-positive lovers have begun to attend positive support group meetings of sex workers.

DISCUSSION

Sex work focused interventions have been introduced in India as a response to a large sex work industry and a high rate of HIV infection among female sex workers. The cornerstones of such interventions include IEC (information, education, and communication), condom promotion, referrals regarding STIs, and creating enabling environments (Amin 2004: 13; Brahme et al. 2006: 107). However, evidence demonstrates that such individual-level interventions have not been effective and there has been a move to focus on "environmental-structural" interventions, which concentrate on community-level factors and examine sex work within the sociocultural setting in which it takes place (Blanchard et al. 2005: S139; Kerrigan et al. 2006: 120). The demonstration projects described in this chapter were designed with traditional female sex workers in rural Rajasthan and Karnataka in an attempt to address the contextual factors that contribute to HIV/AIDS and the continued marginalization of these women within their communities. Similar to the model implemented in Kolkata, the issues relating to the epidemic were articulated as being the responsibility of the community, versus the burden of the individual, which is a relatively novel approach to HIV prevention (Jana et al. 2004: 407), especially among this unique group of sex workers in India.

Premised on the belief that the intervention would only work if the women were supported in ways that enhanced their empowerment and development as a collective group, the projects described here represent significant achievements towards that goal. However, the problems encountered along the way are also significant, as they help illustrate some of the pragmatic realities involved with designing and implementing HIV prevention projects among this highly marginalized group. These data also highlight the complex dynamics involved with the empowerment approach, which has long been a "buzz word" (Asthana and Oostvogels 1996: 136) in HIV prevention research and policy, and has been revealed here to be an infinitely more complicated approach to develop and implement.

Involving the larger community in the projects was one of the most crucial objectives of the demonstration projects. Reaching out to adolescents, retired sex workers, and older active sex workers reflected an awareness of how embedded traditional sex workers are within their communities, which is unique in India and elsewhere. In Rajasthan, *spandan* (for adolescent girls and boys) and *sparsh* (for retired sex workers) are activities in the "habitat" areas, which provide education for youth and small income-generating projects for older women. In Karnataka, the joint participation of SWDP staff with those involved in the RDP provided an opportunity for the women to share resources and gain valuable skills that they used to extend their service coverage, and to help motivate non-Collective members to become involved in the project.

Encouraging the participation of other community groups helped generate wider participation of the sex workers and it engendered a greater sense of ownership over the project. It also represented an attempt to alleviate the stigma surrounding HIV and sex work through recognizing their value to the project as women who are part of a community, versus women who are members of a "high-risk" group. In doing so, the focus was not on individual women but on their place within the larger context of community stakeholders, such as male leaders, youth, and retired sex workers, all of whom have important economic and social roles in the make-up and organization of the sex trade (Chattopadhyay and McKaig 2004: 166; Jana et al. 2004: 407).

Involving the women's lovers was another particularly valuable component. These men provide *Devadasis* with social support, often act as fathers for their children, and they are integral to the women's sexual health because they typically have the last word with regard to condom use. Since the women's lovers often live nearby and were easily accessible by outreach workers, many became directly involved in workshops, some as program facilitators; which is a unique and important outcome of the intervention. Indeed, although long identified as an essential component of HIV prevention, it has not been adequately addressed in India and elsewhere (Brahme et al. 2006: 111).

Another theme that emerged during the implementation of these projects is the importance of reflexivity based on research evidence in program design. It is a given that field conditions and other developments necessitate programmatic changes to ensure project success and applicability. During phase three of the *Saksham* project in Rajasthan, when new evidence emerged that required adapting the program to local conditions, the organizational structure of the project was altered to establish a stronger and more decentralized field presence. The situation in Karnataka was characterized by a series of challenging situations whereby the Collective members refused to cooperate through the programmatic channels ICHAP had initially developed, citing mistrust of ICHAP, fear of failures, and major hesitation about moving from the trusted BIRDS structure into a more unfamiliar model. These difficulties were effectively addressed when the SWDP joined forces with the RDP and when the women grew to trust the RDP employees with whom they worked.

One of the most instructive outcomes of these projects was the creation of alternative prevention methods to educate and encourage the women, which strayed from standard approaches used with female sex workers, such as written IEC materials, self-help groups, literacy training, and rather formulaic activities like condom demonstrations and education sessions (Amin 2004: 16). In Rajasthan the use of referral slips, health diaries, and locally developed visual aids were effective tools with which to communicate HIV/AIDS prevention messages. They were particularly well received by the women and the outreach workers because they were relatively easy to administer in demanding field situations, but also because they represented collaborative efforts on the part of both the women and the outreach workers in their creation. Other significant activities were the joint visits with the Collective in Ahmedabad, Gujurat, and the attendance of outreach workers and team members at important social functions (e.g., birthday celebrations, marriages, funerals), which signified the team's compassion and genuine concern for the wellbeing of the women and their families. The project activities in Karnataka tended to be more standard than those in Rajasthan, and included self-help groups and literacy training. These approaches were not novel, but the observation that the women's motivations for such programs may have had less to do with their actual interests than their desire to conform to their perceptions of project expectations is an important comment on the implications of importing standard prevention/outreach tools.

Another particularly important finding relates to the issue of partnering with the women and their respective Collectives. *Saksham Mahila Ekai* in Tonk and *Saksham Mahila Samiti* in Alwar have been registered, which represents an important achievement for the Rajasthani women and an opportunity to take greater control over their organizations. The women in Jaipur, however, have not been able to form a registered Collective, in part because of the continuing resistance of the *Nat* community leader and the male functionaries associated with him who remain concerned about perceived threats to their local economies. In Karnataka, the projects dealt directly with the Collectives and provided the leadership to develop them as institutions, which was identified as an influential source of social capital in the empowerment process. Embedding the SWDP within the RDP was another crucial factor which engendered vital partnerships between the groups and helped ensure that the women were able to access many mainstream services that may not have been available to them otherwise.

A final cluster of issues pertain to the particular impact that traditional sex work has on program development. With respect to mobilizing the women, the *Devadasis* were able to mobilize with relative ease, due to their established identity as sex workers and the attendant confidence levels and leadership abilities they have gained through their involvement with BIRDS and ICHAP. However, the situation in Rajasthan was markedly different and the *Nat* women had more difficulty coming together as a united force, which is in part due to the influence of male caste and community leaders and their more disparate organization across sex work places, "habitats," and economic destinations.

The influence of male leaders in the control over and organization of the sex trade also plays a powerful role in traditional sex work communities, especially in the case of the *Nat*. The original premise guiding the intervention in Rajasthan was that the male caste leaders and community members would be the primary conduit to reach the sex workers, and that their support would be essential to a successful project. However, it became clear that the concerns of these male leaders related more to the confidentiality of certain information, mainly the monetary returns garnered from sex work, than about the protection or empowerment of the sex workers in their communities. While the SWDP in Karnataka was less affected by male community members, mainly because of the traditional leadership organization practiced by *Devadasi* women for centuries, it was still important to gain the support of these men to ensure wider community support for the women's activities, especially the development of the Collectives.

The projects in Rajasthan and Karnataka demonstrate the importance of addressing HIV prevention among sex workers as a community-based issue, which is particularly relevant in settings in which sex work has traditionally been the socioeconomic underpinning of communities. This experience underscores the importance of empowerment as a profoundly political process, one which involves recognizing the group dynamics in which sex work occurs, the cultural and gender constraints that can impede women's basic human rights, and the fundamental importance of group action and collective identity (Chattopadhyaya and McKaig 2004: 166; Gooptu 2002: 229).

ACKNOWLEDGMENT

We would like to acknowledge the significant contributions of R.C. Swarankar, Alok Mathur, Priyamvada Singh and Parinita Bhattacharjee to the ICHAP projects and the development of this chapter.

NOTES

1. The women from such communities may be referred to as rural, traditional female sex workers (RTFSW) or traditional female sex workers (TFSW), and both acronyms are used in this document to avoid repetition.
2. The Hindi term for "business" that is used throughout India to refer to sex work.
3. An illustration of the women's uncertainties came in the form of one community's refusal to visit the physicians the team had brought in. A previous NGO took blood samples without their permission and then published the results pertaining to HIV and STIs in local newspapers, and the women were afraid that ICHAP was going to do the same. Consequently, the team decided not to bring doctors to this particular sex work place unless they requested us to do so.
4. These contain condoms, a referral slip, illustrations of symptoms of various infections, and a list of physicians in the district.
5. Which place young girls (aged 12–16) at risk of infection, because the first client ceremony is conducted without condoms, often with men who are significantly older than the girls.
6. The others being Maharashtra, Tamil Nadu, Andhra Pradesh, Manipur, and Nagaland, three of which border Karnataka.
7. High volume—more than 10 clients a week; medium volume—5 to 9 clients a week; low volume—less than 4 clients a week.

REFERENCES AND FURTHER READING

Amin, Avni. *Risk, Morality, and Blame: A Critical Analysis of Government and U.S. Donor Responses to HIV Infections Among Sex Workers in India.* Takoma Park, MD: Center for Health and Gender Equity (CHANGE), 2004.

Asthana, Sheena, and Robert Oostvogels. "Community participation in HIV prevention: problems and prospects for community-based strategies among female sex workers in Madras." *Social Science and Medicine* 43(2) (1996): 133–148.

AVERT.ORG. "HIV and AIDS in India." From http://www.avert.org/aidsindia.htm, 2006.

Bhave, Geeta, Christina Lindan, Esther Hudes, Seema Desai, Usha Wagle, Shrivam Tripathi, and Jeffrey Mandel (1995). "Impact of an intervention on HIV, sexually transmitted diseases, and condom use among sex workers in Bombay, India." *AIDS* 9 (Supplement 1) (1995): S21–S30.

Blanchard, James, John O'Neil, B.M. Ramesh, Parinita Bhattacharjee, Treena Orchard, and Stephen Moses. "Understanding the social and cultural contexts of female sex workers in Karnataka, India: implications for prevention of HIV infection." *Journal of Infectious Diseases* 191 (Supplement 1) (2005): S139–146.

Brahme, Rakhika, Shruti Mehta, Seema Sahay, Neelam Joglekar, Manisha Ghate, Smita Joshi, Raman Gangakhedkar, Arun Risbud, Robert Bollinger, and Sanjay Mehendale. "Correlates and trend of HIV prevalence among female sex workers attending sexually transmitted disease clinics in Pune, India (1993–2002)." *Journal of Acquired Immune Deficiency Syndrome* 41(1) (2006): 107–113.

Chattopadhyay, Amit, and Rosemary McKaig. "Social development of commercial sex workers in India: an essential step in HIV/AIDS prevention." *AIDS Patient Care and STDS* 18(3) (2004): 159–168.

Deccan Herald (November 28, 2003).

Gooptu, Nandini. "Sex workers in Calcutta and the dynamics of collective action: political activism, community identity, and group behaviour." In *Group Behaviour and Development: Is the Market Destroying Cooperation?* edited by J. Heyer, F. Stewart, and R. Thorp. Oxford: Oxford University Press, 2002.

Jana, S., Basu, I., Rotherham-Borus, M.J., and Newman, P.A. "The Sonagachi Project: A sustainable community intervention program." *AIDS Educ Prev.* 16(5) (2004): 405–414.

Jordan, Kay. "Devadasi reform: driving the priestesses or the prostitutes out of Hindu temples?" In *Religion and Law in Independent India*, edited by R. Baird. New Delhi: Manohar Publishers and Distributors, 1993.

Karnataka State AIDS Prevention Society (KSAPS), Government of Karnataka, and India–Canada Collaborative HIV/AIDS Project (ICHAP). "Karnataka HIV Status Reports: Report on HIV Sentinel Surveillance 2004." Bangalore: KSAPS and ICHAP, 2004.

Kerrigan, D., Moreno, L., Rosario, S., Gomez, B., Jerez, H., Barrington, C., Weiss, E., and Sweat, M. "Environmental–structural interventions to reduce HIV/STI risk among female sex workers in the Dominican Republic." *Am J Public Health* 96(1) (2006): 120–125.

Kersenboom, Saskia. *Nityasumangali: Devadasi Tradition in South Asia*, New Delhi: Motilal Banarsidass Publishers, 1987.

Levine, Philippa. *Prostitution, Race and Politics: Policing Venereal Disease in the British Empire.* London: Routledge, 2003.

Mane, Purnima, and Peter Aggleton. "Gender and HIV/AIDS: what do men have to do with it?" *Current Sociology* 49(6) (2001): 23–37.

Marglin, Frederique Apffel. *Wives of the God-King. The Rituals of the Devadasis of Puri.* New Delhi: Oxford University Press, 1985.

NACO. *Monthly Updates on AIDS*, July, 31 2005.

Nagelkerke, N.J., P. Jha, and S.J. de Vlas. "Modelling the HIV epidemics in India and Botswana: the impact of interventions to prevent transmission." *Bull World Health Organ* 80 (2002): 89–96.

O'Neil, John, Treena Orchard, R.C. Swarankar, James Blanchard, Kaveri Gurav, and Stephen Moses. "Dhandha, dharma, and disease: traditional sex work and HIV/AIDS in rural India." *Social Science and Medicine* 59 (2004): 851–860.

Orr, Leslie. *Donors, Devotees, and Daughters of God. Temple Women in Medieval Tamilnadu.* New York: Oxford University Press, 2000.

Population Division of the Department of Economic and Social Affairs of the United Nations Secretariat. "World population prospects: the 2002 revision," *Highlights*, New York, February 2003, 78–90.

Rao, Asha, Moni Nag, Mishra Kingshuk, and Arati Dey. "Sexual behaviour pattern of truck drivers and their helpers in relation to female sex workers." *Indian Journal of Social Work* 55(4) (1994): 603–615.

Shankar, Jogan. *Devadasi Cult: A Sociological Analysis.* New Delhi: Ashish Publishing House, 1990.

Sleightholme, Carolyn and Indrani Sinha. *Guilty Without Trial. Women in the Sex Trade in Calcutta.* Calcutta: Stree, 1996.

Swarankar, R.C. "A short note on *nat*: a nomadic community of Eastern Rajasthan." *Man and Life* 25(3–4) (1999a): 215–221.

Swarankar, R.C. "Tradition, tourism and AIDS in Rajasthan." In *Rajasthan*, edited by M.K. Bhasin and R. Kamla. New Delhi: Enterprises, 1999b.

Swarankar, R.C. "From nomadism to prostitution (an ethnographic study of *Nat* community in Rajasthan)." In *The Science of Man in the Service of Man*, edited by M.K. Bhasin and S.L. Malik. New Delhi: University of New Delhi, Department of Anthropology, 2001.

Tarachand, K.C. *Devadasi Custom. Rural Social Structure and Flesh Markets.* New Delhi: Reliance Publishing House, 1991.

UNAIDS. *2006 Report on the Global HIV Epidemic.* Geneva: UNAIDS, 2006.

Zenilman, Jonathan. "Behavioral interventions—rationale, measurement, and effectiveness." *Infect. Dis. Clin. N. Am* 19(2) (2005): 541–562.

CHAPTER 6

The Challenges of HIV/AIDS in Ukraine

Olena Hankivsky[1]

ABSTRACT

This chapter summarizes the history and currently severe HIV/AIDS epidemic in Ukraine. It discusses key issues and challenges regarding reducing the impact of HIV for vulnerable Ukrainian groups, particularly women, by developing gender-sensitive approaches. The Ukrainian HIV epidemic continues to disproportionately affect those who are marginalized, but recently has spread among the heterosexual, non-drug-using population, and those not involved in commercial work, particularly teenage girls. A sustained focus on increasing the knowledge and capacity of policymakers and government officials about HIV/AIDS and strengthening inter-sectoral response is urgently needed.

OVERVIEW

Ukraine, the second largest country in Europe, is struggling with the explosive public health care challenge of HIV/AIDS. It is the worst affected country in Europe and an epicenter of one of the fastest-growing HIV/AIDS epidemics in the world (UNAIDS/WHO 2005). Although the epidemic began largely with injection drug users, it is now spreading to the general population, and this has resulted in a substantial increase in HIV among women and children born to them. In response, the government of Ukraine has developed what can be considered as generally sound legislation and policies. However, these are not always effectively implemented or adequately resourced. Moreover, the lack of awareness and correct information about the disease, as well as continuing stigma and discrimination against those who are diagnosed with HIV/AIDS, have impeded prevention and intervention efforts. Given the current situation, Human Rights Watch has concluded that "Ukraine stands at an important crossroads in its effort to contain the deadly HIV/AIDS epidemic" (2006: 3).

The purpose of this chapter is to provide a brief overview of the history and current HIV/AIDS situation in Ukraine, including key legislation and policies, recent initiatives by non-governmental organizations, public/charitable organizations and international donors to deal with this pressing public health challenge. The chapter will also analyze key issues and challenges for moving forward on the fight against HIV/AIDs, including the need for targeted prevention and intervention efforts for vulnerable groups in Ukrainian society, especially the need for developing gender-sensitive approaches that respond to the unique and growing needs of HIV-positive women—an increasingly growing segment of the affected population.

OVERVIEW OF THE SITUATION

Prior to 1987, HIV/AIDS was virtually nonexistent in Ukraine. However, by 1994, the average rate of infection increased by 33 percent and by 1997 Ukraine had over 25,000 reported cases—over 50 percent of the overall total of all Eastern Europe (Dehne et al. 1999). Between 2000 and 2004, the number of registered cases in the country doubled (International HIV/AIDS Alliance in Ukraine and World Bank 2006). Currently there are 100,403 HIV cases registered in Ukraine (Transatlantic Partners Against AIDS 2006). In reality, however, these numbers may be gross underestimates because infection rates among marginalized and vulnerable populations are difficult to ascertain. Similarly, Amon notes, "official statistics in Ukraine simply do not reflect the current status of the epidemic, and more importantly, the likely future course of the epidemic (2003: 263). According to UNAIDS' Global Report published in 2004, the number of people living with HIV/AIDS exceeded 400,000, or just over 1 percent of the population between the ages of 15 and 49. In 2006, Human Rights Watch reported that this number had increased to as many as 419,000 Ukrainians—or 1.7 percent of the same population group. The worst-hit regions are Donetsk, Dnipopetrovsk, Odessa, and Mykolayiv located in the southeast and south of Ukraine. Growing infections are being recorded in the capital of Kyiv. The average death rate among AIDS patients is 50 percent (Sherbinska 2005).

The epidemic can be seen as driven by high levels of migration and transnational sex, widespread stigma and discrimination, inadequate health and other services, rising rates of tuberculosis, sexually transmitted infections, substance abuse, and a general lack of information about risky behaviors (USAID 2004) Early rapid transmission through the injecting drug use (IDU) community was caused by the distrust of the health care sector, including the fact that disclosure to a health professional requires "obligatory registration and confinement for treatment, possible job loss, loss of one's driving license, and criminal prosecution" (Amon 2003: 263). The epidemic continues to disproportionately affect those who are marginalized, are at higher risk of police violence and those who experience abusive treatment in the health care system (Human Rights Watch 2006).

Although initially contained within the IDU population, the epidemic is now spreading through heterosexual transmission, including sex work, which currently accounts for nearly one third of new cases. As Trifonov, Jackson, and Bega argue, "the HIV/AIDS epidemic is no longer confined to specific marginalized communities; it has of late spread increasingly among the heterosexual, non-drug using population, not involved in commercial work, particularly among teenage girls" (2005: 1). To illustrate, between 1999 and 2003 only 14 percent of new cases were caused by heterosexual transmission. In the first six months of 2006, the figure rose to over 35 percent (Ministry of Health Ukraine et al. 2006). Moreover, according to 2005 surveillance, 8 percent of female sex workers in Kyiv were found to be HIV infected; 25–29 percent were infected in the cities of Poltava, Odessa, Lutsk, and Donetsk, and 32 percent in the city of Mykolayiv (Ministry of Health Ukraine et al. 2006). It is also thought that Ukraine has the highest number of HIV-positive youths in the Eastern Europe/Central Asia Region (http://www.ifrc.org/docs/news/05/05051701/). Significantly, two-thirds of new cases are among young people between the ages of 20 and 24 (International HIV/AIDS Alliance in Ukraine and World Bank 2006).

The pandemic is increasingly gendered. In 2003, 67 percent of all new cases infected through heterosexual sex were women (UNDP 2003: 8). By the end of 2005, it was estimated that there were 200,000 HIV-positive women in Ukraine (http://www.globalhealthreporting.org/countries/ukraine). The increase in official rates is at least partly due to changes in HIV testing practices, especially HIV testing among pregnant women that was introduced in 1996 as part of preventative mother–child transmission programs. According to the Ministry of Health, HIV prevalence among pregnant women is among the highest in Europe: 0.31 percent in 2006 (Ministry of Health Ukraine et al. 2006). Currently, over 40 percent of those infected with HIV/AIDS in Ukraine are women in their prime reproductive years and this number is expected to rise (EuroHIV 2006). The World Bank has stated that "AIDS may become the leading cause of deaths in females aged 15–49 by 2010" (2006: 12).

The future outlook for this epidemic is quite bleak. The International HIV/AIDS Alliance in Ukraine and the World Bank suggest that the problem is worsening and that, by 2014, there will be between 478,500 and 820,400 HIV-positive persons in Ukraine (2006: viii). Moreover, by 2014, they estimate that the total annual AIDS medical care expenditure will be between 41 and 62 million hryvnia (UAH), direct budget revenue losses will be in the range of 263–418 million UAH, and budget expenditures associated with this epidemic will be between 139 and 255 million UAH (1 U.S.$ = 5 UAH) (International HIV/AIDS Alliance in Ukraine and World Bank 2006). These costs will undoubtedly "divert resources from education, science and social welfare, not to mention other health care priorities" (Transatlantic Partners Against AIDS 2005: 8). In sum, the HIV/AIDS pandemic threatens the future of Ukraine's national security, economic development, health and social welfare of its citizens, especially those who are vulnerable and marginalized.

GOVERNMENT RESPONSES

The Ukrainian government has developed a multi-pronged approach to responding to this health epidemic. The Ukrainian AIDS Prevention and Response Center (established in 1989) coordinates the activities of all the Oblast AIDS Prevention Centers, including the development of HIV/AIDS guidelines and protocols for the Centers. Currently, thirty-five regional AIDS centers coordinate a variety of preventative, diagnostic, medical, and counseling services under the supervision of the Ukrainian AIDS Center. The AIDS Center also conducts important epidemiological surveillance of the pandemic. Its clinical base is located at the Lavra AIDS Clinic at the Gromashevsky Research Institute of Epidemiology and Infectious Diseases in Kyiv. The Ministry of Health, through the National AIDS Prevention Center, oversees policy, programming and management and is involved in prevention, care, and treatment services throughout the country's regional Centers. Presently, there are approximately 487 HIV testing sites in Ukraine.

Two years after the AIDS Prevention Center was established, a law "On Prevention of Acquired Immune Deficiency Syndrome (AIDS) and Social Protection of the Population" was passed in 1991. In 1992 a National AIDS Committee was established and, in 1999, this body was replaced by the National AIDS Control Coordinating Council, which mandated that all regions in Ukraine establish HIV prevention programs. In May 2005 a new National Coordination Council on HIV AIDS (NCC) was established by the Cabinet of Ministers. Its objectives are to "coordinate the activities of ministries, other central and local executives authorities and relevant international and public organizations to ensure effective and uniform policy and consolidated disbursement, implementation and monitoring of system for HIV/AIDS activities" (WHO 2005). The Council oversees health education policy development and the coordination of multisectoral plans-monitoring and implementation of control strategies. The Ministry of Health also assists in these efforts by providing management and coordination functions.

In November 2000, the Ukrainian government recognized HIV/AIDS as an epidemic and national emergency. A number of Presidential Decrees—*Urgent Measures to Prevent HIV/AIDS* (November 1, 2000), *Declaring 2002 the Year to Fight AIDS in Ukraine* (June 22, 2001) and *Additional Measures to Strengthen the Response to HIV/AIDS* (August 28, 2001)—were intended to increase public education, improve a variety of preventative initiatives and medical treatment of affected persons, and encourage NGOs and other organizations to continue their work in the area of prevention. In 2001, the Governmental Commission on Response to HIV/AIDS was established. The present Commission is responsible for the coordination and political management of the nation's response to the epidemic.

In addition, two international framework agreements—the *UN International Guiding*

Principles on HIV/AIDS and Human Rights, and the *UN Declaration of Commitment on HIV/AIDS*, Ukraine's *National Law on AIDS*, last amended in 2001—commit the government of Ukraine to the following: continuous epidemiological monitoring of HIV infection in Ukraine, free access of PLWHA (People Living with HIV/AIDS) to all necessary health care, including antiretroviral medicines and individual means of prevention; free access to voluntary and anonymous testing and pre- and post-test counseling on HIV/AIDS; confidentiality of HIV test results; public education on HIV/AIDS, including mass media awareness campaigns and the inclusion of HIV/AIDS in secondary, high-school, college and university curricula; public programs on prevention of sexual transmission of HIV; and prevention of HIV transmission among injection drug users, including the establishment of needle and syringe exchange programs (Trifonov et al. 2005). HIV/AIDS affected persons are also protected under the Ukrainian Labour Code, which makes it illegal for employment to be contingent on HIV testing.

To date, the government has put forward five different national AIDS plans. The first program (1992–1994) focused on the safety of the nation's blood supply. The second (1995–1997) continued to focus on blood safety but expanded to include research and the establishment of treatment and prevention networks. The third (1999–2000) dissolved the National AIDS Prevention Committee. These early programs "failed to provide for activities, except repressive ones, to prevent HIV transmission among the very groups where the epidemic was most serious: injecting drug users, sex workers and others." (UNDP 2003: 15). In 2001, a fourth national plan for combating HIV/AIDS (*HIV/AIDS Control Program for Ukraine for 2001–2003*) was introduced, targeting information/education programs for children and teenagers, educational medial campaigns, reducing the risk among specific groups, donor look safety, treatment and care, and improved prevention and monitoring (UNDP 2003). The latest plan, *National Program for Preventive Measures against HIV Infection, Support and Treatment of People Living with HIV/AIDS for 2004–2008*, has been critiqued because 1) it was developed by a variety of implementing sectors with no needs assessment, budget analysis, or measurement outcomes, and 2) it lacks an implementation plan with appropriate government agency roles and responsibilities (Trifonov et al. 2005).

Confronted by the growing crisis, President Viktor Yuschenko has called on all key stakeholders—government, NGOs, and the business community—to "focus attention and resources on the country's surging epidemic" (Houmenyuk et al. 2006: 5). For his part, in November 2005, Yuschenko announced a presidential decree that established a reference laboratory at the National AIDS Center. In March 2006, the President signed a bill to improve the fight against tuberculosis (TB), a significant development because TB is the most common infection suffered by HIV-positive persons. In December of 2006, the Ukrainian government adopted a resolution to establish a national tuberculosis and HIV/AIDS coordinating council consisting of representatives from the Ministry of Health, the Ministry of the Interior, and the National Security Service. The resolution requires regional administrators to encourage the establishment of local councils. The government also intends to develop a three-year TB and HIV prevention program that will reach approximately 50,000 people with medical assistance and treatment.

INTERNATIONAL INITIATIVES

As of January 2006, international support of Ukraine's fight against HIV/AIDS exceeded U.S.$100 million (Human Rights Watch 2006). It is important to note that most of the funding for HIV/AIDS initiatives comes from foreign governments and international organizations and, according to UNDP, "funds from international donors make a significant contribution to Ukraine's HIV/AIDS efforts" (2003: 16). Several international donors, however, are important to highlight such as the Global Fund to Fight AIDS, World Bank, United States Agency for International Development (USAID), the Joint United Nations Programme on HIV/AIDS (UNAIDS), the United Nations Children's Fund (UNICEF), British Council, International HIV/AIDS Alliance and the International Renaissance Fund, United Kingdom's Department for International Development (DFID), Swedish International Development Agency (SIDA), and Dutch Development Agency (MATRA).

A small number of examples include the 2000 EC–USAID HIV/AIDS Prevention and Awareness Programme for Ukraine that was aimed at developing a coordinated and systematic strategy for HIV prevention involving key stakeholders from the government and NGO sectors. Also worth noting is the program supported by UNICEF, "Prevention of HIV Transmission from Mother to Child for 2001–2003," which assisted the government in developing a national system to monitor HIV transmission from HIV-positive mothers to their children. An evaluation in 2003 found that programme reduced transmission from 27 percent in 2000 to 10 percent in 2004. Ukraine's preventing mother-to-child transmission (PMTCT) response is now recognized as a best practice model in the region and the original programme been renewed for the period of 2004–2010 (http://www.unicef.org/ukraine/activities_4942.html).

Moreover, in 2002, the Global Fund to Fight AIDS, Tuberculosis and Malaria (GFATM) committed close to $90 million over five years to assist in HIV control efforts, including ARV (antiretroviral) drugs for persons living with HIV/AIDS. In January 2004, the fund suspended its grant agreement and one month later appointed the International HIV/AIDS Alliance (Alliance) situated in Kyiv the recipient and steward of the Global Fund activities. On March 15, 2004, the Global Fund entered into an agreement with the Alliance under which the Alliance agreed to provide stewardship and management services in regard to the sum of activities formerly commenced under earlier grant agreements which are now suspended. These arrangements were extended to the end of September 2005. This source of funding has been invaluable; between April 2004 and December 2005 2,600 people began antiretrovirals under this program (Human Rights Watch 2006). Ukraine was invited to apply for continued funding to this program in the spring of 2005 and, through a renewed partnership between government, international donor agencies and NGOs, Ukraine's National Coordination Council was created, with a mandate that is focused on treatment, care, and prevention.

Also in 2002, the Academy for Educational Development, with funding provided by the United States Department of Labor, established SMARTWork/Ukraine, focused on workplace strategies including training and workshops for developing effective HIV/AIDS programs and policies. The program has also produced country profiles and needs assessments, and provided legislative technical assistance to the government (http://www.smartwork.org/programs/ua.shtml). In 2003, using a $60 million loan from the World Bank (with U.S.$17 million national match from Ukraine), the government also initiated a comprehensive HIV-transmission prevention and support program dedicated to harm reduction programs, awareness activities, improving medical facilities, and medicine. This program was suspended in April 2006 because of the Ukrainian government's "failure to launch the program and distribute funds." Indeed, the government had spent only 2 percent of the allocated funds which were intended for medicines, training for health care workers, and other prevention measures targeted high-risk groups including injection drug users, commercial sex workers, and prison inmates. In May 2006, the Ukrainian Ministry of Health agreed to meet all the World Bank requirements for the reinstatement of funds, including the establishment of a working group between the two bodies. In November 2006, the World Bank formally announced that it will reinstate its project in Ukraine and the resumed funding will go toward medical services, medications, equipment, diagnostic systems, and education programs.

Since 2004 the Regional Care Knowledge Hub for the care and treatment of HIV and AIDS in Eurasia has been working with the government of Ukraine to develop and implement Ukraine's national antiretroviral therapies (ART) plan. This has included training care providers in the management of ART and creating appropriate curricula and improving training capacity. In this same year, the United States Agency for International Development launched a U.S.$8.2 million project—SUNRISE. SUNRISE is a project to scale up and strengthen prevention work with communities most vulnerable to HIV/AIDS in Ukraine implemented by Alliance. On January 28, 2005 UNAIDS announced, with the support of the United Kingdom Department for International Development (DfID), an initiative to assist the government of Ukraine in achieving "The Three Ones: Principles for the coordination of national AIDS responses." This model entails: 1) an agreed HIV/AIDS Action Framework that provides the basis for coordinating the work of all partners; 2) a National AIDS Coordinating Authority, with a broad-based multi-sectoral mandate; and 3) a Country-Level Monitoring and Evaluation System. In December 2006, Canada announced financial support for Ukraine as part of its program to fund civil society organizations and governments to implement country strategies in key areas such as HIV/AIDS. Because Canada recognizes that Ukraine is one of the countries most affected by this disease, it has pledged C$3 million to the Open Society Institute to train and develop local organization capacity in harm reduction measures.

NON-GOVERNMENTAL ORGANIZATIONS

Over 150 NGOs are involved in prevention activities in Ukraine. Their work includes pre- and post-test counseling, HIV-related education, public campaigns, rehabilitation of HIV/AIDS affected persons and their families, self-help groups, home care, health promotion, and legal advice. The largest is the All-Ukrainian Network of People Living with HIV/AIDS, which provides support and care for people living with HIV and undertakes advocacy campaigns to change policy and bring about best practices. In August 2006, at the 16th International AIDS Conference, the Network was awarded the Red Ribbon Award for its outstanding contribution of the frontline responses to HIV and AIDS, in particular for addressing stigma and discrimination. Other noteworthy organizations include Transatlantic Partners Against AIDS, AIDS Foundation East West, International Renaissance Foundation, Substance Abuse and AIDS Prevention Foundation, and Ukrainian Harm Reduction Association. Without doubt, NGOs have filled an important role in terms of government lobbying, and information dissemination to the international press (DeBell 2004). They have also filled gaps in education (e.g., training health professionals), prevention and intervention and especially in terms of targeting marginalized populations. The growing access these populations have to prevention and care services is largely being achieved through the development of the nongovernmental sector stimulated by the process of transition (International HIV/AIDS Alliance 2006b). Lekhan et al. similarly argue, "In practice, some of the most effective measures, albeit on a small scale in relation to the scale of the epidemic, have been undertaken by the nongovernmental sectors" (2004: 64).

KEY ISSUES

The involvement of all sectors and key stakeholders has been invaluable in terms of developing responses to HIV/AIDS in Ukraine. However, at all levels, substantial challenges remain for there to be an effective national response; indeed, the complex dimensions of this pandemic—political, economic, and sociocultural—are not well understood and have not been adequately addressed. Moreover, inadequate attention has been paid to the most at-risk groups, including new emergent vulnerable groups, such as women in the country's HIV/AIDS policies, programs, and services.

Legislation and Political Issues

First, there are serious challenges with Ukraine's HIV/related legislation. The

Transatlantic Partners Against AIDS has observed that government legislation is "a) inadequately implemented and poorly enforced; b) frequently ignored by certain government agencies and public-funded institutions (e.g., law enforcement, medical facilities, etc.); c) not enabled by officially approved ministerial guidelines and instructions; or d) significantly underfunded" (2005: 3). Indeed, the lack of political support and implementation issues are of paramount importance. For example, according to the Human Rights Watch, Ukraine's success in combating HIV/AIDS depends on the following actions:

> Ukrainian political leaders must speak out strongly in favour of HIV prevention, care and treatment services for drug users and take urgent steps to hold accountable those responsible for committing abuses. They must also implement the broad protections already in Ukrainian law and policy, and thus give meaning to the range of human rights protections for people living with and at high risk of HIV/AIDS and to which Ukraine has committed itself on paper. (Human Rights Watch 2006: 6)

Another serious issue is the lack of funding dedicated to HIV/AIDS. In 2005, total funding for the National HIV/AIDS Program from public and donor sources was approximately U.S.$40 million, far below the actual need. The WHO has estimated that the funding gap for treatment in 2005 is at least U.S.$214 million (WHO 2005, cited in Trifanov et al. 2005: 1). In 2006 the number increased to close to U.S.$59 million; however, only U.S.$11.5 million comes from the state budget (WHO 2005). Not surprisingly, "Ukraine is struggling to meet growing costs and demand for HIV/AIDS prevention and treatment" (Houmenyuk et al. 2006: 6).

Arguably those in positions of power do not appreciate fully the social and economic impact of the disease, seeing it rather as a medical problem confined to a particular population. Undoubtedly, HIV prevention measures among injecting drug users, while in existence, need to be significantly scaled up to reach sufficient numbers of drug users with quality prevention and care services (International HIV/AIDS Alliance 2006a). In the words of Andrij Klepikov, Executive of the International HIV/AIDS Alliance in Ukraine, "We have no alternative but to halt the epidemic by introducing prevention measures, first of all among the most vulnerable populations" (http://www.aidsalliance.org/sw43956.asp). At the same time, however, there should also be more forward thinking in terms of targeting newly affected populations and developing more comprehensive and effective health promoting policies.

In addition, there is little coordination between different levels of government, non-government organizations and the private sector. This is evidenced by a number of recent observations. First, according to the All-Ukrainian Network of People Living with HIV/AIDS the key issue in overcoming the HIV epidemic is "the effective partnership between the community of people living with HIV, national NGOs, the government, international donor institutions, and technical assistance foundation" (Borushek 2006). In December 2006, the Council of Europe's Human Rights Commissioner Thomas Hammarberg advised the government of Ukraine to increase its cooperation with NGOs in its attempts to stem the spread of HIV/AIDS as well as increasing its services to and protection of HIV-infected people (http://www.ukraine-observer.com/). However, despite their invaluable role, the work of NGOs is largely disregarded by the Ministry of Health (DeBell 2004). National NGOs are seriously underfunded and rely on international donors rather than the Ukrainian government for financial support. Moreover, they are not fully involved or integrated into policy decision-making processes. Finally, the epidemic cannot be halted without the active role of the corporate sector. Any coordinated effort requires the business community to work with government and NGOs and invest in workplace education, policies, and prevention programs (Houmenyuk et al. 2006).

Health Care System

Although the tradition of public health is firmly rooted within the health care system, the system itself requires transformation and reform to meet the changing health needs of its population, especially in terms of preventable diseases such as HIV/AIDS. For example, the country does not have a strong concept of health promotion at either the national or regional levels. Furthermore, there is little central government policy focused on the key health risk behaviours that are responsible for HIV/AIDS transmission and related communicable disease infection (DeBell 2004). Consequently, health promotion efforts have in fact failed to reach high-risk populations such as injecting drug users, commercial sex workers, homosexual men, and prisoners, let alone the more general population (Malinowska-Sempruch et al. 2003; Frost and Tchertkov 2002).

There is also a shortage of specialists and specialized treatment and care programs, including psychological care and counseling for affected populations. In addition, there are no comprehensive or widely accessible networks of treatment and care facilities (Transatlantic Partners Against AIDS 2005). This is especially true for the most vulnerable groups who often have limited or no access to appropriate services. The situation is further complicated by the high prevalence of tuberculosis and a variety of sexually transmitted infections, whose treatment is not systematically linked to HIV/AIDS interventions. High-risk groups, including IDUs (injection drug users), have limited access to prevention services such as harm reduction centers, needle exchange programs, or substitution therapy. Only 10 percent of drug users in Ukraine are covered by harm reduction programs (Balakireva et al. 2003). This appears to be changing; in 2006 the government provided U.S.$1.7 million to the Ministry of Family, Youth and Sport for prevention services for IDUs. Moreover, methadone programs are now underway.

Further, there is limited access within the system to appropriate medicines, including ART treatment. Procurement of ARTs still depends heavily on international donor financial support. In addition, the government of Ukraine has been criticized for overpaying for ARTs due to non-transparency of tenders. The availability and costs of ARTs services aside, "capacity building of health care professionals and institutions is imperative" (Shabarovska et al. 2006) so that the country's national plans and HIV/AIDS treatment and care are effectively implemented. Approximately 7 percent of the infected population is receiving antiretroviral therapy (UNAIDS and WHO 2006). This is in large part due to the prohibitive cost of such therapy which is "beyond both the public purse and almost all private incomes" (Neil et al. 2005: 336). An exception to this general pattern is the treatment of HIV-infected pregnant women, 91.3 percent of whom received antiretroviral prophylaxis during pregnancy and delivery in 2002 (DeBell and Carter 2005: 218). Also worth noting is that there is very little palliative care available in the country. According to Lekhan et al. "the hospice movement in Ukraine is still in its infancy, with only very few meeting the considerable need for palliative care, which is growing rapidly with the spread of AIDS" (2004: 81).

Surveillance of the disease is extremely poor, undermining population targeting and the development of effective prevention and intervention strategies. Accurate epidemiological data has been difficult to obtain until recently, mainly because 1) the disease has been under-researched, and 2) there is little effective communication between university departments, scientific institutes, and government bodies (DeBell 2004). Appropriate monitoring is necessary to support evidence-based policy decision-making and the requirements of donors who are important financiers of the HIV/AIDS response. The *Ukraine National Health Accounts HIV/AIDS Subanalysis 2003–2004* is the country's first attempt to systematically track HIV/AIDS financial flows. Despite some progression on this front, Ukrainian decision-makers report needs more data on the epidemic and more data on the effectiveness of prevention programs and other response activities (UNDP 2005). This is especially important for those officials who have the power to shape and influence the country's HIV/AIDS related legislation and policy.

Another formidable challenge in dealing with HIV/AIDS in Ukraine is the low awareness of the disease and its risks, including correct knowledge about prevention, transmission, disease trajectory, and treatment (DeBell and Carter 2005). A major factor contributing to this situation is the lack of information reaching the general public. While DeBell and Carter have argued that "Ukraine has no public health information service, no sexual health education in schools, and no national information dissemination strategy for HIV/AIDS" (2005: 216), in reality educational training is undertaken by social services for youth in the school system. However, most public education efforts remain concentrated on blood safety measures, surveillance, and treatment, with little attention given to focused prevention activities. Education media is typically paid for by international donors and NGOs and the government has been criticized for not doing enough to support media campaign initiatives. The almost complete lack of investment in prevention activities targeting the vulnerable populations is also widely criticized (International HIV/AIDS Alliance 2006a).

To illustrate: in 2004, the Ukrainian government reported that only 14 percent of young people between the ages of 15 and 25 had a comprehensive understanding of HIV/AIDS (World Bank 2005). Many continue to engage in high-risk behaviors; only 69 percent reported using condoms with non-regular partners (Ukraine Government's UNGASS Report 2006). Surveyed human resource managers in the private sector also demonstrate a clear lack of understanding when it comes to the threat of HIV/AIDS: 48 percent incorrectly believe that it may be possible to contract HIV when someone coughs or sneezes, 70 percent believe that they may be at risk if their co-workers are HIV positive, and 74 percent think there may be a risk of infection from eating in a cafeteria where an HIV-positive individual works (Houmenyuk et al. 2006: 10). Even those charged with policy in this area erroneously believe that HIV infection through homosexual relations is more prevalent than through vertical transmission. According to a recent poll with public servants, "building up or strengthening of information needs of decision makers still remains very relevant, especially with regards to the HIV/AIDS situation and epidemic activities" (UNDP 2005). This includes contextualizing the pandemic and confronting the stigma and discrimination that undermine effective prevention and intervention.

The Socioeconomic Context of HIV/AIDS

Those affected with HIV/AIDS are often living in poverty, with already deteriorating health status. For example, the estimated average earnings of affected persons is U.S.$4,650 (World Bank, cited in DeBell and Carter 2005). Since its independence in 1991, Ukraine has undergone unprecedented political and socioeconomic changes which have left the country in transition, more vulnerable to the spread of HIV/AIDS, and made it more difficult for effective responses to be developed. The country has seen a dramatic rise, for example, in cross-border movement for temporary work, commercial sex work, intravenous drug use, substance use, and unprotected sexual activity. In Ukraine, the gap between the wealthy and poor has widened and this development has also created greater health implications. Moreover, as a transitioning country, community ties and family bonds have weakened and legal and illegal migration has increased (UNDP 2003).

Nevertheless, the government is not adequately tackling the social and economic dimensions which are at the root of the spread of this disease. Until recently, other issues such as impoverishment of the population, unemployment, and decline of social safety net were seen as higher priorities than HIV/AIDS and the links of this disease to the current socioeconomic situation were not recognized (UNDP 2005). Moreover, because the disease was initially—and to a large extent still is—concentrated among injecting drug users and sex workers, it is not systematically approached as a priority issue for the entire population of Ukraine, including the next wave of at-risk persons.

Stigma and Discrimination

HIV carries serious social stigma in Ukraine (DeBell and Carter 2005), which has caused both widespread discrimination and has undermined effective responses across the country to the pandemic. For example, in a 2005 survey of decision-makers in Ukraine, including members of the Verkohvna Rada, local councilors, top officials in ministries, state departments, and committees, 32 percent "agree" or "rather agreed than disagreed" with the statement "People with HIV/AIDS are to be blamed themselves for their misfortune" and 29 percent with the statement "AIDS is God's punishment for drug addition" (UNDP 2005: 27). Ukraine has a law that criminalizes non-disclosure of HIV status when seeking medical care and, as such, cultural attitudes towards those who use drugs, engage in sex work, have same sex relationships, are new immigrants, and those with communicable diseases remain punitive (DeBell 2004). Describing her emotionally damaging interactions with the health care system, one HIV-positive woman explains: "After visiting my doctor I need half a day or the whole day to come to collect myself psychologically" (EngenderHealth/UNFPA 2006: 47).

There is now substantial evidence that the rights of HIV-positive persons, in terms of privacy, confidentiality, access to appropriate information, services, and treatment, are undermined. Human Rights Watch has thus argued that "donors who support HIV interventions in Ukraine should voice concern that their investments are being undermined by widespread human rights abuse against those living with and at highest risk of HIV" (2006: 6). In a 2004 survey of persons living with HIV/AIDS, 42 percent reported "violations of their rights related to employment, education, or privacy because of their HIV status" (http://www.aidsalliance.kiev.ua/cgi-bin/index.cgi?url=/en/library/our/policy5/index.htm). In the same year, a survey with forty HIV-positive women reported that more than one third felt they had been more poorly treated than HIV-negative women in labor and delivery settings and more than half reported that their health care providers assumed they were injection drug users (Ukrainian Institute for Social Research 2004). Not surprisingly, UNDP has argued that "stigma and discrimination can only be surmounted if open, intensive and reasoned debated is carried out on a national scale, and if a concerted effort is made to enshrine human rights for all citizens, both in law and in practice" (2003: 25).

Similarly, Human Rights Watch found discrimination against high-risk groups and those living with HIV/AIDS by health care providers, despite the protections afforded by Ukraine's national AIDS law. According to their 2006 report "Rhetoric and Risk: Human Rights Abuses Impeding Ukraine's Fight Against HIV/AIDS:"

> People living with HIV/AIDS and injection drug users were turned away from hospitals, summarily discharged when their HIV status became known, or provided poor quality care that was both dehumanizing and debilitating to their already fragile health status. Ambulances refused to transport drug users and people living with HIV/AIDS. In some cases, care could only be negotiated through payment for service that should have been provided free of charge. Denial of care was identified by people living with HIV/AIDs, physicians specializing in AIDS care, and AIDS service workers as a particular problem for people seeking treatment at tuberculosis clinics. Tuberculosis is widespread in Ukraine, easily transmitted, and a major cause of death for people living with HIV/AIDS; refusal to treat people living with HIV/AIDS for tuberculosis threatens to jeopardize their lives and the health of thousand of other Ukrainians. (2006: 4)

To further illustrate, one respondent in the study reported that upon hearing of his HIV status, a doctor said, "Why do you come here and make more problems for us? You are guilty yourself for this. You are dragging yourself to your own destruction." And another HIV-positive woman reported that, when she was in labor, "Several people refused to admit me. It was only when I said

'How much' that they took me in. I paid 1,1000 hryvna [U.S.$200] and my daughter was born a few minutes later. If I hadn't paid, I would have given birth in the waiting room" (Human Rights Watch 2006).

Without doubt, those with HIV-positive status are often considered outcasts of Ukrainian society (EngenderHealth/UNFPA 2006). This affects the willingness of people to seek information, go for testing, reveal their positive status to others or try to find necessary services to which they are entitled. For women, in particular, the stigma and discrimination is especially pervasive; HIV status is thought to be caused by behaviors and lifestyle choices (e.g., promiscuity and drug use) that violate traditional gendered norms and expectations of what it means to be a good and respectable female citizen. There are some indications that attention is starting to be paid to the issues of stigma and discrimination through public events such as World AIDS Day. However, the gendered dimensions of HIV/AIDS in Ukraine, and the specific needs of girls and women among whom the rate of HIV infections have been increasing at alarming rates, have not been front and center.

Gendered Dimensions of HIV/AIDS

The World Health Organization (WHO) has concluded that "the effectiveness of HIV/AIDS programs and policies is greatly enhanced when gender differences are acknowledged, the gender-specific concerns and needs of women and men are addressed, and gender inequities are reduced" (2003: 6). To date, in Ukraine, there has been no systematic gendered analysis of the issue, nor has there been any formal policy developed to promote such an analysis. Attention has been focused on IDUs, sex workers, those infected with TB, those living with HIV without adequate recognition of how these are affected or shaped by gender. Ukraine has lagged behind other countries and international organizations in recognizing the significance of sex and gender in relation to HIV/AIDS. Commenting on the current situation in Ukraine, USAID has observed that "one of the factors potentially contributing to the increase in the number of women infected with HIV is the insufficient targeting and appropriate coverage of this group with HIV prevention programs, information and services" (USAID 2006).

The lack of a gendered analysis of the phenomenon is therefore extremely problematic given women's higher vulnerability for contraction physiologically, socially, economically and culturally. In the words of Dr. Alla Scherbinskaya, Head of the Ukrainian AIDS Center: "Looking at the forces behind the epidemic, we see that women and girls are most vulnerable due to their physiology and to socio-economic reasons" (UN 2006). Indeed, worldwide, for reasons of biology, gender, and cultural norms, females are more susceptible than males to HIV infection. Biologically, the risk of infection during unprotected sex is two to four times higher for women than men (Royce et al. 1997). And of course this has gendered implications in terms of mortality. For example, in Ukraine, it is expected that the life of expectancy of women will be shortened by three to five years as a result of the epidemic; for males, it is two to four years (Transatlantic Partners Against AIDS 2005). And by 2014 it is estimated that AIDS will be responsible for 60 percent of all deaths among women as compared to 30 percent among men (Ministry of Health, as cited in Transatlantic Partners Against AIDS 2005).

Among all women, however, female sex workers are at the most heightened risk of HIV infection. This is significant because of the numbers of Ukrainian women who engage in sex work to supplement their incomes. For instance, in a 2001 survey by the State Institute for Family and Youth Issues, more than 50 percent of women support their children and families through sex work (cited in UNDP 2003). This reality necessitates consideration of how prevention initiatives can be effective with this specific population. First, the vulnerability of sex workers must be understood as resulting from forced or coerced sex, including physical trauma which increases risk of transmission, limited capacity to negotiate condom use with clients, and a variety of abuses by police. According to the UNDP, "HIV/AIDS prevention programs aimed at sex workers have the best results when the women are treated as people capable of protecting both themselves and their clients from HIV transmission. For this to happen, the legal situation of sex workers, and programs that work for them, have to be modified" (2003: 26). In addition, more attention needs to be paid to general social policy, the economy, and developing appropriate health interventions.

In terms of gendered research done to date, the 2005 USAID-funded project "Scaling up the National Response to HIV/AIDS through information services (SUNRISE), conducted and published by International HIV/AIDS Alliance in Ukraine," demonstrated that female IDUs in Ukraine are potentially more vulnerable to HIV/AIDS than men. This is because female drug users often are dependent on not only illicit drugs but men who provide them with drugs and involve them in commercial sex. WHO reports that most heterosexual cases are among female partners of drug users, and that a significant proportion of HIV positive pregnant women are either partners of injectors, or injectors themselves (Donoghoe et al. 2005). Moreover, help-seeking of this group is undermined by the fact that many such women will not disclose their use of drugs because the status of a drug user "goes against expected, traditional female roles and is therefore condemned by society even more so than in the case of females" (USAID 2006).

Participants of the SUNRISE study reported needing women-specific consultations, female self-help groups, humanitarian and basic financial aid for children from low-income families, antiretroviral therapy for their children, high-quality formula/nutrition for babies, and cultural and educational opportunities for children. The women also indicated that they needed better information during pregnancy and childbirth and during HIV testing. Indeed, most women in Ukraine do not know they are HIV positive until they become pregnant. While USAID is undertaking a project to train obstetricians and midwives in voluntary counseling and testing services in the cities of Mykolayiv, Odessa, and Sevastopol, and is funding a maternity hospital that works with HIV-positive mothers, there is no national program for counseling around HIV testing among pregnant women. From research done to date, HIV-positive women are calling for pre- and post-test counseling and also peer counseling. As put by one such woman, "I wanted to talk to the same person as I was" (Okromoshenko et al. 2006).

And although testing is generally on the increase, Human Rights Watch has concluded that "Ukraine's public health system fails to adequately protect the rights of pregnant women living with HIV/AIDS" (2006: 54). Few women have information about the actual testing and their right to refuse an HIV test. Health professionals often release test results to family members without having the woman's consent, fail to inform women about effective prevention practices, exaggerate the risk of HIV transmission to fetuses or try to influence a woman's choice of whether to continue with their pregnancy, often pressuring them to have abortions (Human Rights Watch 2006). This is further evidenced by a 2006 EngenderHealth/UNFPA study examining the sexual and reproductive health needs of women and adolescent girls living with HIV in Ukraine. According to one respondent, "One day I came to the gynecologist for a medical examination. I was pregnant and they said that the child would be HIV positive and that an abortion had to be done . . . This is connected with the fact that they don't want to see HIV-positive people, and they forbid HIV positive to deliver," and in the words of another respondent, "Their attitudes towards those who are HIV positive must be changed and then, maybe, people will come to see the doctor more often" (EngenderHealth/UNFPA 2006: 43, 45).

There is also a general lack of information among the female population surrounding the disease. In 2002, UNICEF, UNAIDS, and WHO reported that only 9 percent of young women could identify three methods of HIV prevention and that nearly 80 percent held one or more misconceptions about HIV/AIDS (UNICEF, UNAIDS, and WHO 2002). According to results presented in the

National Report on Declaration of Commitment on HIV/AIDS Implementation, only 14 percent of the young women questioned know all routes of HIV transmission. The lack of information also extends to the existing health infrastructure and available services. As one woman puts it, "Honestly speaking the majority of HIV positive women know very little about what services exist and where they can receive them" (EngenderHealth/UNFPA 2006: 47). It is therefore very difficult for an HIV-positive woman in Ukraine to get the medical care she needs (Okromoshenko et al. 2006).

The fear of health professionals interacting with HIV-positive female patients has also been noted. According to Dr. Semenenko of USAID's HIV/AIDS program, "infected women are placed in separate maternity wards, as part of an extraordinary and baseless system of protecting the rest of the population" (http:stories.usaid.gov). Another physician respondent in the above-mentioned EngenderHealth/UNFPA study explained: "Well everyone is subconsciously afraid of being infected in the process of any procedures" (2006: 46). And in the words of an HIV-positive woman, "Having learnt my status, the midwife refused to examine me. She said that such women should be examined at the cemetery" (Okromoshenko et al. 2006).

Although a gender analysis of the epidemic is required at all levels of government legislation and policy, especially in the health sector, the problem is also cultural. Gender is after all a cultural construct and this must be reflected in any attempts at transforming current responses. For instance, numerous misconceptions remain about the relative status and power of Ukrainian women. When Ukraine was still a part of the former Soviet Union, women enjoyed relative gender equality in education, health, and in the employment sector. Not only has independence undermined such equality, it has failed to transform traditional gender stereotypes, especially in terms of what are considered appropriate and acceptable gender roles. For example, according to a 2003 UNDP report *Ukraine and HIV/AIDS: Time To Act*, "while extramarital relations are considered a norm for men, women are expected to be faithful wives and responsible mothers" (2003: 12) Ironically, then, a woman's risk of HIV infection depends less on her lifestyle, moral principles or number of sexual partners than on her ability to insist on condom use by her partner (2003: 12).

HIV-positive women report refraining from using condoms because of a lack of understanding of risk, preference for sex without a condom, perception of mistrust, and the difficulty in discussing issues of sexuality (EngenderHealth/UNFPA 2006: 48). Women report fearing their partners' reaction and judgment, and fear being abandoned (EngenderHealth/UNFPA 2006). Once a woman becomes infected, the stigma is overwhelming As one participant in the Human Rights study put it, once a woman reveals her HIV status, it is typical that "the husband leaves them, and parents say you are not our daughter any more, don't come home anymore" (2006: 55). HIV-positive women report feeling abandoned by their families, communities, and government and wanting changes so that their rights and health needs are acknowledged and respected.

In the final analysis, then, while targeting specific at-risk populations remains a priority, a strong case can also be made for developing a gender-inclusive approach to HIV/AIDS in Ukraine. Ideally, a gendered approach to the pandemic would include "specifically addressing women in prevention and care programs, focusing on their increasing vulnerability to infection, and their difficulty in negotiating safer sex with their partner" (UNDP 2003: 26). Moreover, any adequate gender analysis would also necessitate linking the socioeconomic situation in the country to the spread of HIV/AIDS and addressing the cultural norms and stereotypes that make women more susceptible to infection and prevent them from receiving timely, proper, and gender-appropriate services. Moreover, any gender-sensitive response should ensure that the voices of women as users of services be included in the development, implementation, and evaluation of HIV/AIDS legislation and policy.

CONCLUSION

In the final analysis, the HIV/AIDS pandemic in Ukraine requires attention to a number of interrelated issues. Legislation that is in place must be systematically implemented. More attention needs to be paid to raising the political and financial commitments to HIV/AIDS, including policymaking and budgeting processes. Moreover, a sustained focus on increasing the knowledge and capacity of policymakers and government officials about HIV/AIDS and strengthening inter-sectoral coordination in responding to the problem are urgently needed (Transatlantic Partners Against AIDS 2005). Stigma and discrimination must also be confronted through increasing education and awareness. Most importantly, however, the groups currently most affected, as well as those who are becoming increasingly affected, require the immediate attention of all sectors, especially those in government and in the health care sectors who have the power to determine future legislation and policy directions; and to keep in line with the knowledge and promising practices of other jurisdictions and to respond to the changing face of the growing epidemic. Ukraine also needs to develop an appropriate gender analysis of the phenomenon. This will be an important step in ensuring appropriate, timely, and effective prevention and intervention initiatives for *all* at-risk populations.

NOTE

1. The author gratefully acknowledges the helpful comments of Anna Dovbakh—Head of Team: Program and Resource Development International HIV/AIDS Alliance in Ukraine—on an earlier draft of this chapter.

REFERENCES AND FURTHER READING

Amon, J.J. (2003) "The HIV/AIDS Epidemic in Ukraine: Stable or Still Exploding." *Sexually Transmitted Infections*, 79: 263–264.

Balakireva, O. et al. (2003) *The Prospects for Development of HIV Prevention Programs among Injecting Drug Users*. UNICEF, UNAIDS, Social Monitoring Center. Kiev.

Borushek, I. (2006) *Scaling up Access to Substitution Treatment—Lessons from Ukraine All-Ukrainian Network of PLWHAs/International AIDS Alliance*, 16th International AIDS Conference, Toronto, August 13–18, 2006.

Buskey, Megan (2005) "Life After the Trash Can." *Transitions Online*, September 19, http://www.tol.cz/look/TOL/article.tpl?IdLanguage=1&IdPublication=4&NrIssue= 133.

DeBell, D. (2004) *Research as a Tool in Policy Formation for HIV/AIDS Educational and Prevention in Ukraine*. Global Forum for Health Research Forum 8, Mexico City, November 2004.

DeBell, D. and R. Carter. (2005) "Impact of Transition on Public Health in Ukraine: Case Study of the HIV/AIDS Epidemic." *BMJ*, 331(23): 216–218.

Dehne, K.L, L. Khodakevich, F.F. Hamers, and B. Schwartländer. (1999) "The HIV/AIDS Epidemic in Eastern Europe: Recent Patterns and Trends and Their Implications for Policy-Making." *AIDS*, 13: 741–749.

Demchenko, I., M. Varban, and N. Salabai. (2005) *Factors Contributing to National Policy Development on HIV/AIDS: Analytical Report Based on the Survey of Decision Makers in Ukraine, Kyiv*. United Nations Development Programs, Governance of HIV/AIDS Project.

Donoghoe, M.C, J.V. Lazarus, and S. Matic. (2005) "HIV/AIDS in the Transitional Countries of Eastern Europe and Central Asia." *Clinical Medicine* 5:487–490.

EngenderHealth/UNFPA. (2006) *Sexual and Reproductive Health Needs of Women and Adolescent Girls Living with HIV: Research Report on Qualitative Findings from Brazil, Ethiopia and the Ukraine*, United Nations, Geneva.

EuroHIV. (2006) *HIV/AIDS Surveillance in Europe: End Year Report 2005*, no. 73. Saint Maurice, Institut de Veille Sanitaire.

Fisher, I. (2002) "Stigma of AIDS Strong in Ukraine." *New York Times*, January 23, http://query.nytimes.com/gst/fullpage.html?sec=health&res.

Frost, L. and V. Tchertkov. (2002). "Prisoner Risk Taking in the Russian Federation." *AIDS Educ Prev* 14 (Supplement B): 7–23.

Glazkova, E. (2005) "Interview with KORRESPONDENT Magazine," *Korrespondent* 17 (156), April 7, http://www.antiAIDS.org/en/about/publications/554/1540. Accessed on June 16, 2006.

Houmenyuk, O., T. Bylik, and T.U. Yavorska, (2006) *Why HIV/AIDS is a Threat to Business in Ukraine and What Should be Done about It*. Kyiv, Transatlantic Partners Against AIDS.

Human Rights Watch. (2006) *Rhetoric and Risk: Human Rights Abuses Impeding Ukraine's Fight against HIV/AIDS*." New York, Human Rights Watch.

International HIV/AIDS Alliance (2006). *Strengthening the Response to the HIV Epidemic in Ukraine: Positive Sides of Economic Transition*. http://www.AIDSalliance.org/sw29482.asp.

International HIV/AIDS Alliance in Ukraine. (2006a) *Program Overcoming HIV/AIDS Epidemic in Ukraine*. http://www.AIDSalliance.kiev.ua/cgi-bin/index.cgi?url=/en/gfund/index.htm. Last accessed June 19, 2006.

International HIV/AIDS Alliance in Ukraine. (2006b). *Supporting Community Action on AIDS in Developing Countries: Ukraine*. http://www.AIDSalliance.org/sw7229.asp?usepf=true. Last accessed June 12, 2006.

International HIV/AIDS Alliance in Ukraine and World Bank. (2006) *Socioeconomic Impact of HIV/AIDS in Ukraine*. Washington DC, World Bank.

Lekhan, V., V. Rudiy, and E. Nolte. (2004) *Health Care Systems in Transition: Ukraine*. Copenhagen, WHO Regional Office for Europe on behalf of the European Observatory on Health Systems and Policies.

Lowry, J. and E. Nyanenkova. (2005) "Ukrainian Red Cross and Eurovision come closer." http://www.ifrc.org/docs/news/05/05051701/. Last accessed June 25, 2006.

Malinowska-Sempruch, K., J. Hoover, and A. Alexandrova. (2003). *Unintended Consequences: Drug Policies Fuel the HIV Epidemic in Russia and Ukraine*. New York: Open Society Institute, 2003.

Ministry of Health Ukraine. (2006) *Ukraine: National Report on the Follow-up to the UNGASS Declaration of Commitment on HIV/AIDS—Reporting Period January 2003–2005*. Kyiv. Ministry of Health.

Ministry of Health Ukraine et al. (2006) *HIV-Infection in Ukraine*: Information Bulletin no. 26. Kyiv, Ministry of Health of Ukraine, Ukrainian AIDS Center, L.V. Gromashevskogo Institute of Epidemiology, and Central Sanitary Epidemiological Station of the Ministry of Health of Ukraine.

Namjilsuren, T. (2004) "Positive Women in Ukraine: Living with Denial, Discrimination and HIV/AIDS." http://www.who.int/3by5/news19/en/print.html. Last accessed April 3, 2006.

Neil, L., O. Zalata, and R. Coker. (2005) "On the European Union New Eastern Border: Health Promotion, HIV and Ukraine." *European Journal of Public Health* 15(4): 336–338.

Okromoshenko, S., N. Zaika, I. Mogilevkina, A. Bishop, and K. Stekhnin. (2006) Needs of HIV Positive Women in Ukraine. Poster presentation at the 16th AIDS Conference in Toronto, Canada, August 13–18, 2006.

Royce, R. et al. (1997). "Sexual Transmission of HIV/AIDS." *New England Journal of Medicine* 336(15): 1072–1078.

Rudiy, V. (2004) *Ukrainian Anti-HIV/AIDS Legislation: Current State and Ways of Improvement*. Kyiv: Sfera.

Shabarovska, A., O. Kostyuk, A. Sherbinska, and S. Antoniak. (2006) The Regional Knowledge Hub's Strategy to Build Human Resource Capacity for Rapid Scale-Up of Ukraine's Ability to Provide Antiretroviral Therapy to PLWHA. Poster presentation at the Eastern European and Central Asian AIDS Conference, Moscow, May 2006.

Sherbinska, A. (2005) *National Plan of ART Scale Up in Ukraine, Presented at the Human Capacity Building Strategy to Support ART Scale Up in Ukraine*. Kyiv, KMAPE Meeting, September 26, 2005.

Transatlantic Partners Against AIDS (2005) "The HIV/AIDS Epidemic in Ukraine." *Transatlantic Partners Against AIDS*, Vol. 2, No. 2.

Trifonov, D., J-M Jackson, and A. Bega. (2005) *Strengthening Ukraine's Response to HIV/AIDS: Eliminating Gaps Between Legislation and Implementation*, Policy brief 2 (2), Transatlantic Partners Against AIDS.

Trifonov, D., V. Lyubarevich, J.M. Jackson. (2006) "Effective Management of Ukraine's HIV/AIDS Epidemic: A Policy Blueprint for the New President," *Transatlantic Partners Against AIDS* 3(1).

Ukraine Government. (2006) *National Report on the Follow-Up to the UNGASS Declaration of Commitment on HIV/AIDS, Reporting Period: January 2003–December 2005*. Kyiv.

Ukrainian AIDS Center. (2005) *Minutes from the "Human Capacity Building Strategy to Support ART Scale Up in Ukraine" Meeting with the Regional Knowledge Hub for Care and Treatment of HIV/AIDS*, Eurasia, September 26, 2005. http://www.AIDSknowledgehub.org/about/approaches/249/. Last accessed on June 19, 2006.

Ukrainian Institute for Social Research, Ukrainian AIDS Center, Ministry of Health of Ukraine, Youth NGO "Life Plus," and POLICY Project. (2004) *Access of HIV-Positive Women to Quality Reproductive Health and Maternity Services*, Kyiv.

"Ukraine Celebrates Progress on World AIDS Day." http://www.AIDSalliance.org/sw43956.asp. Last accessed June 12, 2006.

UN. (2005) "5,000 Race for Life in Downtown Kyiv." http://www.un.kiev.ua/en/pressroom/news/589/. Last accessed June 25, 2006.

UN. (2006) "Women of Ukraine take a lead in tackling HIV/AIDS." http://www.un.kiev.ua/en/pressroom/news/322/. Last accessed June 25, 2006.

UNAIDS/WHO. (2005) *Epidemiological Fact Sheet—2004 Update*. http://www.who.org.

UNAIDS/WHO. (2006) *AIDS Epidemic Update*. Geneva, Switzerland: UNAIDS. http://www.unAIDS.org/en/HIV_data/epi2006/.

UNDP. (2003) *Ukraine and HIV/AIDS: Time to Act*, Kyiv, Ukraine Human Development Report. Special edition.

UNDP. (2005) *Factors Contributing to National Policy Development on HIV/AIDS: Analytical Report Based on the Survey of Decision Makers in Ukraine*. Kyiv, UNDP.

UNICEF. (2004) "Ukraine Fights Rising HIV/AIDS Infection Rate." http://www.unicef.org/infobycountry/ukraine_fights_AIDS.html. Last accessed on June 12, 2006.

UNICEF, UNAIDS, and WHO. (2002). *Young People and HIV/AIDS: Opportunities in Crisis*, New York: UNICEF. http://www.unicef.org/publications/index_4447.html

USAID. (2004) *Health Profile: Ukraine. HIV/AIDS*, Washington DC, USAID.

USAID. (2006) "Gender Study Gains a Better Understanding of Needs of HIV-Positive People," *USAID Insight*, 3:3–4.

WHO (2003) *Integrating Gender into HIV/AIDS Programs: A Review Paper*. Geneva: World Health Organization: Department of Gender and Women's Health, Family and Community Health.

WHO (2004) *Ukraine: Summary Country Profile for HIV/AIDS Treatment Scale up*. Geneva, World Health Organization.

WHO (2005) *Ukraine Summary Country Profile for HIV/AIDS Treatment Scale up*. Geneva, World Health Organization.

World Bank. (2005) *Ukraine*. http://web.worldbank.org/WBSITE/EXTERNAL/COUNTRIES/ECAEXT/0,,contentMDK:20657882~pagePK:146736~piPK:146830~theSitePK:258599,00.html

World Bank. (2006) *HIV/AIDS in Ukraine*. Washington DC, World Bank.

"World Bank, Ukraine Health Ministry to Establish Working Group on TB, HIV/AIDS Project Grant." (2006) http://kaisernetwork.org/daily_reports.cfm?DR_ID=37736&dr_cat=4. Last accessed June 12, 2006.

CHAPTER 7

Homosexual Repression and AIDS in Post-Soviet Central Asia

Laëtitia Atlani-Duault[1]

ABSTRACT

Very limited information is available regarding male homosexuality and AIDS in Central Asia. This chronological analysis is divided into four parts: 1) the 19th century and particularly the October Revolution of 1917, 2) the repressive turn of events in the 1930s, 3) the glasnost period of the 1980s, and 4) finally the independence of the Central Asian republics in 1991 and the subsequent influence of international aid. This chapter concludes that international developments, particularly in defense of sexual minorities in the fight against HIV/AIDS, has provoked significant social change in Central Asia, including the decriminalization of homosexuality and the legalization of local homosexual NGOs.

Gay men were in the forefront of AIDS activism from the start, virtually at the same time as the discovery of the strange new syndrome. As the disease was first detected in a cohort of homosexual men, gay men and their allies, often with no familiarity with medicine or the health system, coalesced into grassroots organizations, mobilized volunteers, and looked for answers. They constructed innovative peer-led models of popular education, helped the sick outside the usual channels and upended the traditional dominance of physicians and government health experts. In doing so, they won considerable if grudging respect from medical and public health establishments and placed themselves at the center of the worldwide epidemic both for their expertise as well as another "community" that required mobilization from within as an essential piece of the overall national response to the complexities of HIV/AIDS as it spread across the globe.

A consensus gradually emerged among the international health agencies and donor entities that direct efforts led by gay or homosexual men themselves were a welcome piece of the ideal national response to HIV/AIDS. In addition, the stigma arising from HIV could only be met by a head-on challenge to cultural homophobia and discrimination as AIDS sufferers turned into "people living with HIV" who ought to be respected in their human rights and offered compassionate and effective medical treatment, whatever the origins of the infection. This implied a direct challenge to legal and cultural sanctions against homosexuality, and international aid often came with these implicitly gay-friendly strings attached. The donor agencies saw that gay-oriented peer education and prevention campaigns would require a tolerant legal and social environment to be successful, to reach into the often clandestine lives of vulnerable men hiding their practices from police, relatives, and the next-door neighbor.

However, the Central Asian republics formerly belonging to the USSR present a particular challenge to this friendly scenario. Although homosexual behavior is rooted in pre-Soviet practices in some cases, the countries can also be exceptionally intolerant and adamant against allowing this particular form of "foreign" influence to take root.

After an analysis of homosexuality in the Soviet era, I will show how the HIV/AIDS epidemic in this understudied part of the world has aggravated prejudice and discrimination in an already strongly homophobic region characterized by powerful state control over all political expressions. Yet, at the same time, it is clear that HIV provided courageous individuals with an extraordinary opportunity to fight for the rights of homosexuals.

This chronological analysis, which takes as its starting point the nineteenth century, will be divided into four parts, each of which deals with a key event in the history of the region's *goluboi*, or "blues," as male Central Asian homosexuals refer to themselves (Russian slang that literally means "light blue")[2]: the October Revolution of 1917, the repressive turn of events in the 1930s, the glasnost period of the 1980s, and finally the independence of the Central Asian republics in 1991 and the subsequent influence of international aid. We will rely both on data in existing literature and on the field studies we have carried out in Central Asia beginning in 1995. The information available on all aspects of sexuality in post-Soviet Central Asia is very limited and even more so in the case of male homosexuality and AIDS.

THE 1917 REVOLUTION: FREEDOM OR REVOLUTIONARY CHAOS?

Before the Russian conquest of Central Asia, it was commonplace to see boys (children and young adolescents) named *batchas, baccá* or *bacheh*[3] used as dancers in cafés and other places dedicated to entertainment, as well as in homes for family occasions like marriages and circumcisions (Baldauf 1998). "These *batchas*, or young dancers, are an institution throughout Central Asia, although they are especially prized in Bukhara and Samarkand" (in what is now Uzbekistan), commented the adventurer Eugene Schuyler in his notebooks in 1876. They were also noticed by Count Palhen, who visited Uzbekistan at the beginning of the twentieth century. He described their dances as particularly lascivious: the boys danced barefoot, wore long hair, and were dressed and made up like women, with their fingernails and toenails painted red. The movements of their bodies aroused carnal desires in the male audience (Schuyler 1876; Palhen 1964). Schuyler and Palhen also confirm the boys' roles as child prostitutes. "Every man of a high social position or rank has to have one in his service; those men with less money at their disposal group together in order to have a *batcha* to amuse themselves during their moments of rest and leisure," noted Schuyler. Initiated to the role at a very young age, these children did not choose their activity but were forced into it by their families. While many lived poor and miserable lives, some managed to become known as gifted artists. In these cases, writes Schuyler (1876: vol. I, 132–133), "They earn as much respect as do our greatest artists and singers. Their every movement is followed and applauded, and I have never seen a more interested public than one excited by *batchas*. The crowd seems to eat the dancers up with their eyes all the while clapping their hands to the rhythm of their feet."

Conquered by the Tsar in the nineteenth century, Central Asia was constrained to adopt Russian legislation. In line with the Russian Criminal Code that came into force in 1832, sexual relations between men (*muzhelozhstvo*) were forbidden. Those found guilty were stripped of their civil and property rights, and deported to Siberia for periods of four to five years. This legislation remained in effect until 1903, when it was replaced by a new criminal code that prescribed prison terms of five to eight years for the same act (Kon 1995). However, the law was rarely applied in Russia and even less frequently in Central Asia.

After the 1917 revolution, parts of Central Asia were gradually absorbed into Soviet territory through conquest. From the revolution up until 1991, a single policy was applied throughout the Soviet Union to control all aspects of social life, including sexuality. Two very different periods characterized Soviet policies towards homosexuality. Immediately after the October Revolution came a time of rupture with the Tsar's policies, as sodomy was decriminalized and a series of liberalizing measures affecting sexual behavior and family life were introduced.

Although this decriminalization has attracted much interest from historians, there are many conflicting opinions as to how this "liberation" actually affected Soviet homosexuals in the 1920s. A heated debate on the subject, heavily influenced by political considerations, took place during the Cold War (Bauml Duberman, Vicinus, and Chauncey 1989; Baer 2002; Healy 2002). According to one group, the Bolsheviks' avant-garde move to decriminalize homosexuality was to be admired, especially given that homosexuality was still illegal in the United States and most European countries at the time (Lauritsen and Thorstad 1974). In this they shared the views of many contemporary Soviet doctors and lawyers who were particularly proud of the move. The latter touted it as an example to follow in international conferences on the subject, such as the meeting organized by the International League for Sexual Reform in Copenhagen in 1928.

A second group argued that homosexuals were victims of discrimination in the Soviet Union even before the Stalinist reaction (Karlinsky 1976, 1977, 1989). They noted that, although sodomy was no longer a criminal act between 1917 and 1921, it was not explicitly permitted—an important distinction within the peculiarities of Soviet law. During this period of war communism, there was no criminal code setting out what was legally permissible and what was not. For authors like Karlinksy (1989) and Schluter (2002), this "legal holiday" seemed to have been interpreted by members of the first group as legalizing sodomy. In reality, where no precise instructions had been given—as in this case—officers were charged with applying the old Tsarist legal code. If the new 1922 Criminal Law Code failed to mention sodomy, this absence could be read as an omission, an omission that was "corrected" by Stalin in 1934 (Karlinsky 1976, 1977).

The debate took a new turn of events after 1991, when some archives were made public for the first time (Engelstein 1992; Naiman 1997; Healey 2001, 2002; Schluter 2002). These documents suggest that the situation for Soviet homosexuals in the 1920s was more complex than previously supposed. Two points are particularly relevant.

First, the decriminalization of homosexuality should be considered in the light of the historical and intellectual context of the 1920s. Following the 1917 revolution and throughout the 1920s, debate raged on the subject of "free love" and the possibility of redefining "sexual morality" for the proletariat in all large towns of the Soviet Union. During these debates Party theorists were divided, as "the Party did not maintain a rigid orthodoxy, and differences were freely expressed, especially regarding such contentious issues as sexual relations, child-rearing, and the need for the family in the transition to socialism" (Goldman 1993: 5; Naiman 1997). Even if they did not explicitly advocate the rights of homosexuals (Goldman 1993; Healey 2002), many jurists, Party members, and renowned feminists such as Alexandra Kollontai did announce the imminent "disappearance of the family" (Clements 1973, 1979; Farnsworth 1980).

Following this line of reasoning, the highest Soviet legislative authority, the Central Executive Committee, ratified in October 1918 a new code on marriage and the family. The aim of this new code was to "make [the family] unnecessary" (Goikhbarg 1918: 4–9). To achieve this goal, housework was to be transferred to the public sphere. Unpaid tasks carried out by women at home would henceforth be taken care of by paid workers (in cafeterias, laundries, crèches for children, and so forth), and these activities were to be financed collectively (Stuchka 1925; Kollontai 1920). In these circumstances, cohabitation would come to replace marriage. Citizens would enter and exit relationships as they chose, freed from the social pressures linked to having offspring. Parents would care for their children outside of any marriage framework with the help of the collective. The family would gradually disappear, leaving in its place fully autonomous individuals, free to choose their partners—and the sex of their partners—in line with the considerations of love and mutual respect. This is the very unique context in which the decriminalization of homosexuality in the

Soviet Union took place following the October Revolution.

However, upon a closer reading of the archives, the contradictory language employed by the Bolsheviks on the subject of homosexuality becomes apparent. Generally, this language changes in line with whether the homosexual practices under discussion are occurring in Slavic regions or in Central Asia or the Caucasus. While homosexual acts amongst supposedly "civilized" Slavic populations were seen as resulting from a disease that could be treated by modern medicine and psychiatry, the same acts were considered "retrograde" and "primitive" when practiced by the distant Central Asian and Caucasian populations. This duality was clearly visible in the *Great Soviet Encyclopaedia* published in 1930, where homosexuality merited two separate entries. The first, by the psychiatrist Mark Sereiskii, gave a biomedical overview of the phenomenon, limited to Europe and the Slavic population of the Soviet Union. The second entry, entitled "An Ethnographical Essay" and written by P. Preobrazhenskii, discussed homosexuality amongst the "non-civilized" peoples of the Far Northern and "Asian" territories in the Soviet Union (Healey 2001, 2002). In these regions homosexual practices were considered to be the result of harmful "indigenous customs," which later became the object of an eradication campaign waged by the Soviet government (Durmanov 1938). To facilitate the task, sodomy was made illegal in Azerbaijan in 1923, in Uzbekistan in 1926 and in Turkmenistan in 1927, while remaining legal in the rest of the Soviet Union.

THE SHIFT OF THE 1930s

In 1934 homosexuality was again criminalized throughout the Soviet Union. Under Article 121 sexual contact between men became a crime punishable by five years' imprisonment. Described by Nicolai Krylenko, the People's Commissioner in charge of justice, as a sign of the bourgeoisie's moral decadence and an anti-proletarian act, homosexuality came to be associated with the old order and was considered "anti-revolutionary" (Kon 1995). Article 121 was a powerful tool for the authorities to target men considered enemies of the regime. This article allowed for the men in question to be discredited, harassed, hauled before the courts, and convicted. It could also be used to extend the incarceration of those already in detention camps. Those in camps for homosexual practices systematically became targets for the other prisoners, and they were pariahs subjected to violence and persecution, including organized sexual violence.

Exact figures as to how many victims were punished pursuant to Article 121 are unknown, as the archives remain closed. However, Sergei Scherbakov, cited by Igor Kon, has estimated this number at around 1,000 men per year. Real figures are probably much higher. Even if the archives are eventually made fully public, the statistics would be complicated by the fact that many Soviet homosexuals were convicted of charges not covered by Article 121, such as "hooliganism" or being a "class enemy" (Gessen 1994; Kon 1995).

A strong means of repression, legal proceedings, examining the merest "*suspicion*" of homosexuality, all this gave a free rein to multiple forms of social harassment. This habitual harassment forced Soviet homosexuals to take refuge in secrecy, in meetings in places quickly uncovered by neighbors and the authorities, where the risk of being unmasked and arrested was ever present. Life in collective apartments was not conducive to intimacy. It was common for families, including children and grandparents, to be allocated a single room in a collective apartment. Here, one or more persons were always charged with surveillance and informing on neighbors for crimes ranging from anticommunist acts, theft, or the organization of groups. Although the number of collective apartments diminished after Nikita Khruschchev's arrival to power in 1954 when many new apartments were built and families were finally entitled to their own apartments, it was rare for a single person to be allocated one.

Even renting a hotel room was difficult from a legal point of view as well as a practical one. A man who was unmarried or had no family ties could not rent a hotel room for more than one person. Renting a hotel room in the town where one lived was also impossible. Nor was it easy to go to another town, as each person had a passport and a residence permit obliging him or her to reside in the place the authorities had designated. People's movements were often monitored, as the Communist Party declared that no Party member should have a secret from the group. Finding a time and place for intimate moments was therefore a real problem. In spite of the control and surveillance exercised, moments could still be snatched in public baths, parks, gardens, cars, film theaters, or on night trains, but always fearfully and on the sly.

This shift in the Soviet policy on homosexuality from the relative "liberalization" of the 1917–1934 period to the toughened stance of the 1930s finds its explanation in the larger context of Soviet policy on sexuality put in place by Stalin in the 1930s. This policy was to set the tone for the next fifty years. Indeed, at the beginning of the 1930s, "the Party broke radically with revolutionary ideals. In a sharp break with the pedagogical and rehabilitative ideals of the revolution, the Party designated the family, along with the militia, the courts, and the procuracy, to enforce social order on the streets. Far from withering away, the family became an indispensable unit in the state's control of its citizenry" (Goldman 1993: 327).[4] Abortions were made illegal in 1936 and remained illegal until 1956. Psychoanalysis became the target of heated ideological criticisms, and Freud's works were forbidden (Etkind 1993). All forms of erotic art were censored. Studies on sexuality were banned, and schools put an end to sexual education, as the Soviet advisor on education at the time, Anton Makarenko, deemed it useless. This qualification was also valid for sexual education within families, and Makarenko recommended parents to skillfully elude questions put to them by their children and turn conversations with adolescents towards the subject of morality.

This apparent turnaround was not just a simple reaction to the disorganized post-revolutionary situation, an argument used by the government to justify its change in attitude. As noted by Igor Kon (1995), repressive sexophobia was essential for totalitarian control of the individual. James Riordan quotes George Orwell: "It was not merely that the sex instinct created a world of its own that was outside the Party's control and which therefore had to be destroyed if possible. What was more important was that sexual privation induced hysteria, which was desirable because it could be transformed into war-fever and leader-worship." Riordan adds: "In all probability it was not a conscious strategy in the beginning but rather a continuation of revolutionary asceticism; people who had renounced everything thought they had the right to force everyone else to do the same."

But over the years this tendency became entrenched. "If a person was first and foremost a productive force working for the universal future of humankind, he or she should produce material commodities during work time and at home at night, produce children. Everything else had to be eradicated" (1993: 24). The situation slowly began to change at the end of the 1960s; however, debates and studies on sexuality (and homosexuality) remained few and far between. Up until the USSR's dying breath, "the Soviet people's sexual behavior is the best kept state secret of all time," as Igor Kon humorously remarked. "The top army command at least knows the whereabouts and staffing of our military bases, but no one has an inkling of our sex lives" (Kon and Riordan 1993: 27).

Given this background of secrecy and homosexual repression, it was impossible for sexual minorities to follow the Western example and form groups defending their basic human rights. There was, however, one exception to this rule. In May 1984, one month before Mikhail Gorbachev came to power, a group of around thirty young people from Leningrad led by Aleksandr Zaremba founded an informal organization of gays and lesbians named the "gay laboratory." With help from the International Gay and Lesbian Association (ILGA) via the Finnish association SETA, they managed to get information to the West testifying to the unenviable conditions facing "blues" in the

USSR (Kon 1995; Schluter 2002). Kept under KGB surveillance and faced with threats and repression, the group was finally dissolved in 1986. Its members were deported to Siberia or forced to emigrate overseas, and Zaremba was put in prison. Any further attempts to set up associations were publicly invisible until the very end of the glasnost period.

GLASNOST

During the first years of glasnost, the situation remained largely unchanged although the popular press did begin to examine the subject of homosexuality.[5] For the first time in the Soviet Union, homosexuality was the subject of a public debate, not only in journalistic articles on the subject but also in letters from homosexuals and their relatives. Many readers discovered for the first time the extent to which homosexuals were discriminated against, the police brutality they faced and the solitude they experienced (Kon 1995). While the debate was launched by a small number of newspapers in favor of fighting homophobia, the subject was also addressed in the largely homophobic conservative press.

Taking advantage of the new atmosphere, a hitherto inconceivable study was carried out by the Soviet Center for Study of the Public Opinion on the subject of homosexuality amongst Soviet citizens in different Republics of the Union. The results spoke for themselves. Homophobia was prevalent throughout the Soviet Union: 64.4 percent of those interviewed showed strong hostility towards homosexuals. When asked what should be done with homosexuals, 33.7 percent stated that they should be killed (or "liquidated," to use the Stalinist term), 30.7 percent said homosexuals should be "isolated from the rest of society," referring to prisons or psychiatric asylums. Another 10.1 percent said they should be "left to themselves," and 6.4 percent said that they should be given "help." Also, as David Schluter rightly underlines, 19.5 percent of people interviewed, or one person in five, chose not to reply (answering "it's difficult to say"). With approximately one out of every three Soviet citizens wishing homosexuals dead, stigmatization was an immense problem (Schluter 2002).

Homophobic prejudices were aggravated by the arrival of HIV/AIDS—*Sindrom Priobretennao Immunodefista* (SPID) in Russian. In 1985, Nikolai Burgasov, the Deputy Minister of Health, declared that "any great increase in HIV/AIDS infection rates is impossible in the Soviet Union as homosexuality is severely punished by our Criminal Law Code" (Burgasov 1986). Despite the familiar echo of AIDS exceptionalism in which government ministers the world over scoffed at the idea of an HIV epidemic in their countries because of the supposed superior moral fiber of their populations, the comment is an extraordinary expression of faith in the State's power to control sexual behavior through law enforcement.

Meanwhile, the policies put in place by the Soviet authorities to fight HIV/AIDS were so vaguely expressed that they allowed blood tests and other proceedings to be forced upon all those suspected of homosexual acts (Atlani-Duault 2005, 2007c). Attempting to take advantage of glasnost, some Soviet doctors and intellectuals tried to protest against this situation and demand the decriminalization of sodomy, but without success (Podkolodny 1989). Attempts to encourage voluntary HIV testing were undermined by the underlying repressive atmosphere, social ostracism, and breaches of confidentiality in the testing process. Soviets engaged in homosexual practices had numerous grounds to fear compulsory HIV testing given that they were almost certain to meet with hostility and stigmatization. Those diagnosed as HIV positive, not surprisingly, were hesitant to reveal their sexual orientation.

A Soviet activist, Roman Kalinin, tells how the address book belonging to the HIV-positive "VK" was confiscated by police. VK's acquaintances were forced to undergo HIV tests, then kept under surveillance by the police and the KGB. They were also victims of blackmail and threatened with public exposure. Under these circumstances the relatively low number of HIV cases attributed to homosexual transmission during the 1990s suggests a serious underestimate (Mikkelsen 1996).

In spite of the violence of the legal repression and rampant homophobia, the relative tolerance characterizing the last years of the Soviet Union led to the creation of the first Soviet homosexual movement in Russia: the Sexual Minorities Association. Founded at the end of 1989, the movement was described as "a human rights organization dedicated to obtaining the complete equality of people of different sexual orientations" (Kon 1995: 252). In its first campaign the organization used the government-owned media to request the withdrawal of Article 121 and to bring about a change in public attitudes towards sexual minorities as well as the country's approach to responding to the HIV/AIDS epidemic. The organization demanded that discriminatory statutes be revoked and that an amnesty be declared for all those condemned under it.

The Sexual Minorities Association quickly split into two groups as a result of internal divisions in 1990. The most radical group, which received the most media attention, was the *Osvobozhdenie* (Freedom) Union. The group's leaders were the highly visible Roman Kalinin and Yevgenia Debryanskaya. The second group, ARGO (*Assotsiatsiya za Ravnopravie Gomosexualistov*—the Asssociation for Equal Rights for Homosexuals), chose a less confrontational route, concentrating its efforts on legal reforms and fighting homophobia through dialogue and lobbying. In Leningrad two further groups were created: the "Tchaikovsky Fund for the Defence of Cultural Initiatives and Assistance to Sexual Minorities," close to the Moscow Union; and the association *Kryla* (first called *Nevskie Berega*, then *Nevskaya Perspektiva*), which was close to the positions of ARGO. Slowly but surely, associations were also set up in other Russian cities, such as Nizhny Tagil, Barnaul, Kaluga, Murmansk, Rostov, and Tomsk, as well as in Ukraine, Byelorussia, and the Baltic States.

However, while the relaxation of laws under glasnost led to the creation of associative homosexual movements in the northern part of the Soviet Union, this was not the case in Central Asia. Indeed, this region was kept under an iron rule by the First Secretaries of the Communist Party in power in each republic, and the relative freedom experienced in the European expanses of the Union did not spread to Central Asia. In this region organized homosexual advocacy groups were still subject to severe repression by the government.

1991 AND THE INDEPENDENCE OF CENTRAL ASIAN REPUBLICS

In 1991 the collapse of the Soviet Union led to the independence of the Central Asian countries of Kazakhstan, Kyrgyzstan, Tajikistan, Turkmenistan, and Uzbekistan. The peoples of Central Asia, who during Soviet times identified with one of the great world powers and enjoyed a relatively high standard of living, found themselves with a new nationality (Kazakh, Kyrgyz, Tajik, Turkmen, or Uzbek). Most experienced a radical decrease in purchasing power as the Soviet economic system was dismantled abruptly with very little to replace it (Poujol 2004). At the same time, the budgets of the new independent states were extremely limited and far inferior to the sums previously allocated to them by Moscow. State spending for education, health, housing, and pensions was drastically reduced.

Most of the Central Asian heads of state were national first secretaries of the Communist Party before 1991 and became presidents of their respective republics either through a vote of the old regime's parliaments in single-candidate elections or through a truly "Soviet" electoral performance like Saparmurat Niazov's 1992 victory in Turkmenistan with 99.5 percent of all votes (Mandrillon 1993). The next decade saw strong personalization of presidential power. Niazov, for example, organized a referendum in 1994 that allowed him to remain in power for five more years, and then in 1999 arranged to be elected Turkmenistan's "President for Life" through a "consultation of the people" (Khal Maslahaty). Similar strategies were used by the Kazakh President Nursultan Nazerbaev in 1995, Tajikistan's President Emomali Rakhmonov in 1999 and 2003, and President

Islam Karimov of Uzbekistan in 1995 and 2002.

International development organizations arrived in Central Asia as the republics became independent. Previously, the region was an almost inaccessible slice of Soviet territory. They came at the request of the region's governments, who wished to tap into the ample resources of these agencies that they hoped would compensate for the loss of direct funding from the central Soviet administration.

They discovered, somewhat to their surprise, that one of the international aid organizations' priorities was to prevent HIV/AIDS as the epidemic exploded in Central Asia just a few years after independence. Currently, Uzbekistan and Kazakhstan have the highest rates of HIV and AIDS in Central Asia—7,757 and 5,440 cases respectively as of December 2005 (UNODC 2005a and b, UNAIDS 2006). The epidemic is less serious in Kyrgyzstan and Tajikistan for the moment, with only 807 and 506 reported cases of HIV infection respectively at the same date. Turkmenistan is a special case: it is impossible to find reliable data on the prevalence of HIV within its borders as public discussion of tuberculosis, dysentery, cholera, hepatitis, and AIDS is forbidden in the country since May 2004. Officially, these diseases do not exist (Anonymous 2003; Rechel and McKee 2005).

Care must be taken when citing official data as real infection rates are probably higher than those declared. The United States Centers for Disease Control suggested in their 2002 estimates that these figures should be multiplied by at least ten to approach the true rate of infection. Perhaps more important than the absolute numbers of infected persons is the explosive increase in HIV incidence (new infections) in Central Asia. For example, Kazakh official statistics show a 238 percent rise in the rate of infection between 2000 and 2001 (CDC/CAR 2002). Real rates of infection are almost certainly higher (Atlani-Duault 2007b).

From the beginning the principal driver of the spread of HIV in the region has been injection drug use (Atlani 1998, 2002; Atlani et al. 2000; Atlani-Duault 2007a, 2007b). Opiates are easily accessible thanks to the proximity to Afghanistan. However, international aid organizations aimed to tackle all possible means of infection, and some of them decided to concentrate on HIV infection among men who have sex with men. Part of their strategy included imposing certain conditions on the distribution of aid in the HIV prevention field. The transfer of funds to Central Asian governments became contingent on the reform of legislation pertaining to homosexuality and on the legalization of local "blue" advocates' groups. When possible, international development workers negotiated changes in Soviet-era legislation on homosexuality before releasing financial aid (Atlani-Duault 2007b).

This pressure had a considerable effect. Three of the five Central Asian Republics—Kazakhstan in 1997, followed by Kyrgyzstan and Tajikistan in 1998—have since decriminalized homosexuality. While the reform was a veritable breath of fresh air in Kazakhstan and Kyrgyzstan, in Tajikistan the change seems merely cosmetic. As for Uzbekistan and Turkmenistan, legal repression is still the norm. Article 120 of the new Uzbek Criminal Code passed in 1995 still allows for sodomy to be punished by three years' imprisonment. In Turkmenistan the law is unclear. The country adopted a new Criminal Code in 1997, but it is impossible to know whether the article making homosexuality a criminal offense was removed from the final document signed by the President.

Once homosexuality was decriminalized in Kazakhstan and Kyrgyzstan, the next step was for active homosexual advocacy groups to register as local NGOs (nongovernmental organizations). This was important because it is very difficult for any non-profit group to obtain official recognition in Central Asia today. Without such registration an NGO cannot receive financial and technical aid from overseas entities. These registered groups were provided some limited financial assistance and training in lobbying, advocacy, marketing, fundraising, and management techniques.

Today, three "blue" NGOs are active in Kazakhstan: one in the city of Almaty and two in the capital of Karaganda, founded in

1997 and 2001 respectively. Encouraged by international donors, they regularly launch campaigns to inform their members of their rights and how to prevent HIV infection. Anonymous and free services are also available: a helpline, psychological support, legal advice, and medical assistance for those with sexually transmitted diseases and HIV/AIDS. In the Kyrgyz capital of Bishkek, an NGO was recognized in 1997 after two years of unofficial existence. First registered as a young people's association to deal with HIV/AIDS, it also works for homosexual rights and has set up information and help lines. Members regularly lobby with reporters and editors to stimulate sympathetic media coverage. They also organize training sessions for policemen, prison guards, and religious groups to promote tolerance and understanding.

Kyrgyz *goluboi* advocates also have attempted to set up activities in provincial areas of Osh and Issyk Kul by training volunteers. They also set up the capital's first "blue" discotheque and nightclub, whose profits support the work of the association. This independence means the association is free to engage in a broad menu of activities, a rare freedom compared to the other associations of the region. Despite the permanent uncertainties it faces, the Kyrgyz association is at least able to withstand the irregularity of project support from international sources and the hostility of mostly homophobic state structures.

However, even in those countries where the law has changed and NGOs are active, discrimination against homosexuals is still strong. In 1998 a study of one hundred men claiming to have sexual relations with other men was carried out in the capital of Kyrgyzstan. Ninety-two percent of the respondents mentioned the homophobic environment. Out of respect for their families and for fear of discrimination, sexual contacts between men were described as limited to closed groups of friends and pursued with extreme care. According to the study, 47 percent of those interviewed were married or in a stable relationship with a woman.

With no really safe meeting places, some areas in large towns or cities have come to be identified as locations for homosexual meetings (*pleshka* in Russian slang). Often, these spots are just stretches of roads with heavy pedestrian traffic, such as a park or square, public toilets, a subway station or bus stops. Hammams and public baths (*banyas*) are very popular, as well as certain cafés and restaurants in large towns. Private apartments and *dachas* are also used as meeting places. A recent phenomenon, the internet, is becoming more and more popular as a means of meeting and talking to other *goluboi*. Meeting on the internet is seen as safer than hanging around areas that are obviously known to the police.[6] Many homosexual men in the region receive anonymous death threats and, if violence follows, the attacks are carried out under the nearly indifferent gaze of the forces of law and order. The region's homosexually active men in the region are generally ill-informed as to their rights, and many in Kyrgyzstan, Kazakhstan and Tajikistan do not know that homosexuality has been decriminalized in their countries. Police sometimes contribute to the confusion and in fact may be unaware of the changes.

The most violent form of discrimination is harassment by the forces of law and order. Often, they rely on the threat of persecution (under Article 121 in those countries where this article is still in force or under laws relating to any other crime such as the "hooliganism" charges popular during the Soviet period) to utilize violence or to extort written confessions. These confessions are then regularly used to obtain bribes and denunciations. If suspects refuse, they can expect prison, where more violence, including violence of a sexual nature, awaits them.

Just as during the Soviet period, persecution can take a political form, such as the case of Ruslan Shapirov. A homosexual Uzbek journalist and the leader of an association defending press freedoms, he was arrested in 2003 after publishing a series of articles denouncing human rights abuses in Uzbekistan. Accused of sodomy and pedophilia, he confessed to these crimes under torture and after death threats. His lawyer, Surat Ikramov, was kidnapped and beaten on his way to a meeting to organize Shapirov's defense. Shapirov was sentenced to five and a half years in prison, reduced to four years on appeal. Supported by numerous international organizations such as Human Rights Watch, Amnesty International, and Reporters Without Borders, Shapirov managed to escape from prison in 2004 and has since obtained political refugee status in the United States.

Given this grim environment, it is hardly surprising that Central Asian homosexuals have difficulty identifying with a "gay community." Indeed, any group identification is almost always considered too dangerous for their personal security and for the security of their families. Beyond this refusal to identify with a group, the very fact of belonging to an NGO fighting for homosexuals' rights can be dangerous. While admirable for the strength and courage of their members, associations fighting for homosexual rights in Central Asia remain subject to strict governmental controls, and members can easily be targeted. For example, at the end of the 1990s volunteers from a now defunct association carried out a small study on the subject of homosexuality in one Central Asian country. Following this research, an extremely hostile article was published in a local newspaper including information gathered during the interviews that should have remained anonymous. Not only did the people targeted become victims of physical and mental harassment, but the organization lost credibility among local homosexual men, who were further discouraged from any form of group activity.

In another incident in 2002 in Kyrgyzstan, three young homosexual men who had volunteered in one of the "blue" NGOs were suspected by the police of murdering another man, also homosexual. Despite the fact that there was no proof against them (Vand der Veur 2004), they were convicted and sentenced to fourteen to fifteen years in prison. Favorable evidence was suppressed, as defense witnesses were considered unreliable due to their sexual orientation. One of the accused has contracted tuberculosis in prison and is in poor health.

CONCLUSION

As this chronological analysis shows, history weighs particularly heavily on the *goluboi* of Central Asia. Although largely unaware of it, the international actors nonetheless provoked significant social change. Their actions were driven by the powerful notion that the defense of sexual minorities was a key link in the fight against HIV/AIDS. While this double "motor" largely ignored the cultural specificities of the populations they were aiding, it was bold enough to effect the changes desired by their local partners, e.g., the decriminalization of homosexuality in some countries or the legalization of local "blue" NGOs.

However, the weight of history has been particularly striking in recent years. While there was a (very) relative "breathing space" during the previous decade partly due to HIV/AIDS, the conditions facing Central Asian homosexuals today are unenviable. In the 1990s their efforts coincided with the tentative opening up of governments following independence and the influence of international agencies pursuing their HIV/AIDS agenda.

Today, after the "colored revolutions" in Georgia, Ukraine, and Kyrgyzstan, leaders of these countries have become extremely suspicious of international humanitarian aid organizations (Atlani-Duault 2007b). Consequently, strong state control of local NGOs receiving assistance from foreign sources has been stepped up. Local organizations must constantly register and re-register themselves and are subject to strict supervision by the forces of law and order. In addition, nationalist claims are more and more common, reviving the homophobic slogans of the past to attack sexual and ethnic minorities and, by implication, their foreign sponsors. The worst may be feared for the region's homosexuals, in particular for those who have had the courage to emerge and attempt to play a political role.

NOTES

1. This article draws on a recently published book, *Humanitarian Aid in Post-Soviet Countries: An Anthropological Perspective* (Routledge 2007). The themes developed in this text have also been discussed, in another perspective and to a different extent, in Atlani-Duault (2007c). I am very grateful to Rhonda Campbell, Tim Frasca, Catherine Poujol, and Andrew Wilson for their helpful comments and advice on an earlier draft of this article.
2. I will use the terms "homosexuals" and "goluboi" when discussing the Soviet Union because this is the term applied at the time. Given the paucity of solid information or direct testimony from the men themselves, it is extremely hard to determine to what extent they had an identity of themselves as "homosexuals" or, alternatively, if they had no such identity and accepted the overwhelming social view that they were perverted or mentally ill. For the purposes of the article, I will say "homosexuals" until dealing with awakening of the modern "gay" emancipation movement and the whole post-Soviet period, because by then some of the men definitely did see themselves in these terms. There remain many types of homosexual behavior in Central Asia and elsewhere that are not properly called "gay," but this is an issue too complex to address in this space.
3. A term probably derived from the Persian word *bacche*, meaning "child."
4. Almost all of those who had participated in writing the previous Family Code, or who had taken part in the debates following its introduction in the 1920s, were sent to psychiatric institutions, imprisoned, or condemned to death.
5. *Moskovsky komsomolets, komsomolskaya pravda, Sobesednik, Molodoi kommunist, Literaturnaya gazeta, Ogonyok, Argumenty y fakty, Spid-info*, amongst others.
6. According to Uzbek informers, the town of Namangan is reputed to be a place where sexual contact between (married) men and sexual contact between (married) women has been happening for generations. As an aside, this town is also considered in the rest of the country as a stronghold of radical Islam.

REFERENCES AND FURTHER READING

Aggleton, P., and Homans, H. (eds.), (1988) *Social Aspects of AIDS* (London: Falmer Press).

Aggleton, P., Hart, G., and Davies, P. (1992) *AIDS: Rights, Risk and Reason* (London: Falmer Press).

Aggleton, P., et al. (1993) "Voluntary Sector Responses to HIV and AIDS: A Framework for Analysis," in P. Aggleton, G. Hart and P. Davies (eds.), *AIDS: Facing the Second Decade* (London: Falmer Press), pp. 131–141.

Altman, D. (1994) *Power and Community: Organizational and Cultural Responses to AIDS* (London: Taylor and Francis).

Anonymous (2003) "Health and Dictatorship: Effects of Repression in Turkmenistan, *Lancet*, 361: 69–70.

Atlani, L. [*See* Atlani-Duault] (1998) "Le Sida se lève à l'Est," *Transcriptase*, 64: 20–24.

Atlani, L. (2002) "Europe de l'Est: aujourd'hui les usagers de drogues, et demain?" *Trancriptase*, 100: 10–14.

Atlani, L. [*See* Atlani-Duault] et al. (2000) 'Social Change and HIV/AIDS in the Former Soviet Union: The Making of an Epidemic,' *Social Science and Medicine*, 50: 1547–1556.

Atlani-Duault, L. (2005) *Au bonheur des autres. Anthropologie de l'aide humanitaire* (Nanterre: Société d'ethnologie).

Atlani-Duault, L. (2007a) *Humanitarian Aid in Post-Soviet Countries. An Anthropological Perspective* (London and New York: Routledge).

Atlani-Duault, L. (2007b) "Goluboi ou la difficulté d'être 'bleu'. Réflexions sur l'homosexualité en Asie centrale soviétique et post-soviétique," *Anthropologie et Sociétés*, in press.

Atlani-Duault, L. (2007c) "Sur les cendres des révolutions de couleur. Drogues et démocratisation en Asie Centrale," *Revue d'Etudes Comparatives Est-Ouest*, 38(1): 29–44.

Baer, B.J. (2002) "Russian Gays/Western Gaze." *GLQ: A Journal of Lesbian and Gay Studies* 8(4): 499–522.

Baldauf, I. (1988) *Die Knabenliebe in Mittelasien: Bacabozlik* (Berlin: Das Arabische Buch).

Bauml Duberman, M., Vicinus M. and Chauncey G. Jr. (eds.) (1989) *Hidden from History: Reclaiming a Gay and Lesbian Past* (New York: New American Library).

Burgasov, N.P. (1986) "Vystuplenie na kruglom stole," *Literaturnaya gazeta*, 7: 15.

CDC/CAR (Centers for Disease Control/Central Asia Region) (2002) "HIV and AIDS Epidemic in Central Asia." Unpublished Report.

Clements, B.A. (1973) "Emancipation through Communism: The Ideology of A.M. Kollontai," *Slavic Review*, 32(2): 323–338.

Clements, B.A. (1979) *Bolshevik Feminist: The Life of Aleksandra Kollontai* (Bloomington: Indiana University Press).

De Jong, B. (1982) "An Intolerable Kind of Moral Degeneration': Homosexuality in the Soviet Union," *Review of Socialist Law* 4: 341–357.

Dowsett, G.W. (1996) *Practicing Desire: Homosexual Sex in the Era of AIDS* (Stanford: Stanford University Press).

Durmanov, N.D. (1938) *Ugolovnoe pravo: Osobennaia chast': Prestupleniia, sostavliaiushchie perezhitki rodogo byta* (Moscow: Iuridicheskoe izd. NKIu SSSR).

Engelstein, L. (1992) *The Keys to Happiness: Sex and the Search for Modernity in Fin-de-Siècle Russia* (Ithaca: Cornell University Press).

Essig, L. (1999) *Queer in Russia: A Story of Sex, Self, and the Other* (Durham: Duke University Press).

Etkind, A. (1993) *Eros nevozmozhnovo. Istoria psikhoanaliza v Rossii* (St. Petersburg: Meduza).

Farnsworth, B. (1980) *Alexandra Kollontai. Socialism, Feminism, and the Bolchevik Revolution* (Stanford: Stanford University Press).

Gessen, M. (1994). *The Rights of Lesbians and Gay Men in the Russian Federation*, report, San Francisco: International Gay and Lesbian Human Rights Commission.

Goikhbarg, A.G. (1918) "Pervyi Kodeks Zakonov RSFST," *Proletarskaia revoliutsiia I pravo*, vol. 7.

Goldman, W. (1993) *Women, the State and Revolution: Soviet Family Policy and Social Life, 1917–1936* (Cambridge: Cambridge University Press).

Healey, D. (2001) *Homosexual Desire in Revolutionary Russia: the Regulation of Sexual and Gender Dissent* (Chicago: University of Chicago Press).

Healey, D. (2002) "Homosexual Existence and Existing Socialism: New Light on the Repression of Male Homosexuality in Stalin's Russia," *GLQ: A Journal of Lesbian and Gay Studies*, 8(3): 349–378.

Karlinsky, S. (1976) "Russia's Gay Literature and History," *Gay Sunshine* 29–30: 1–7.

Karlinsky, S. (1977) "Russia's Gay Literature. Part II: Controversy," *Gay Sunshine* 31: 25–26.

Karlinsky, S. (1989) "Russia's Gay Literature and Culture: The Impact of the October Revolution," in Martin Bauml Duberman, Martha Vicinus, and George Chauncey Jr. (eds.), *Hidden from History: Reclaiming the Gay and Lesbian Past* (New York: New American Library), pp. 348–364.

Klein, L. (2000) *Drugaia liubov* (Saint-Petersburg: Folio-press).

Kollontai, A. (1920) *La Famille et l'Etat communiste* (Paris: Bibliothèque communiste).

Kon, I.S. (1988) *Vvedenie v seksologiyu* (Moscow: Meditsina).

Kon, I.S. (1989) *Psikhologiya rannei yunosti* (Moscow: Prosveshchenie).

Kon, I.S. (1991) *Vkus zapretnovo ploda* (Moscow: Molodaya gvardia).

Kon, I.S. (1992) "Culture and Sexuality in the Former USSR," *Planned Parenthood in Europe* 21(2): 2–4.

Kon, I.S. (1995) *The Sexual Revolution in Russia* (New York: The Free Press).

Kon, I.S. (1998) *Lunnyi svet na zare* (Moscow: Olimp).

Kon, I.S. and Riordan J. (eds.) (1993) *Sex and Russian Society* (London: Pluto Press).

Lauritsen, J. and Thorstad D. (1974) *The Early Homosexual Rights Movement (1864–1935)* (New York: Times Change).

Mandrillon, M.H. (1993) "Des hommes de l'ancien régime," in Ferro M. et Mandrillon M-H., *L'Etat de Toutes Les Russies. Les Etats et les nations de l'ex-URSS* (Paris: La Découverte/IMSECO), pp. 422–423.

Mann, J.M., Tarantola, D.J.M., and Netter, T.W. (eds.) (1995) *AIDS in the World* (Cambridge: Harvard University Press).

Mikkelsen, H. (1996) "Men who Have Sex with Men in the Former USSR," in UNAIDS report, Geneva, unpublished.

Naiman, E. (1997) *Sex in Public: The Incarnation of Early Soviet Ideology* (Princeton: Princeton University Press).

Oostvogels, R. (1997) *Assessment of Men Who Have Sex with Men in Bishkek* (Geneva: World Health Organization), report.

Pahlen, K.K. (1964) *Mission to Turkestan* (London: Oxford University Press).

Parker, R. (1996) "Empowerment, Community Mobilization and Social Change in the Face of HIV/AIDS," *AIDS*, 10 (Sup. 3): S27–S31.

Podkolodny, F. (1989) "The Sin of Sodomy in the Soviet Union," *Journal of Sex Research* 26(4): 549–552.

Poujol, C. (2004) "How Can We Use the Concept of Transition in Central Asian Post-Soviet History? An Attempt to Set a New Approach," in CIMERA (eds.), *The Illusions of Transition: Which Perspectives for Central Asia and the Caucasus?* (Geneva: PSIO/IUHEI).

Rechel, B. and McKee, M. (2005) *Human Rights and Health in Turkmenistan*, London: London School of Hygiene and Tropical Medicine.

Rotikov, K. (1998) *Drugoi Peterburg* (St. Petersburg: Liga Plius).

Schluter, D.P. (2002) *Gay Life in the Former USSR* (New York: Routledge).

Schuyler, E. (1876) *Turkistan: Notes of a Journey in Russian Turkistan, Khokand, Bukhara and Kuldja* (London: Sampson, Low, Marston, Searle and Rivington).

Stuchka, P. (ed.) (1925–1927) *Entsiklopediia gosudarstva i prava* (Izdatel'stvo kommunisticheskoi Akademii).

Tuller, D. (1996) *Cracks in the Iron Closet: Travels in Gay and Lesbian Russia* (Boston: Faber and Faber).

UNAIDS (2006) *Report on the Global AIDS Epidemic.*

UNODC (2005a) "HIV/AIDS midpoint estimates" report: unpublished.

UNODC (2005b) "The Opium Economy in Afghanistan. An International Problem", report: unpublished.

Vand der Veur, D. (2004) *The Country of Human Rights . . . But Not for Homosexuals*. Report.

CHAPTER 8

"African Sexualities" Revisited

The Morality of Sexuality and Gender in the Era of Globalization and AIDS in Tanzania

Hansjörg Dilger

ABSTRACT

This chapter provides a brief overview of the literature and media reports that in the late 1980s and early 1990s shaped discussions on "Sexuality in Africa" in the international arena. This is followed by a description of the sexuality of young people in the rural Mara Region of Tanzania and of the multiple meanings and practices that shape the sexualities of women and men in the context of marriage and kinship dynamics. The chapter then summarizes how sexuality in Africa is imagined by internationally driven AIDS campaigns, and how this fits with the cultural, political, economic, and moral processes that shape the construction of sexualities in specific regions of sub-Saharan Africa.

CONSTRUCTING SEXUALITY IN AN EPIDEMIC OF SIGNIFICATION

As early as 1988, Paula Treichler stated that HIV/AIDS had become an "epidemic of signification" in the U.S.[1] Meanings and metaphors attached to the disease, and to the social and sexual behaviors that were understood to be the cause of HIV infection, had become the essential way U.S. society not only situated the epidemic in its specific historical and cultural settings, but also to a significant degree the way individual and collective responses to the multiple challenges associated with the disease were shaped.

Meanings attached to HIV/AIDS are the result of often contradictory and mutually entangled strategies pursued by different social actors at different societal levels. Manifesting themselves predominantly in language, meanings are created not only by the media, in the discourses of AIDS activists, by conservative religious forces or the "general public." They are also shaped by medical and health professionals who, despite their seemingly scientific and neutral stance, have often reinforced the stigmatization of those who became sick with HIV/AIDS and finally died (Treichler 1999: 19ff.).

Treichler concluded that discourses on HIV/AIDS can *never* be neutral. In contrast to Susan Sontag (1988), who called for a "demystification" and "neutralization" of U.S. society's views of HIV/AIDS, Treichler argued that illness *is* metaphor and that the process of meaning-building is essential for every society's ability to develop socially significant ways of dealing with the epidemic. Moreover, Treichler emphasized that the constructions and meanings surrounding HIV/AIDS have very real effects—on the allocation of funding for research and policymaking, as well as on the situations of those living with the disease. Consequently, she argued that the importance of the social dimension of HIV/AIDS should not be denied in the development of social policies, as this dimension is "far more pervasive than we are accustomed to believe" (Treichler 1999: 15).

Looking at the topic of "AIDS in Africa,"

we find that the process of meaning-building has been even more pervasive than it has been for AIDS in the Western context. While "sexuality in Africa" and "sex with Africans" have always evoked multiple associations in Western societies (Gilman 1985), the HIV/AIDS epidemic highlighted how strongly notions of "African sexuality" are associated with the most exotic forms of human sexual behavior in the Western mind. Similar to the way stereotyped images of the male homosexual body have shaped the epidemic of signification in the U.S.A., excessive fantasies about a specific "African sexuality" represented the black body in Western discourses on AIDS in Africa as insatiable, alien, and deviant.

In Western media reports on AIDS in Africa from the 1980s we find, on the one hand, sensationalistic depictions of a dehumanized and inherently promiscuous sexuality set in brothels and other locations of "degenerate amusement." Characteristic of such a view is the report of a journalist, who in an article for *Vanity Fair* in the 1980s is confronted with the "infamous" and "promiscuous" nightlife of urban Uganda. Late into the night, he goes to a bar in Maska, which he describes as "the most degenerate scene, the closest thing to Sodom I have ever seen. Guys completely bombed, with girls on their laps, etc. Obviously nobody cares about getting AIDS" (quoted in Watney 1989: 87).

On the other hand, and apart from rampant fantasies about prostitution and the red-light districts stretching from Nairobi to Johannesburg and Dakar, the European/North American discourse on sexuality and AIDS in Africa has been fed by images of an enforced, exotic and often violent sexuality said to prevail on the continent: polygyny, female genital mutilation, and especially the (gang) rapes of women and babies in South Africa have made "sexual violence" and "child rape" the main issues for international media reports on AIDS in Africa. It is particularly disturbing, according to these reports, that the current "child rape crisis" in South Africa is driven by traditional healers, who—because of the belief that HIV/AIDS can be prevented (or even healed) through sexual intercourse with a virgin—are said to have laid the foundation for a perverted violence directed at babies and infants.[2]

Having outlined some of the issues that have figured prominently in Western media and popular discourse on sex and AIDS in Africa since the 1980s, this chapter will *not* be concerned so much with how stereotyped debates in the media have foreclosed a more differentiated discussion on crucial issues such as prostitution, child abuse, or sexual violence in African countries. This text will also *not* attempt to analyze the striking continuity that connects postcolonial fantasies about a "black African sexuality" to the discourse of colonial state powers, who in the early twentieth century decried the "immoral and uncontrollable (sexual) behaviors" said to prevail especially among African women as the cause of the spread of syphilis (Vaughan 1991: 129–154).[3]

In this chapter I want to argue that there is no such thing as a unitary or monomorphous "African sexuality," but that sexuality in Africa (as elsewhere) has to be read as "many different things depending on the contexts it is part of" (Helle-Valle 2004: 195). As Philip Setel has argued intriguingly for northwest Tanzania, sexual relationships in Eastern Africa are "[f]ar from operating in a mode of sexual chaos," but are based on differentiated ideas about the rights and values, as well as the social, moral, and material implications of these relationships. The diversity of sexuality and sexual behaviors prevailing in a specific historical and social setting, Setel argues, can consequently only be described by addressing their respective material, symbolic, and moral dimensions (1999: 141f.).

In the following sections I will draw on studies on sexuality in Africa, as well as on my own fieldwork in Tanzania, and argue that the sexual lives of women and men in Eastern Africa are shaped not only by (globally driven) political-economic processes and structural constraints such as poverty or socioeconomically produced gender hierarchies. Their sexualities must also be analyzed in light of age- and gender-specific concepts of trust, kinship, reproduction, and marriage, and finally with regard to illness and illness causation. In conclusion, I will summarize how sexuality in Eastern and

Southern Africa has been imagined by international AIDS campaigns, and how this fits together with the political, economic, and cultural-moral processes that shape the constructions of sexuality in specific regions of sub-Saharan Africa.

SEXUALITIES IN CONTEMPORARY AFRICA

Sexuality as a discrete concept came into being in post-Enlightenment Europe when the rising bourgeoisie claimed control over their sexual practices and relationships that until then had been subject to the strict regulations of an aristocratic society. As Diane Jeater (1993: 39) has described with regard to Great Britain, this process was intimately tied to newly arising ideas about physical health and sexual (ab)normality: "The idea that physical health and sexual 'normality' were inextricably linked emanated from the middle classes and grew in influence during the [nineteenth] century. Unable to claim purity of blood, being excluded from the aristocratic classes, the rising nineteenth-century bourgeoisie claimed purity of body, instead." In this newly constituted framework, married couples were granted more privacy rights. The regulation of family relations and sexual relationships were increasingly withdrawn from the bonds of kinship networks and the public sphere and became a matter of individualized responsibility. Under these circumstances, the violation of moral codes and norms (for instance, in the case of "adultery") was regarded as "immoral" and ground for a "guilty conscience." At the same time, however, the transgression of moral codes was also considered "natural" and somehow "human." It was only the *obviously* deviant sexual practices in this context—such as homosexuality or the exotic sexual practices of African men and women—that were classified as "perverse" or "diseased."

Ideas of an individualized and self-responsible sexuality as they were crafted in post-Enlightenment Europe—and which have been further transformed in the 1960s and 1970s when sexual liberation led to an increasing separation of sex from marriage, reproductive processes, and partly also from "love" (cf. Giddens 1992)—have only been of limited value for the analysis of sexuality in the often agriculture-based societies of Southern and Eastern Africa. As many recent publications on HIV/AIDS emphasized, sexual cultures in sub-Saharan Africa are strongly determined by structural constraints, insofar as urbanization, migration, structural adjustment policies, or poverty all have an important impact on gender relations and thus on the sexual lives of men and women in the region (cf. Schoepf 1992; Haram 1995; Baylies 2000). Moreover, many anthropologists argued that the sexuality of women and men in Africa has to be situated in the very broad social and cultural contexts of a group or a society as sexual behaviors and relationships depend on a wide range of sociocultural ideas and practices of kinship, gender, the person, trust, and morality (cf. Ahlberg 1994; Heald 1995; Setel 1999; Dilger 2003; Helle-Valle 2004).

That sexuality can be experienced very differently in one and the same society—and that sexualities are determined by a number of factors relating to individual agency and structural constraints—is exemplified by recent studies on HIV/AIDS in South Africa. Catherine Campbell (1997) has shown that sexual behaviors among gold-mine workers in KwaZulu Natal are embedded not only in a self-overestimating masculine identity, but also in the everyday working and living conditions in the rural mines. While the often life-threatening working conditions in the mines have created a feeling of powerlessness among the workers—compared to which HIV infection is perceived as a comparatively small problem—unsafe sex with prostitutes gives the workers a feeling of closeness and trust. In the context of the mines, where there is not much space for close social or emotional ties, this is often of considerable importance for men living far away from their families and wives/partners.[4]

Compared to the sexualities of workers in the gold mines, the ideas and practices evolving around sexual identities and lifestyles in South Africa's *urban* centers look rather different. According to Deborah Posel (2005: 130), the discourses and modes of talking about sex in the post-apartheid era have produced "a series of discrete discursive nodes, each nested in and shaped in particular ways by recent global economic positionings, national processes of class and status formation . . ., the acceleration of the AIDS epidemic, as well as the strategies and powers of new social movements." Posel identifies four discrete fields that determine the way sexuality is perceived in contemporary South Africa: First, President Thabo Mbeki's reaction to international discourses on "African AIDS" and "African sexuality," which he argued were shaped by racist and stigmatizing ideologies; second, the emergence of new social movements that draw on the state's progressive gender policies and the international human rights discourse on the freedom of sexual choice (for instance, the gay and lesbian movement); third, the introduction of neoliberal policies which have not only broadened access to consumer goods from the global economy, but have also led to the emergence of a black youth consumer culture that celebrates "sexual freedom" and is consciously breaking with the segregation policies of the apartheid state; and finally, a discourse on "romantic" and "true" love among young people according to which partners talk openly about sexuality and birth control, as well as about the protection from STDs (sexually transmitted diseases) such as HIV/AIDS.

This latter discourse on romantic and true love draws on globalized images and values, as they can also be found among other young

Exhibit 8.1 "True Love"

Uko katika
mapenzi
ya kweli?
ARE YOU TRULY IN LOVE?

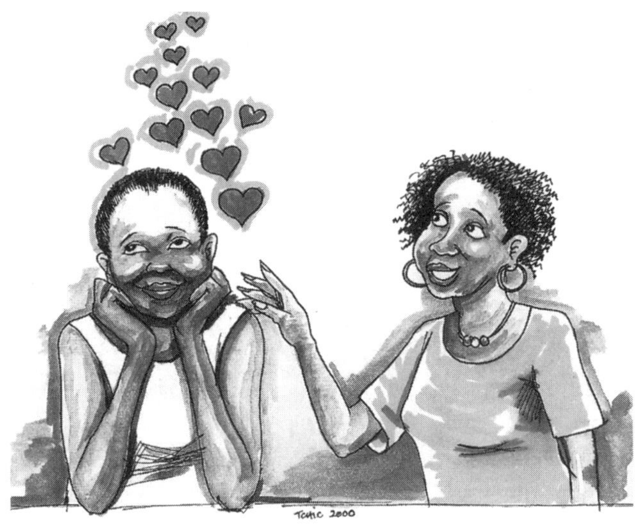

Source: Femina, February-April 2000, Dar es Salaam

Exhibit 8.2 The young couple decides—after a longer discussion—to use condoms: "Condoms protect, love doesn't," says the young woman, and her partner agrees: "It's true." Interestingly, the Kiswahili term for condom is "*buti*," which means "trunk, boot." This term fits into a wider metaphorical network that connects perceptions of sexuality and HIV/AIDS to images of technology, mobility, and modernity. In rural Tanzania, young people often told me that "AIDS is an accident on the road that cannot be avoided" (Dilger 2000).

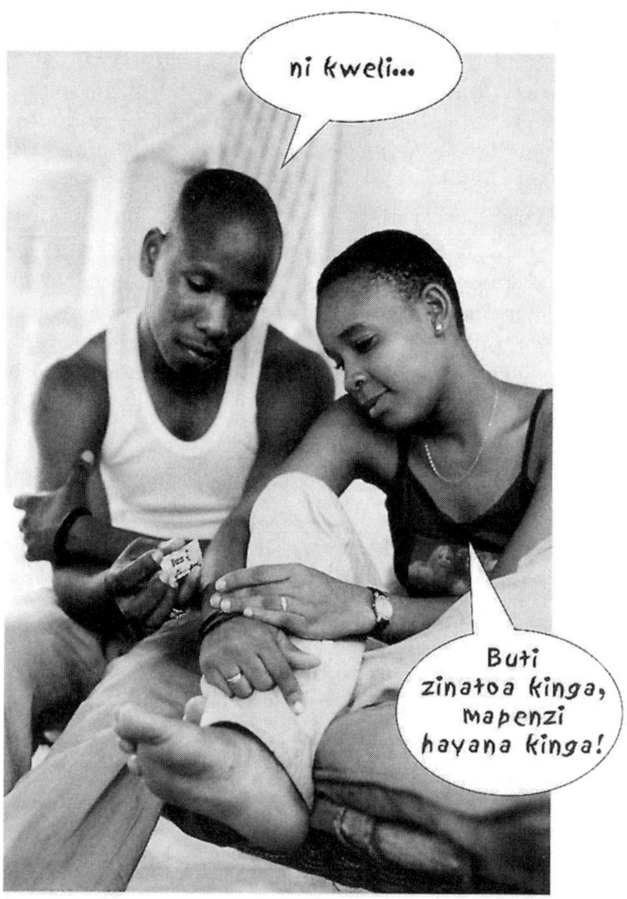

Source: Femina, February-April 2000, Dar es Salaam

people in Southern and Eastern Africa, who form part of a newly constituting urban middle class in the region. In urban Tanzania, this group of young people is sometimes called the "condom generation"—and in a broader sense it can indeed be understood as an answer to the challenges of the HIV/AIDS epidemic insofar as these young people have become the target of numerous internationally funded campaigns. "True love," (Exhibit 8.1) as discussed and promoted by advice columns and picture stories run by fashionable, lifestyle magazines like *Femina*,[5] is based not solely on sexual attraction or satisfaction, but rather on values like friendship, loyalty, trust, respect, and finally tenderness (*Femina* 2000: 20). The use of condoms in this context is seen by both partners not as a sign of "lack of trust" (Dilger 2003: 39–41) but as an expression of mutual esteem and of acknowledging responsibility for the partner's health (Exhibit 8.2). That this implies an acknowledgment of responsibility to one's self for one's *own* health—and that safe sex can therefore be "cool" (Posel 2005: 133)—is expressed in the statement by 22-year-old Shaban, the male character in a picture story in *Femina* (2000: 25). He says,

"If you want to be a winner in the game of love and pleasure, you have to go for condoms."

SEXUALITIES IN RURAL TANZANIA

Discourses concerning "true love" (Kiswahili: *mapenzi ya kweli*) and "mutual trust" (*kuaminiana*) are also quite popular among unmarried young men and women in rural Tanzania. My field studies in Northwestern Tanzania showed, however, that young people there only rarely used condoms for protection against HIV/AIDS or other STDs.[6] The young people I interviewed during my research were between 16 and 23 years old and had mostly finished their primary education, and some had completed, or were still attending, secondary school—often in a region far from their home villages. Those who had finished their primary schooling were working as farmers or fishermen or, as in the case of most of the young women, they were engaged in some kind of small-scale trade or business.

The majority of the young men and women I talked to were highly aware of HIV/AIDS and how to avoid HIV infection. However, only very few of them thought that HIV/AIDS (or any other STD) presented a *personal* threat. Young men, in particular, described the use of condoms as lust-hindering. Furthermore, many of them told me that among male peers impregnating a girl is a sign of virility and "honor" (*sifa*). Babu, a 21-year-old fisherman, said:

> If [a boy] has made a girl pregnant he will see that he is a real man who is doing real work.

Young women, on the other hand, were not merely passive victims of their partners—many of them expressed very similar disinclinations towards condoms as their male counterparts. As Adoyo, an 18-year-old seamstress, put it:

> A girl or a woman feels happier than about anything else in this world when a man ejaculates into her and when she receives the man's sperm. But if you use a condom you cannot feel good.

Most of the young people I interviewed felt that it was morally contemptible to insist on the use of condoms, especially in more stable relationships. An important issue in this discourse is the gift-giving that young men are "traditionally" supposed to engage in with their female partners. Both sexes agreed that such presents are an important and desirable part of sexual relationships; however, they also said that there was a very thin boundary between presents given as an expression of "love" and presents given as "payment" (*malipo*). Young men, in particular, were often convinced that *because of* their presents they had the right to make *all* decisions in a sexual relationship. Manuel, a 23-year-old fisherman, said:

> Let's just say you've given money to a girl. Now it is up to you, the boy, if you want the condom or not. Because now you will talk about *money* and not about *love*. (Emphasis added)

Young women, on the other hand, found themselves in a dilemma. Fearing that their boyfriends could take them for "prostitutes" (*malaya*), they didn't want to appear too demanding—neither with regard to presents nor the use of condoms. While my female interviewees were often afraid of HIV infection (and even more so of an unwanted pregnancy, which they perceived as an even greater threat), all of them associated condom use with "immoral behavior" and did not consider their use an important means of health protection.

As a result of these various gender-specific conflicts, young women and men in Mara designated "trust in their partner" as the most effective way to protect themselves from HIV infection. This trust was often based on the partner's perceived lifestyle and physical health. As Tembo, a 21-year-old secondary school student put it:

> I trusted [my girlfriend] because of her character. We were in the same school and she was somehow different from her friends. *They* want money from you and then you go with them. But my girlfriend wanted no money. She said that she loved me with her heart. (Emphasis added)

Exhibit 8.3 Brochure on premarital HIV-testing in Tanzania that plays on the idea of "testing love" by means of modern technology

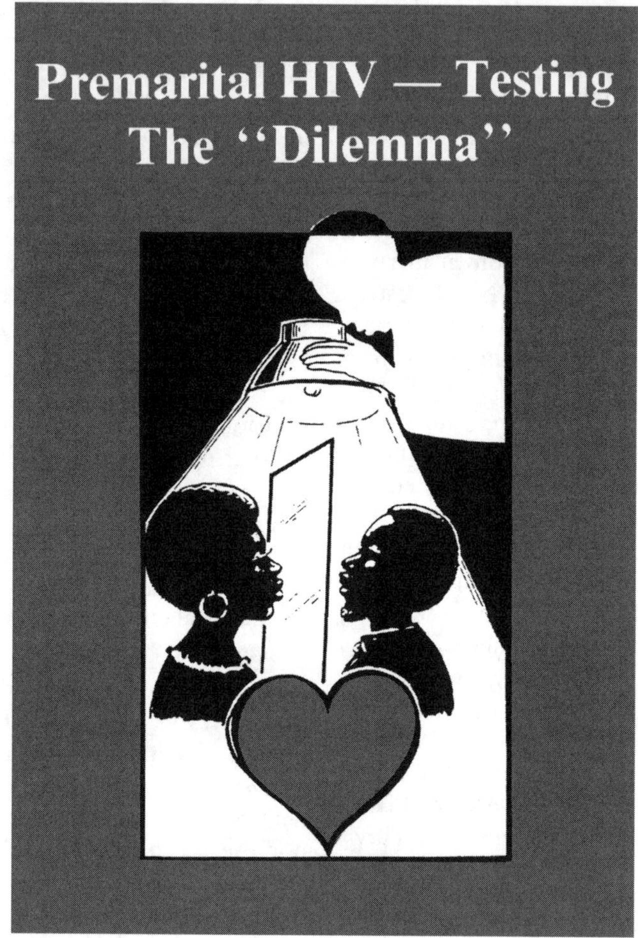

Source: Ministry of Health, National AIDS Control Programme, Tanzania

On the other hand, many youths were aware that they put their "trust in love" over their "trust in health." Consequently, some called their readiness to trust a "belief of darkness" (*imani ya giza*), or a "deceptive belief" (*imani ya uongo*). Juma (male, 23) shared these doubts; yet, paradoxically, "trust" was his primary criterion for protecting himself against HIV, and he called for a "microscope for testing trust" without even mentioning the medical testing facilities at the local hospital:

> The trust we have is based on our words. If we had a microscope for mutually testing our trust then we could have certainty. . . . You sleep with a girl and then she tells you "You are the only one." But the next day you meet her with another boy. This is a deceptive belief and it is not real.

Kinship, Fertility, and Reproduction

Conflicts resulting from divergent perceptions of trust or protection against HIV may also play an important role among *married* partners. At the same time, however, sexuality in a marriage is embedded—even more so than in the case of unmarried youths—in a cultural praxis of fertility and reproduction, which is not only an individual matter concerning the married couple but may also involve their extended families.[7]

A "functioning marriage" in rural Tanzania means, on one hand, that it is a "fertile" relationship, i.e., that it bears offspring. As

Ute Luig (1997: 251) has argued for Zambia, children in African agricultural societies are often factors in power relations. Children are not only important for increasing the numerical size of a lineage; human labor is also the most important condition for agricultural work. Finally, children are held responsible for the care of elderly parents and for maintaining relations with the family's ancestors. Thus a large number of offspring is the basic precondition for the *material* as well as the *spiritual* survival of a lineage. In this context, the use of condoms is a delicate issue, as it is diametrically opposed to these core values of social, spiritual, and physical reproduction.

On the other hand, a marriage in rural Mara is thought to function well if married partners uphold the numerous ritual prescriptions regulating sexual behavior in crucial phases of life—for example, on the occasions of birth, death, farming, and other matters of domestic reproduction. The observance of these prescriptions is of elementary importance as negligence may result in an illness named *chira*. *Chira* (pronounced "tshira") may affect not only the married couple but often also their children or—if their children are already grown up—*their* respective partners and offspring. Thus, if the potentially lethal *chira* is not treated with a specific herbal medicine (Dholuo: *manyasi*), it may lead to illness and death of whole families. The flipside of this is, however, that the correct observance of ritual prescriptions is vitally important for a lineage's continuity and success in daily life.

The existence of ritual prescriptions for sexual behavior by no means implies that all lineage or community members in rural Mara observe these restrictions *at all times*. On the contrary, the *negligence* and ignorance of ritual prescriptions concerning sexuality have become an integral part of contemporary life in the region, which is marked by mobility, outward migration, and increasingly individualized lifestyles. Ritual prescriptions *do* become the subject of individual and familial discussions, however, when a young man or woman becomes gravely sick and the family starts searching for the causes of his or her illness. Especially if the illness is suspected to be HIV/AIDS-related, the probability that it is *also* related to *chira*—a wasting disease very similar to HIV/AIDS in its symptoms—is high (Dilger 2005: 144ff., 2006).

The close connection people in Mara make between HIV/AIDS and *chira* makes clear how strongly marital sexuality is embedded in wider social and kin relations. Ritual prescriptions associated with *chira* refer to *prohibitions* on sexual intercourse during burial festivities, the mourning period, pregnancy, menstruation, and the breastfeeding period. On the other hand, there are specific *prescriptions* for periods in which it is of vital importance to have sexual intercourse in order to avoid *chira*. The latter apply mainly to the formal ending of mourning periods, agricultural work, house-building, or the move into a new home. In the case of farming activities, for instance, my interviewees said that the owner of a compound must have sexual intercourse with his first wife before he can start harvesting or sowing. Only then should grown-up sons, who are married but have not yet founded their own compound, have intercourse with their wives and start farming.[8]

If a young man or woman in Mara gets sick today and cannot be successfully treated at the local hospital, his or her family is very likely to suspect that he or she might be infected with HIV. Moreover, the search for treatment will often give rise to far-reaching family discussions on whether the illness was possibly caused by *chira*, and what specific violations of traditional requirements have occurred. In these debates, which often spread throughout the rural communities via rumors and gossip (cf. Dilger 2005: 309ff.), *who* had sex with *whom* and *on what occasion* (and, often even more importantly, who did *not*) are not the only issues. Changes in kinship relations may also become the subject of intense debate, as they are often seen as the deeper cause for the non-observance of sexual prescriptions and prohibitions leading to *chira*. Rural–urban migration and the sometimes long absences of husbands and wives from their respective compounds have rendered almost impossible the observance of *all* sexual prescriptions and prohibitions that would have helped to avoid *chira*.

OUTLOOK: FROM "AFRICAN SEXUALITY" TO SEXUAL DIVERSITY IN AFRICA

The story of "Sexuality and HIV/AIDS in Africa" has been written by a variety of actors, including politicians, the media, health professionals, international development organizations, and, most importantly, communities. In particular, this story has drawn on images and fantasies that have their origin in a colonial past and that were for many years perpetuated even by academic writings.[9]

In this chapter I have emphasized that sexualities in Africa can take very different shapes and are experienced in very different ways—depending on locality (especially rural/urban), gender, age, educational, and cultural background, and an individual's marital status. In conclusion, I would like to argue that the diversity of sexualities cannot be adequately addressed by the uniform ABC campaigns that have become very popular throughout the region. A basic problem of these campaigns is that the message "**A**bstain, **B**e Faithful, or Use **C**ondoms" is based on Westernized notions of sexuality, gender, and health (prevention) that are often contradictory to the structural conditions as well as to the social and cultural processes that have shaped everyday life in African communities over the last decades. With the ongoing processes of globalization and Westernization, sexual behaviors and identities in Africa have admittedly become subject to processes of individualization and "self-fashioning" (cf. Foucault 1990). Particularly, the many NGOs (nongovernmental organizations) that have mushroomed in Southern and Eastern Africa over the last few years have presented sexuality as a "site of rational, individual choice and agency—an opportunity for empowerment and 'healthy positive living'" (Posel 2005: 134). What the ABC approach tends to neglect, however, is that, while decisions concerning sexuality may often be individual, they are more often than not also embedded in the wider social, economic, and political relationships that shape daily life in contemporary Africa.

That sexual decisions in Southern and Eastern Africa are not always made individually or as a result of a consensual agreement between equal sex partners—and that HIV/AIDS prevention in Africa is thus not "as easy as ABC" (Heald 2002)—is obvious in those social contexts that are shaped by excessive poverty, prostitution, or comprehensive violence (e.g., in civil wars). Furthermore, however, the close connection between sexual decisions and acts and the social and cultural context has become visible in the empirical example from rural Mara. Young men and women are not only confronted with almost insurmountable dilemmas and conflicts that challenge their sexual decisions with regard to issues of trust, honor, shame, and, not least, the morality of economics. Marital sexuality is also shaped by concepts of fertility and reproduction, and in its association with *chira* is subject to very strict moral obligations and prescriptions embedded in the wider social and kinship relations. In this latter regard, sexuality in Mara has become ambivalent, as it is not only the *precondition* for physical and social continuity; at the same time, it is *dangerous*, as the nonobservance of ritual prescriptions may lead to illness and even death (cf. Heald 1995). All these ideas and practices—that may *all* become part of the sexual lives of women and men in and from Mara over their lifetime—have become uncertain in the era of AIDS and globalization, and often also loaded with fear.

To conclude, I would argue that future HIV/AIDS prevention campaigns should pay closer attention to the diverse social and cultural contexts that shape sexualities in Southern and Eastern Africa and that may lead to contradictions and conflicts in sexual decision-making, which have to be resolved by individual actors in flexible, and sometimes also non-consistent, ways (Helle-Valle 2004; Dilger 2003: 45f.). A particular challenge for future HIV/AIDS work will be to understand how different modes of sexuality are being shaped and transformed by processes of globalization and by international AIDS programs, including the abstinence and anti-abortion programs that are currently promoted by the U.S. Presidential Emergency Plan for AIDS Relief (PEPFAR). While the

Exhibit 8.4 HIV/AIDS poster showing a woman who insists—despite the presents that she is offered by her partner—on "safe sex." She says: "I don't sell my body for *pochi*! Let's use a condom."[10]

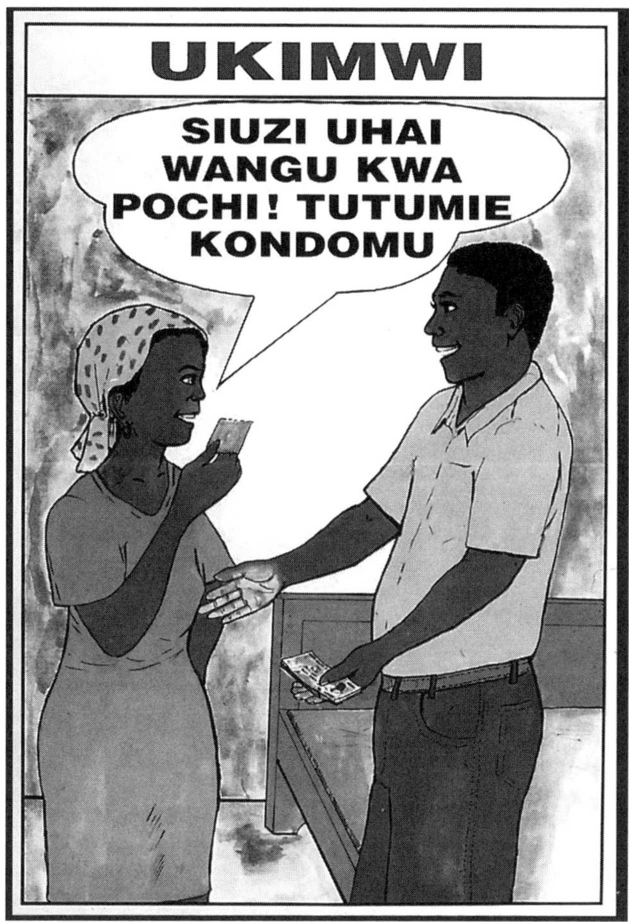

Source: AMREF, GTZ and other development organizations

heavily funded PEPFAR initiative may find strong support from Pentecostal and other rapidly growing fundamentalist movements in sub-Saharan Africa (cf., Dilger 2007), it will also represent a sharp contradiction to other AIDS programs in the region that have been established by other international actors and that promoted comprehensive sex education and condom distribution as major strategies for prevention. Second, the issue of "masculinity" and "male sexuality" in prevention and care programs should be more thoroughly addressed. Over the last few years it has been emphasized that culturally shaped ideals and expectations of masculinity put young men under increasing sexual pressure, thus making them more vulnerable to HIV infection. Men do not represent only "the problem" in the epidemic; they often live within a gender structure of male cultural and socioeconomic privilege which can also be disadvantageous—not least with regard to their health (Baylies 2000).

Finally, the discussion of sexuality and HIV/AIDS in Africa requires a more critical reflection on the discourses, images, and fantasies that have shaped perceptions of "African sexuality" in the context of international development work. It is true that poverty, prostitution, and gender-specific violence have become part of how sexuality is experienced and lived in contemporary Africa and elsewhere. However, in order to arrive at a more differentiated way of dealing

Exhibit 8.5 Poster advocating that closer communication between parents and their children could help young people to resolve conflicts related to sexuality and HIV/AIDS: "If parents don't talk with us about sex, who will?"[11] In addition, the poster's imagery addresses the more general conflicts facing young women and men in Tanzania in everyday life—conflicts that result from tightly interwoven tensions between tradition and modernity, the local and the global, village and town life, older and younger generations.

Wazazi wasipoongea nasi kuhusu kujamiiana nani atafanya hivyo?
If parents don't talk with us about sex, who will?

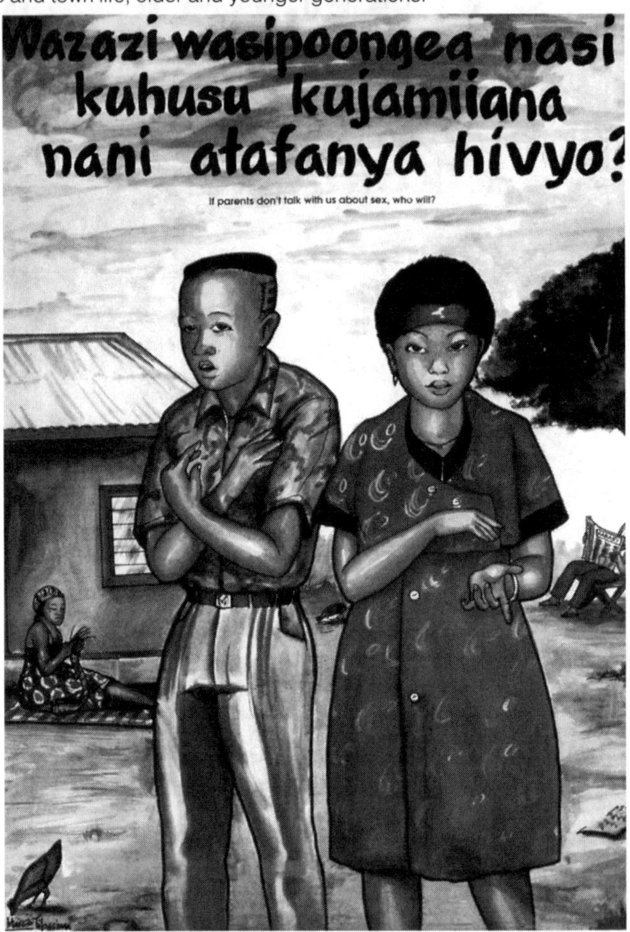

Source: Kuleana, Mwanza

with sexualities on the continent—and in order to adapt HIV/AIDS prevention efforts to the social and historical contexts in which they take place—it is necessary to acknowledge the close relationship that exists between sexual ideas, behaviors, and identities, and the social, economic, and cultural settings from which they emerge. While detailed ethnographic research on sexuality may be time-consuming and also "embarrassing" for researcher and respondents, it is essential so that "our ideas about our own and others' sexual behavior will [no longer] continue to be based more on impressions, images and prejudices than on facts" (Sabatier 1988: 75). In the words of Paula Treichler (1999: 39), we need an "epidemiology of meaning"—a "comprehensive mapping and analysis of [the] multiple meanings" that have become the basis for the formulation of policies in the realm of sex education and prevention in Africa.

NOTES

1. Treichler (1988). A revised version of the text was published in the reader *How to Have Theory in an Epidemic: Cultural Chronicles of HIV* (Treichler 1999). Throughout this text I refer to the revised version.
2. http://archives.cnn.com/2001/WORLD/africa/11/26/safrica.rape/ http://news.bbc.co.uk/1/hi/world/

africa/1703595.stm (both accessed on September 12, 2005).

3. A good example of this revivalism of colonial categories in the context of HIV/AIDS was Princess Gloria von Thurn und Taxis, who—during a TV appearance in 2001—attributed the spread of HIV/AIDS in Africa to the fact that "the black man" simply likes "*Schnakseln*" too much (*Schnakseln*: colloquial word, in the Austrian dialect, for having sex). Also, numerous HIV/AIDS campaigns in sub-Saharan Africa did not shy away from perpetuating the colonial legacy of condemning polygynous unions and the ritual cleansing of widows through sexual intercourse as "harmful practices," thus stigmatizing them as the major "cultural barriers" for the successful prevention of HIV/AIDS in Africa (Gausset 2001: 510). For the continuities between colonial and postcolonial framings of sexuality in Africa—and for the multiple gendered fantasies, anxieties, and desires of those who produced these discourses—see Gilman (1985), Bibeau and Pedersen (2002), and Arnfred (2004).
4. In addition, in the 1930s and 1940s *same sex* relationships also played an important role in the mining context and often developed into marriage-like bonds (Moodie et al. 1990).
5. *Femina* was founded in 1999 and today 92,000 copies are printed every three months. The magazine is distributed to secondary schools and NGOs in Tanzania, and furthermore sold in the country's urban centers. It is funded by the Swedish and the Norwegian development agencies SIDA and NORAD.
6. Fieldwork in rural and urban Tanzania (Mara Region/Dar es Salaam) was carried out between 1995 and 2003. Research questions concerned gender relations, intergenerational relations and youth sexuality in the context of modernity, and at a later stage the social and familial networks of people with HIV/AIDS in the context of rural–urban migration (cf. Dilger 1999, 2003, 2005, 2006).
7. In most cases I observed, the extended families of a husband and his wife had a say not only in the choice of the respective partner, but also how the whole marriage process was organized. In addition, the husbands' families often provided part of the "brideprice" (*mahari*) given to the bride's family and therefore had a legitimate interest in the maintenance of a "functioning marriage" (Dilger 1999).
8. These prescriptions apply only to agricultural products (e.g., maize or sorghum), the sowing and harvesting of which are closely connected to periods of rain or dryness, but not to staple foods such as cassava, which is continually worked in the fields.
9. It is impossible here to discuss in detail the scholarly arguments made for a distinct "African Sexuality," which in comparison to a "Eurasian" model of sexuality was said to be characterized by loose morals, a weaker marriage bond, and the sexual liberty of African women (Caldwell et al. 1989). According to Bibeau and Pedersen (2002), these and other theories that focused on environmental and/or genetic explanations for the spread of HIV/AIDS in Africa were "a descriptive voyeuristic sightseeing tour of African sexuality, based on a highly selective (and biased) reading of the existing literature." For further critique of the "African sexuality thesis," see Ahlberg (1994), Heald (1995), and Arnfred 2004.
10. The depiction of *pochi* as a banknote is misleading: the correct translation of *pochi* is "chain bangle."
11. It should be remarked, however, that in many parts of Africa discussions of sex take place by way of preference between grandparents and grandchildren.

REFERENCES AND FURTHER READING

Ahlberg, Beth Maina. "Is There a Distinct African Sexuality? A Critical Response to Caldwell." *Africa* 64/2 (1994): 220–242.

Arnfred, Signe. "'African Sexuality'/Sexuality in Africa: Tales and Silences." In *Re-Thinking Sexualities in Africa*, edited by Signe Arnfred. Uppsala: The Nordic Africa Institute, 2004. 59–76.

Baylies, Carolyn. "Perspectives on Gender and AIDS in Africa." In *AIDS, Sexuality and Gender. Collective Strategies and Struggles in Tanzania and Zambia*, edited by Carolyn Baylies and Janet Bujra (with the Gender and AIDS Group). London: Routledge, 2000. 1–24.

Bibeau, Gilles, and Duncan Pedersen. "A Return to Scientific Racism in Medical Social Sciences." In *New Horizons in Medical Anthropology. Essays in Honour of Charles Leslie*, edited by Mark Nichter and Margaret Lock. London: Routledge, 2002. 141–171.

Caldwell, John C., Pat Caldwell, and Pat Quiggin. "The Social Context of AIDS in Sub-Saharan Africa." *Population and Development Review* 15/2 (1989): 185–234.

Campbell, Carole A. "Male Gender Roles and Sexuality: Implications for Women's AIDS Risks and Prevention." *Social Science and Medicine* 41/2 (1995): 197–210.

Campbell, Catherine. "Migrancy, Masculine Identities and AIDS: The Psychosocial Context of HIV Transmission on the South African Gold Mines." *Social Science and Medicine* 45/2 (1997): 273–281.

Dilger, Hansjörg. *Besser der Vorhang im Haus als die Fahne im Wind. Geld, AIDS und Moral im ländlichen Tanzania*. Münster: Lit Verlag, 1999.

Dilger, Hansjörg. "AIDS ist ein Unfall. Metaphern und Bildlichkeit in AIDS-Diskursen Tanzanias." *Afrika Spectrum* 35/2 (2000): 165–182.

Dilger, Hansjörg. "Sexuality, AIDS, and the Lures of Modernity: Reflexivity and Morality among Young People in Rural Tanzania." *Medical Anthropology* 22/1 (2003): 23–52.

Dilger, Hansjörg. *Leben mit AIDS. Krankheit, Tod und soziale Beziehungen in Afrika. Eine Ethnographie.* Frankfurt am Main: Campus, 2005.

Dilger, Hansjörg. "The Power of AIDS. Kinship, Mobility and the Valuing of Social and Ritual Relationships in Tanzania." *African Journal of AIDS Research* 5/2 (2006): 109–121.

Dilger, Hansjörg. "Healing the Wounds of Modernity: Community, Salvation and Care in a Neo-Pentecostal Church in Dar es Salaam, Tanzania." *Journal of Religion in Africa* 37/1 (2007): 59–83.

Femina (February–April 2000), Tanzania.

Foucault, Michel. *The History of Sexuality*, Vol. 2, *The Use of Pleasure*. New York: Random House, 1990.

Gausset, Quentin. "AIDS and Cultural Practices in Africa: The Case of the Tonga (Zambia)." *Social Science and Medicine* 52(4) (2001): 509–518.

Giddens, Anthony. *The Transformation of Intimacy: Sexuality, Love and Eroticism in Modern Societies.* London: Polity Press, 1992.

Gilman, Sander. *Difference and Pathology. Stereotypes of Sexuality, Race, and Madness.* Ithaca: Cornell University Press, 1985.

Haram, Liv. "Negotiating Sexuality in Times of Economic Want: The Young and Modern Meru Women." In *Young People at Risk. Fighting AIDS in Northern Tanzania*, edited by Knut-Inge Klepp, Paul M. Biswalo, and Aud Talle. Oslo: Scandinavian University Press, 1995: 31–48.

Heald, Suzette. "The Power of Sex: Some Reflections on the Caldwells' 'African Sexuality' Thesis." *Africa* 65/4 (1995): 489–505.

Heald, Suzette. "It's Never as Easy as ABC: Understandings of AIDS in Botswana." *African Journal of AIDS Research* 1/1 (2002): 1–11.

Helle-Valle, Jo. "Understanding Sexuality in Africa: Diversity and Contextualised Dividuality." In *Re-Thinking Sexualities in Africa*, edited by Signe Arnfred. Uppsala: The Nordic Africa Institute, 2004. 195–207.

Jeater, Diana. *Marriage, Perversion and Power. The Construction of Moral Discourse in Southern Rhodesia 1894–1930.* Oxford: Oxford University Press, 1993.

Luig, Ute. "Ethnographische Anmerkungen zum Verhältnis von Fruchtbarkeit, Geschlecht und Macht in Afrika." In *Begegnungen und Einmischungen. Festschrift für Renate Rott*, edited by Marianne Braig, Ute Ferdinand, and Martha Zapata. Stuttgart: Heinz, 1997. 247–267.

Moodie, T. Dunbar (with Vivienne Ndatshe and British Sibuyi). "Migrancy and Male Sexuality on the South African Gold Mines." In *Hidden From History: Reclaiming The Gay and Lesbian Past*, edited by Martin Duberman, Martha Vicinus, and George Chauncey, Jr. New York: Penguin, 1990. 411–425.

Posel, Deborah. "Sex, Death and the Fate of the Nation: Reflections on the Politicization of Sexuality in Post-Apartheid South Africa." *Africa* 75/2 (2005): 125–153.

Sabatier, Renée. *Blaming Others. Prejudice, Race and Worldwide AIDS.* London: Panos Institute, 1988.

Schoepf, Brooke G. "Women at Risk: Case Studies from Zaire." In *The Time of AIDS. Social Analysis, Theory, and Method*, edited by Gilbert Herdt and Shirley Lindenbaum. Newbury Park: Sage, 1992. 259–286.

Setel, Philip. *A Plague of Paradoxes: AIDS, Culture, and Demography in Northern Tanzania.* Chicago: University of Chicago Press, 1999.

Sontag, Susan. *AIDS and its Metaphors.* New York: Farrar, Straus and Giroux, 1988.

Treichler, Paula A. "AIDS, Homophobia, and Biomedical Discourse: An Epidemic of Signification." *Cultural Studies* 1(3) (1988): 263–305.

Treichler, Paula A. *How to Have Theory in an Epidemic. Cultural Chronicles of AIDS.* Durham: Duke University Press, 1999.

Vaughan, Megan. *Curing their Ills. Colonial Power and African Illness.* Cambridge: Polity Press, 1991.

Watney, Simon. "Missionary Positions: AIDS, 'Africa', and Race." *Differences. A Journal of Feminist Cultural Studies* 171 (1989): 83–100.

CHAPTER 9

Best Practice Example from the Philippines

A Low-Level Prevalence Country and the Male "Bridge" Population

Taigy Thomas, Lianne Urada, Donald Morisky, and Robert Malow

ABSTRACT

If the chain of HIV/AIDS transmission is to be interrupted in seemingly low-risk female populations, reducing male risk behavior would seem critical. The Philippines is one such country that has done this. Utilizing the assets of its history, culture, and political infrastructure, the Philippines continues to have a low incidence of HIV/AIDS, proving the success of its multilevel, multisectorial efforts. This chapter highlights these efforts while providing a detailed description of a longitudinal research program. Readers will: 1) identify the importance of combinations of educational strategies directed at individual and organizational determinants of behavior change; and 2) recognize the utility of a strong methodological approach to assess the relative effectiveness of the program.

OVERVIEW

Men who have sex with men (MSM), commercial sex workers (CSWs), and injection drug users (IDUs) have historically been high-risk subpopulations for HIV infection. However, rates of HIV are no longer confined to these populations. In fact, sex between a male and female now accounts for the majority of transmission worldwide. As of May 2006, 90 percent of all adolescent and adult HIV/AIDS infections were a result of heterosexual intercourse (NIAID 2006). In Eastern Europe, Asia, Latin America, and sub-Saharan Africa, for example, an estimated 60 percent of all new HIV/AIDS cases are female.

Often the causes of transmission are beyond the women's control and unrelated to "risk" behaviors, such as engaging in unprotected intercourse with multiple sex partners. Indeed, the cause is frequently related to the behaviors of others, particularly their male partners, to whom they typically remain monogamous. However, the same cannot be said for the partner. For example, a Tanzanian study (Yahya-Malima et al. 2007) revealed that close to 50 percent of men had multiple partners, and 78 percent of the population never used a condom. A typical chain of transmission, therefore, may begin with a male who infects a female CSW, who infects a male client, and who in turn infects the unsuspecting wife or girlfriend.

Evidence of such "bridging" is found in many countries worldwide. Indonesia, for example, remained a low HIV/AIDS incidence country in the early stage of the Global HIV/AIDS epidemic. With the steady increase of IDUs, Indonesia suffered increasing HIV/AIDS rates, first focused in the IDU population and then later in commercial sex workers (Sugihantono et al. 2003; Ruxrungtham et al. 2004). Finally, Indonesian HIV/AIDS rates escalated in the general population and subsequently among females. Parts of Myanmar (Gillieatt and Talikowski 2005), Vietnam (Des Jarlais et al. 2005),

Cambodia (Gorbach et al. 2000), and Thailand (Podhisita et al. 1994) are seeing the same bridging phenomena. Thus, such *bridge* populations serve as an important driver of the epidemic, with a typical pattern being that HIV/AIDS is initially spread most among high-risk network members within a given population (CSWs, IDUs). Then, at some point, persons outside of this network become exposed (Ruxrungtham et al. 2004). Since the wives/girlfriends often hold marital ideals of mutual intimacy, sharing, and sexual pleasure, they become prime candidates for infection, as these ideas are not supportive of safer sex practices to stem the rapid viral spread (such as using a condom or non-penetrative sex).

Beyond marital ideas, economic, social, and biological circumstances are also considered to increase transmission of HIV/AIDS from men to women. Young women are especially at risk of acquiring STIs (sexually transmitted infections) and HIV/AIDS because "the reproductive tracts of young women are susceptible to injury during intercourse" (Jujemay and Awit 2007). In many developing countries, females are economically dependent on their male partners, and therefore may have trouble halting their partners' promiscuous behavior (Jujemay and Awit 2007). The Remedios Aids Foundation notes that many female CSWs in the Philippines find it difficult to negotiate condom use with clients. Additionally, the Foundation finds that the illegality of the sex trade sometimes prohibits sex workers from being truthful to their customers about hygiene (for example, infection status) for fear of being exposed and punished (Jujemay and Awit 2007).

COMPONENTS OF PREVENTION EFFORTS FOR LOW-RISK FEMALE POPULATIONS

If the chain of HIV/AIDS transmission is to be interrupted in seemingly low-risk female populations, prevention strategies to reduce male risk behavior would seem critical. Such prevention must acknowledge the epidemic's new direction—that low-risk female populations are principally being infected. Prevention efforts must also consider the following components when targeting HIV risk in male populations.

Use a Multisystems-Level Approach

One of the seminal findings of the last two decades of HIV/AIDS research and prevention is that individuals cannot always control their own behavior; that is, individuals may not always be able to dictate their knowledge levels or personal beliefs, and thus cannot control their subsequent HIV vulnerability. A number of factors exogenous to the individual influence the effectiveness of prevention.

This finding is in stark contradiction to the many individual-level models which focused on intrapsychic, or personal, factors only. These models—namely the Health Belief Model (HBM), the Theory of Reasoned Action (TRA), the Transtheoretical Model, and Social Learning Theory (SLT)—collectively assess the likelihood of a particular individual acting in a specified manner. Individual-level factors alone, however, are not apt to reduce HIV/AIDS risk and thus taken alone these models are limited in the fight against HIV/AIDS (Susser 1994; Diez-Roux et al 2002; Aral and Holmes 1999; Barnett and Whiteside 1999; Burris et al. 2004).

Link and Phalen (2000: 84) argue that, when public health interventions control individual-level risk factors, "social inequalities in the distribution of disease are perpetuated because the contexts in which risk are taken and the fundamental social causes of self harm" remain unchanged. In other words, individual-level frameworks may not reduce HIV/AIDS risk, as they ignore the context in which risk occurs. Contextual factors are usually the source of HIV/AIDS risk behaviors and often overshadow individual-level influences. Thus, individual-level interventions may not be sufficient in helping individuals sustain newly adopted prevention behaviors when countervailing influences are present (DiClemente et al. 2005; Ashton and Seymour 1988; Pickett and Pearl 2001; Susser and Susser 1996; Diez-Roux

1998). In countries in conflict or war, for example, condom use may not be sustained when at odds with the basic human need for survival (i.e., needing money for shelter or food). An individual's choice to have unprotected sex may be based on his or her overarching economic condition. It is, therefore, important to understand and address the larger contextual factors influencing risk behavior (Aral et al. 2007). This may include prevention efforts for: 1) individual thoughts, perceptions, and behaviors (individual-level); 2) interpersonal factors such as face-to-face interactions with family and friends (network-level); 3) community-level efforts; and 4) efforts that impact the broader society, such as policies.

It is also important to maintain a multisectorial response in a low prevalence country. Low HIV/AIDS prevalence sometimes translates to governments assigning a low priority to HIV/AIDS prevention, especially given the competing health, education, economic development, and defense concerns typical among most developing countries. Since HIV/AIDS is invisible in its early stages and early epidemics place few demands on the health sector, there are few readily apparent reasons to initiate a response or turn limited human resources and budgets to prevention.

Give It Time

Governments and philanthropic societies have turned towards an "evidence-based" ideology. This ideology emphasizes the use of contemporaneous research findings as the basis of decision-making (Rosenberg and Donald 1995; McKibbon 1998). Although adopting an ideology that attempts to utilize rigorously evaluated research programs to inform funding and strategic planning seems intuitive, a downfall is that funding or attention is withdrawn if evidence does not show improvements. Interventions take a considerable amount of time to reach a goal of behavior change and governments and funding agencies should not solely look to short-term evidence-based efforts.

Use Community-Based Participatory Approach

A participatory approach is an endorsed belief that community ownership and participation is essential for program sustainability and population-level changes. In participatory action research (PAR), or user participation, community members are encouraged to participate in the planning, implementation, and management of health interventions (Parry et al. 2001; Gillies 1998). Communities are allowed to identify priorities, intervention strategies, and community assets. Outsiders (e.g., researchers) alone cannot tap into the cultural or social strengths existing in a given environment that can aid in making prevention efforts successful.

Major public health initiatives that have applied this model include "Healthy Cities" initiatives throughout the world. In 1988, for example, California developed the first domestic state-wide "Healthy Cities" program (Twiss 2001). The goal for participating cities was to raise health as a priority in decision-making processes in local governments. The California Healthy Cities project required local governments to lead in the initiatives due to their responsibility for many of the functions related to the root causes of morbidity and mortality (e.g., poor housing, unsafe parks and recreation, inadequate transportation).

BEST PRACTICE EXAMPLE

Several countries can serve as "best practices" examples that target and deter male high-risk behaviors. Still, with most programming being established in homosexual populations, only a few countries serve as tenacious examples of *"best practices"* in heterosexual populations. The Philippines is one such country. Utilizing the assets of its history, culture, and political infrastructures, the Philippines continues to have a low incidence of HIV/AIDS, proving the success of its multilevel, multisectorial efforts.

HIV in the Philippines

Similar to conditions in nations with high HIV/AIDS prevalence (e.g., Thailand), all of the ingredients for a potential HIV/AIDS epidemic currently exist in the Philippines. The Philippines continues to have poor economic conditions and high-risk sentinel surveillance groups (sex workers, migrant workers, IDUs). Globalization during the past decade has attracted international terrorists and human and child sex trafficking in the region. Other risk factors include: inconsistent or "infrequent use of condoms during paid sex, high levels of non-ulcerative STIs in some population groups, and high rates of needle-sharing among drug injectors in some areas (77 percent in Cebu)" (Abdool et al. 2007; Mateo et al. 2004; WHO 2006). Additionally, empirical studies show that risk may be increasing.

Compared to prior HIV/AIDS rates in the country, there has been a dramatic rise in HIV/AIDS cases. In fact, the rates have increased from 6,000 to 9,000 (Philippines Department of Health 2000), with an estimated 12,000 cases (Abdool et al. 2007). The ten sentinel surveillance sites in the Philippines showed an increase in HIV/AIDS prevalence in three cities for sex workers, and in one city for IDUs (Zablan and Ogena 2003). The Philippines Health Secretary Francisco Duque III blamed the increase on "sustained high prevalence of sexually transmitted diseases or STIs, high rates of unprotected sex, and the growing community of injecting drug users." He warned that the epidemic is "gaining momentum" (*Philippines Star* 2006). The *Philippines Country Report* (Remedios 2006) reveals continuing problems with dissemination of HIV/AIDS/STIs, the lack of adequate baseline data of populations at risk, and inadequate information on religious and cultural barriers to prevention. People living with HIV/AIDS still fear stigma and discrimination if they seek services, so that reaching a critical mass of people who have disclosed their HIV/AIDS status is problematic. The Philippines surveillance risk assessments identified sexual conservatism, which can result in unwillingness to discuss sex and promote condom use, low and incorrect condom use, gender inequity, and invisibility of the epidemic as current risk factors (Barnett and Whiteside 2006).

Despite the virus being prevalent in the country for a long period among certain traditionally high-risk groups (e.g., CSWs, IDUs, MSM), few in the general Filipino population are infected (Abdool et al. 2007).[1] Specifically, since its initial detection in 1984, HIV/AIDS is still only thought to have infected 12,000 people (UNAIDS 2006). Even among higher-risk groups, HIV/AIDS prevalence remains low. For example, among injecting drug users in Cebu City in 2005, the HIV/AIDS prevalence was estimated at 1 percent. Additionally, among female commercial sex workers, the HIV/AIDS infection rate is also below 1 percent. A low-level prevalence can be attributed to many natural factors, such as geography and culture, but it is also attributed to *social factors and sociopolitical factors*.

Geography

Physical spatial locations are prime factors for infectious disease spread. Several studies have found that HIV is geographically clustered (Law et al. 2004; Zenilman et al. 1999). Particularly, as people migrate, as populations become mobile, and as urbanization ensues, HIV/AIDS increases. For the Philippines, however, the physical-spatial location, or geography, serves as a protective factor decreasing the spread of HIV/AIDS (as does its history with social hygiene clinics). The Philippines is an archipelago of over 7,000 islands. The archipelago is comprised of 81 provinces. Provinces are further subdivided into cities (*lungsod*) and municipalities (*bayan*). The provinces also are grouped or aggregated into 17 regions based on geographical, cultural, and ethnological characteristics. Moreover, the islands within the archipelago are noncontiguous, making migration or overseas fusion minimal. Additionally, most roads are unpaved. Thus, travel by land is less convenient than in other countries. The geography of the Philippines, therefore, serves to help to stem transmission.

Culture

Despite ongoing political instability and possible corruption, high social cohesion is a cultural factor credited with keeping HIV/AIDS rates low in the Philippines. Socially, women and men traditionally have equal roles. Both are vested in the Filipino values of authoritarianism and small-group centeredness (Bulatao 1966). This translates to close kinships and strong family ties. In Filipino households, authoritarianism is seen in both men and women, who are strong in child-rearing and discipline (Barnett and Whiteside 2006). Discipline in the form of parental monitoring and less permissiveness are associated with delays in sexual debut, decreased frequent sexual activities, less risky sexual behavior, fewer sexual partners, and increased condom use among adolescents (Li et al. 2000; Miller et al. 1999).[2] Social cohesion translates into strong group relations and cooperation with group norms, values, or activities. As such, the Philippines has: 1) a high proportion of monogamous relationships; 2) a high proportion of male circumcision; 3) a low number of IDUs; 4) a relatively low number of full-time sex workers; 5) a low number of sex worker clients per night; 6) low rates of anal sex; and 7) a low prevalence of ulcerative STIs in the population. All of these are protective factors against HIV/AIDS transmission. (Barnett and Whiteside 2006; National Economic and Development Authority 2000; Mateo et al. 2004)

Social Factors

In the Philippines, there are several social factors serving as protective factors. Equality in education, for example, is a primal protective factor in the Philippines. Approximately 96 percent of the Philippines population is literate, and literacy is about equal between males and females (Barnett and Whiteside 2006). Policies against sexism, stigmas, and discrimination also exist. This does not negate the fact that lack of employment opportunities and a struggling economy may help to make women more vulnerable to sex work and, consequently, STIs and HIV/AIDS than men. In fact, many females migrating from the poorest provinces become indirect entertainers in legal establishments or direct freelancers, streetwalkers, or workers in illegal brothels. Sex workers often lack power in negotiating safer sex (e.g., using condoms) with high-risk partners, such as with military men, transportation drivers, and drug users. Still, the low rate of HIV/AIDS even among this high-risk group might be attributed to the protective effect of most social factors.

Sociopolitical Factors

Before the bifurcation from the United States in 1946, the Philippines established a National Sexually Transmitted Disease Control Program in 1945. Social hygiene clinics, which now number 180, were created by a congressional act. They are primarily in urban and rural areas where commercial sex establishments are located. The social hygiene clinics, which target high-risk CSW groups and their clients, are thought to be a protective factor within the country.

In the 1980s, the Philippines established an early surveillance system which assessed sero-prevalence rates in "high-risk" groups (e.g., CSWs, IDUs, and MSM). The country later established an HIV/AIDS Registry in 1991 and a National HIV/AIDS Sentinel Surveillance System (NHSSS) in 1993 that shed light on the modes of transmission, age, and gender of people infected and most at risk. The Philippines government further created a Philippines National AIDS Council (PNAC) under the Department of Health in 1992 that oversees an integrated and comprehensive approach to HIV/AIDS prevention and control (Republic Act No. 8504, Philippines AIDS Prevention and Control Act of 1998, accessed on Chan Robles Virtual Law Library). An NHSSS Behavioral Sentinel Surveillance, added in 1997, examined the knowledge and sexual behaviors of high-risk groups in ten cities. These early systems are governmental or structural venues by which comprehensive nationwide educational and information campaigns were established.

Early policies also helped to establish a comprehensive strategy. Policies in the 1990s, specifically the Republic Act No.

8504, or the Philippines AIDS Prevention and Control Act of 1998, were instrumental in the fight against HIV. With the 1998 Act, the government devolved authority to local government units. Local units were then mandated to incorporate HIV/AIDS education into the school curriculum at intermediate grades, secondary and tertiary levels, including non-formal and indigenous learning systems. Local units are also to provide information in the health sector and workplace. Local officials such as the provincial governor, city or municipal mayor, or the city (*barangay*) captain are to coordinate campaigns among concerned government agencies, nongovernment organizations and church-based groups. The Act calls for universal precautions in practices and procedures that carry the risk of HIV/AIDS transmission. The Act prohibits compulsory testing, except for overseas workers and military personnel.[3] The Act also prohibits discrimination against people living with HIV/AIDS. The Act further provides basic health and social services for individuals living with HIV/AIDS. In addition, informational aids or materials on the cause, modes of transmission, prevention, and consequences of HIV/AIDS infection are provided at all international ports of entry and exit.

Although prostitution is illegal in the Philippines, many local city governments continue to regulate the entertainment establishments of female bar workers through targeted testing and counseling. Targeted counseling and testing (Holtgrave 2007; Valdiserri 2007) are part of a national plan for prevention. Individuals are also given post-test advice on how to keep their negative status or, in cases where they are positive, how to keep from infecting others (Valdiserri 2007). Besides targeting high-risk groups, Filipino counseling and testing services focus on geographic areas (e.g., cities) with high risk of HIV/AIDS infection. Services such as the government-run social hygiene clinics in the Philippines provide specialized services for groups with less routine access to health care.

Female entertainment workers in disco and karaoke bars, beer gardens, and massage parlors are also mandated to attend a government social hygiene clinic for STI check-ups on a weekly or bimonthly basis. In the Philippines, the rate of STIs and other diseases sometimes associated with HIV/AIDS (e.g., tuberculosis and malaria) are high. The Philippines has an extremely high rate of tuberculosis (seventy-five deaths per day, according to the Department of Health). Tuberculosis, easier to detect than HIV/AIDS, is often associated with HIV/AIDS/AIDS in other nations (e.g., South Africa.) Malaria is also important and in the Philippines there were an estimated 43,644 cases in 2003, according to the World Health Organization. Targeted testing and counseling of establishment-based sex workers (Bellis et al. 2007; Jeal and Salisbury 2007) are supported by case studies globally. For example, in Liverpool, the city created a zone where 96 percent of sex workers agreed to work where they could adhere to established regulations and gain access to health services (Bellis et al. 2007).

The Philippines Department of Health (DOH) recognized the value of collaboration with other government agencies, international organizations, nongovernment organizations, civil societies, co-members in the Philippines National AIDS Council and research institutions (Asian Development Bank 2007). For example, from 1994 to 2003, a series of prevention efforts were implemented in the Philippines by the School of Public Health at the University of California, Los Angeles and the College of Public Health at the University of the Philippines, Manila. Morisky and colleagues from the University of California at Los Angeles (UCLA) in collaboration with Tiglao and colleagues of the University of the Philippines at Manila, collected longitudinal data from female bar workers, potential male customers, and establishment managers in the southern Philippines.

A major aspect of Morisky's collaborative research in the Philippines utilized a participatory approach; training managers and peer educators from approximately 110 different establishments. The study 1) implemented an educational policy on HIV/AIDS prevention in all intervention sites and met with City Health Officials at the usual care site to identify important recommendations that were found to have a significant effect on condom-use behavior and reduction of STIs; 2) coordinated all intervention activities with the National AIDS Council of the Philippines, and worked closely with Regional Health Departments and City Health Departments in the four respective study sites; and 3) expanded this initial program to address the educational needs of populations which female bar workers identified as usual customers (military, transportation drivers, factory workers, high-risk communities).

Using data collected from this collaboration, Morisky et al. (2006) examined how variations in social influence impacted condom use and sexually transmitted infections among female bar workers in the southern Philippines. Guided by Social Influence Models, combining Social Cognitive Theory and Socio-Structural Theories, Morisky and collaborates implemented three conditions which varied on a social influence dimension: peer influence only, manager influence only, and combined peer–manager influences. Female bar workers receiving structural peer and establishment interventions reported more positive condom attitudes, more establishment policies favoring condom use, and fewer STIs (Morisky et al. 2006) than the peer-only intervention group or control group. Those receiving manager-only interventions had fewer STIs, but fewer condom attitudes, knowledge, and higher perceived risk than the peer-only intervention.[4] The peer-mediated intervention studies with high-risk males yielded significant increases in self-reported condom usage, knowledge about HIV/STI transmission, and attitudes towards condoms from baseline to post-test to follow-up (Morisky et al. 2004; Morisky et al. 2005b).

Other studies have reinforced Morisky's finding about conditions in the Philippines that reduced sexual risk among sex workers. For example, in one study, sexually transmitted infections declined among sex workers and their clients in the Philippines, following outreach, one-time presumptive treatment, and regular screening of sex workers (Wi et al. 2006). In the study, peers and non-government organizations mobilized both registered and unregistered sex workers in Angeles City for the treatment. Only 5 percent of the clients among brothel-based sex workers reported condom use at last sexual contact with their regular non-commercial partners. Lower STIs among sex workers and a 50 percent reduction among the male bridge population resulted from presumptive treatment, but were only temporary if continuing interventions were not sustained (Wi et al. 2006).

CONCLUSION

Strengthening prevention efforts to stem the HIV epidemic requires a serious reflection of the new-fangled course of the disease. Low-risk female populations are principally being infected. Components of prevention efforts for low-risk female populations include addressing the male bridge population through a *multisystems-level approach*. Other components include *time* and use of a *participatory approach* in prevention and research efforts.

This chapter aimed to improve the effectiveness of national and local responses to the epidemic among groups currently at risk by utilizing the Philippines response as a best practices response. Through this example, governments and communities should be able to develop strategies to reduce harm caused by the disease and test those strategies with methodologically sound approaches.

NOTES

1. Five populations in the Philippines have primarily been at risk: women, young adults, MSM, CSWs, and oversees Filipino workers (OFWs) (Remedios Aids Foundation Inc. 2006). Among the high-risk groups overseas workers are more likely to serve as bridge populations. The Philippines has one of the highest overseas worker populations in the world. Workers often contract HIV/AIDS abroad and return to their home country. Among OFWs, those infected were "seafarers (33 percent), domestic helpers (17 percent), employees (nine percent), entertainers (eight percent), and health workers (six percent) (Jujemay and Awit 2007)."

Lack of accurate knowledge about how HIV/AIDS is contracted and transmitted is cited as a major reason for susceptibility among overseas Filipino workers (Jujemay and Awit 2007). Barriers to assisting overseas Filipino workers include "inadequate referral systems and still limited access to HIV/AIDS services, such as voluntary counseling and treatment (Asian Development Bank 2007)." Additionally, many studies show "low knowledge of HIV/AIDS, low condom use, poor health-seeking behavior, and little preparation for loneliness, cultural adaptations and difficult living and working conditions abroad (Jujemay and Awit 2007)." This results in approximately thirty percent of HIV/AIDS-infected individuals in the Philippines contracting the virus as overseas workers (Philippines DOH 2006, www.fhi.org 2004). In April 2007, 81 percent of new HIV/AIDS cases in the Philippines were males between the ages of 25 and 39 years (HIV/AIDS National Epidemiology Center; Jujemay and Awit 2007).

2. It is, however, important to note, according to the Young Adult Fertility and Sexuality Study by the University of the Philippines Population Institute, that many youth think that AIDS can be cured (27.8 percent) and that only those with multiple sex partners get AIDS (78.5 percent). The study also shows that young people's practice of premarital (23.2 percent) and unprotected commercial sex (50 percent of sexually active young men), coupled with misconceptions, puts them at risk of STIs (Jujemay and Awit 2007; Young Adult Fertility and Sexuality Study 3, 2002).
3. All overseas Filipino workers and diplomatic, military, trade, and labor officials and personnel assigned overseas must undergo or attend a seminar on the cause, prevention and consequences of HIV/AIDS. This effort is coordinated by the Department of Labor and Employment or the Department of Foreign Affairs, the Department of Tourism and the Department of Justice through the Bureau of Immigration, in collaboration with the Department of Health, and the mandatory testing of Filipinos going overseas may explain why rates of HIV/AIDS are detected most among this group.
4. Using the data from this collaboration, Morisky and his collaborates have published several other articles relevant to this chapter, which are summarized below. For example, Morisky et al. (1998) reported that over 50 percent of the female bar workers thought condoms hurt when they used condoms. Sneed and Morisky (1998) observed that attitudes and norms are predictive of condom use, as mediated by intentions. Morisky et al. (2002b) found a decrease in STIs when karaoke bar workers were mandated by the city to attend the social hygiene clinic. The managers of the establishments formed an association and began a loan program to increase the compliance of female bar workers to take medication for STIs. Morisky et al. (2002a) reported both personal and situational factors were important influences on female bar workers' condom use. Substance use of male clients increased STIs among female bar workers, and regular partners of the female bar workers lowered the STIs (Chiao and Morisky 2007; Chiao et al. 2006).

REFERENCES AND FURTHER READING

Abdool-Karim, S., Abdool-Karim, Q., Gouws, E. and Baxter, C. (2007). "Global epidemiology of HIV/AIDS-AIDS." *Infectious Disease Clinics of North America*, 21(1):1–17.

Aral, S., Douglas, J., and Lipshutz, JlM. (2007). *Behavioral Interventions for Prevention and Control of Sexually Transmitted Diseases*. Springer U.S.

Aral, S. and Holmes, K. (1999). *Social and Behavioral Determinants of the Epidemiology of STDs; Industrialized and Developing Countries in Sexually Transmitted Diseases*. J. Wasserheit, Editor, McGraw-Hill: New York. pp. 39–76.

Ashton, S. and Seymour, H. (1988). *The New Public Health: The Liverpool Experience*. Open University Press.

Asian Development Bank (March 7, 2007). *ADB Supporting Philippines in Combating Spread of HIV/AIDS*. Press release retrieved July 21, 2008, from http://www.adb.org/Media/Articles/2007/11996-philippines-combating-hiv-aids/default.asp.

Barnett, T. and Whiteside. A. (1999). "HIV/AIDS and development: Case Studies and a Conceptual Framework." *European Journal of Development Research*, 11:200–234.

Barnett, T. and Whiteside, A. (2006). *AIDS in the Twenty-First Century: Disease and Globalization*. Second Ediction. London: Palgrave Macmillan.

Bellis, M., Watson, F., Hughes, S., Cook, P., Downing, J., Clark, P. and Thomson R. (2007). "Comparative Views of the Public, Sex Workers, Businesses and Residents on Establishing Managed Zones for Prostitution: Analysis of a Consultation in Liverpool," *Health Place*. September, 13(3):603–16.

Bulatao, J. (1966). *Split-Level Christianity*. Manila, Quezon City: Ateneo de Manila University Press.

Burris, S., Blankinship, K., Donoghoe, M., Sherman, S., Blankenship, K., Vernick, J., Case, P., Lazzarini, Z. and Koester S. (2004). "Addressing the 'Risk Environment' for Injection Drug Users; the Mysterious Case of the Missing Cop." *The Milbank Quarterly* 82(1):125–156.

Center for Health Research, University of Indonesia (2000). *Results of the 1996–1999 Behavioral Surveillance Surveys in Jakarta, Surabaya, and Manado*. Jakarta: Center for Health Research, University of Indonesia.

Chiao, C. and Morisky, D. (2007). "The Role of Regular Sex Partner in Sexually Transmitted Infections and Re-infections: Results from the Study of Female Entertainment Establishment Workers in the Philippines." *Sexual Transmitted Diseases*, 8:534–540.

Chiao, C., Morisky, D., Ksobsech, K., Rosenberg, R., and Malow, R. (2006). "The Relationship Between HIV/Sexually Transmitted Infection Risk and Alcohol Use During Commercial Sex Episodes: Results From the Study of Female Commercial Sex Workers in the Philippines." *Substance Use and Misuse* 41(10–12):1509–1533.

Des Jarlais, D., Johnston, P., Friedmann, P., Kling, R., Liu, W., Ngu, D., Chen, Y., Hoang, T., Donghua, M., Van, L., Tung, N., Binh, K., and Hammett, T. (2005). "Patterns of HIV Prevalence Among Injecting Drug Users in the Cross-Border Area of Lang Son Province, Vietnam, and Ning Ming County, Guangxi Province, China." *BioMedical Central Public Health*, August 24(5):89.

DiClemente, R., Salazar, L., Crosby, R., and Rosenthal, S. (2005). "Prevention and Control of Sexually Transmitted Infections Among Adolescents: The Importance of a Socio-Ecological Perspective—A Commentary." *Journal of the Royal Institute of Public Health*, 119:825–836.

Diez-Roux, A. (1998). "Bringing Context Back into Epidemiology: Variables and Fallacies in Multilevel Analysis." *American Journal of Public Health*. 88:216–222.

Diez-Roux, A., Schwartz, S., and Susser, E. (1998). "Ecologic Studies and Ecological Variables in Public Health Research." In *The Oxford Textbook of Public Health*, edited by R. Fan, Conner, and Villarreal. AIDS Science and Society. Jones and Bartlett Publishers.

Diez-Roux, A., Schwartz, S., and Susser, E. (2002) "Ecologic Studies and Ecological Variables in Public Health Research." In *The Oxford Textbook of Public Health*, R. Detels, et al., Editors. London: Oxford University Press. pp. 493–507.

Gillieatt, L., and Talikowski, S. (2005). "Female Sex Work in Yangon, Myanmar." *Sexual Health* 2(3):193–202.

Gillies, P. (1998). "The Effectiveness of Alliances or Partnerships for Health Promotion." *Health Promotion International*, 13:99–120.

Gorbach, P., Sopheab, H., Phalla, T., Leng, H., Mills, S., Bennett, A., and Holmes, K. (2000). "Sexual Bridging by Cambodian Men: Potential Importance for General Population Spread of STD and HIV Epidemics." *Sexually Transmitted Diseases*, 27(6):320–326.

Holtgrave, D. (2007). "Costs and Consequences of the U.S. Centers for Disease Control and Prevention's Recommendations for Opt-Out HIV/AIDS Testing." *Public Library of Science Medicine* 4(6):e194. doi:10.1371/journal.pmed.0040194.

Jeal, N. and Salisbury, C. (2007). "Health Needs and Service Use of Parlour-Based Prostitutes Compared with Street-based Prostitutes: A Cross-Sectional Survey." *British Journal of Obstetrics and Gynecology*, 114(7):875–881.

Jujemay, G. and Awit, J.G. (June 15, 2007), "Editorial: *Sexual Jeopardy.*" *Sun Star Cebu*. http://www.sunstar.com.ph/static/ceb/2007/06/18/oped/editorial.html.

Law, D., Serre, M., Christakos, G., Leone, P., and Miller, W.C. (2004). "Spatial Analysis and Mapping of Sexually Transmitted Diseases to Optimize Intervention and Prevention Strategies." *Sexually Transmitted Infections*. 80:294–299.

Li, X., Stanton, B., and Feigelman, S. (2000). "Impact of Perceived Parental Monitoring on Adolescent Risk Behavior over 4 Years." *Journal of Adolescent Health* 27:49–56.

Link, B. and Phalen, J. (2000). "Evaluating the Fundamental Causes Explanation for Social Disparities in Health." In *The Handbook of Medical Sociology*, 5th edition, edited by C. Bird, P. Conrad, and A. Freemont, Upper Saddle River, NJ: Prentice Hall. pp. 33–46.

McKibbon, K. (1998). "Evidence Based Practice." *Bulletin of the Medical Library Association*. 86(3): 396–401.

Mateo, R., Sarol, J., and Poblete, R. (2004). "HIV/AIDS in the Philippines." *AIDS Education Prevention*, 16 (3 Supplement A):43–52.

Miller, K., Forehand, R., and Kotchick, B. (1999). "Adolescent Sexual Behavior in Two Ethnic Minority Samples: The Role of Family Variables." *Journal of Marriage and the Family*, 61:85–98.

Morisky, D. Ang, A., Coly. A., Tiglao. T. (2004). "A Model HIV/AIDS/AIDS Risk Reduction Program in the Philippines: A Comprehensive Community-Based Approach through Participatory Action Research." *Health Promotion International*, 19:69–76.

Morisky, D., Ang, A. and Sneed, C. (2002a). "Validating the Effects of Social Desirability on Self-Reported Condom Use." *AIDS Education and Prevention*, 14:351–360.

Morisky, D., Chiao, C., Stein, J.A., and Malow, R. (2005a). "Impact of Social and Structural Influence Interventions on Condom Use and Sexually Transmitted Infections among Establishment-Based Female Bar Workers in the Philippines." *Journal of Psychology and Human Sexuality*, 17:45–63.

Morisky, D.E., Nguyen, C., Ang, A., Tiglao, T.V. (2005b). "HIV/AIDS prevention among the Male Population: Results of a Peer Education Program for Taxicab and Tricycle Drivers in the Philippines." *Health Education and Behavior*, 32(1):57–68.

Morisky, D., Peña, M., Tiglao, T. and Liu, K. (2002b). "The Impact of the Work Environment on Condom Use among Female Bar Workers in the Philippines." *Health Education and Behavior*, 29:461–472.

Morisky, D.E., Stein, J., Chiao, C., Ksobiech, K., Malow, R. (2006). "Impact of a Social Influence Intervention on Condom Use and Sexually Transmitted Infections among Establishment-Based Female Sex Workers in the Philippines: A Multilevel Analysis." *Health Psychology*, 25(5):595–603.

Morisky, D., Stein, J., Sneed, C., Tiglao, T., Tempongko, S., Baltazar, J., Detels, R. and Liu, K. (2002c). "Modeling Personal and Situational Influences on Condom Use Among Establishment-Based Commercial Sex Workers in the Philippines." *AIDS and Behavior*, 6:163–172.

Morisky, D., Tiglao, T., Sneed, C., Tempongko, S., Baltazar, J., Detels, R, and Stein, J. (1998). "The

Effects of Establishment Practices, Knowledge and Attitudes on Condom Use among Filipina Sex Workers." *AIDS Care*, 10:213–220.

National Economic and Development Authority (NEDA) (2000). *Living with HIV/AIDS: Case Study on Filipinos Living with HIV/AIDS*. Produced by the Health Action Information Network for NEDA with the support of the UNDP.

National Institute of Allergy and Infectious Diseases (NIAID) (2006). *HIV Infection and AIDS: An Overview*. Office of Communications and Public Liaison National Institute of Allergy and Infectious Diseases National Institutes of Health Bethesda, MD.

Parry, O., Gnich, W., and Platt., S. (2001). "Principles in Practice: Reflections on a 'Postpositivist' Approach to Evaluation Research." *Health Education Research*, 16(2):215–226. Oxford University Press

Philippines Department of Health (2000). *Consensus Report on STI, HIV and AIDS Epidemiology Philippine*. World Health Organization, Geneva.

Philippines Department of Health (2003). *Overview of HIV/AIDS, TB and Malaria in Philippines*. Statistical data provided by the UN, World Bank, WHO, UNAIDS. http://www.theglobalfund.org/programs/countrystats.aspx?CountryId=PHL&lang= (accessed July 22, 2008).

Philippines National AIDS Council (2005). *4th AIDS Medium Term Plan, 2005–2010, Philippines*, UNAIDS, Geneva.

Philippines Star (02/01/2006), Manila, Philippines. "9,000 Filipinos Positive for HIV." http://www.philstar.com/philstar/News200602010404.htm. Accessed on February 1, 2006.

Pickett, K., and Pearl, M. (2001). "Multilevel Analyses of Neighborhood Socioeconomic Context and Health Outcomes: A Critical Review." *Journal of Epidemiology and Community Health*, 55(2):111–122.

Podhisita, C., Morris, M., and Wawer, M. (1994). "Bridge Populations in the Spread of HIV/AIDS in Thailand International Conference on AIDS." 10: 298 (abstract no. PC0120). Institute for Population and Social Research, Mahidol University, Thailand.

Remedios (2006). *Philippines Country Report*. http://www.remedios.com.ph/fhtml/country_report_2006_iii.htm.

Rosenberg, W. and Donald, A. (1995). "Evidence Based Medicine: An Approach to Clinical Problem Solving." *British Medical Journal*, 310 (6987):1122–1126.

Ruxrungtham, K., Brown, T. and Phanuphakb, P. (2004). "HIV/AIDS in Asia." *Lancet*, 364; 9428(3): 69–82.

Sneed, C.D. and Morisky, D.E. (1998). "Applying the Theory of Reasoned Action to Condom Use Among Sex Workers". *Social Behavior and Personality* 26(4):317–328.

Sugihantono, A., Slidell, M., Syaifudin, A., Pratjojo, H., Utami, I., Sadjimin, T. and Mayer, K. (2003). "AIDS Patient Care and STDs. Syphilis and HIV Prevalence among Commercial Sex Workers in Central Java, Indonesia: Risk-Taking Behavior and Attitudes that May Potentiate a Wider Epidemic." *AIDS Patient Care and STDs*. 17(11):595–600.

Susser, E., (1994). "The Logic in Ecology." *American Journal of Public Health*. 84:830–835.

Susser, M, and Susser, E. (1996). "Choosing a Future for Epidemiology: I. Eras and Paradigms." *American Journal of Public Health*, 86(5): 668–673.

Sweat, M. and Denison, J. (1995). "Reducing HIV/AIDS in Developing Countries with Structural and Environmental Interventions." *AIDS*, 9 (Supplement A): S251–S257.

Tiglao, T., Morisky, D., Tempongko, S., Baltazar, J., and Detels, R. (1996). "A Community Participation Action Research Approach to HIV/AIDS/AIDS Prevention among Sex Workers." *Promotion and Education*, 25–28.

Twiss, J. (2001). "Cities and Partners in Community based Public Health: Policy and Practice." *Partnership for the Public's Health: A collaboration of the California Endowment and the Public Health Institute* Issue 2: November.

UNAIDS (2006). *Report on the Global AIDS Epidemic*. United Nations, Geneva.

Valdiserri, R. (2007). "Late HIV/AIDS Diagnosis: Bad Medicine and Worse Public Health." *Public Library of Science Medicine* 4(6):e200. doi:10.1371/journal.pmed.0040200.

Wi, T., Ramos, R., Steen, T., Esguerra, M., Roces, M., Lim-Quizon, M., Neilsen, G., and Dallabetta, G. (2006). "STI Declines among Sex Workers and Clients Following Outreach, One Time Presumptive Treatment and Regular Screening of Sex Workers in the Philippines." *Sexually Transmitted Infections*, 82(5):386–392.

World Health Organization (2006). *UNAIDS/WHO Global HIV/AIDS Online Database*. Geneva and New York. http://www.who.int/globalatlas/default.asp.

Yahya-Malima, K., Matee, M., Evjen-Olsen, B. and Fylkesnes, K. (2007). "High Potential of Escalating HIV/AIDS Transmission in a Low Prevalence Setting in Rural Tanzania." *BioMedical Central Public Health*, 7(1):103–112.

Young Adult Fertility and Sexuality Study (YAFS 3) (2002). *Youth, Sex, and Risk Behaviors in the Philippines*. Quezon City, Philippines: Demographic Research and Development Foundation, Inc. and the UP Population Institute, University of the Philippines, Diliman.

Zablan, Z., and Ogena, N. (2003). *Drivers of the HIV Epidemic Among Female Sex Workers in the Philippines*. Demographic Research and Development Foundation, Inc, Quezon City, Philippines. Abstract published on the 16th International AIDS Conference, Toronto, website http://www.cdc.gov/hiv/conferences.htm.

Zenilman, J., Ellish, N., Fresia, A., and Glass, G. (1999). "The Geography of Sexual Partnerships in Baltimore: Applications of Core Theory Dynamics Using a Geographic Information System." *Sexually Transmitted Diseases*, 56:75–81.

SECTION 3

Critical Intersections between Biomedicine, Behavior, and HIV

Sex workers and tourism politics in the Philippines

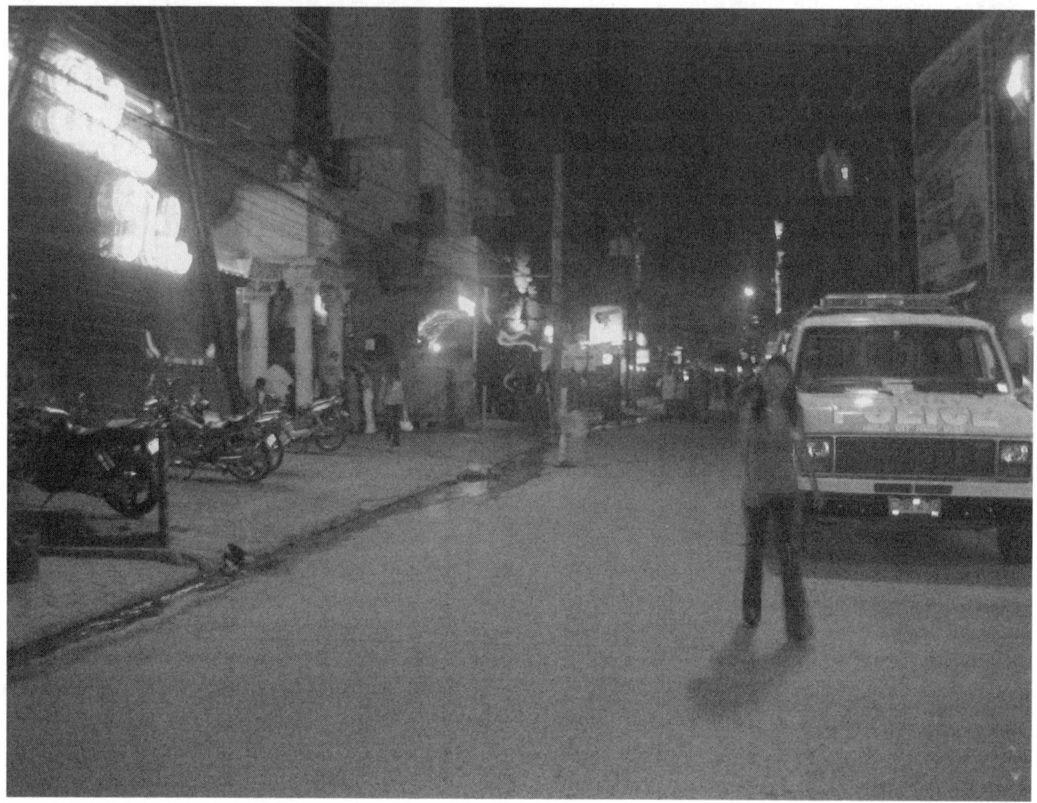

Source: Photo courtesy of Lianne Urada

Looking Inside the Pill Bottle

The Evolution of HIV Antiretroviral Combination Drug Therapy

Sande Gracia Jones

In June 1981 the first description of what would become known as AIDS was reported in a publication by the Centers for Disease Control (CDC). Cases of HIV infection soon became reported around the U.S.A. and the world, and the rapidness of the spread of HIV was staggering. By October 1981 the CDC was calling HIV an epidemic (Bennett 2003). The first European case of HIV was reported in France in July 1981. Soon afterward, cases were reported in other European countries, the Caribbean, and Central Africa. By the mid-1980s, at least 100,000 people across five continents had been infected. The AIDS pandemic assumed major proportions and by 1992 was described as a global epidemic that was out of control.

HIV/AIDS still remains a global health problem. But for those with access to them, powerful antiretroviral (ARV) drug combinations have improved survival rates dramatically. ARV drug therapy has changed the prognosis for HIV from "dying with AIDS" to living with a chronic disease.

This chapter will take a look inside the ARV pill bottle and will present an overview of how HIV replicates within the body and how HIV ARV drugs work to suppress the virus; describe the evolution of HIV drug therapy from AZT to HAART, from a historical perspective, and from the perspective of both researchers and persons living with HIV; explore past and current issues related to ARV drug resistance and medication adherence; and conclude with a brief discussion of HIV drug therapy in the twenty-first century.

OVERVIEW: HIV AND DRUG THERAPY

HIV: Attack on the Body

In 1982 the Centers for Disease Control and Prevention (CDC) used the term "AIDS" to denote that AIDS was the severe end of a clinical syndrome composed of a wide range of constitutional symptoms, opportunistic illness, and hematological and neurological impairment. AIDS in the 1980s was viewed as a highly acute illness with a short survival period, and infection with HIV was considered "an automatic death sentence."

By 1986 two types of virus that caused AIDS were isolated and identified, and the virus that caused AIDS in the U.S.A. was given the name of Human Immunodeficiency Type-1 Virus (HIV). Scientists found that HIV was a retrovirus. Retroviruses have some unique properties, differing from other viruses. Their genes are encoded in two single-stranded RNA (ribonucleic acid); transcription of genetic material is reversed (RNA to DNA (deoxyribonucleic acid) versus DNA to RNA); and reverse transcriptase enzyme is needed for transcribing RNA into DNA. Scientists also discovered that HIV was spread through infected body fluids.

Once inside the body, HIV was attracted to the CD4 cells (T-helper cells of the white blood cells) of the immune system. HIV's entry into the host cell initially occurred when the HIV virion bound with the CD4 molecule, utilizing chemokine coreceptor molecules (CXCR4 or CCR5) on the surface of the target cell. Entry of HIV-1 into the target cell was mediated by two viral envelope glycoproteins, gp120 and gp41, which formed complexes that facilitated entry of HIV into the host cell.

Once attached to a receptor on the cell surface, HIV injected the cell with the virus's genetic material, HIV RNA. The reverse transcriptase enzyme then helped convert HIV RNA into DNA. Once the HIV RNA became incorporated into the genetic material of the CD4 cell, the CD4 cell changed into an HIV-producing cell. The infected cell would now produce many new HIV cells before dying. Another enzyme, the protease enzyme, then reshaped the newly generated HIV cells (called virions), which facilitated their movement out of the infected cell, into the bloodstream. HIV replication involved finding new CD4 cells to infect and convert into HIV-producing cells. Once in the bloodstream, the HIV virions sought out uninfected CD4 cells to infect. Although the body manufactured many new CD4 cells each day, over time the number of uninfected CD4 cells would become less than the amount of HIV-infected cells, and the CD4 cell count would begin to decline.

This attack on the body's immune system crippled the body's ability to fight infection. The weakened immune system left the body vulnerable to numerous health problems, including lethal opportunistic infections that would otherwise not develop in an individual with a healthy immune system. The normal CD4 count in a cubic millimeter of blood is 800–1,200 cells. When the attack on the immune system resulted in a decrease of the CD4 cell count down to 200 cells or less, the HIV-positive person was now said to have developed AIDS. Without treatment, people at this stage of the illness were prone to opportunistic infections, such as PCP (Pneumocystis *carinii* pneumonia), and malignancies, such as Kaposi's sarcoma, a skin cancer denoted by a distinct dark purplish lesion.

HAART: Attack on HIV

Understanding how HIV works to replicate within the body has facilitated the development and evolution of drug therapy for HIV care. Current HIV drug treatment utilizes sophisticated and powerful antiretroviral (against a retrovirus; ARV) drugs, working in combination to attack HIV by interrupting viral replication. The success in 1996 of initial clinical drug trials using a combination of HIV drugs has spearheaded research in the twenty-first century on a variety of new HIV drug categories and new medications.

In 1996 researchers at the World AIDS Conference announced dramatic success with HIV treatment by using powerful new antiretroviral drugs from different drug categories. Combining drugs from different HIV drug categories into a "drug cocktail" or drug regimen showed initial success at slowing viral replication. The following drugs from different drug categories worked inside infected $CD4^+$ cells by inhibiting the action of enzymes necessary for HIV replication:

1. Non-nucleoside analog reverse transcriptase inhibitor drugs (NNRTIs) attached to the reverse transcriptase enzyme, preventing the enzyme from converting HIV RNA into DNA.
2. Nucleoside analog reverse transcriptase inhibitors (NRTIs) worked by becoming part of HIV's DNA, thus derailing the HIV building process. Once damaged, HIV DNA could not work to take control of the cell's DNA.
3. Protease inhibitors (PIs) worked at a later stage in the replication process. The PI drugs worked by preventing the protease enzyme from effectively cutting HIV viral proteins into virions. The defective virions were then unable to infect other $CD4^+$ cells.

Working together in combination, the drugs from different antiretroviral categories were able to block HIV at several points in its replication, slowing its spread in the body. This strategy became known as highly active (or highly aggressive) antiretroviral therapy (HAART). Largely because of HAART, the death rate from AIDS in the United States dropped almost 66 percent between 1996 and 1998.

However, the powerful new drugs had side effects. Patients complained of nausea, inability to focus, and a general feeling of "feeling lousy" (Jones 2002). More severe side effects included fat redistribution (lipodystrophy and lipoatrophy) and elevated serum cholesterol and triglycerides, which could indicate an increased risk for cardiac disease. Another concern with HAART was the increased risk for lactic acidemia and acidosis, especially with NRTI drugs.

Prolonged elevated levels of lactic acid can lead to liver problems, multiple organ failure, coma, and death. Questions began to be raised about the long-term effects of the drugs. AIDS activists began to ask whether HAART is a cure for AIDS, or just a further problem for persons with AIDS? Discussion and debate ensued over the new drug therapy.

HISTORICAL PERSPECTIVE-HIV/AIDS DRUG THERAPY

AZT and OI Drugs

From 1981 to 1986 treatment of HIV and AIDS focused on therapies to treat the opportunistic infections (OIs) caused by organisms from protozoa, parasite, bacterial, and viral families, such as *Candida*, *Toxoplasmosis*, *Histoplasmosis*, *Cryptococcus*, and *Coccidioides*. However, there was no drug that could halt or alter the progression of HIV in the body. AIDS activists loudly insisted on the need for a drug that would fight the virus; if not cure it, then at least halt the virus's progressive attack on the body.

In 1986, persons infected with HIV gleaned renewed hope for survival when the Food and Drug Administration (FDA) approved the use of an experimental drug, zidovudine (AZT; ZDV; Retrovir), for the treatment of HIV/AIDS. AZT was a nucleoside analog reverse transcriptase inhibitor (NRTI) drug that had originally been developed for the treatment of cancer, but had so many toxicities in animal studies that it was withdrawn from further study. However, AZT became one of the first drugs tested in HIV clinical drug trials, and initial results showed great promise of efficacy. Over the next ten years, AZT would become a household word, singularly associated with a deadly disease called AIDS (Burkett 1995).

People taking AZT began to report a variety of side effects, such as anemia and fatigue, and drug toxicity became a concern. The AZT dosage initially recommended was replaced with a lower and less toxic dosage. However, a new problem arose. Some patients became drug resistant after six to eighteen months of AZT therapy (Rabkin et al. 1994). Hope for a cure began to fade in the AIDS community, and questions began to be raised about the safety and efficacy of AZT. At this point, researchers began to study medication adherence in HIV care.

Adherence to AZT

As previously described, patients on AZT were also taking multiple drugs for HIV symptom management and prevention of OIs. These medication regimens involved taking multiple medications two to three times a day. Although several studies were conducted to look at factors involved in HIV medication adherence, a review of the literature revealed that most studies looked at adherence to AZT versus adherence to a multi-drug HIV medication regimen.

More adherent participants were found to depend upon a significant other for a wide range of social, economic, and emotional support (Morse et al. 1991). Factors that facilitated adherence included taking the drug twice a day, better adaptive coping, belief in ability to adhere to therapy, being likely to take medications when at home, and a history of prior opportunistic infection (Eldred et al. 1998; Singh et al. 1996). One study found five variables associated with AZT adherence: (a) belief that AZT prolongs life, (b) no history of IV (intravenous) drug use, (c) taking one to three other drugs along with AZT, (d) a diagnosis of AIDS, and (e) use of a medication timer (Samet et al. 1992).

Belief in AZT therapy was noted in other studies. One study found that participants who terminated AZT therapy believed that taking the drug was harmful, were skeptical about its ability to prevent illness, and felt that physicians' directives about medication usage in general could be disregarded (Smith et al. 1997). However, another study revealed that, although over 95 percent of participants reported believing AZT to be life-prolonging, participants took only 75 percent or less of their prescribed AZT doses (Frick et al. 1998). Other reported predictors of AZT non-adherence included taking four or more other medications along with AZT, three-times-a-day dosing schedules, depression, and problems taking the medications (Eldred et al. 1998; Freeman et al. 1996; Singh et al. 1996; Muma et al. 1995). In summary, while there were conflicting findings on factors related to adherence, non-adherence to AZT was a common finding.

HIV Drug Therapy: Losing Hope

In 1990 researchers announced a promising new drug, fialuridine (FIAU). Hope that this could be the sought-after cure for an end to the death sentence of AIDS was renewed throughout AIDS communities. Fifteen people were started in a clinical drug trial for the new medication in July 1993. Two months later, many were on the verge of death. Seven patients needed liver transplants. Five patients died before they could acquire a new liver. The clinical drug trial was immediately stopped, and hope faded (Burkett 1995).

On October 9, 1991, a new NRTI drug, didanosine (Videx; ddI), was approved by the FDA, followed by approval of the NRTI drug zalcitabine (Hivid; ddC) on June 19, 1992. However, patients taking the new drugs began to exhibit some serious side effects, such as pancreatitis and peripheral neuropathy.

In 1993 findings from the Concorde AZT drug trial studies were presented at the World AIDS Conference, the international AIDS conference that brings leading scientists, clinical researchers, and AIDS care providers together to share their scientific findings. The results were grim. The investigators concluded that, after reviewing the outcomes of three years of clinical trials, the result was that the use of prophylactic AZT in symptom-free patients neither prolonged life nor delayed AIDS onset.

Once again, hope for survival faded in the AIDS community. On June 24, 1994, the FDA approved a new drug, the NRTI stavudine (Zerit; d4T). However, peripheral neuropathy was again experienced as a side effect of the drug. On November 24, 1995, the 500,000th American died of AIDS (Burkett 1995).

Regaining Hope: HAART for HIV

Hope for survival resurfaced in 1995. After a decade of limited drug treatment, HIV/AIDS drug therapy dramatically changed. In September 1995, clinical studies on new drug therapies were presented at the 5th European Conference on Clinical Aspects and Treatment of HIV Infection (Churchill 1996). These studies reported promising clinical data on the effectiveness of two- and three-drug combination regimens in reducing the amount of HIV that was present and replicating in the blood (called the HIV viral load). Additionally, the simultaneous administration of AIDS drugs from different categories appeared to help reverse the effect of HIV on the immune system, by causing an increase in the CD4 T-cell levels (CD4 count) in the body. An increase in the CD4 count in HIV-infected patients impeded life-threatening OIs from invading and causing disease, and improved the health status of persons infected with HIV.

Encouraged by the initial study results, in late 1995 the FDA approved lamivudine (Epivir), a nucleoside analog reverse transcriptase inhibitor (NRTI) drug, and saquinavir (Invirase), the very first of a new class of drugs called protease inhibitors (PIs).

In early 1996, a panel of international AIDS experts convened to draft guidelines on the use of antiretroviral (ARV) therapy (Carpenter et al. 1996). The decisions made at this meeting heralded the advent of a new era in treatment of HIV/AIDS. For the first time since the start of the HIV/AIDS epidemic, the expert panel recommended that the preferred initial drug therapy would be regimens that included a combination of different nucleoside reverse transcriptase inhibitor (NRTI) drugs. Multiple drug therapy became the standard of care, and monotherapy, or the use of only one drug, such as AZT, was seen as an ineffective and outdated mode of therapy. Therapy was recommended based on the client's CD4 cell count and clinical status, along with the results of a new laboratory test, the HIV viral load test, that measured the amount of HIV in the blood. The panel of experts, recognizing that they were experiencing a time of groundbreaking therapy for the treatment of HIV/AIDS, stated that therapeutic approaches would need to be updated as outcomes of studies on protease inhibitor (PI) drugs became available, and as new drugs continued to emerge.

On March 4, 1996, the FDA approved the PI ritonavir (Norvir). By July 1996 two more drugs had been approved; another PI, indinavir (Crixivan), and nevirapine (Viramune), a drug in the new category of non-nucleoside reverse transcriptase inhibitor (NNRTI) agents. Quantification of HIV through tests for HIV viral load became the recommended standard of care to determine the effectiveness of the new treatment regimes.

The Department of Public Health and Human Services in the United States also met in 1996 and issued new guidelines for HIV occupational exposure (Dobkin 1996). Although still emphasizing the small numbers of health care workers who had become infected with HIV through occupational exposure, the new guidelines recognized the potential threat of HIV infection from exposure to contaminated body fluids. The new guidelines recommended that health care workers who had suffered a high-risk exposure to HIV, should begin post-exposure prophylaxis (PEP), consisting of a triple drug combination therapy regimen, including a protease PI drug, as soon as possible post-exposure.

HAART: The New "Drug Cocktail"

Reports of success from the 11th International AIDS Conference held in June 1996 in Vancouver, Canada, heralded the advent of hope for a cure for HIV, through the simultaneous administration of two and three different HIV drugs, often from different categories of HIV medications. Physicians, scientists, and pharmaceutical companies began to use the term "drug cocktail" to describe the multi-drug therapy regime. The "drug cocktail" became the buzzword in HIV/AIDS care, and held out the promise of a cure for AIDS that had heretofore eluded the scientific community (McBride 1997). Word of the breakthrough quickly spread throughout AIDS communities. Using the term "drug cocktail" was an effective marketing strategy, seen as an alluring promise by some persons with HIV (Burkett 1995: vii).

> By the age of 46, Ivan had lived under the dark cloud of HIV infection for 14 years . . . he had been a substance abuser for many years . . . Six months earlier he'd started taking the new wonder drugs touted in Vancouver as the miraculous "drug cocktail." He loved their use of the word cocktail—"so user-friendly, so reassuring for people like me," he said.

Researchers at the 36th Interscience Conference on Antimicrobial Agents and Chemotherapy, held in New Orleans in September 1996, summarized their progress in conquering HIV during the previous year as having outstripped that of the past decade. The new HIV "drug cocktail" was seen as the hope of ending AIDS. On September 28, 1996, Dr. Robert

Gallo announced at an AIDS conference in Miami that a cure for AIDS "may be here by the end of the century."

A&U: America's AIDS Magazine and *POZ* were consumer journals that discussed HIV from the perspective of people living with HIV. A random review of the journals from 1995 to 1996 revealed that a majority of the paid commercial advertisements were from viatical companies (financial companies that buy life insurance policies)—"sell your life insurance policy to get money now"—and from companies that produced drugs and nutritional supplements for AIDS wasting. By 1997, however, the focus of advertisements began to change. The ARV drug advertisements increased, and pictured a new promise to people with HIV. The advertisements depicted handsome young Caucasian and African-American men engaged in physical activities—biking, climbing mountains, and sailing. The advertisements promoted the wonderful effects of the new HIV drugs on personal health and stamina, and appeared to mirror the promise of a new and renewed life. By 1998, the advertisements changed to also feature women and heterosexual couples, which reflected the changing demographics of HIV/AIDS.

The Reality of Taking HAART

Between 1997 and 1999, five more drugs received FDA approval: the NNRTI drugs delavirdine (Rescriptor) and efavirenz (Sustiva); the NNRTI drug abacavir sulfate (Ziagen); and the PI drugs nelfinavir (Viracept) and amprenavir (Agenerase). New guidelines were drafted for the treatment of HIV. Combination therapy, using a combination of one to three drugs from two or three different drug categories, including protease inhibitors, became the recognized standard of care, and the use of highly aggressive antiretroviral therapy (HAART), initiated as soon as an HIV diagnosis was confirmed, was expected to be effective in stopping and eradicating HIV infection.

However, the recommended HIV drug regimens required people to take a minimum of twelve pills per day, with some regimens requiring up to twenty pills per day. Each medication had specific food, fluid, and/or dosage timing requirements. A potential concern about medication adherence was voiced by leading AIDS researchers, who wondered, "Can theory be reduced to practice?" This related to the fact that clients enrolled in clinical drug trials, under close scrutiny, did fairly well in terms of adhering to the strict regimens of the medication protocols. The question remained whether medication adherence behaviors, exhibited by participants in clinical drug trials, could be replicated by persons in "the real world" of everyday life and activities.

Several of the HIV medications had specific dosage timing intervals and/or dietary requirements. Some drugs needed to be taken on empty stomachs, while others needed to be taken with high-fat meals. Some medications required a minimum of sixty-four ounces of water a day, to prevent kidney stones. Some medications needed to be taken every eight hours to maintain therapeutic levels of the medication, in order for the medication to attack and suppress the virus and viral replication. Several medications needed an alkaline environment for bio-absorption, so could not be co-administered with medications that had an acidic pharmacological composition (alkaline and acidic incompatibilities). Twenty medications commonly used to treat cardiac, gastrointestinal, and other conditions, were contraindicated for patients who were also taking protease inhibitors (PIs), because of the potential for drug–drug interaction which could result in lethal cardiac arrhythmias and electrolyte imbalance (Dykeman et al. 1996).

Articles in *POZ* began to feature information on various HIV drug therapies and about living life on medications. Adherence and dealing with side effects were topics frequently discussed. In one article, AIDS activist Mary Fischl discussed what it was like for her, as a woman infected with HIV, to attempt to take the new drug therapies (Martin 1997: 103).

> It is not the AIDS virus, exactly, that has kept me away . . . it is the therapy that we are employing to fight it. I'm wrestling with prescriptions that may save my life and with side effects of those prescriptions which make me wonder if life is worth saving. I am weary beyond imagination, frustrated to the point of rage, and discouraged . . . How do I tell a young person "Come into the system. You don't feel bad now, but let's get you on medication, and then you'll really feel horrible?" Everyone's saying that protease inhibitors are the cure, but it's just not that simple.

By 1997, continued clinical studies revealed that the new drugs would not cure HIV/AIDS. However, the new drugs had a dramatic impact on the health of people living with AIDS. In 1996, the United States death rate from AIDS dropped for the first time since the peak in 1995, when there were 49,895 deaths of persons with AIDS (HHS News 1997). In 1996, there were only 37,221 deaths of persons with AIDS. The downward trend continued in 1997, with only 21,445 deaths. By 1998 the rate had fallen to 17,171 deaths. HIV patients had 71,000 fewer hospitalizations in 1997 than 1995, resulting in 878,000 fewer days of hospital care for HIV patients (National Center for Health Statistics 1999). Hospital admissions for AIDS patients had such a dramatic decrease that specialty inpatient AIDS units throughout the United States began to close due to lack of patients (Morrison 1998; Napper 1998).

HIV Drug Resistance

By 1997, a potential barrier to long-term success with HAART drug therapy was discovered. Once again, drug resistance was a concern in AIDS care. Research studies presented at the 1997 Annual Antiretroviral Conference demonstrated that HIV viral suppression could be achieved by the use of "drug cocktails," combining a variety of potent protease inhibitor (PI) drugs with reverse transcriptase inhibitor drugs. However, the challenges of managing these multi-drug combinations were immense, and included the problem of strict patient compliance with a rigorous food and drug schedule. If patients stopped taking their medication, or took a decreased dose of medication, the patient's virus could mutate and become resistant to the medication, and this could occur within a two-week period. "Partial" adherence and "drug holidays" were as big a problem as total non-adherence.

Adherence to the medication regimens involved a major commitment to strict adherence of drug schedules. Antiretroviral (ARV) medications were found to be most effective when taken at full doses in relationship to meals (Katzenstein et al. 1997). Maintaining maximum antiretroviral potency required meticulous adherence to demanding medication regimens, including adhering to specific instructions regarding dosing timing intervals and food requirements for medication administration (Williams 1999).

HIV therapy was unforgiving, in comparison to drug therapies for other chronic diseases, which are often forgiving of lapses in adherence (Altice and Friedland 1998). A medication adherence rate of nearly 100 percent (ratio of medication doses taken to doses prescribed) was needed for HIV viral suppression. A medication adherence rate of 80 percent, acceptable in other chronic diseases, did not produce complete suppression of viral replication (Williams 1999). Thus the issue of adherence and drug resistance, along with how to facilitate adherence to the rigorous medication schedules, became the leading concern in HIV/AIDS care.

Adherence: Patient–Provider Relationships

Lerner, Gulick, and Dubler (1998) discussed the concepts of HIV non-adherence from a historical perspective, noting that physicians and public health officials had for a long time noted non-adherence to treatment among patients with tuberculosis (TB), diabetes, and hypertension. Patients who were unable or unwilling to follow prescribed regimens had been called *ignorant*, *vicious*, *recalcitrant*, and *noncompliant*. However, history provided two major lessons regarding non-adherence. First, labels such as "non-adherent" overemphasized the practitioner's role in determining who should receive treatment and how it should be administered. Second, the ability to predict non-adherence in individual patients remained elusive. Given these findings, Lerner et al. (1998) advocated revisiting the longstanding tendency to reflexively categorize patients as either adherent or non-adherent. Instead, an approach that discouraged labeling and emphasized active patient participation in therapy would avoid judgmental and inaccurate assessments of patient behavior. The authors concluded that this approach might help patients take HIV medications more successfully.

In their 1994 book *Good Doctors, Good Patients: Partners in HIV Treatment*, Rabkin, Remien, and Wilson discussed how the traditional paternalistic doctor–patient relationship changed in the era of HIV. The more assertive HIV-positive person, initially while healthy, was likely to consider the physician a consultant or advisor, helping to determine the treatment plan, and the patient might even consult with more than one physician as part of the process. This concept of egalitarian relationships between physicians and patients was fairly new and was practiced "perhaps nowhere as earnestly as in HIV medicine."

The authors noted that this change was derived from the philosophies, attitudes, and assumptions about authority and responsibility of activists within the gay community. The early activisists were smart, well educated and often held high-level positions in businesses and various professions. In the face of slow governmental response and inadequate provision of medical and social service, gay men initiated research, provided social services, and, by becoming politically active, promoted necessary medical services for people with HIV illness (Rabkin, Remien and Wilson 1994: 49):

> They were fighting for their lives and the survival of their community. In this context, gay men with AIDS were not willing to assume the traditional docile, passive patient role: they demanded, and generally were granted, more participation in their medical care. This proactive stance is now being adopted by other people living with AIDS, as well as patients with such diseases as breast cancer.

Adherence Challenges

Estimated rates of non-adherence to HAART ranged from 50 percent to 70 percent (Chesney 2000). Therefore, understanding factors involved in medication adherence was once again an important issue in HIV/AIDS care. Additional research was needed to identify psychological, physiological, sociocultural, and environmental factors associated with HIV medication non-adherence in various populations (Chesney et al. 2000).

The advent of the new "drug cocktails" had brought new hope for life, but the rigor of following the requirements of the medication schedule had a negative impact on quality of life. From the client's perspectives, the competing world of work and play were factors that led to non-adherence. Additionally, the side effects of the medications impacted dramatically on health status. A person with HIV but no symptoms of illness (HIV-positive asymptomatic) would now begin to feel ill after starting on the medication regimen. Patients on regimens containing protease inhibitors (PIs), which had strict dietary and fluid requirements, were also challenged to take these medications when outside of home or the controlled setting of the clinical drug trial group. Even specialized hospital AIDS units had problems adjusting routine medication and meal schedules to meet the timing and dietary requirements of the HIV combination drug regimen (Jones and Holloman 2000).

As noted by Chesney, psychological, physiological, sociocultural, and environmental factors could affect adherence. One qualitative study explored the experience of taking HIV medications from the perspective of HIV-positive women with a history of substance abuse (Jones 2003). Factors that helped the women with adherence included the provision of psychological and sociocultural services, such as social support, methadone, and antidepressant therapy. The study found that taking and having AIDS drugs could potentially reveal women's HIV-positive status, which could lead to rejection, social isolation, and possible domestic violence or physical abuse. The women reported hiding their HIV medications in bottles of Midol or prenatal or children's vitamins, so no one would see their medications. As one woman stated, "Everyone, even people on the street, knows that if you take AZT, you got AIDS."

Other Factors in Adherence

The review of literature found additional factors that impacted adherence to HIV combination drug therapy. Gifford et al. (2000) found that confidence in medication-taking ability, or perceived self-efficacy, and convenience of the medication regimen, or "fit" with routine and daily activities, was associated with greater medication adherence. Self-efficacy and social support were also noted in a study by Catz, Kelly, Bogart, Benotsch, and McAuliffe (2000). Roberts (2000) found six main facilitators of adherence: "making a commitment," health beliefs, "routinizing," social support, professional support, and mechanical devices. Other related factors included reminders and cues, planning, response to HIV/AIDS, interactions with others, patient characteristics, and HIV medication characteristics (Kemppainen et al. 2001).

Factors related to tolerability of the HIV medications were also important. A study of didanosine (Dodge et al. 1998) found that patients' preference of formulation was related not only to palatability but also to defined gastrointestinal (GI) side effects of the drug. In another didanosine study (Reynolds et al. 1999), participants described engaging in a variety of self-devised strategies to attenuate difficult and inconvenient aspects of adhering to the medication regimen.

In one study participants discussed the burden of taking pills and their resentment of the need to make medications the focus of their lives (Stone et al. 1998). Erlen and Mellors's (1999) adherence study revealed the metaphor of "balancing the hardships and the blessings." Bunting, Bevier and Baker (1999) noted that adherence may have a developmental component, as clients overcame their resistance to the burden of taking large quantities of medicine with their accompanying side effects. Thus, while many studies noted adherence barriers and facilitators, most researchers concluded that further research was needed to determine what would facilitate successful long-term adherence with prescribed HIV combination drug therapy.

Along with tolerability of the medications, "pill burden" affected adherence. Pill burden related to the burden of taking numerous pills, several times a day; in essence, the pills for life become a burden for life. Finding a better way to administer HIV medications was needed.

The start of a new era in ARV therapy quietly began in September 1997, when the FDA approved Combivir, a pill that contained a combination of two NRTI drugs: lamivudine (Epivir) and zidovudine (Retrovir). Both drugs were owned by the same pharmaceutical company. Because the two medicines were frequently prescribed together, the manufacturer combined them into one tablet. This was one of the first advances in an "easier" administration method for ARV therapy. One concern was that the doses were pre-set or "fixed" in the pill. If a patient needed to take a larger dose of one of the two medications, the patient would have to go back to the original method of taking two separate pills. In spite of this concern, the success of Combivir would lead to more co-packaged, fixed-dose combination (FDC) drugs in the twenty-first century.

Adherence: Health Care Workers and PEP

Although the potential development of drug resistance underlied the necessity of strict adherence to the HIV medication regimen, the process of medication adherence was, and is still, not well understood. Research studies have conflicting findings as to predictors of adherence, and findings vary between specific groups and populations. However, further insights on adherence and the experience of taking HIV medication regimens has been gained by studying non-experimental "real-life" case studies of health care workers taking HIV medications as post-exposure prophylaxis (PEP) for an occupational exposure to HIV.

The 2005 updated Public Health Service (PHS) guidelines for the management of PEP emphasizes adherence to HIV PEP when it is indicated for an exposure, along with expert consultation in management of exposures, follow-up of exposed workers to improve adherence to PEP, and monitoring for adverse events. The emphasis on PEP adherence is important, because studies have found that many health care workers do not adhere to the recommended four weeks of a triple-drug HIV medication regimen.

Concerns have been raised regarding the high incidence of non-adherence in persons who are educated and trained to provide health care and health promotion education to others. What motivates a health care worker to take or not take PEP? In a study of HIV medication adherence, a nurse described her up-and-down experience taking a PEP regimen of AZT, Epivir, and Crixivan for an occupational exposure to HIV. She was 28, had only been out of nursing school for a few months, and was a single mother with two young children. After giving an injection to a dying AIDS patient, she accidentally stuck herself with the used needle. Concerned about becoming infected with HIV, and the impact it would have on her children, she decided to take PEP (Jones 2002):

> The Crixivan (indinavir) made me so sick, incredibly nauseous. They gave me Compazine, but it made me drowsy, so I couldn't take it and work at the same time. So I threw up six times a day for that entire month. My life was to take those pills and try to wait an hour until I threw up again. But I kept it up. It was worth it if it would prevent me from getting HIV.

Ironically, her adherence and perseverance to the PEP regimen did not pay off. Eight months later she was hospitalized with a life-threatening respiratory infection. Her bloodwork revealed that she had sero-converted (went from a state of being HIV negative to HIV positive), making her one of the first cases in which taking PEP did not prevent HIV, just prolonged the onset of acute symptoms of HIV. Further bloodwork also revealed that, along with HIV, she had contracted hepatitis C from the needle-stick.

Tolerability of the HIV medications in relation to side effects may be an overwhelming deterrent to PEP adherence. Urbshott (1999) described his personal experience attempting to comply with his PEP regimen. An AIDS clinical drug trial research nurse, Urbshott realized upon reflection that his own personal assumptions were that non-adherence to HIV/AIDS treatment meant two things to him: lack of respect for personal health, and disregard for the health of fellow humans by playing with the resistance of an infectious agent. On a subconscious level, there was a feeling of superiority about adherence, the feeling that "This would never be the case with me."

Because of an occupational exposure, Urbshott was placed on a moderate-level PEP regimen (no PI), a twenty-eight-day regimen of zidovudine (AZT) and lamivudine (Epivir) twice a day. Trying to stay on the post-exposure regime was a demanding, exhausting journey. By Day 4 he was constantly nauseous, and was having dry retches by Day 5. He then began to experience agitation, restlessness, and cognitive impairment. He felt too ill to work, or to study. Even though he knew that these were the side effects of AZT, he felt as if he was methodically losing control. On Day 12, after intense thinking and reflection, Urbshott made the decision to discontinue PEP. As a health care provider, this was an emotional and reflective moment.

> I made a decision. On Day 12 I stopped taking my medications. It was a very carefully thought-out decision. It was not an easy one. I felt tremendous remorse and failure at not having been strong enough to finish the course of treatment. I felt less than the nurse I believed I should represent. And perhaps the most important emotion from this experience was that of guilt for having subconsciously or silently judged those about whom I actually knew so little: my patients.

Urbshott wrote that this experience would forever change his life and his practice as a nurse. He learned that non-adherence is not a decision made lightly; it may be the difference between life and quality of life. In conclusion, he asked other health care workers to carefully consider their own biases and assumptions when talking about adherence issues to clients and other care providers.

HIV DRUG THERAPY IN THE TWENTY-FIRST CENTURY

The twentieth century ended with complicated HAART regimens, and adherence and resistance issues. HIV drug therapy in the twenty-first century has become somewhat simplified, but at the same time has become more complex. The advent of fixed-dose combination (FDC) drugs has dramatically decreased the number of pills that need to be taken each day. The success of HIV antiretroviral (ARV) combination drug therapy has been demonstrated by decreased AIDS mortality in developed countries of the world. But the expense of these medications has been one of the deterrents to global access of these drugs.

New HIV Drugs and New Drug Categories

As of 2008, the Food and Drug Administration (FDA) has approved over thirty medications or pre-packaged fixed-dose combination (FDC) drugs for the treatment of HIV. In November 2000, the FDA approved Trizivir, which includes three NRTI drugs: abacavir sulfate (Ziagen), lamivudine (Epivir), and zidovudine (Retrovir). Because these three medicines frequently are prescribed together, the manufacturer combined them into one tablet. The recommended dosage of Trizivir is one tablet (300 mg of abacavir sulfate, 150 mg of lamivudine, and 300 mg of zidovudine) taken twice a day. In August 2004 the FDA approved two more co-formulated drugs: Epzicom, a combination drug containing the NRTI drug: abacavir sulfate (Ziagen) and lamivudine (Epivir), and Truvada, another NRTI combination drug containing emtricitabine (Emtriva) and tenofovir disoproxil fumarate (tenofovir DF or Viread).

A historic event occurred in 2006 when the FDA approved Atripla tablets, a fixed-dose combination of three ARV drugs, in a single tablet taken once a day, alone or in combination with other ARV drugs. Atripla became the first approved HIV one-pill, once-a-day product. Additionally, Atripla is the first combination to contain drugs from two different drug categories. Atripla combines three drugs into one pill: the NNRTI Sustiva (efavirenz) with the NRTIs Emtriva (emtricitabine) and Viread (tenofovir disoproxil fumarate). Different pharmaceutical companies own the three drugs. The companies formed a joint venture for Atripla, a first of its kind of collaboration in the field of HIV/AIDS.

Besides the three drug categories previously mentioned, the FDA also approved another HIV drug category, the entry and fusion inhibitors. Fusion inhibitors work by blocking HIV in the bloodstream from binding to receptors (such as the CCR5 receptor) and entering uninfected CD4 cells. The injectible drug enfuvirtide (Fuzeon) was joined in this category by a new tablet drug, mariviroc (Selzentry), which received FDA approval in August 2007. In October 2007, the FDA also approved raltegravir (Isentress), the first drug in a new category, the integrase inhibitors. Integrase inhibitors work by blocking integrase, a protein that HIV needs to insert its viral genetic material into the genetic material of an infected cell. In January 2008 the FDA also approved a new NNRTI drug, etravirine (Intelence).

Initial HIV drug regimens usually include a combination of an NNRTI drug or a boosted (includes ritonavir) PI with an NRTI (Bartlett 2007). For example, 2008 guidelines from the Department of Health and Human Services (DHHS) panel on Antiretroviral Guidelines recommend starting with the NNRTI drug efavirenz (Sustiva) or one of the following PI drugs: atazanavir (Reyataz)/ritonavir, fosamprenavir (Lexiva)/ritonavir or lopinavir/ritonavir (Kaletra) plus one of the following NRTI drugs: abacavir sulfate plus lamivudine (Epzicom) or tenofovir DF + emtricitabine. An alternative regimen would be the NNRT nevirapine (Viramune) or one of the following PIs: atazanavir (Reyataz), fosamprenavir (Lexiva), and ritonavir (Kaletra), or saquinavir and ritonavir. This regimen can be combined with either zidovudine plus lamivudine (Combivir: ordidanosine plus either emtricitabine (Emtriva) or lamivudine (Epivir). However, the drug combination that is selected and prescribed by the provider will depend on many factors, including the extent of HIV disease progression and previous HIV medication history.

HIV drug guidelines continue to be developed by expert panels from various AIDS groups, such as the International AIDS Society, or federally sponsored groups, such as DHHS. HIV drug guidelines are continually re-evaluated and revised, based on new data from clinical drug trials or post-marketing studies.

Global Issues: Access to Care

In the twenty-first century HIV remains a global health issue. In 2002, the United Nations (UN) met in a historical Special Session on the global impact of HIV. This was the first time the UN had ever convened a Special Session on a health issue. The goal of the session was to endorse a Declaration of Commitment, outlining the key goals, action, and targets needed to successfully contain HIV/AIDS and dramatically reduce its spread and impact. Leaders from around the world gathered to discuss what was happening around the world, and to develop a global agreement on improving HIV prevention and care. Access to drugs was a major concern of many of the underdeveloped nations.

Ambassadors and delegates from 149 countries attended the three-day meeting. The opening speech by UN Secretary General Kofi Annan focused attention on the death and devastation wrought by the global epidemic of HIV/AIDS. This thought was echoed by each of the speakers who followed. Each country was allowed five minutes to address the session and describe how AIDS had impacted their country. Delegates from the African nations spoke out against the cost of AIDS therapy, and expressed the need to circumvent international patent laws in order to make affordable drug therapy accessible to the developing countries of the world, which have been hardest hit by the epidemic. Other major topics included further research on vaginal microbicides for HIV prevention for women, and more money for the development of AIDS vaccines.

The issue of generic drugs was discussed at the UN Special Session. Controversy at first developed when countries, such as Cuba, Brazil and India, announced that they would fight HIV by manufacturing generic HIV drugs, at low cost, for distribution in their countries. Pharmaceutical companies declared that this was an infringement of patent law, trade agreements, and intellectual property rights. Over time the controversy was resolved, and the FDA now approves generic HIV drugs that are manufactured and distributed in other countries. The FDA has now approved more than twenty treatments to be used as part of the President's Emergency Plan for AIDS Relief program (PEPFAR), initiated in 2003 to fight the international HIV/AIDS pandemic. Issues have arisen, however, regarding how to implement global HIV drug therapy to all who are affected.

Looking inside the pill bottle, in the twenty-first century HIV drug therapy is not a cure for AIDS, but is helping win the battle against death from AIDS. However, other types of medications, such as vaccines and microbicides that are currently in clinical trials, may help prevent HIV infection. In the future, these types of medications may actually win the war against AIDS by preventing HIV infection from ever occurring again.

REFERENCES AND FURTHER READING

Altice, F.L. and Friedland, G.H. "The era of adherence to HIV therapy." *Annals of Internal Medicine* 129:6 (1998): 503–505.

Bartlett, J. *2007 Pocket Guide, Adult HIV/AIDS Treatment.* Johns Hopkins University, 2007.

Bennett, J. "Historical Overview of the HIV Pandemic." In *ANAC's Core Curriculum for HIV/AIDS Nursing*, 2nd edition, edited by C. Kirton. Thousand Oaks, CA: Sage Publications, 2003.

Bunting, S.M., Bevier, D.J. and Baker, S.K. "Poor women living with HIV: self-identified needs." *Journal of Community Health Nursing*, 16:1 (1999): 41–52.

Burkett, E. *The Gravest Show on Earth: America in the Age of AIDS.* Boston: Houghton Mifflin, 1995.

Carpenter, C., et al. "Antiretroviral therapy for HIV infection in 1996." *JAMA* 276:2 (1996): 146–154.

Catz, S.L., Kelly, J.A., Bogart, L.M., Benotsch, E.G. and McAuliffe, T.L. "Patterns, correlates and barriers to medication adherence among persons prescribed new treatments for HIV disease." *Health Psychology* 19:2 (2000): 124–133.

CDC. *HIV/AIDS Statistics.* Rockville, MD: Centers for Disease Control, 1999.

Chesney, M.A. "Factors affecting adherence to antiretroviral therapy." *Clinical Infectious Diseases*, Supplement 2 (2000): S171–S176.

Chesney, M.A., Ickovics, J.R., Chambers, D.B., Gifford, A.L., Neidig, J., Zwicki, B. and Wu, A.W. "Self-reported adherence to antiretroviral medications among participants in HIV clinical trials: the AACTG adherence instruments. Patient Care Committee and Adherence Working Group of the Outcomes Committee of the Adult AIDS Clinical Trials Group (ACTG)." *AIDS Care* 12:3 (2000): 255–266.

Churchill, S. "Protease inhibitors: implications for HIV research and treatment." *Journal of the International Association of Physicians in AIDS Care* (1996): 13–18.

Department of Health and Human Services. 2008. "Guidelines for the use of antiretroviral agents in HIV-1-infected adults and adolescents January 29, 2008." http://aidsinfo.nih.gov/contentfiles/AdultandAdolescentGL.pdf. Retrieved February 18, 2008.

Dobkin, J.F. "New needlestick guidelines." *Infectious Medicine* 13:7 (1996): 536.

Dodge, R.T., Shipp, K.W. and Miralles, G.D. "Improved gastrointestinal tolerance and palatability of didanosine in adults by the use of pediatric powdered formulation." *Journal of the Association of Nurses in AIDS Care* 9:5 (1998): 27–31.

Dykeman, M.C., Wallace, R., Ferrell, P., Jasek, J. and Tortorice, P.V. "Drug interactions: how they affect people living with HIV/AIDS." *Journal of the Association of Nurses in AIDS Care* 7:4 (1996): 67–79.

Eldred, L.J., Wu, A.W., Chaisson, R.E. and Moore, R.D. "Adherence to antiretroviral and Pneumocystis prophylaxis in HIV disease." *Journal of Acquired Immune Deficiency Syndrome Human Retrovirology* 18:2 (1998): 117–125.

Erlen, J.A. and Mellors, M.P. "Adherence to combination therapy in persons living with HIV: balancing the hardships and the blessings." *Journal of the Association of Nurses in AIDS Care* 10:4 (1999): 75–84.

Freeman, R.C., Rodriguez, G.M. and French, J.F. "Compliance with AZT treatment regimen of HIV-seropositive injection drug users: a neglected issue." *AIDS Education and Prevention* 8:1 (1996): 58–71.

Frick, P.A., Gal, P., Lane, T.W., and Sewell, P.C. "Antiretroviral medication compliance in patients with AIDS." *AIDS Patient Care* 12:6 (1998): 463–470.

Gifford, A.L., Bormann, J.E., Shively, M.J., Wright, B.C., Richman, D.D. and Bozzette, S.A. "Predictors of self-reported adherence and plasma HIV concentrations in patients on multidrug antiretroviral regimens." *Journal of Acquired Immune Deficiency Syndrome* 23:5 (2000): 386–395.

HHS News. 1997. "Vital statistics report shows significant gain in health." http://www.cdc.gov/nchs/pressroom/97news/mortgain.htm. Retrieved February 18, 2008.

Jones, S. G. "The other side of the pill bottle: the lived experience of HIV^{+} nurses on HIV combination drug therapy." *Journal of the Association of Nurses in AIDS Care* 13:3 (2002): 22–36.

Jones, S. G.. "Life in a pill bottle: the experience of taking HIV medications." *International Journal of Human Caring* 7:2 (2003): 57–65.

Jones, S.G. and Holloman, F. "Continuous quality improvement project: decreasing the potential for the development in the inpatient setting of drug resistance by improving nursing practice for HAART administration." *Journal of the Association of Nurses in AIDS Care* 11:2 (2000): 76–86.

Katzenstein, D.A., Lyons, C., Mologhan, J.P., Ungvarski, P., Wolfe, G.S. and Williams, A. "HIV therapeutics: confronting adherence." *Journal of the Association of Nurses in AIDS Care* 8: Supplement (1997): 46–58.

Kemppainen, J.K., Levine, R.E., Mistal, M. and Schmidgall, D. "HAART adherence in culturally diverse patients with HIV/AIDS: a study of male patients from a Veteran's Administration Hospital in northern California." *AIDS Patient Care and STDS* 15:3 (2001): 117–127.

Lerner, B.H., Gulick, R.M. and Dubler, N.N. "Rethinking nonadherence: historical perspectives on triple-drug therapy for HIV disease." *Annals of Internal Medicine* 129:7 (1998): 573–578.

McBride, S.H. "The AIDS cocktail." *Managed Health Care* 7:11 (1997): 39–41.

Martin, M. "Mary Fisher gets mad." *POZ*, December 1997, 103–104.

Morrison, C. "HIV/AIDS units: is there still a need?" *Journal of the Association of Nurses in AIDS Care* 9:6 (1998): 16–18.

Morse, E.V., Simon, P.M., Coburn, M., Hyslop, N., Greenspan, D., and Balson, P.M. "Determinants of subject compliance within an experimental anti-HIV drug protocol." *Social Science Medicine* 32:10 (1991): 1161–1167.

Muma, R.D., Ross, M.W., Parcel, G.S. and Pollard, R.B. "Zidovudine adherence among individuals with HIV infection." *AIDS Care* 7:4 (1995): 439–447.

Napper, R.L. "Census trends in AIDS specialty units." *Journal of the Association of Nurses in AIDS Care* 9:6 (1998): 42–46.

National Center for Health Statistics. 1999, June 9. "New data show AIDS patients less likely to be hospitalized." Centers for Disease Control and Prevention. http://www.cdc.gov/od/oc/media/pressrel/r990608.htm. Retrieved February 18, 2008.

Rabkin, J., Remien, R. and Wilson, C. *Good Doctors, Good Patients: Partners in HIV Treatment*. New York: NCM Publishers, Inc., 1994.

Reynolds, Nancy R., Neidig, J.L. and Brashers, D.E. "Patient appraisal of mandarin orange didanosine: implications for adherence and well-being." *Journal of the Association of Nurses in AIDS Care* 10:1 (1999): 35–41.

Roberts, K.J. "Barriers to and facilitators of HIV-positive patients' adherence to antiretroviral treatment regimens." *AIDS Patient Care and STDs* 14:3 (2000): 155–168.

Samet, J., et al. "Compliance with zidovudine therapy in patients infected with HIV, type 1: a cross-sectional study in a municipal hospital clinic." *American Journal of Medicine* 92:5 (1992): 495–502.

Singh, N., Squier, C., Sivek, C., Wagener, M., Nguyen, M.H. and Yu, V.L. "Determinants of compliance with antiretroviral therapy in patients with human immunodeficiency virus: prospective assessment with implications for enhancing compliance." *AIDS Care* 8:3 (1996): 261–269.

Smith, M.Y., Rapkin, B.D., Morrison, A. and Kammerman, S. "Zidovudine adherence in persons with AIDS: the relation of patient beliefs about medication to self-termination of therapy." *Journal of General Internal Medicine* 12 (1997): 216–223.

Stone, V.E., et al. "HIV/AIDS patients' perspectives on adhering to regimens containing protease inhibitors." *Journal of General Internal Medicine* 13:9 (1998): 586–593.

Urbshott, G.B. "Reflections on HIV, adherence and objectivity." *Journal of the Association of Nurses in AIDS Care* 10:6 (1999): 99–100.

U. S. Public Health Service. 2005. "Updated U.S. Public Health Service Guidelines for Management of Occupational Exposures to HIV: Recommendations for Postexposure Prophylaxis." http://www.cdc.gov/mmwr/preview/mmwrhtml/rr5409a1.htm. Retrieved February 18, 2008.

Williams, Ann B. "Adherence to highly active antiretroviral therapy." *Nursing Clinics of North America* 34:1 (1999): 113–129.

This Belize City billboard shows that in many cases, due to poverty, if girls do not exchange sexual acts for money they cannot pay their school fees

Have you heard me today?
No sex... No school.
That's the choice I face.
Equality for women helps fight AIDS.

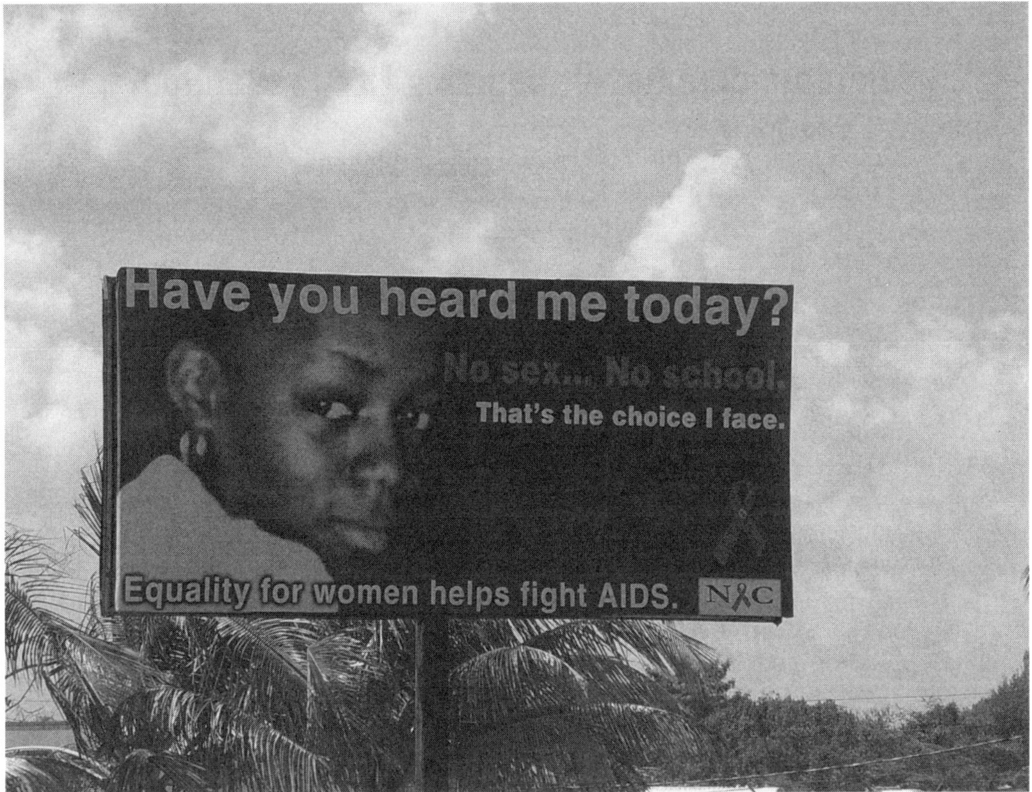

Source: Photo courtesy of Cynthia Pope (2007)

CHAPTER 10

Microbicides: Revolutionizing HIV Prevention?

Laurie Sylla and Clair Kaplan

ABSTRACT

Microbicides have the potential to revolutionize HIV prevention for women as dramatically as "the pill" transformed women's options and protections. While microbicides will not be a substitute for challenging systemic gender inequity, and first generation products are likely to be less efficacious than condoms, microbicides will increase women's power to reduce their risks of HIV/AIDS. This chapter provides several strategies that need to be implemented to make microbicides a viable and universally accessible option for helping to control HIV in women. Microbicide research investment needs to increase dramatically, including creation of research infrastructure in the global south, where large-scale effectiveness trials will need to be carried out.

THE URGENT NEED

As other authors in this volume note (see Rao and Weiss; Durvasula et al.; Ibembe), social, cultural, and biological vulnerability to HIV has led to women becoming an ever-increasing proportion of those living with HIV/AIDS. Heterosexual transmission is the main mode of spread of HIV, and in many parts of the world the primary risk factor for women becoming infected is marriage (International Partnership for Microbicides 2005a; UNAIDS/WHO 2005; Shattock and Solomon 2004). In 2005, women and girls accounted for 46 percent of adolescents/adults around the globe living with HIV/AIDS (Alfsen 2004; International Partnership for Microbicides 2005a; UNAIDS/WHO 2005). Seventeen million women were living with HIV/AIDS; about a million more than in 2003. In sub-Saharan Africa, home to two-thirds of the epidemic, women and girls comprise 57 percent of individuals living with HIV/AIDS and 65 percent of new infections (UNAIDS/WHO 2005: 1–98). Epidemiological studies have found young women and girls (15–24) three to six times more likely than their male peers to be infected at the same age, and married girls are more likely than their unmarried counterparts to be infected (Glynn et al. 2001; Kelly et al. 2003).

After more than 20 years of intensive condom promotion, worldwide condom adoption has dramatically increased; however, usage is still inadequate and unevenly distributed (UNAIDS 2005). Condom use remains low in many countries, even in casual partnerships. For example, in Madagascar, a country with rising HIV prevalence, only 12 percent of boys and five percent of girls aged 15–24 reported using a condom during their last intercourse (Direction Générale de la Lutte contre le SIDA and et al. 2005). Numerous studies have found that in many parts of the world, including Bangladesh, Yemen, Pakistan, Jakarta, Peru, and parts of India, sex workers frequently used condoms less than half of the time with their paying partners, and in many instances were unaware that condoms offered protection from HIV/AIDS, or even that condoms existed. Injection drug users throughout

Eastern Europe and Asia who purchased or sold sex were even less likely than non-drug users to use condoms (UNAIDS 2005).

In primary partnerships, condom use is even lower, placing married women at very high risk (Meehan and et al. 2004; UNAIDS/WHO 2005; UNAIDS 2005). For example, one study found that married women in a rural farming region in Nicaragua were twice as likely as sex workers in the region to have HIV (UNAIDS 2005).

Current prevention strategies are insufficient. They stress behavioral choices that are not feasible for the world's most vulnerable. Additional options, particularly those that are user-controlled and do not require partner participation, are clearly needed. This has led many to call for investment in the development of a safe, effective, affordable microbicide (Alfsen 2004; D'Cruz and Uckun 2004; Elias and Coggins 2001; Grown, Gupta, and Pande 2005; Harrison, Rosenberg, and Bowcut 2003; Heise, McGrory, and Wood 1998; Howett and Kuhl 2005; International Partnership for Microbicides 2005a; Lewis 2004; UNAIDS 2005).

Microbicides are designed to be self-administered topically to mucosal surfaces such as the vagina or rectum to help prevent transmission of HIV and possibly other sexually transmitted infections (STIs). They may be produced as gels, creams, suppositories, or in innovative forms such as slow-release rings. While the emphasis is on compounds that will prevent HIV infection, researchers are also assessing the efficacy of these compounds for reducing STI transmission and protecting against pregnancy (Bird et al. 2004; Braunstein and van de Wijgert 2005; Elias and Coggins 2001; Scholand, DeSimone, and Pomerantz 2005; Shattock and Solomon 2004). They may be used as sole agents, or in conjunction with physical barriers such as diaphragms and cervical caps, as well as with female and male condoms, thus increasing efficacy (Bird et al. 2004; Braunstein and van de Wijgert 2005). Microbicides are unique in that they can be used by women without partner cooperation, consent or, in some instances, even knowledge (Elias and Coggins 2001). Ideally, microbicides will provide protection for both partners.

There are currently several dozen candidate microbicides in various stages of active investigation, including pre-clinical trials where the bulk of the products in the pipeline are, Phase I and II safety trials, and Phase III effectiveness trials, but the drug development process can take a decade or more from initial discovery to final regulatory approval. Estimates on the soonest a microbicide could be available somewhere in the world range from within the next three to five years to significantly later, depending on how the forerunners fare in large-scale efficacy trials (Alfsen 2004; Shattock and Solomon 2004; Smith et al. 2005). As of December 2005, five products had begun large-scale effectiveness trials. By February 2008, trials of two of these products had been suspended early. A third large-scale effectiveness trial was completed, but could not demonstrate product efficacy, perhaps in part due to low product adherence. Only two products remain in late-stage trials. At this time, there is great interest in using reformulated antiretrovirals (medications used to treat HIV) as microbicides. These products would target HIV specifically, and likely be more efficacious than broader spectrum products, but raise concerns about resistance (Rosenberg 2008).

New drug development is very costly and most agents that enter the pipeline fail at various steps before safe, efficacious, and usable compounds emerge. Increases in international public and private sector funding, coordination of efforts, and sharing of expertise could help speed the process (Alfsen 2004). Advocacy groups, such as the Alliance for Microbicide Development, the Global Campaign for Microbicides, and the International Partnership for Microbicides, have been instrumental in pushing for increased investment from government, and academic and other non-profit institutions, as well as for support from the pharmaceutical industry (Harrison 2000; International Partnership for Microbicides 2005a). For a variety of reasons, including an uncharted global regulatory environment, market uncertainties, large upfront development costs, and low expectations for microbicide profitability, the pharmaceutical industry is unlikely to invest significant resources in product development until a first generation efficacious product has been discovered, thus increasing the need for public investment (Cobb et al. 2002).

In addition to being efficacious, microbicides will need to be acceptable to users, nontoxic, affordable, and physically stable in a range of settings and temperatures (Mantell et al. 2005). Acceptability will be affected by product characteristics, timing of use, gender norms and interpersonal relationship dynamics, personal feminine hygiene practices, social meanings of using any type of protection, and differing cultural norms and personal preferences regarding lubrication during sexual activity (Braunstein and van de Wijgert 2005; Elias and Coggins 2001; Weeks et al. 2004). Acceptability is as important as efficacy, because acceptability will lead to use, and use will be the driving factor in determining effectiveness (Smith et al. 2005). Efficacy is defined as the power or capacity to produce a desired effect, whereas effectiveness is determined by efficacy modified by how consistently and correctly a product is used.

Women's biological vulnerability to HIV —in other words, the fact that HIV is more readily transmitted from males to females than from females to males—may be tied to vaginal and rectal micro-abrasions from penetrative sex, the increased duration of exposure to infectious seminal fluids by susceptible vaginal, cervical, and rectal mucosal tissue, larger surface area of the vagina and rectum as compared to the penile urethral opening, and the nature of the cervix and the rectum as thin and fragile cellular structures (Miller and Shattock 2003). Adolescent females are even more vulnerable because of cervical cellular changes, called ectopy, which increase biologic vulnerability (Heise and Wood 2005). The presence of other sexually transmitted infections (STIs) can further compromise tissue defenses and increase susceptibility to infection. STIs like syphilis or herpes may manifest with external as well as undetected internal lesions, increasing access for HIV to target cells. Whether lesions are present or not, STIs typically increase white blood cells in the area in an attempt to fight off infection. These same cells are targets for HIV, providing more sites for the virus to infect (Harrison, Rosenberg, and Bowcut 2003; Turmen 2003).

Vaccines, the best technology for preventing infectious disease, have virtually wiped out smallpox and nearly eradicated other lethal or debilitating infectious diseases such as polio. While the vigorous search for a safe, effective vaccine protective against HIV continues, experts caution that, for reasons too complex to delineate here, successful product development is many years away (Johnston and Flores 2001; Spearman 2003).

In the absence of an effective vaccine, only behavioral means are currently available for preventing sexual transmission of HIV. These include abstaining from sexual activity, being mutually monogamous with an uninfected partner, and using male or female condoms. However, each of these methods has inherent problems.

Abstinence is rarely a lifelong choice that most individuals would willingly embrace, and moreover—as Stephen Lewis, UN Special Envoy on AIDS in Africa, has pointed out—abstinence in marriage is generally neither feasible nor desirable (Lewis 2004). Behavioral data from country after country continues to demonstrate high prevalence of unprotected sexual activity from puberty onward (UNAIDS 2005). The emphasis on "abstinence *only*" can leave young people, especially girls, at increased risk if they do not know how to protect themselves when vows of abstinence are broken (Dailard 2003).

Mutual monogamy can be effective, provided both partners are uninfected, but many people do not know their own or their partner's HIV status. In the global south, where the majority of HIV infection is concentrated, limited testing is available and most people do not seek out testing in the absence of treatment. Individuals may be monogamous and believe they are protecting themselves and each other, yet they may have been infected by a previous partner. Another limitation of relying on mutual monogamy is that the only person whose monogamy can be counted on is one's own. In the United States, a country where marital fidelity is strongly held as a social value, current or previous marital infidelity has been reported by a third of currently married males and a quarter of currently married females, and by 56 percent of currently divorced males and 59 percent of currently divorced females (Janus and Janus 1993; Rouse 2002). Male polygamy is a common and accepted practice in many parts of the world. Given that the majority of HIV-infected women in the world report being infected by their only partner, their husbands, relying on partner monogamy is clearly a risky method of protection (UNAIDS/WHO 2005).

Male condoms have been one of the cornerstones of HIV prevention since the beginning of the epidemic and, while their promotion and adoption has been far more limited, female condoms have also demonstrated significant effectiveness in preventing HIV transmission. Despite overwhelming evidence of effectiveness, condoms are used in only a relatively small percentage of sexual acts, and use is lowest in primary partnerships. Barriers to consistent, effective condom use include cultural mores, religious teaching, timing of use, ignorance of correct use, perceived diminished sensation, available supply, perceived interference with intimacy, cultural meanings regarding condom use and trust, discomfort with asking partners to wear condoms, partner refusal, women's inability to insist on their use by their partners, and their contraceptive activity (Dunkle et al. 2004; Lichtenstein 2005; Macaluso et al. 2000; Mosack et al. in press; Saul et al. 2004; Severy et al. 2005; Weeks et al. 2004).

Abstinence and barrier methods, when used consistently and correctly, are effective for preventing HIV and STI transmission and also conception. In all the discourse on HIV prevention, little attention has been paid to the meaning and value of motherhood, either to the social, economic, and cultural pressures on women to become mothers, or to the personal desire and yearning to become a parent. A non-contraceptive microbicide could, for the first time, allow women to take action to protect themselves from sexual transmission of infection yet still become pregnant. This would be revolutionary.

Microbicides will contribute to the ability of individuals around the globe to exercise their sexual and reproductive rights. Sexual rights include the rights of all individuals to: 1) decide freely and responsibly on all aspects of their sexuality, including protecting and promoting their sexual and reproductive health; 2) be free of discrimination, coercion, or violence in their sexual lives and in all sexual decisions; and 3) expect and demand equality, full consent, mutual respect, and shared responsibility in sexual relationships (World Association of Sexual Health 2006). Reproductive rights rest on the recognition of the basic right of all couples and individuals to freely decide the number, spacing, and timing of their children. These rights include access to the information and means to make reproductive choices, the right to attain the highest standard of sexual and reproductive health, and the ability to make decisions concerning reproduction free of discrimination, coercion, and violence (UNFPA 2006).

Microbicides fit into this sexual and reproductive rights framework by offering a new user-controlled method for preventing disease transmission, potentially supplementing existing disease prevention methods with a non-contraceptive option. In most cultures around the world, where women are not free to determine the circumstances under which they will have intimate relationships or engage in sexual activity, the ability to use a product without partner negotiation, cooperation, consent, or even knowledge, is an important step toward sexual freedom.

THE SCIENCE

Microbicides may work through multiple mechanisms of action. One class of agents under investigation works by nonspecific surface action against membranes or outer viral envelopes, thus disrupting the virus. Products in this class are both spermicidal and non-spermicidal, offering hope of a non-contraceptive microbicide. A variety of products under development work to enhance vaginal defense mechanisms against infection, many of them utilizing lactobacilli and promoting favorable and balanced vaginal environments. Another class of products inhibits the viral life cycle and replication, and another prevents entry into mucosal cells.

Many of these products also demonstrate activity against other sexually transmitted pathogens (D'Cruz and Uckun 2004; Harrison, Rosenberg, and Bowcut 2003; Howett and Kuhl 2005; Scholand, DeSimone, and Pomerantz 2005; Weber, Desai, and Darbyshire 2005).

In addition to the urgent need for vaginal microbicides, there is also a need for a rectal microbicide. A microbicide that provides protection during anal intercourse would be an important protective tool for both heterosexuals and for men who engage in anal intercourse with other men. Anal intercourse is the most efficient route of sexual transmission of HIV, and is a common, yet underreported practice of both heterosexuals and homosexuals. In the United States, the number of women who report engaging in receptive anal sex is seven times the number of men who report engaging in receptive anal sex with other men (Gorbach 2004). Development of a safe and effective rectal microbicide will be even more challenging than development of a vaginal microbicide. It cannot be assumed that a product that is safe and effective for the vagina will be safe or effective in the rectum. Studies of nonoxynol-9 (N-9), a licensed contraceptive that was an early microbicide candidate, found that it increased the likelihood of HIV transmission, even as it was being widely recommended by public health agencies and clinicians (Newell et al. 2004).

In addition, the rectal environment is more fragile than the vaginal environment. Only a single layer of epithelial cells serves as protection against pathogens, and this surface is easily damaged. The colorectal mucosa is the largest site of lymphocytes in the body, and is also heavily populated with langerhans cells, dendritic cells, and macrophages, making it a prime site for both acquiring and transmitting HIV infection (Di Stefano et al. 2001: 637–643). Because it a long, open tube rather than a closed pouch like the vagina, understanding how much product is needed and where it must reach remains under study (Fuchs et al. 2005). Additionally, it is politically more challenging to obtain public research dollars to study rectal safety and efficacy of candidate products, despite the urgent need to protect both men and women from HIV transmission during anal intercourse.

THE IMPACT

Scientific challenges notwithstanding, discovery of even a modestly efficacious microbicide could have tremendous impact. Researchers at the London School of Hygiene and Tropical Medicine have developed a mathematical model for assessing the impact of introducing microbicides of varying effectiveness into different populations whose epidemics are at different stages of development. Using conservative assumptions, they estimate that introducing a 60 percent-efficacious microbicide into 73 lower income countries could avert 2.5 million HIV infections over three years if it is used by only 20 percent of people who currently have contact with a health care system during half of the sex acts in which they don't use condoms. Averting this number of infections translates into cost savings of $2.7 billion in health care costs and $1 billion in productivity benefits (Watts et al. 2002). Smith et al. (2005) used mathematical modeling to come to the conclusion that daily risk of HIV acquisition for female sex workers would be reduced by 19 percent or 28 percent, respectively, if a microbicide of 30–50 percent efficacy or 50–80 percent efficacy were available.

While some worry about the availability of a microbicide having a negative impact on condom use, historical data from family planning demonstrates that introducing any new method into the prevention mix increases the total utilization of any prevention methodology. Modeling studies of individual risk have also shown that, if an individual is using a microbicide, substantial reductions in condom use could be tolerated among inconsistent condom users without increasing that individual's risk of contracting HIV. In fact, if individuals used a microbicide that was 50 percent efficacious during half of the sexual acts where they didn't use condoms, individuals who currently use condoms a quarter of the time could cease using condoms altogether without increasing their risk of infection. Only individuals who are already consistent condom users (more than 70 percent use) would increase their personal risk if they reduced their condom use and used the microbicide less than half of the time when they did not use condoms (Foss et al. 2003; Watts et al. 2002).

The impact of microbicides goes beyond simply interrupting the chain of HIV infection. Young uninfected children are three times more likely to survive if their mothers are living than if their mothers are dead. For children with HIV, the difference is even greater (Newell et al. 2004). Preventing women from acquiring HIV will increase child survival and help stem the rising tide of AIDS orphans, who number more than 12 million in sub-Saharan Africa alone (UNAIDS 2005). Quality of family life, ability of children to attend school, access to food, and household economics are all affected by the presence of a living mother. Sero-discordant couples who want to protect the uninfected partner but who desire children would also have new options. Aside from the very real survival benefit a microbicide will provide, the sense of control many women will feel at having *something* they can do to protect themselves, and the sense of empowerment that will be created for some women is incalculable. Microbicides could be the biggest breakthrough in reproductive health since the pill, and could revolutionize HIV prevention in similar ways (Forbes 2002).

Numerous studies have demonstrated women's desire for and willingness to use microbicides (Darroch and Frost 1999; Elias and Coggins 2001; Hammett et al. 2000; Hill 2001; Mantell et al. 2005; Morar et al. 2004; Mosack et al. in press; Rwabukwali et al. 2004; Weeks et al. 2004). A twelve-country marketing study carried out by the European Union found great demand for microbicides and a willingness by women to pay triple what they would pay for a condom for a microbicide (Hill 2001). High-risk inner-city women who participated in a two-week microbicide simulation trial in Hartford, Connecticut, in the United States, reported strong interest in using a highly efficacious microbicide with their primary partner (98.8 percent), casual partners (100 percent), and paying partners (100 percent) (Mosack et al. in press; Weeks et al. 2004). Authors of a nationwide phone survey concluded that an estimated 21.3 million U.S. women would be potentially interested in using a microbicide (Darroch and Frost 1999). While a modestly efficacious microbicide will make an enormous difference to millions of women who feel that they have no other option to protect themselves, microbicide efficacy may need to approach condom efficacy for uptake by women who are accustomed to having access to condoms and making decisions about their use.

Although microbicides may be a method that can be "female-controlled," they will be used in the context of women's lives that are still often controlled by men. For widespread microbicide adoption, products will have to be acceptable to men as well as women. Male resistance is one of the barriers to more widespread condom use. Microbicides will need to be experienced by male partners as neutral, pleasure-enhancing, or non-detectable (Heise and Wood 2005; Koo et al. 2005; Pool et al. 2000; Rwabukwali et al. 2004; Severy and Newcomer 2005; Severy et al. 2005; UNAIDS 2005; Weeks et al. 2004). Initially it was thought that "stealth use" would be of primary importance to women, necessitating a product that would be undetectable by male partners. While this will be of importance to a significant subset of women, both clinical trial and acceptability research has shown that the majority of women with primary partners disclose product use to their partners (Hammett et al. 2000; Mosack et al. in press; Pool et al. 2000; Weeks et al. 2004; Woodsong 2004). Greater understanding of the social and cultural meanings of microbicide use within primary partnerships will help guide design of products and programs that foster widespread adoption (Koo et al. 2005; Mantell et al. 2005; Morar et al. 2004; Mosack et al. in press; Rwabukwali et al. 2004; Severy and Newcomer 2005; Severy et al. 2005; Weeks et al. 2004).

THE ETHICAL CHALLENGES

It is critical that any product that appears to be virucidal in vitro (in a test tube) be subjected to rigorous clinical trials that assess safety and efficacy in people; however, conducting clinical trials of microbicides requires negotiating many ethical conundrums. Since it isn't known if any of the products being tested offer protective benefit, ethical conduct requires that everyone who participates in microbicide trials must be provided with prevention counseling, male (and sometimes female) condoms, and STI treatment or referral (Heise and Wood 2005; Heise, McGrory, and Wood 1998; de Zoysa, Elias, and Bentley 1998). Since HIV transmission is a relatively rare event and trial endpoints will be determined by comparisons of transmission rates in each study arm, large-scale effectiveness trials need to be conducted in geographic areas with significant incidence rates and in populations that don't use intravenous drugs. These conditions are generally found only in resource-limited settings, such as sub-Saharan Africa. Within these settings, there is typically little or no pre-existing research infrastructure, a general unfamiliarity within the study population of research concepts such as randomization or placebos, severely limited health care access, and little or no antiretroviral treatment (ART) for HIV (Heise and Wood 2005).

Ethical issues in research are rooted in the principles of respect for persons, beneficence, and justice (Beauchamp and Childress 2001; Council for International Organizations of Medical Sciences 2002; Heise and Wood 2005; Heise, McGrory, and Wood 1998; Lo and Groman 2003; MacQueen, Karim, and Sugarman 2003; Shapiro and Benatar 2005; World Medical Association 2004). Respect for persons includes respecting the autonomy of individuals to make informed decisions about voluntarily participating in trials. Beneficence requires that vulnerable individuals are assured protections and that benefit is maximized while risk is minimized. The principle of justice requires that the benefits and burdens of the research are distributed fairly among participants and society (Beauchamp and Childress 2001; Council for International Organizations of Medical Sciences 2002; Heise, McGrory, and Wood 1998; Lo and Groman 2003; MacQueen, Karim, and Sugarman 2003; Slack et al. 2005; World Medical Association 2004). Challenges arise when attempting to meet these principles in a world that is fundamentally unjust, a quality in this instance characterized by inequitable distribution of resources, including life-saving HIV treatment (Heise and Wood 2005).

Respect for persons has generally been upheld via informed consent, but securing this can be quite complex in these settings. When research is conducted in settings with high illiteracy rates and a scarcity of health care, therapeutic misconception (the belief that the product being given *must* be therapeutically beneficial) is common. When multiple languages are spoken and there are no local words to portray research concepts, extra diligence is required by researchers to assure that participants understand the study, randomization, the possibility of not receiving an actual microbicide, the possibility that the microbicide might not confer protection, and potential risks of participation. Researchers conducting clinical trials on vaccines and microbicides have come to view informed consent as a process that needs to be revisited throughout the study, rather than as a static event (Heise and Wood 2005; MacQueen, Karim, and Sugarman 2003). Ethical issues also arise regarding consent of male partners who may be exposed to the trial product. Women may have more than one partner during the course of the trial, and partners may work and be unable to make it to the clinic, making their consent impractical. Some women may only be able to participate if they conceal their participation from male partners who might not approve of the testing, or even of the concept of the method. To manage this, penile tolerance studies are being done during Phase I and Phase II testing to assure that exposure to the product will be safe for male partners of women enrolled in effectiveness trials. Participants are often given information to share with partners if they choose to disclose it to them (Elias and Coggins 2001; Heise and Wood 2005).

Another group that presents ethical, practical, and legal challenges is adolescents, who are typically treated as "children" for research purposes. As such, they are defined as a vulnerable group possibly unable to give fully informed consent and needing special protections. At a meeting of international stakeholders brought together by the Global Campaign for Microbicides (GCM) in 2003, a group of ethicists, microbicide research experts, and advocates came to the consensus that, given the disproportionate brunt of the epidemic being borne by adolescent girls, the significant differences in biological vulnerability between adolescent and adult women, the potential benefits and harms of a microbicidal product, and their likelihood of comprising a substantial group of users, there is need to assess the safety and efficacy of microbicides in teenage girls (Heise and Wood 2005).

Another difficult issue arises around what should be provided for those who become infected with HIV during a trial (Heise and Wood 2005; MacQueen, Karim, and Sugarman 2003; Slack et al. 2005). In actuality, trial participants are less likely to contract HIV than comparable individuals not participating in a prevention study, because they receive intensive HIV prevention counseling and provision of condoms. However, new infections will still occur. With the plummeting cost of HIV treatment, many advocates insist that those who become infected during the trial should be entitled to lifelong antiretroviral treatment (ART), which is the highest standard of care available. Others say that it may not always be possible to get ART in a particular setting, that only a few people will receive that benefit, and that there are other services that may be more immediately beneficial to either everyone in the trial or the broader community, such as reproductive health care or STI treatment. The logistical challenges of promising ART to study subjects who seroconvert during the trial are significant because they may not need medications for several years, and by that time the study will be finished, study personnel will be gone, and funds will have expired. Complex tracking systems and systems for managing medical treatment would need to be in place and operated by someone in the host country (Forbes 2006). Some worry that it could become impossible to find trial sponsors if this standard were imposed, slowing research, or that creating access to treatment for a select few could amount to "undue inducement." International documents that guide the ethical conduct of research offer conflicting and loosely defined guidance (Council for International Organizations of Medical Sciences 2002: 17–23; Heise and Wood 2005: 1–75; MacQueen, Karim, and Sugarman 2003: 340; World Medical Association 2004; de Zoysa, Elias, and Bentley 1998: 571–575).

The challenges of competing concerns are exacerbated by inequitable study partnerships and unclear lines of responsibility among researchers, the trial sponsors, and local governments. Trial staff are likely to be present for only a few years and then leave when the trial is finished. Questions that arise around provision of trial benefits include: What package of benefits should be given to whom? Who should provide the benefit? What mechanisms exist for providing benefits other than directly through the trial? How will providing benefits exacerbate local inequities? Will potential subjects take risks they wouldn't normally take because of "undue inducements" created by trial benefits? Should the benefits provided by the trial be sustainable after the trial is ended? Is it feasible for the trial benefits to be sustainable? How can trial benefits be used to ratchet up local capacity? What input should the community have in determining trial benefits and who in the community should be involved in the negotiation and decision-making process? What are the obligations of the trial sponsor to provide for the health and care needs of trial participants? How do the benefits provided address the ethical principles of distributive justice? What are the responsibilities of host country governments to assume responsibility for making HIV treatment available to their citizens? (Heise and Wood 2005).

UNAIDS and the World Health Organization have held several international ethics consultation meetings around these issues, seeking consensus among sponsors, investigators, and host countries. The process continues to evolve as changes are seen in the scientific, political, and socioeconomic factors influencing the epidemic. The Global

Campaign for Microbicides consensus is that microbicide trials cannot, in and of themselves, correct the enormous inequities in global health, but should be used as an opportunity to build local capacity, improve the local standard of care, and minimize inequities (Forbes 2006; Heise and Wood 2005).

Future ethical dilemmas will emerge as trials are designed to refine products once partial efficacy is determined. Questions of whether it is more ethical to test a new product against a placebo arm or against both placebo and older-product arms could complicate further recruitment and funding (Heise and Wood 2005). Another future challenge will be assuring that those most in need of a microbicide, including those who have participated in clinical trials, will have access once efficacious products are approved. Historically, new innovations in public health, such as discovery of novel vaccines, take decades to trickle to less wealthy countries (McGrory and Gupta 2002), yet, in this case, study subjects from these countries will have been indispensable to the development process and have the most pressing need for the product. Planning and preparation for product introduction are needed prior to product approval. Assuring accessibility will include creating supportive policy and social environments that encourage microbicide adoption. This will include: addressing manufacturing, distribution, storage, and import/export systems to assure there is a continuous adequate product supply; exploring incentives, tariff reductions, manufacturing innovations, and subsidies that will keep products affordable; and preparing country regulatory authorities for product approval and licensing. Regulatory bodies need to set standards for product approval and licensure in their respective countries. The World Health Organization is providing guidance to countries that do not have experienced regulatory agencies such as the Food and Drug Administration. Lessons learned from introduction of the female condom, tampons, other contraceptive technologies, popular market goods, and vaccines should be analyzed and applied to microbicide introduction.

Commitments from bilateral and international donors, such as USAID, DFID, and the World Bank, to subsidize microbicide marketing and distribution costs need to be obtained now. The free market has failed to meet the needs of those most vulnerable to infection and disease. Global initiatives are currently transforming research, development, and distribution of public health goods and commodities to address these failures. Steps should be taken to ensure that microbicide development benefits from these changes (McGrory and Gupta 2002). Exploratory research to understand women's preferences for access to products (e.g., via local markets, family planning/prenatal clinics, local healers, etc.) will help inform successful introduction.

THE FUTURE

Much progress has been made in the microbicide field in recent years. Annual U.S. investment in microbicides has increased dramatically from $35 to $142 million in the past five years, but a doubling of current microbicide research expenditure is needed to keep the pipeline of new products moving and to develop expanded trial capacity in the global south (Harrison et al. 2005). Vocal, visible advocacy will be key to increasing resources for microbicide research and promotion.

Microbicides will not be a magic bullet. Removing structural barriers that contribute to women's risk, confronting gender inequity at the policy and individual level, keeping girls in school, promoting use of male and female condoms, and continuing vaccine research are all critical to reducing HIV risk. But large scale change typically occurs slowly and incrementally. With 8,000 women a day becoming newly infected, we cannot sit back and do nothing until the day that gender power imbalances are rectified. The current HIV mantra of ABC—Abstain, Be faithful, or use Condoms—is miserably failing women the world over. It is failing their partners as well. While condoms, abstinence, and fidelity will continue to be crucial to HIV prevention, they are inadequate in and of themselves. Adding new prevention technology, such as safe and effective vaccines and microbicides,

Exhibit 10.1 Seven things you can do to make microbicides a reality

- Learn more about microbicides.
- Talk to friends, family, and colleagues about microbicides.
- Contact your Congressional Representatives and political leaders and ask them to increase microbicides funding.
- Ask your local organization to host a microbicides program.
- Find out if there is a microbicides advocacy group where you live. Get involved if there is one!
- Participate in a microbicides trial if there is one near you.
- Ask your community group or workplace to endorse the Global Campaign for Microbicides.

will increase the capacity of many of the world's most vulnerable individuals to protect themselves. Microbicides should be seen as fitting a niche within a continuum of HIV harm reduction options. Even if only partially effective, with consistent use they have the potential to prevent millions of infections and to put power in women's hands.

REFERENCES AND FURTHER READING

Alfsen, A. "Environmental Factors in HIV/AIDS Epidemic Development: New Perspectives for Gender Equity and Global Protection Against HIV Transmission." *Annals of the New York Academy of Sciences* 1023 (2004): 164–174.

Beauchamp, T. L., and J. F. Childress. *Principles of Biomedical Ethics*. 5th ed. Oxford: Oxford University Press, 2001.

Bird, S. T., S. M. Harvey, J. E. Maher, and L. J. Beckman. "Acceptability of an Existing, Female-Controlled Contraceptive Method that could Potentially Protect Against HIV: A Comparison of Diaphragm Users and Other Method Users." *Women's Health Issues* 14, no. 3 (2004): 85–93.

Braunstein, S., and J. van de Wijgert. "Preferences and Practices Related to Vaginal Lubrication: Implications for Microbicide Acceptability and Clinical Testing." *Journal of Women's Health* 14, no. 5 (2005): 424–433.

Burger, H., and B. Weiser. "Biology of HIV-1 in Women and Men." *Clinical Obstetrics and Gynecology* 44, no. 2 (2001): 137–143.

Centers for Disease Control and Prevention. *HIV/AIDS Surveillance Report, 2004*. Atlanta, GA: U.S. Dept of Health and Human Services: Centers for Disease Control and Prevention, 2005.

Cobb, P., T. Robinson, S. Shah, D. Upmalis, J. Vail, M. Walker, K. Whaley, K. White, and G. Brown. *The Economics of Microbicide Development, A Case for Investment: A Report of the Pharmaco-Economics Working Group of the Rockefeller Microbicides Initiative*. New York: Rockefeller Foundation, 2002.

Cohen, J. "HIV/AIDS in India. Till Death do Us Part." *Science* 304, no. 5670 (2004): 513.

Council for International Organizations of Medical Sciences. "International Ethical Guidelines for Biomedical Research Involving Human Subjects." *Bulletin of Medical Ethics* no. 182 (2002): 17–23.

Dailard, Cynthia. "Understanding 'Abstinence': Implications for Individuals, Programs, and Policies." *The Guttmacher Report on Public Policy* 6, no. 5 (2003): 4–6.

Darroch, J. E., and J. J. Frost. "Women's Interest in Vaginal Microbicides." *Family Planning Perspectives* 31, no. 1 (1999): 16–23.

D'Cruz, O. J., and F. M. Uckun. "Clinical Development of Microbicides for the Prevention of HIV Infection." *Current Pharmaceutical Design* 10, no. 3 (2004): 315–336.

de Zoysa, I., C. J. Elias, and M. E. Bentley. "Ethical Challenges in Efficacy Trials of Vaginal Microbicides for HIV Prevention." *American Journal of Public Health* 88, no. 4 (1998): 571–575.

Di Stefano, M., A. Favia, L. Monno, P. Lopalco, O. Caputi, A. C. Scardigno, G. Pastore, J. R. Fiore, and G. Angarano. "Intracellular and Cell-Free (Infectious) HIV-1 in Rectal Mucosa." *Journal of Medical Virology* 65, no. 4 (2001): 637–643.

Direction Générale de la Lutte contre le SIDA, et. al. *Enquête Nationale ANC Madagascar. Direction Générale de la Lutte Contre le SIDA, Ministère de la Santé et Laboratoire National de Référence VIH/SIDA*. 2005.

Dunkle, K. L., R. K. Jewkes, H. C. Brown, G. E. Gray, J. A. McIntryre, and S. D. Harlow. "Gender-Based Violence, Relationship Power, and Risk of HIV Infection in Women Attending Antenatal Clinics in South Africa." *Lancet* 363, no. 9419 (2004): 1415–1421.

Elias, C., and C. Coggins. "Acceptability Research on Female-Controlled Barrier Methods to Prevent Heterosexual Transmission of HIV: Where have we been? Where are we Going?" *Journal of Women's Health and Gender-Based Medicine* 10, no. 2 (2001): 163–173.

Forbes, Anna. "Demanding Microbicides: An Invisible Condom in Your Future?" http://www.thebody.com/content/art16571.html (2003).

Forbes, Anna. "Moving Toward Assured Access to Treatment in Microbicide Trials." *PLoS Medicine* 3, no. 2 (2006).

Foss, A. M., P. T. Vickerman, L. Heise, and C. H. Watts. "Shifts in Condom Use Following Microbicide Introduction: Should we be Concerned?" *AIDS* 17, no. 8 (2003): 1227–1237.

Fuchs, E. J., R. Wahl, K. Macura, J. Leal, L. Grohskopf,

and C. W. Hendrix. "Imaging the Distribution of a Rectal Microbicide Gel and Semen Surrogate in the Lower Gastrointestinal Tract." *Clinical Pharmacology and Therapteutics* 77, no. 2 (2005): P60.

Global Coalition on Women and AIDS. "Stop Violence Against Women Fight AIDS." http://womenandaids.unaids.org/themes/docs/UNAIDS%20VAW%20Brief.pdf. Cited 2005.

Glynn, J. R., M. Carael, B. Auvert, M. Kahindo, J. Chege, R. Musonda, F. Kaona, A. Buve, and Study Group on the Heterogeneity of HIV Epidemics in African Cities. "Why do Young Women have a Much Higher Prevalence of HIV than Young Men? A Study in Kisumu, Kenya and Ndola, Zambia." *AIDS* 2001 Aug. 15, Suppl. 4: S51–S60.

Gorbach, Pamina. *Epidemiology of Anal Sex*. London ed.2004.

Grown, C., G. R. Gupta, and R. Pande. "Taking Action to Improve Women's Health through Gender Equality and Women's Empowerment." *Lancet* 365, no. 9458 (2005): 541–543.

Gupta, Geeta Rao. *Briefing: Voices from the Community: Taking Action on Health and Wealth Disparities*. Washington DC: Kaiser Family Foundation, 2004.

Hammett, T. M., T. H. Mason, C. L. Joanis, S. E. Foster, P. Harmon, R. R. Robles, H. A. Finlinson, R. Feudo, S. Vining-Bethea, G. Jeter, K. H. Mayer, P. Doherty-Iddings, and G. R. Seage III. "Acceptability of Formulations and Application Methods for Vaginal Microbicides among Drug-Involved Women: Results of Product Trials in Three Cities." *Sexually Transmitted Diseases* 27, no. 2 (2000): 119–126.

Harrison, P. F. "Microbicides: Forging Scientific and Political Alliances." *AIDS Patient Care and Stds* 14, no. 4 (2000): 199–205.

Harrison, P., G. Lamourelle, J. Rowley, and M. Warren. *Tracking Funding for Microbicide Research and Development: Estimates of Annual Investments 2000 to 2005*. UNAIDS HIV Vaccines and Microbicides Resource Tracking Working Group, 2005.

Harrison, P. F., Z. Rosenberg, and J. Bowcut. "Topical Microbicides for Disease Prevention: Status and Challenges." *Clinical Infectious Diseases* 36, no. 10 (2003): 1290–1294.

Heise, L., C. E. McGrory, and S. Wood. *Practical and Ethical Dilemmas in the Clinical Testing of Microbicides: A Report on a Symposium*. New York: International Women's Health Coalition, 1998.

Heise, Lori, and Susan Wood. *Rethinking the Ethical Roadmap for Clinical Testing of Microbicides: Report on an International Consultation*. Washington, DC: Global Campaign for Microbicides, 2005.

Hill, R. "Assessment of the Potential Market: A Summary of Survey Results from 11 European and Developing Countries." *AIDS* Suppl. 1, no. 15 (2001): S23.

Hillier, S. L., T. Moench, R. Shattock, R. Black, P. Reichelderfer, and F. Veronese. "In Vitro and in Vivo: The Story of Nonoxynol 9." *Journal of Acquired Immune Deficiency Syndromes: JAIDS* 39, no. 1 (2005): 1–8.

Howett, M. K., and J. P. Kuhl. "Microbicides for Prevention of Transmission of Sexually Transmitted Diseases." *Current Pharmaceutical Design* 11, no. 29 (2005): 3731–3746.

International Partnership for Microbicides. *Developing HIV Prevention Options for Women Worldwide, 2004 Annual Report*. http://www.ipmmicrobicides.org/pdfs/highlights/policy_k_092005.pdf ed. Silver Spring, MD: International Partnership for Microbicides, 2005a.

International Partnership for Microbicides. *Microbicides: An Essential HIV Prevention Strategy for Achieving the Millennium Development Goals*. Silver Spring, MD: International Partnership for Microbicides, 2005b.

Janus, S., and C. Janus. *The Janus Report on Sexual Behavior*. Indianapolis, IN: John Wiley and Sons, 1993.

Johnston, M. I., and J. Flores. "Progress in HIV Vaccine Development." *Current Opinion in Pharmacology* 1, no. 5 (2001): 504–510.

Kelly, R. J., R. H. Gray, N. K. Sewankambo, D. Serwadda, F. Wabwire-Mangen, T. Lutalo, and M. J. Wawer. "Age Differences in Sexual Partners and Risk of HIV-1 Infection in Rural Uganda." *Journal of Acquired Immune Deficiency Syndromes: JAIDS* 32, no. 4 (2003): 446–451.

Koo, H. P., C. Woodsong, B. P. Dalberth, M. Viswanathan, and A. Simons-Rudolph. "Title: Context of Acceptability of Topical Microbicides: Sexual Relationships." *Journal of Social Issues* 61, no. 1 (2005): 67–93.

Lewis, Stephen H. *Keynote Address: 11th Conference on Retroviruses and Opportunistic Infections*. San Francisco, CA ed.2004.

Lichtenstein, B. "Domestic Violence, Sexual Ownership, and HIV Risk in Women in the American Deep South." *Social Science and Medicine* 60, no. 4 (2005): 701–714.

Lo, B., and M. Groman. "NBAC Recommendations on Oversight of Human Subject Research." *Seton Hall Law Review* 32, no. 3 (2003): 493–512.

McGrory, E., and G. R. Gupta. *Preparing for Microbicide Access and Use: A Report by the Access Working Group of the Microbicide Initiative Funded by the Rockefeller Foundation*. New York: Rockefeller Foundation, 2002.

MacQueen, K. M., Q. A. Karim, and J. Sugarman. "Ethics Guidance for HIV Prevention Trials." *BMJ* 327, no. 7410 (2003): 340.

Macaluso, M., M. J. Demand, L. M. Artz, and E. W. Hook III. "Partner Type and Condom use." *AIDS* 14, no. 5 (2000): 537–546.

Mantell, J. E., L. Myer, A. Carballo-Dieguez, Z. Stein, G. Ramjee, N. S. Morar, and P. F. Harrison. "Microbicide Acceptability Research: Current Approaches and Future Directions." *Social Science and Medicine* 60, no. 2 (2005): 319–330.

Meehan, A., et. al. "Prevalence and Risk Factors for HIV in Zimbabwean and South African Women." *15th International AIDS Conference. Abstract MoPeC3468* Bangkok. 11–16 July (2004).

Miller, C. J., and R. J. Shattock. "Target Cells in Vaginal

HIV Transmission." *Microbes and Infection* 5, no. 1 (2003): 59–67.

Morar, Neetha S., Qwabe N. Dladla, S. Gumede, and G. Ramjee. "Acceptability of Microbicides among Male Partners of the COL1492 Trial Participants, Abstract #02311." London ed. London: *Microbicides 2004* (2004): xxx.

Mosack, K., M. Weeks, L. N. Sylla, and M. Abbott. "High-Risk Women's Willingness to Try a Simulated Vaginal Microbicide: Results from a Pilot Study." *Women and Health* 42, no. 2 (in press).

National Coalition Against Domestic Violence. "Domestic Violence Facts." http://www.ncadv.org/files/DV_Facts.pdf. Cited 2005.

Newell, M. L., H. Coovadia, M. Cortina-Borja, N. Rollins, P. Gaillard, and F. Dabis. "Mortality of Infected and Uninfected Infants Born to HIV-Infected Mothers in Africa: A Pooled Analysis." *Lancet* 364, no. 9441 (2004): 1236–1243.

Ojikutu, B. O., and V. E. Stone. "Women, Inequality, and the Burden of HIV." *New England Journal of Medicine* 352, no. 7 (2005): 649–652.

Patton, D. L., Y. T. Cosgrove Sweeney, L. K. Rabe, and S. L. Hillier. "Rectal Applications of Nonoxynol-9 Cause Tissue Disruption in a Monkey Model." *Sexually Transmitted Diseases* 29, no. 10 (2002): 581–587.

Phillips, D. M., C. L. Taylor, V. R. Zacharopoulos, and R. A. Maguire. "Nonoxynol-9 Causes Rapid Exfoliation of Sheets of Rectal Epithelium." *Contraception* 62, no. 3 (2000): 149–154.

Pool, R., J. A. Whitworth, G. Green, A. K. Mbonye, S. Harrison, J. Wilkinson, and G. J. Hart. "An Acceptability Study of Female-Controlled Methods of Protection Against HIV and STDs in South-Western Uganda." *International Journal of STD and AIDS* 11, no. 3 (2000): 162–167.

Rosenberg, Z., *Recent Developments in Microbicide Clinical Trials: A Statement on the Carraguard and PRO-2000/5 HIV Prevention Trials*, http://www.global-campaign.org/clientfiles/Carraguard%20PRO%202000%20ZR%20Statement,%202-20-08.doc.pdf. Silver Spring, MD: International Partnership for Microbicides. Accessed February 19, 2008.

Rouse, L. *Marital and Sexual Lifestyles in the United States; Attitudes, Behaviors and Relationships in Social Context*. Binghamton, NY: Haworth Press, 2002.

Rwabukwali, C. B., J. W. McGrath, R. A. Salata, S. A. Rundall, and D. Akurut. "Anticipated Acceptability of a Vaginal Microbicide among Men Attending the Mulago STD Clinic in Kampala, Uganda, Abstract #02131." *Microbicides 2004* (2004): 127.

Saul, J., J. Moore, S. T. Murphy, and L. C. Miller. "Relationship Violence and Women's Reactions to Male- and Female-Controlled HIV Prevention Methods." *AIDS and Behavior* 8, no. 2 (2004): 207–214.

Scholand, S. J., J. A. DeSimone, and R. J. Pomerantz. "Anti-HIV-1 Microbicides—'Chemical Condoms' Designed to Limit the Scourge of the HIV-1 Pandemic." *Current Pharmaceutical Design* 11, no. 29 (2005): 3747–3756.

Severy, L. J., and S. Newcomer. "Critical Issues in Contraceptive and STI Acceptability." *Journal of Social Issues* 61, no. 1 (2005): 45–65.

Severy, L. J., E. Tolley, C. Woodsong, and G. Guest. "A Framework for Examining the Sustained Acceptability of Microbicides." *AIDS and Behavior* 9, no. 1 (2005): 121–131.

Shapiro, K., and S. R. Benatar. "HIV Prevention Research and Global Inequality: Steps Towards Improved Standards of Care." *Journal of Medical Ethics* 31, no. 1 (2005): 39–47.

Shattock, R., and S. Solomon. "Microbicides—Aids to Safer Sex." *Lancet* 363, no. 9414 (2004): 1002–1003.

Slack, C., M. Stobie Milford, G. Lindegger, D. Wassenaar, A. Strode, and C. Ijsselmuiden. "Provision of HIV Treatment in HIV Preventive Vaccine Trials: A Developing Country Perspective." *Social Science and Medicine* 60, no. 6 (2005): 1197–2208.

Smith, R. J., E. N. Bodine, D. P. Wilson, and S. M. Blower. "Evaluating the Potential Impact of Vaginal Microbicides to Reduce the Risk of Acquiring HIV in Female Sex Workers." *AIDS* 19, no. 4 (2005): 413–421.

Spearman, P. "HIV Vaccine Development: Lessons from the Past and Promise for the Future." *Current HIV Research* 1, no. 1 (2003): 101–120.

Turmen, T. "Gender and HIV/AIDS." *International Journal of Gynaecology and Obstetrics* 82, no. 3 (2003): 411–418.

UNAIDS. "Intensifying HIV Prevention." Geneva, Switzerland, August 2005. http://www.unaids.org/NetTools/Misc/DocInfo.aspx?LANG=en&href=http://gva-doc-owl/WEBcontent/Documents/pub/Governance/PCB04/pcb_17_05_03_en.pdf. Cited 2005.

UNAIDS/WHO. *AIDS Epidemic Update December 2005*. Geneva, Switzerland: UNAIDS, 2005.

UNFPA. "International Conference on Population and Development (ICPD) Programme of Action." New York. http://www.unfpa.org/icpd/icpd_poa.htm#ch7. Cited 2006.

Watts, C., L. Kumaranayake, P. Vickerman, and F. Terris-Prestholt. *The Public Health Benefits of Microbicides in Lower-Income Countries: Model Projections. A Report by the Public Health Working Group of the Microbicide Initiative Funded by the Rockefeller Foundation*. New York: The Rockefeller Foundation, 2002.

Weber, Jonathan, Kamal Desai, and Janet Darbyshire. "The Development of Vaginal Microbicides for the Prevention of HIV Transmission." In PLoS Med database online. http://bll.epnet.com/externalframe.asp?tb=0&_ug=sid+265D8CAB%2D983F%2D41E0%2D8BAA%2DA189CFC0BDB0%40sessionmgr5+3BAB&_us=hd+True+SLsrc+ext+or+ Date+828E&_usmtl=ftv+True+137E&_uso=hd+False+db%5B0+%2Daph+1BEE&fi=aph_17179354_AN&lpdf=true&pdfs=&tn=&tp=PC&es=cs%. Cited May 31, 2005.

Weeks, M. R., K. E. Mosack, M. Abbott, L. N. Sylla, B. Valdes, and M. Prince. "Microbicide Acceptability among High-Risk Urban U.S. Women: Experiences and Perceptions of Sexually Transmitted HIV Prevention." *Sexually Transmitted Diseases* 31, no. 11 (2004): 682–690.

Woodsong, C. "Covert use of Topical Microbicides: Implications for Acceptability and use." *Perspect. Sex.Reprod.Health* 36, no. 3 (2004): 127–131.

World Association of Sexual Health. "Declaration of Sexual Rights." http://www.worldsexology.org/about_sexualrights.asp. Cited 2006.

World Medical Association. "World Medical Association Declaration of Helsinki: Ethical Principles for Medical Research Involving Human Subjects." http://www.wma.net/e/policy/b3.htm. September 10, 2004. Cited 2006.

CHAPTER 11

Current Perspectives on the Neuropsychology of HIV

Ramani S. Durvasula, Lisa R. Norman, and Robert Malow

ABSTRACT

It is well documented that HIV directly infects the central nervous system (CNS) and this is accompanied by a pattern of neuropsychological (NP) decline in a large proportion of HIV-infected persons. The advent of highly active antiretroviral therapy (HAART) has impacted the NP functioning of persons with HIV and AIDS, and this has reduced the NP deterioration observed in persons living with HIV (PLWH). Nonetheless, the subtle HIV-associated cognitive slowing, memory impairments, and executive dysfunction in conjunction with the direct and indirect psychiatric sequelae of HIV can compromise decision-making, functional capacity, and overall quality of life in PLWH. Controversial and contemporary issues are spotlighted, including the impact of HAART on NP performance in HIV, methodological issues, co-infection with hepatitis C, and the NP of HIV in the developing world.

INTRODUCTION

HIV/AIDS continues to be a global epidemic, with estimates of over 40 million people living with HIV (PLWH) (UNAIDS 2006). In the U.S.A., HIV has disproportionately affected women and ethnic minority groups. In the mid-1990s, the advent of highly active antiretroviral therapy (HAART) regimens has changed the face of the epidemic, particularly in developed nations, and has extended life expectancy for most HIV-infected individuals. As such, much of the empirical work conducted in the pre-HAART era may need to be recast in light of the changing demography, epidemiology, and clinical management of this disease, particularly work relating HIV to neuropsychological (NP) dysfunction. There is a sizable literature documenting the cognitive, behavioral, and psychiatric changes that often affect PLWH, which have ramifications for clinical management and functional impairment. In addition, this pattern of NP deterioration may be differentially impacted by other co-morbid conditions and sociodemographic co-factors.

NEUROPSYCHOLOGY OF HIV AND AIDS

HIV has direct and indirect effects on the central nervous system (CNS) (Brew et al. 1988; Ho et al. 1985; McArthur 1987). These effects can manifest through a variety of neuropsychiatric symptomatology. Exhibit 11.2 illustrates the HIV neurobehavioral disturbances that occur within the context of HIV infection (Grant 2007).

These CNS changes are often manifested as progressive NP decline in a sizable proportion of persons with HIV and AIDS. Immunocompromise associated with HIV/AIDS often leads to CNS opportunistic infections such as toxoplasmosis, which result in moderate to severe NP dysfunction. However, HIV also exerts direct effects on the brain, and can result in NP deficits that

Exhibit 11.1 Abbreviations used throughout the chapter

AIDS	Acquired Immunodeficiency Syndrome
ARV	Antiretroviral Therapy
CNS	Central Nervous System
CSF	Cerebrospinal Fluid
HAART	Highly Active Antiretroviral Therapy
HADC	HIV-Associated Dementia Complex
HCV	Hepatitis C Virus
HDS	HIV–Dementia Scale
HIV	Human Immunodeficiency Virus
MCMD	Minor Cognitive Motor Disorder
NIH	National Institutes of Health
NIMH	National Institute of Mental Health
NP	Neuropsychological
OI	Olfactory Identification
PLWH	Persons Living with HIV
PML	Progressive Multifocal Leukoencephalopathy
WAIS	Wechsler Adult Intelligence Scale

range from mild cognitive symptomatology to dementia. The cardinal NP symptomatology includes cognitive and motor slowing, attentional disruption, executive dysfunction, and memory impairment (Grant and Heaton 1990; Heaton et al. 1995; van Gorp et al. 1993). Language, visuoperception, and overall cognitive functioning are generally intact, with significant changes in these domains observed with the onset of dementia. Apraxia, agnosia, and aphasia, or other symptoms of cortical dementias are not observed as a direct effect of HIV, but rather as a result of opportunistic infections such as toxoplasmosis, cryptococcal meningitis, cytomegalovirus or neoplasms (Fernandez et al. 2004). While dementia is a relatively uncommon occurrence among PLWHs, a pattern of milder NP deficits in the domains listed above is observed in up to half of persons who are symptomatic or who have AIDS (McArthur et al. 1994; Heaton et al. 1995). The study findings presented in Exhibit 11.3 illustrate the distribution of neurocognitive disorders by stage of HIV disease (Grant 2007).

Shortly after the discovery that HIV could directly infect the CNS, and produce neurological complications that accom-

Exhibit 11.2 HIV neurobehavioral disturbances

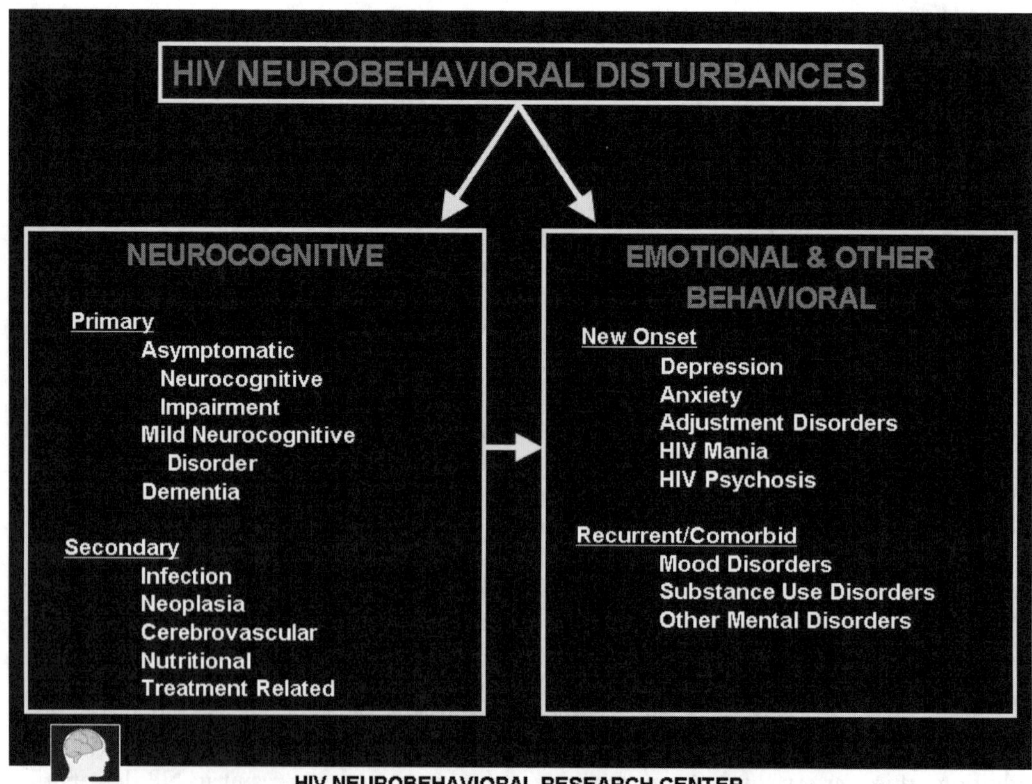

Exhibit 11.3 Prevalence of neurocognitive disorders by stage of HIV disease

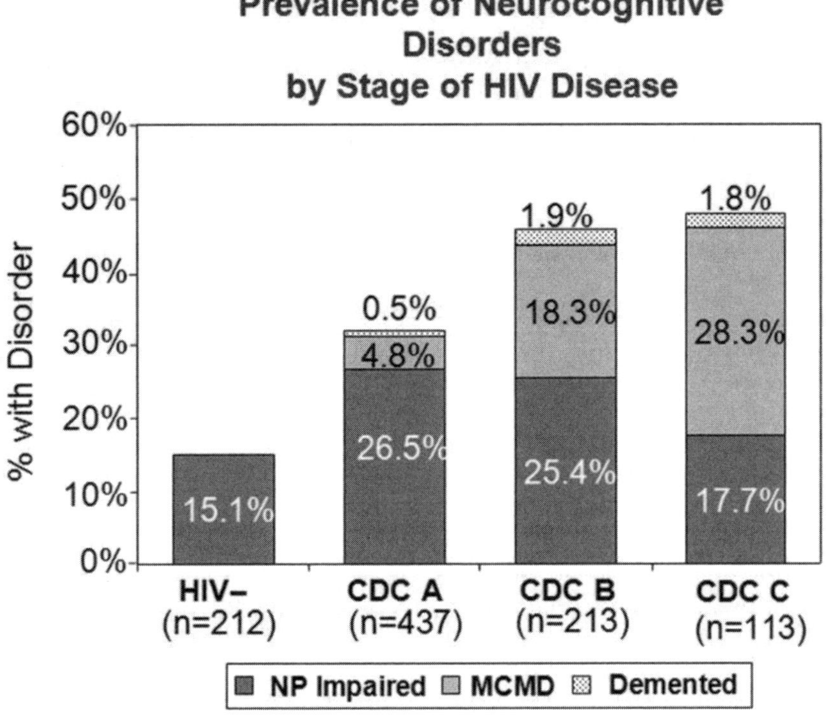

Source: I Grant and R Heaton, HNRC, UCSD

panied AIDS, the collection of cognitive and behavioral changes that was observed in a subset of patients with advanced disease was termed AIDS Dementia Complex (Navia et al. 1986a). Significant immunosuppression was considered a co-requisite for AIDS Dementia Complex and was observed almost exclusively in those with late-stage AIDS. The onset of this neurocognitive symptomatology was insidious and the progression gradual, though systemic illness could facilitate progression or augment the symptomatology. Forgetfulness, concentration difficulties, and general cognitive slowing were typical initial symptoms. Behavioral changes were also relatively common, particularly apathy and social withdrawal. In general, the HIV-related dementias are conceptualized as subcortical dementias due to the early prominence of psychomotor slowing and white matter changes, and the absence of typical cortical syndromes such as aphasia or apraxia until much later stages (Navia et al. 1986a, 1986b)

NEUROPSYCHOLOGICAL ASSESSMENT OF HIV ASSOCIATED COGNITIVE DECLINE

Given that the cardinal symptoms of HIV-associated cognitive impairment are psychomotor and motor slowing, reaction time deficits, memory impairment, and executive dysfunction, test batteries which include multiple measures of these domains are optimal. To date there is no single "test" that can diagnose dementia, though screening measures such as the HIV Dementia Rating Scale (HDS) (Power et al. 1995) can suggest whether further assessment may be warranted. The HDS consists of four brief subtests, and has low sensitivity and modest specificity. Measures of psychomotor speed which assess divided attention (e.g., Trail Making Test Part B) are often most sensitive to the types of impairments observed in persons with HIV. Computerized reaction time tasks are exceptionally sensitive to the types of slowed processing observed in HIV, and may be useful with asymptomatic patients for whom NP deficits are likely to be quite subtle. Memory assessment may be best measured via delayed recall (e.g., California Verbal Learning Test—II—delayed recall) as this subset of memory is most profoundly affected, particularly relative to tests that assess recognition. In addition, assessment of memory should optimally include both verbal and nonverbal measures. Assessment of executive functioning should incorporate measures of set shifting and hypothesis formation (e.g., Wisconsin Card Sorting Test), abstraction (e.g., WAIS [Wechsler Adult Intelligence Scale] Similarities), and inhibition (e.g., Stroop Interference Trial). As with any NP assessment, a detailed clinical interview which assesses demographic information, psychiatric history, medical history (particularly neurological history, current and past drug and alcohol use, current medications, social and occupational history, and any functional impairments or ecological manifestations of NP dysfunction) should also be employed (Fernandez et al. 2004). Records on viral load, CD4, history of CNS opportunistic infections (OIs), and antiretroviral regimen are also critical when conducting such assessment and diagnosis.

Deconstruction of the attentional and information-processing changes observed in persons with HIV has been attempted through the use of cognitive and experimental paradigms. Computerized assessments of attention, reaction time, and working memory have revealed that relative to automatic processing, controlled attentional processing is more impaired in PLWH (Hinkin et al. 1999; Hinkin et al. 2000; Martin et al. 1995). This level of specificity is often not possible with traditional NP tests and, as such, employment of finer-grained computerized assessments is of utility in characterizing HIV-associated cognitive deficits.

The NIMH (National Institute of Mental Health) Workgroup on Neuropsychological Assessment Approaches (Butters et al. 1990) proposed a battery of tests which provides comprehensive assessment of not only the types of subtle neurocognitive changes observed secondary to HIV, but also to detect any focal CNS disturbances such as opportunistic infections or neoplasms. The proposed battery includes assessment of the following domains: a) premorbid intelligence; b) attention; c) speed of processing; d) memory; e) abstraction; f) language; g) visuospatial; h) construction abilities; i) motor abilities; j) psychiatric assessment. In clinical practice, the type and number of tests used is best guided by the patient history and presenting complaints.

ONGOING CHALLENGES IN THE NEUROPSYCHOLOGICAL ASSESSMENT OF HIV

The face of HIV has changed significantly since the onset of the AIDS epidemic in the United States. Much of our knowledge on the progression of HIV-related cognitive decline was generated in the pre-HAART era. In addition, other issues in HIV have also been evolving, such as the impact of comorbid Hepatitis C infection among HIV-infected drug abusers. As HIV continues to proliferate at staggering rates in developing nations, where many patients do not have access to HAART or adequate medical care, the picture of NP decline must be revisited. The epidemiology of HIV in the United States has been shifting, and rates of infection are increasing most rapidly in ethnic minority group members, and among persons of lower socioeconomic status (CDC 2007). As such, other co-factors that may contribute to the NP picture of HIV must be considered. HIV infection does not occur in a vacuum. Persons with HIV are more likely to have histories of substance use, and those with limited economic resources are also more likely to have lower levels of education, greater exposure to environmental toxicities, histories punctuated by violence and attendant injury, and poorer access to health care. Substance use and poverty represent markers for variables that weaken the cognitive substrate and decrease cognitive reserve (Satz 1993; Satz et al. 1993). As such, in the face of CNS insults such as HIV and/or substance use, the threshold for the onset of cognitive impairments in persons with such risk factors drops, and they are more vulnerable to earlier onset of, and more significant NP impairments. Ongoing work with such cohorts must carefully characterize cohorts on the basis of ethnicity, socioeconomic status, and neurological and health histories.

HAART AND NEUROPSYCHOLOGICAL PERFORMANCE

The advent of highly active antiretroviral therapies (HAART) has changed the face of HIV/AIDS. In 1993, AIDS was the leading cause of death in adults ages 25–44 years old, but has since shifted to the fifth leading cause of death in that age group (Selik et al. 1993; Minimo and Smith 2001). As early as 1987 the effects of nucleoside analogues, particularly zidovudine, were reported (Yarchoan et al. 1987) and were followed by reports of declines in the incidence of AIDS-related dementias (Portegies et al. 1989). Even among those already diagnosed with HADC (HIV-Associated Dementia Complex), improvements in NP and neurological functioning were reported upon initiation of AZT treatment (Portegies 1994). Much of what we have learned about NP performance and HIV has been learned in the era prior to the advent of HAART. The advent of HAART has resulted in a significantly lower incidence of HIV-related neurobehavioral disorders (Sacktor et al. 1998; Sacktor et al. 2001, 2002, Deutsch et al. 2001). However, a second "spike" of NP dysfunction will likely again be observed as the HIV-infected population ages, and the convergence of neuropsychological disorders attributable to aging and the direct effects of HIV are observed (Dore et al. 1999).

The prevalence of HADC has increased, though there has been an attendant drop in incidence, a trend which is likely attributable to greater life expectancy with the use of HAART (Dore et al. 1999). While incidence rates are dropping, minor neurological impairments continue to persist even in the face of HAART treatment (Tozzi et al. 2001). It is estimated that in HAART recipients, 40–60 percent of PLWH still have some measurable HIV neurocognitive deficits (McArthur 2007).

In general, however, studies examining the impact of HAART on cognitive functioning have reported a positive effect on NP performance (Ferrando et al. 1998; Letendre et al. 2004; Schrooten et al. 2004; Tozzi et al. 1999; Deutsch et al. 2001; Ellis et al. 2002). Deutsch et al. (2001) found that twice as many subjects in a pre-HAART cohort developed NP impairment when compared to a post-HAART cohort. In addition, CSF (cerebrospinal fluid) penetrance of antiretroviral drugs is also an important consideration. Individuals whose antiviral regimen included greater numbers of CSF-penetrating drugs showed a greater reduction in CSF viral load, which corresponded to greater cognitive improvement (Ellis et al. 2002). It is currently unclear whether specific classes of HAART afford greater protection, but it is assumed that at least some level of protection of cognitive function is mediated by HAART-related improvement in immunological function (Deutsch et al. 2001).

In the era of HAART, some have suggested that duration of disease may be the primary risk factor for NP dysfunction, independent of CD4 count (Brew 2004). Traditionally, severe immunosuppression was considered a requisite for HADC; however, a proportional increase in HADC was observed even among those with CD4 counts in the 201–350 range after the advent of HAART. This shift, with severe immunosuppression no longer a necessary condition for the onset of HADC, and the manifestation of HADC in relatively healthy patients may in part be due to the poor penetration of antiretroviral agents into the brain, a reservoir for HIV from the outset. As such, some of the biological markers that were once useful red flags for clinicians monitoring HADC (e.g., plasma CD4), have lost some of their utility. Recent research reveals that immunosuppression is associated with greater prevalence and sustenance of NP impairment, and that restoration of immunocompetence is accompanied with a greater likelihood of NP recovery (Robertson et al. 2007). In the post-HAART period, HADC is believed to develop in approximately 15 percent of those with AIDS and MCMD (minor cognitive motor disorder) in nearly 40 percent (Sacktor et al. 2002), thus NP assessment of this patient population is still a necessary clinical issue. Because of the evolving changes in the onset and natural history of NP dysfunction in HIV due to HAART, alternative taxonomies for HIV dementias have been proposed. McArthur et al. (2003) suggest three subtypes: chronic active, chronic inactive, and subacute progressive, with the subacute progressive category most consistent with the clinical picture of HIV dementia in the pre-HAART era.

If there is a qualitative difference in the NP deficits observed in the pre- and post-HAART era, it is possible that prolonged disease duration permits the neuropathological changes to spread to previously spared areas of the brain. Some have argued that the introduction of HAART has resulted in either "inactive" or "chronic" forms of HADC (Brew 2004). This suggestion emerged from work examining the efficacy of abacavir for treatment of HADC. In this study, over half (56 percent) of the mild–moderate HADC subjects had low plasma viral loads (HIV-1 RNA levels < 100 copies/ml) at baseline, and a large majority (83 percent) had very low CSF microglobulin levels, which suggests that even in the face of adequate viral management NP impairments continue to emerge (Brew 2004). Brew suggested that those with the "inactive" or "fixed" form of HADC, for whom the viral markers were low, may have responded maximally to HAART prior to beginning the trial of abacavir. For these patients, additional treatment with HAART would not confer any additional benefit or concomitant improvements in NP functioning. In contrast, those with the "chronic" form of infection harbor the virus in their brains for many years, with continuous damage to neurons in a manner that is undetectable via traditional markers (i.e., CSF and plasma viral load). This may occur because HAART does not bring all CSF parameters back to normal. For example, one study investigated the effectiveness of combination HAART therapy in decreasing levels of beta-2 microglobulin and neopterin, two biomarkers used for predicting HADC. They found that neuropsychologically normal HIV-infected individuals can have mild elevations of neopterin despite normal levels of beta-2 microglobulin and HIV-1 RNA in both plasma and CSF (Abdulle et al. 2002). This dissociation may be indicative of an ongoing inflammatory immune response in the brain. Thus, despite the appearance of control of HIV, subtle neuropathological change continues even in the post-HAART era.

The adherence demands of HAART result in a bi-directional relationship between neurocognition and adherence. On the one hand, neurocognitive deficits, particularly memory impairment and executive dysfunction, have been linked to poor adherence (Hinkin et al. 2002; Hinkin et al. 2004; Solomon and Halkitis 2007), while poor adherence can result in more rapid disease progression which can result in greater NP impairment. HIV-positive drug abusers may be at particularly high risk for suboptimal adherence (Freeman et al. 1996; Malow et al. 1998; Ferrando et al. 1996), with some work indicating that current substance abusers are four times more likely to be poor adherers than drug-free subjects (Mason et al. 2002). Substance use, particularly methamphetamine use, can deleteriously impact the efficacy of HAART, which can result in more rapid disease progression and a greater likelihood of NP deficits. This is particularly notable, given that HIV disease progression in general is more rapid among drug abusers (Khalsa and Royal 2004). Furthermore, identification of NP complications may help in managing HIV-positive patients and enhance their ability to adhere to complex medical regimens (Hilsabeck and Malek-Ahmadi 2004).

Current clinical belief and practice still hold that accurate adherence is important, and there is evidence suggesting that cognitive functioning plays an important role in medication adherence. Studies have shown that "forgetting" is a primary cause of HAART non-adherence (Chesney et al. 2000). Specific associations between poor adherence and memory, attention and executive dysfunction have also been observed (Albert et al. 1999; Durvasula et al. 1998; Hinkin et al. 2002). The relationship between neurocognitive integrity and medication adherence has been found to be mediated by the complexity of the medication regimen

(Hinkin et al. 2002). This research has found that participants with executive dysfunction and who were on a three-times-per-day dosing schedule were significantly less likely to adhere to HAART than those on simpler dosing schedules.

HEPATITIS C CO-INFECTION

Approximately one third of all individuals with HIV are co-infected with Hepatitis C virus (HCV), with rates significantly higher (60–90 percent) among injection drug users (Verucchi et al. 2004). The increasing rates of Hepatitis C co-infection in persons with HIV have been associated with an increased risk of NP impairment (Perry et al. 2007; Cherner et al. 2005; Hilsabeck, Castellon, and Hinkin 2005; Hinkin et al. in press; Letendre et al. 2005). A possible synergistic effect of HIV/HCV co-infection has been suggested, with co-infected individuals demonstrating significantly slower reaction times than those with either HIV or HCV alone. Von Giesen et al. (2004) observed that a greater proportion of HIV/HCV co-infected persons met criteria for AIDS dementia than did those with advanced HIV only. Some dissociation between the two disease processes has been observed, with HCV-only infected persons showing slowed information processing while HIV-only infected persons evidenced more executive impairment on a Stroop reaction time task.

The neuropathologic basis for neurocognitive deficits in co-infection is still not entirely clear. It is possible that it may reflect the additive burden of two concurrent disease processes. However, a possible synergistic mechanism may derive from evidence that HCV replication occurs in the same cells as HIV (e.g., monocytes/macrophages and T and B lymphocytes) and some preliminary evidence that HIV facilitates HCV replication in monocytes/macrophages (Laskus et al. 2004). Increased neurocognitive deficits in co-infection may also be related to diminished liver function, as HIV has been demonstrated to hasten fibrosis progression in persons with HCV (Benhamou et al. 2004). HIV and HCV share neurometabolic similarities, including elevated creatine in fronto-striatal regions. Disentanglement of the myriad factors that may contribute to greater NP compromise in co-infected persons—immune processes, liver function, CNS changes, and drug use history—is a complex enterprise. However, clinicians working with co-infected clients must remain aware of the heightened likelihood of cognitive compromise.

AGING AND HIV

The attendant decrease in morbidity and mortality due to HIV and AIDS has resulted in a population of HIV-infected persons that is getting older. Persons over 55 represent nearly 18 percent of the total number of AIDS cases in the U.S. (CDC 2007). In the U.S., HIV-related hospital admissions fell 40 percent between 2000 and 2004; however, increasingly persons with HIV were being admitted for treatment of age-related illnesses such as heart disease (Hellinger 2007). Older HIV-positive persons experience a briefer duration between initial seroconversion and AIDS diagnosis, higher mortality following AIDS diagnosis, and briefer latency between AIDS diagnosis and onset of dementia and death (Butt et al. 2001; Chen et al. 1998; Martin et al. 1995; McArthur et al. 1993; Goetz et al. 2001).

As such, NP assessment of older HIV-infected persons has to account for the independent contributions of normal aging on both cognition and immunological functioning as well as the impact of HIV on the brain. In addition, other dementing processes such as Alzheimer's disease, cerebrovascular disease and other pathological processes associated with aging will contribute to NP decline in older cohorts. Older HIV-positive adults have evidenced higher rates of NP deficits, with those over 50 having a 50 percent or greater likelihood of cognitive impairment (Hinkin et al. 2001; Goodkin et al. 2001, Valcour and Paul 2006; Justice et al. 2004; Valcour et al. 2004). One study found that among older participants (those older than 50 years of age) dementia was the more common classification (23 percent), whereas among younger participants a milder form of cognitive impairment was more prevalent (22 percent) (Becker et al. 2004).

In addition, immunological changes such as declining T-cell proliferation and T-cell dysfunction that are part of HIV are also part of the normal aging process (Miller et al. 1990; Sansoni et al. 1993; Effros et al. 1994). Appay and Rowland-Jones (2002) have hypothesized that because of the similar immunological profiles of younger HIV-positive individuals and uninfected normal elderly, HIV infection causes accelerated aging of the immune system. To examine whether normal aging may potentiate the deleterious NP effects of HIV, Hardy et al. (1999) examined aging and cognition in 601 HIV seropositives (who were divided on the basis of AIDS diagnosis) and 227 HIV negatives. There was a greater percentage of impaired individuals among the older (older than 50 years) AIDS participants compared to the other groups with 87 percent of older AIDS patients performing 1.5 standard deviations or greater in the impaired direction on two or more tests. Reaction time is particularly affected among older HIV-positive adults, especially for more demanding and complex task conditions (Hardy et al. 2004; Goodkin et al. 2003).

HIV IN WOMEN

Epidemiology statistics reveal that women clearly comprise a lower percentage of persons with HIV/AIDS (less than 20 percent), though rates of infection in women continue to hold steady (CDC 2007). As a result, far less of the literature examining the NP sequelae of HIV has examined cohorts of women, and in those studies employing gender-mixed cohorts, women tend to comprise a very small percentage of the sample; thus the applicability of findings to HIV seropositive women as a whole is limited. Similar to studies that have employed entirely male cohorts or gender-mixed cohorts, NP studies of HIV-infected women have revealed deficits in psychomotor speed, attention, and memory (Durvasula et al. 2001; Mason et al. 1998; Cohen et al. 2001; Richardson et al. 2001). In general, women appear to evidence NP deficits that are similar to those observed in men, though little longitudinal work has been done to examine the onset of such deficits as a function of disease progression. Women tend to present with more advanced disease at the time of HIV diagnosis; as such they are likely to receive HAART later in disease progression, a factor that could result in more rapid NP deterioration secondary to HIV. Infected women typically have less education, poorer access to treatment, and fewer socioeconomic resources than their male counterparts (Ickovics and Rodin 1992), all of which can place them at greater risk for neuropsychiatric complications of HIV. Morrison et al. (2002) found higher rates of major depression as well as greater symptoms of anxiety and depression in HIV seropositives compared to HIV seronegative controls. In addition, consideration of other gender specific hormonal factors is important, particularly given the possible neuroprotective effects of both exogenous and endogenous estrogen (Asthana et al. 1999). One study found that that estrogen protects against the synergistic toxicity by HIV proteins, methamphetamine, and cocaine (Turchan et al. 2001). A more recent study found that estrogen attenuates gp120 and tat1-72-induced stress and prevents loss of dopamine transporter function among postmenopausal women who are living with HIV (Wallace et al. 2006).

DEVELOPING NATIONS—IMPLICATIONS OF NEUROAIDS RESEARCH

HIV has been increasing at alarming rates in many developing nations. It is estimated that two-thirds of the 40 million PLWH reside in sub-Saharan Africa (UNAIDS 2006). Insufficient access to antiretroviral (ARV) medication, nutritious food, and other basic needs remains a chronic issue and can contribute to increased NeuroAIDS complications as well as morbidity and mortality. Given these conditions, many of the pre-HAART-era studies may best inform our understanding of the patterns of NP compromise observed in PLWH from developing nations. With the ARV access now available in developed nations, NP research in the U.S. and Europe is more focused on detection of subtle impairments, ecological validity (e.g. work performance), and, as such, is less relevant for developing countries. There are some indications that neurological expression of HIV may be different around the world. Shankar et al. (2003) observed that PML (Progressive Multifocal Leukoencephalopothy), an OI that can have significant NP effects, is rarely reported in India and Africa, a finding they attribute to differences in viral strains.

NeuroAIDS research in developing nations presents numerous challenges ranging from cultural appropriateness to linguistic/translational issues. Cultural differences also complicate assessment of psychopathology. Western diagnostic categories such as depression and anxiety often do not translate well and symptom expression via somatic complaints is more likely to be observed. One multisite study of particular relevance is the WHO Neuropsychiatric AIDS study. This study was conducted in the pre-HAART era in the early 1990s in high-seroprevalence regions (e.g., Bangkok, Thailand; São Paulo, Brazil; Kinshasa, Zaire; and Nairobi, Kenya) The major finding was that subtle cognitive deficits were observed in the asymptomatic phase of infection, but that these deficits were not associated with neurological changes or changes in social functioning (Maj et al. 1994).

Only a handful of other studies have examined HIV-associated dementia in the developing world and these have observed relatively high rates of neurological problems and AIDS dementias. In one study of hospitalized patients in Nairobi, 21 percent of patients had neurological complications, with CNS opportunistic infections most prevalent (e.g., cryptococcal meningitis, toxoplasmosis) (Jowi et al. 2007). HADC was found to be relatively common in HIV seropositives in Uganda, with older age and greater immunosuppression as indexed by CD4 associated with a greater likelihood of dementia (Wong et al. 2007). NP tests such as the finger-tapping test have revealed poorer performance in HIV seropositives compared to negatives on finger tapping in a sample of community resident HIV seropositives and seronegatives (Clifford et al. 2007). A study of neurocognitive consequences of HIV in southern India was recently published and indicated that, when compared to healthy controls, treatment naive HIV-positive individuals revealed significant differences on most cognitive tests, with lower performances obtained by the HIV-positive individuals (Yepthomi et al. 2006). The results suggest that, among individuals with the clade C virus in India, as many as 56 percent of the patients with advanced HIV meet the criterion for impairment in two cognitive domains. Researchers in other countries such as China are conducting descriptive studies of AIDS dementia (Wu et al. 2007). However, to date, NP investigations in developing nations are very preliminary, and the need for assessment instruments that can capture the cardinal symptoms of HADC and MCMD in samples diverse with respect to language and education is critical. Infected persons and those most vulnerable to infection are often very poor, with histories characterized by low education, malnutrition, poor health care, and a greater likelihood of exposure to violence, environmental toxins, or other environmental conditions that contribute to CNS injury. As such, the threshold for the onset of cognitive impairment among HIV-infected persons in developing nations is likely to be quite low and the attendant functional impairments that accompany such cognitive changes are likely to onset more severely and rapidly. This may have far-reaching clinical and cultural implications, particularly for women in such settings, as they often have young children in their care, or remain responsible for the care of ailing husbands and other family members. Well-designed NeuroAIDS studies using culturally appropriate and fair NP test materials are critical to addressing NeuroAIDS in developing nations.

Of the many health complications engendered by HIV, the NP decline and conditions such as dementia may be among the most clinically and personally challenging. The loss of freedom and control that accompany such disorders, and the attendant distress for both the patient and significant others can be overwhelming. While the advent of HAART has helped to mitigate more severe cognitive symptomatology, subtle deficits still proliferate, and the aging HIV-positive population will have to face the double jeopardy of the normal aging process and HIV particularly (Justice et al. 2004). Our understanding of the CNS changes observed in HIV and AIDS are well developed, though we still are attempting to understand the wide variance in the severity, onset, and progression of NP symptomatology across patients. As imaging technologies evolve, more precise understanding of the structural and metabolic mechanisms that underlie the NP deterioration observed in HIV will be made clear. In addition, understanding the real-world validity of these NP changes is needed to maximally benefit HIV seropositive patients. However, as the epidemic rages in the developing world, new challenges abound as we attempt to capture the picture of cognitive decline in socioeconomically and culturally diverse infected men, women, and children around the world.

DESIGN OF ART AND ADJUNCTIVE TRIALS FOR HADC—CLINICALLY RELEVANT QUESTIONS AND CHALLENGES

There are a number of questions that arise as a result of neurocognitive disabilities and HIV.

Exhibit 11.4 presents some of these questions that need to be addressed in future research initiatives.

A number of challenges exist for the NeuroAIDS community. It is imperative to identify neurological priorities for NIH (National Institutes of Health), and national AIDS organizations. It is equally important to continue to follow the prevalence of HADC and MCMD and to develop clinically useful predictive and surrogate markers. Well-designed clinical trials which address the impact of HAART and other adjunctive therapies on HADC and MCMD are needed, and implementation of such trials is complicated by issues such as the impact of "burnt out" inactive HADC (Brew et al. 2007). It is also important to recognize the limitations of current definitional criteria. Lastly, it is important to develop therapies and outcome measures that can be applied in resource-limited settings (McArthur 2007).

Exhibit 11.4 Clinically relevant questions

- How reversible is HADC, and when should treatment start?
- If virological suppression is complete, will this protect against HADC?
- What is needed to close the treatment gap?
- What are the determinants of treatment response?
- How can we dissect comorbidities?
- Can we improve outcome measures to reduce variability and sample size?

REFERENCES AND FURTHER READING

Abdulle, S., Hagberg, L., Svennerholm, B., Fuchs, D., Gisslen, M. 2002. "Continuing intrathecal immunocactiation despite two years of effective antiretroviral therapy against HIV-1 infection." *AIDS*, 16(16): 2145–9.

Albert, S.M., Weber, C.M., Todak, G., et al. 1999. "An observed performance test of medication management ability in HIV: relation to neuropsychological status and medication adherence outcomes." *AIDS Behav.*, 3:121–8.

Appay, V., Rowland-Jones, S.L. 2002. "Premature ageing of the immune system: the cause of AIDS?" *Trends Immunol.*, 23(12):580–5.

Asthana, S., Craft, S., Baker, L.D., Raskind, M.A., Birnbaum, R.S., Lofgreen, C.P., Veith, R.C., Plymate, S.R. 1999. "Cognitive and neuroendocrine response to transdermal estrogen in postmenopausal women with Alzheimer's disease: results of a placebo-controlled, double-blind, pilot study." *Psychoneuroendocrinology*, 24(6):657–77.

Becker, J.T., Lopez, O.L., Dew, M.A., Aizenstein, H.J. 2004. "Prevalence of cognitive disorders differs as a function of age in HIV virus infection." *AIDS*, 18(Suppl. 1):S11–S18.

Benhamou, Y., Bochet, M., DiMartino, V., et al. 1999. "Liver fibrosis progression in human immunodeficiency virus and hepatitis C virus coinfected patients." *Hepatology*, 30: 1054–8.

Benhamou, Y., Bonyhay, L. (2004). "Treatment of hepatitis B virus infection in patients coinfected with HIV." *Gastroenterol Clin North Am.* 33(3): 617–27.

Benhamou, Y., Di Martino, V., Bochet, M., Colombet, G., Thibault, V., Liou, A., Katlama, C., Poynard, T., MultivirC Group. 2001. "Factors affecting liver fibrosis in human immunodeficiency virus-and hepatitis C virus-coinfected patients: impact of protect inhibitor therapy." *Hepatology*, 34(2):283–7.

Brew, B.J. 2004. "Evidence for a change in AIDS dementia complex in the era of highly active antiretroviral therapy and the possibility of new forms of AIDS dementia complex." *AIDS*, 18 Suppl. 1:S75–S78.

Brew, B.J., Halman, M., Catalan, J., Sacktor, N., Price, R.W., Brown, S., Atkinson, H., Clifford, D.B., Simpson, D., Torres, G., Hall, C., Power, C., Marder, K., McArthur, J.C., Symonds, W., Romero, C. 2007. "Factors in AIDS dementia complex trial design: results and lessons from the abacavir trial." *PLoS Clin. Trials*, 2(3):e13.

Brew, B.J., Rosenblum, M., Price, R.W. 1988. "AIDS dementia complex and primary HIV brain infection." *J Neuroimmunol.*, 20(2–3):133–40.

Butt, A.A., Dascomb, K.K., DeSalvo, K.B., Bazzano, L., Kissinger, P.J., Szerlip, H.M. 2001. "Human immunodeficiency virus infection in elderly patients." *South Med. J.*, 94(4):397–400.

Butters, N., Grant, I., Hazby, J., Judd, L.L., Martin, A., McClelland, J., Pequegnat, W., Schacter, D., Stover, E. 1990. "Assessment of AIDS-related cognitive changes: recommendations of the NIMH Workgroup on neuropsychological assessment approaches." *J. Clin. Exp. Neuropsychol.*, 12(6):963–78.

Centers for Disease Control and Prevention (CDC). 2007. *HIV/AIDS Surveillance Report*, 17.

Chen, H.X., Ryan, P.A., Ferguson, R.P., Yataco, A., Markowitz, J.A., Raksis, K. 1998. "Characteristics of acquired immunodeficiency syndrome in older adults." *J. Am. Geriatr. Soc.*, 46(2):153–6.

Cherner, M., Letendre, S., Heaton, R.K., Durrelle, J., Marquie-Beck, J., Gragg, B., Grant, I., HIV Neurobehavioral Research Center Group. 2005. "Hepatitis C augments cognitive deficients associated with HIV infection and methamphetamine." *Neurology*, 64(8):1343–7.

Chesney, M.A., Ickovics, J.R., Chambers, D.B, Gifford, A.L., Neidig, J., Zwickl, B., Wu, A.W. 2000. "Self-reported adherence to antiretroviral medications among participants in HIV clinical trails: the AACTG adherence instruments. Patient Care Committee and Adherence Working Group of the Outcomes Committee of the Adult AIDS Clinical Trials Group (AACTG)." *AIDS Care*, 12(3):255–66.

Clifford, D.B., Mitike, M.T., Mekonnen, Y., Zhang, J., Zenebe, G., Melaku, Z., Zewde, A., Gessesse, N., Wolday, D., Messele, T., Teshome, M., Evans, S. 2007. "Neurological evaluation of untreated human immunodeficiency virus infected adults in Ethiopia." *J Neurovirol.*, 13(1):67–72.

Cohen, R.A., Boland, R., Pual, R., Tashima, K.T., Schoenbaum, E.E., Celentano, D.D., Schuman, P., Smith, D.K., Carpenter, C.C. 2001. "Neurocognitive performance enhanced by highly active antiretroviral therapy in HIV-infected women." *AIDS*, 15(3):341–5.

Deutsch, R., Ellis, R.J., McCuthcan, J.A., Marcotte, T.D., Letendre, S., Grant, I. HNRC Group. 2001. "AIDS-associated mild neurocognitive impairment is delayed in the era of highly active antiretroviral therapy." *AIDS*, 15(14):1898–9.

Dore, G.J., Correll, P.K., Li, Y., Kaldor, J.M., Cooper, D.A., Brew, B.J. 1999. "Changes to AIDS dementia complex in the era of highly active antiretroviral therapy." *AIDS*, 13(10):1249–53.

Durvasula, R.S., Golin, C., Stefaniak, M. 1998. "Determination of medication adherence in HIV+ women: a pilot investigation." Conference Record of the 12 World AIDS Conference, Geneva: Marathon Multimedia: 665.

Durvasula, R.S., Miller, E.N., Myers, H.F., Wyatt, G.E. 2001. "Predictors of neuropsychological performance in HIV positive women." *J. Clin. Exp. Neuropsychol.* 23(2):149–63.

Effros, R.B., Boucher, N., Porter, V., Zhu, X., Spaulding, C., Walford, R.L., Kronenberg, M., Cohen, C., Schachter, F. 1994. "Decline in CD8 t cells in centenarians and in long term t-cell structures: a possible cause for both in vivo and in vitro immunosenescence." *Experimental Gerontology*, 29:601–9.

Ellis, R.J., Moore, D.J., Childers, M.E., Letendre, S., McCutchan, J.A., Wolfson, T., Spector, S.A., Hsia, K., Heaton, R.K., Grant, I. 2002. "Progression to neuropsychological impairment in human immunodeficiency virus infection predicted by elevated cerebrospinal fluid levels of human immunodeficiency virus RNA." *Arch. Neurol.*, 59(6):923–8.

Fernandez, F., Maldonado, J., Ruiz, J. 2004. "Neuropsychiatric aspects of HIV-1 infection." In *Substance Abuse: A Comprehensive Textbook*, 4th ed., J. Lowinson, P. Ruiz, R.B. Millman (eds). Philadelphia: Lippincott, Williams and Wilkins.

Ferrando, S., Van Gorp, W., McElhiney, M, Goggin, K., Sewell, M., Rabkin, J. 1998. "Highly active antiretroviral treatment in HIV infection: benefits for neuropsychological function." *AIDS*, 12(8):F65–F70.

Ferrando, S.J., Wall, T.L., Batki, S.L., Soresen, J.L. 1996. "Psychiatric morbidity, illicit drug use and adherence to zidovudine (AZT) among injection drug users with HIV disease." *Am. J. Drug Alcohol Abuse*, 22(4):475–87.

Freeman, R.C., Rodriquez, G.M., French, J.F. 1996. "Compliance with AZT treatment regiment of HIV-seropositive injection drug users: a neglected issue." *AIDS Educ. Prev.*, 8(1):58–71.

Goetz, M.B., Boscardin, W.J., Wiley, D.M., Alkasspooles, S. 2001. "Decreased recovery of CD4 lymphocytes in older HIV-infected patients beginning highly active antiretroviral therapy." *AIDS*, 15(12):1576–9.

Goodkin, K., Heckman, T., Siegel, K., Linsk, N., Khamis, I., Lee, D., Lecusay, R., Poindexter, C.C., Mason, S.J., Suarez, P., Eisdorfer, C. 2003. " 'Putting a face' on HIV infection/AIDS in older adults: a psychosocial context." *J. Acquire. Immune. Defic. Syndr.*, 33 Suppl 2:S171–S184.

Goodkin, K., Wilkie, F.L., Concha, M., Hinkin, C.H., Symes, S., Baldewicz, T.T., Asthana, D., Fujimura, R.K., Lee, D., Van Zuilen, M.H., Khamis, I., Shapshak, P., Eisdorfer, C. 2001. "Aging and neuro-AIDS conditions and changing spectrum of HIV-1-associated morbidity and mortality." *J. Clin. Epidemiol.*, 54 Suppl. 1:S35–S43.

Grant, I. 2007. "HIV, meth and the brain: implications for HIV risk." Oral presentation given at NIDA conference, Bethesda, MD: May.

Grant, I., Heaton, R.K. 1990. "Human immunodeficiency virus—Type 1 (HIV-1) and the brain." *J. Consult. Clin. Psychol.*, 58:22–30.

Hardy, D.J., Castellon, S.A., Hindin, C.H. 2004. "Perceptual span deficits in adults with HIV." *J. Int. Neuropsychol. Soc.*, 10(1):135–40.

Hardy, D.J., Hinkin, C.H., Satz, P., Stenquist, P.K., van Gorp, W.G., Moore, L.H. 1999. "Age differences and neurocognitive performance in HIV infected adults." *NZ J Psychol.* 28:94–101.

Heaton, R.K., Grant, I., Butters, N., White, D.A., Kirson, D., Atkinson, J.H., McCutchan, J.A., Taylor, M.J., Kelly, M.D., Ellis, R.J., Wofson, T., Velin, R., Marcotte, T.D., Hesselink, J.R., Jernigan, T.L., Chandler, J., Wallace, M., Abramson, I., HIV Neurobehavioral Research Center 1995. "The HNRC 500—neuropsychology of HIV infection at different disease stages. HIV Neurobehavioral Research Center." *J. Int. Neuropsychol. Soc.*, 1 (3): 231–51.

Hellinger, F.J. 2007. "The changing pattern of hospital care for persons living with HIV: 2000–2004." *J Acquir Immune Defic Syndr.*, 45(2):239–46.

Hilsabeck, R.C., Castellon S.A., Hinkin, C.H. 2005. "Neuropsychological aspects of coinfection with HIV and hepatitis C virus." *Clin. Infect. Dis.*, 41 Suppl. 1:S38–S44.

Hilsabeck, R., Malek-Ahmadi, P. 2004. "Neurobehavioral correlates of chronic hepatitis C." *J. Psychopathol. Behav. Assess.*, 26 (3):203–10.

Hinkin, C.H., Castellon, S.A., Atkinson, J.H., Goodkin, K. 2001. "Neuropsychiatric aspects of HIV infection among older adults." *J.Clin. Epidemiol.*, 54 Suppl. 1:S44–S55.

Hinkin, C.H., Castellon, S.A. Hardy, D.J. 2000. "Dual-task performance in HIV-1 infection," *J. Clin. Exp. Neuropsychol.*, 22:16–24.

Hinkin, C.H., Castellon, S.A., Hardy, D.J., Granholm, E., Siegle, G. 1999. "Computerized and traditional Stroop task dysfunction in HIV-1 infection." *Neuropsychology*, 13:111–21.

Hinkin, C.H., Castellon, S.A., Levine, A.J., Barclay, T.R., Singer, E.J. (in press). "Neurocognitive performance in individuals co-infected with HIV and Hepatitis C." *Journal of Addictive Disorders*.

Hinkin, C.H., Hardy, D.J., Mason, K.I., Castellon, S.A., Durvasula, R.S., Lam, M., Stefaniak, M. 2004. "Medication adherence in HIV-infected adults: effect of patient age, cognitive status, and substance abuse." *AIDS*, 18:S19–S25.

Hinkin, C.H., Hardy, D.J., Mason, K.I., Castellon, S.A., Lam, M.N., Stefaniak, M. 2002. "Verbal and spatial working memory performance among HIV-infected adults." *J. Int. Neuropsychol. Soc.*, 8:532–8.

Ho, D.D., Rota, T.R., Schooley, R.T., Kaplan, J.C., Allan, J.D., Groopman, J.E., Resnick, L., Felsenstein, D., Andrews, C.A., Hirsch, M.S. 1985. "Isolation of HTLV-III from cerebrospinal fluid and neural tissues of patients with neurologic syndromes related to the acquired immunodeficiency syndrome." *N. Engl. J. Med.*, 313:1493–7.

Ickovics, J.R., Rodin, J. 1992. "Women and AIDS in the United States: epidemiology, natural history, and mediating mechanisms." *Health Psychol.*, 11(1):1–16.

Jowi J.O., Mativo, P.M., Musoke, S.S. 2007. "Clinical and laboratory characteristics of hospitalized patients with neurological manifestations of HIV/AIDS at the Nairobi hospital." *East Afr. Med. J.*, 84(2):67–76.

Justice, A.C., McGinnis, K.A., Atkinson, J.H., Heaton, R.K., Young, C., Sadek, J., Madenwald, T., Becker, J.T., Conigliaro, J., Brown, S.T., Rimland, D., Crystal, S., Simberkoff, M., The Veterans Aging Cohort 5-Site Study Project Team. 2004. "Psychiatric and neurocognitive disorders among HIV-positive and negative veterans in care: veterans aging cohort five-site study." *AIDS*, 18 Suppl. 1: S49–S59.

Khalsa, J.H., Royal, W. 2004. "Do drugs of abuse impact on HIV disease?" *J. Neuroimmunol.*, 147(1–2):6–8.

Laskus, T., Bardowski, M., Jablonska., Kibler, K., Wilkinson, J., Adair, D., Rakela, J. 2004. "Human immunodeficiency virus facilitates infection/replication of hepatitis C virus in native human macrophages." *Blood*, 103(10):3854–9.

Letrendre, S.L., Cherner, M., Ellis, R.J., Marquie-Beck, J., Graff, B., Marcotte, T., Heaton, R.K., McCutchan, J.A., Grant, I., HNRC Group. 2005. "The effects of hepatitis C, HIV, and methamphetamine dependence on neuropsychological performance: biological correlates of disease." *AIDS*, 2005, 19 Suppl. 3:S72–8.

Letrendre, S.L., McCutchan, J.A., Childers, M.E., Woods, S.P., Lazzaretto, D., Heaton R.K., Grant, I., Ellis, R.J., HNRC Group. 2004. "Enhancing antiretroviral therapy for human immunodeficiency virus cognitive disorders." *Ann. Neurol.*, 56(3):416–23.

Maj, M., Satz, P., Janssen, R., Zaudig, M., Starace, F., D'Ellia, L., Sughondabirom, B., Mussa, M., Naber, D., Nedeti, D. 1994. "WHO Neuropsychistriatric AIDS Study, cross-sectional phase II. Neuropsychological and neurological findings." *Arch. Gen. Psychiatry*, 51(1):51–61.

Malow, R.M., Baker, S.M., Klimas, N., Antoni, M.H., Schneiderman, N., Penedo, F.J., Ziskind, D., Page, B., McMahon, R. 1998. "Adherence to complex combination antiretroviral therapies by HIV-positive drug abusers." *Psychiatr. Serv.*, 49(8):1021–2, 1024.

Martin, E.M., Pitrak, D.L., Pursell, K.J., Mullane, K.M., Novak, R.M. 1995. "Delayed recognition memory span in HIV-1 infection." *J. Int. Neuropsychol. Soc.*, 1(6):575–80.

Mason, K.I., Campbell, A., Hawkins, P., Madhere, S., Johnson, K., Takushi-Chinen, R. 1998. "Neuropsychological functioning in HIV-positive African American women with a history of drug use." *J. Nat. Med. Assoc.*, 90(11): 665–74.

Mason, K., Thrasher, D., Castellon, S., Lam, M., Hardy, D., Stefaniak, M., Durvasula, R., Hinkin, C. 2002. "Neurocognitive and neuropsychiatric predictors of adherence in HIV+ men and women." Presented at the 30th Annual Meeting of the International Neuropsychological Society, Toronto, CA. Abstract in *Journal of the International Neuropsychological Society*, 8:159.

McArthur, J.C. 1987. "Neurologic manifestations of AIDS." *Medicine*, 66(6):407–37.

McArthur, J.C. 2007. "Neuro-AIDS in drug users." Oral presentation given at NIDA conference, Bethesda, MD, May.

McArthur, J.C., Haughey, N., Gartner, S., Conant, K., Pardo, C., Nath, A., Sacktor, N. 2003. "Human immunodeficiency virus-associated dementia: an evolving disease." *J. Neurovirol.*, 9(2):205–21.

McArthur, J.C., Hoover, D.R., Bacellar, H., Miller, E.N., Cohen, B.A., Becker, J.T., Graham, N.M., McArthur, J.H., Selnes, O.A., Jacobson, L.P. 1993. "Dementia in AIDS patients: incidence and risk factors. Multicenter AIDS Cohort Study." *Neurology*, 43(11):2245–52.

McArthur, J.C., Selnes O.A., Glass, J.D., Hoover, D.R., Bacellar, H. 1994. "HIV dementia. Incidence and risk factors." *Res. Publ. Assoc. Res. Nerv. Ment. Dis.*, 72:251–72.

Miller, E.N., Selnes, O.A., McArthur, J.C., Satz, P., Becker, J.T., Cohen, B.A., Sheridan, K., Machado, A.M., Van Gorp, W.G., Visscher, B. 1990. "Neuropsychological performance in HIV-1 infected homosexual men: the Multicenter AIDS Cohort Study (MACS)." *Neurology*, 40(2):197–203.

Minimo, A.M., Smith, B.L. 2001. "Deaths: preliminary data for 2000." *National Vital Statistics Report*, 49(12):25–6.

Morrison, M.F., Petitto, J.M., Ten Have, T., Gettes, D.R., Chaippini, M.S., Weber, A.L., Brinker-Spence, P., Bauer, R.M., Douglas, S.D., Evans, D.L. 2002. "Depressive and anxiety disorders in women with HIV infection." *Am. J. Psychiatry*, 159(5):789–96.

Navia, B.A., Cho, E.S., Petito, C.K., Price, R.W. 1986a. "The AIDS dementia complex: II. Neuropathology." *Ann. Neurol.*, 19(6):625–35.

Navia, B.A., Jordan, B.D., Price, R.W. 1986b. "The AIDS dementia complex: I. Clinical features." *Ann. Neurol.*, 19(6):517–24.

Perry, W., Hilsabeck, R.C., Hassanein, T.I. 2007. "Cognitive dysfunction in chronic hepatitis C: a review." *Dig. Dis. Sci.*, Aug [Epub ahead of print].

Portegies, P. 1994. "AIDS dementia complex: a review." *J. Acquir. Immune. Defic. Syndr.*, 7 Suppl 2:S38–S48.

Portegies, P., De Gans, J., Lange, J.M., Derix, M.M., Speelman, H., Bakker, M., Danner, S.A., Goudsmit, J. 1989. "Declining incidence of AIDS dementia complex after introduction of zidovudine treatment." *BMJ.*, 299(6703):819–21.

Power, C., Selnes, O.A., Grim, J.A., McArthur, J.C. 1995. "HIV dementia scale: a rapid screening test." *J Acquir Immune Defic Syndr Hum Retrovirol* 8(3): 273–8.

Richardson, J., Barkan, S., Cohen, M., Back, S., Fitz-Gerald, G., Feldman, J., Young, M., Palacio, H. 2001. "Experience and covariates of depressive symptoms among a cohort of HIV-infected women." *Soc Work Health Care*, 32(4):93–111.

Robertson, K.R., Smurzynski, M., Parsons, T.D., Wu, K., Bosch, R.J., Wu, J., McArthur, J.C., Collier, A.C., Evans, S.R., Ellis, R.J. 2007. "The prevalence and incidence of neurocognitive impairment in the HAART era." *AIDS*, 21(14):1915–21.

Sacktor, N., McDermott, M.P., Marder, K., Schifitto, G., Selnes, O.A., McArthur, J.D., Stern, Y., Albert, S., Palumbo, D., Kieburtz, K., De Marcaida, J.A., Cohen, B., Epstein, L. 2002. "HIV-associated cognitive impairment before and after the advent of combination therapy." *J. Neurovirol.*, 8(2):136–42.

Sacktor, N., Skolasky, R., Lyles, R., et al. 1998. "Highly active antiretroviral therapy (HAART) improves cognitive impairment in HIV+ homosexual men." *J. Neurovirol.*, 4:365.

Sacktor, N., Tarwater, P.M., Skolasky, R.L., McArthur, J.C., Selnes, O.A., Becker, J., Cohen, B., Miller, E.N., Multicenter for AIDS Cohort Study (MACS). 2001. "CSF antiretroviral drug penetrance and the treatment of HIV-associated psychomotor slowing." *Neurology*, 57(3):542–4.

Sansoni, P., Cossarizza, A., Brianti, V., Fagnoni, F., Snelli, G., Monti, D., et al. 1993. "Lymphocyte subsets and natural killer cell activity in healthy old people and centenarians." *Blood*, 82:2767–73.

Satz, P. 1993. "Brain reserve capacity on symptom onset after brain injury: A formulation and review of evidence for threshold theory." *Neuropsychology*, 7:273–95.

Satz, P., Morgenstern, H., Miller, E.N., Selesn, O.A., McArthur, J.C., Cohen, B.A., Wesch, J., Becker, J.T., Jacobson, L., D'Elia, L.F. 1993. "Low education as a possible risk factor for cognitive abnormalities in HIV-1: findings from the Multicenter AIDS Cohort Study (MACS)." *J. Acquir. Immune. Defic. Syndr.*, 6(5):503–11.

Schrooten, W., Florence, E., Dreezen, C., Van Esbroeck, M., Fransen, K., Alonso, A., Desmet, P., Colebunders, R., Kestens, L., De Roo, A. 2004. "Five year immunological outcome of highly active antiretroviral treatment in a clinical setting: results from a single HIV treatment centre." *Int. J. STD AIDS*, 15(8): 523–8.

Selik, R.M., Chu, S.Y., Buehler J.W. 1993. "HIV infection as leading cause of death among young adults in U.S. cities and states." *JAMA*, 269(23):2991–4.

Shankar, S.K., Satishchandra, P., Mahadevan, A., Yasha, T.C., Nagaraja, D., Taly, A.B., et al. 2003. "Low prevalence of multifocal leukoencephalopathy in India and Africa: is there a biological explanation?" *J. Neurovirol.*, 9:S59–S67.

Solomon, T.M., Halkitis, P.M. 2007. "Cognitive executive functioning in relation to HIV medication adherence among gay, bisexual, and other men who have sex with men." 2007. *AIDS Behav.*, 17 [Epub ahead of print].

Tozzi, V., Balestra, P., Galgani, S., Narciso, P., Ferri, F., Sebastián, G., DiAmato, C., Affricao, C., Pigornini, F., Pau, F.M., De Felici, A., Benedetto, A. 1999. "Positive and sustained effects of highly antiretroviral therapy on HIV-1 associated neurocognitive impairment." *AIDS*, 13(14):1889–97.

Tozzi, V., Balestra, P., Galgani, S., Narciso, P., Sampaolesi, A., Antinor, A., Guilanelli, M., Serraino, D., Ippolito, G. 2001. "Changes in neurocognitive performance in a cohort of patients treated with HAART for 3 years." *J. Acquir. Immune. Defic. Syndr.*, 28(1):19–27.

Turchan, J., Anderson, C., Hauser, K.F., Sun, Q., Zhang, J., Liu, Y., Wise, P.M., Kruman, I., Maragos, W., Mattson, M.P., Booze, R., Nath, A. 2001. "Estrogen protects against the synergistic toxicity by HIV proteins, methamphetamine and cocaine." *BMC*

Neuroscience, 2:3. http://www.biomedcentral.com/1471-2202/2/3. Retrieved October 30, 2007.

UNAIDS, 2006. *AIDS Epidemic Update—December 2006*. Joint United Nations Programme on HIV/AIDS, Geneva, Switzerland.

Valcour, V.G., Shikuma, C.M., Watters, M.R., Sacktor, N.C., 2004. "Cognitive impairment in older HIV-1 seropositive individuals: prevalence and potential mechanisms." *AIDS*, 18 Suppl. 1: S79–S86.

Valcour, V., Paul, R. 2006. "HIV infection and dementia in older adults." *Clin. Infect. Dis.*, 42(10):1449–54.

Van Gorp, W.G., Lamb, D.G., Schmitt, F.A. 1993. "Methodologic issues in neuropsychological research with HIV-spectrum disease." *Arch. Clin. Neuropsychol.*, 8(1):17–33.

Verucchi, G., Calza, L., Mafredi, R., Chiodo, F. 2004. "Human immunodeficiency virus and hepatitis C virus coinfection: epidemiology, natural history, therapeutic options and clinic management." *Infection*, 32(1):33–46.

Von Giesen, H.J., Heintges, T., Abbasi-Boroudjeni, N., Kucukkoylu, S., Koller, H., Haslinger, B.A., Oetter, M., Arendt, G. 2004. "Psychomotor slowing in hepatitis C and HIV infection." *J. Acquir. Immune. Defic. Syndr.*, 35(2):131–7.

Wallace, D.R., Dodson, S., Nath, A., Booze, R.M. 2006. "Estrogen attenuates gp120- and tat1-72-induced oxidative stress and prevents loss of dopamine transporter function." *Synapse*, 59(1):51–60.

Wong, M.H., Robertson, K., Nakasujja, N., Skolasky, R., Musisi, S., Katabira, E., McArthur, J.C., Ronald, A., Sacktor, N. 2007. "Frequency of and risk factors for HIV dementia in an HIV clinic in sub-Saharan Africa." *Neurology*, 68(5):350–5.

Wu, Y.C., Zhao, Y.B., Tang, M.G., Zhang-Nunes, S.X., McArthur, J.C. (2007). "AIDS dementia complex in China." *J. Clin. Neurosciences*, 14(1):8–11.

Yarchoan, R., Masur, H., Broder, S. 1987. "Therapy of acquired immunodeficiency syndrome." *Cancer Chemother. Biol. Response Modif.*, 9:200–25.

Yepthomi, T., Paul, R., Vallabhaneni, S., Kumarasamy, N., Tate, D.F., Solomon, S., Flanigan, T. 2006. "Neurocognitive consequences of HIV in southern India: a preliminary study of clade C virus." *J. Int. Neuropsychol. Soc.*, 12(3):424–30.

CHAPTER 12

Overview of Adherence to Antiretroviral Therapies

Jane Simoni, K. Rivet Amico, Cynthia Pearson, and Robert Malow

ABSTRACT

Antiretroviral medications (ARV) have enhanced longevity and health among people living with HIV, yet challenges to their full implementation and success remain. Notable, their requirement of near-perfect adherence has been difficult to achieve. In this chapter, we overview the barriers to achieving optimal levels of ARV adherence, theoretical conceptualizations of these barriers and the factors facilitating ART (antiretroviral therapies) adherence, and, finally, research on the behavioral strategies evaluated to promote adherence. We pay particular attention to global issues in ARV adherence, including problems in fully accessing these life-saving regimens and the unique barriers of resource-constrained settings. Issues relevant to pediatric HIV infection also are considered.

In the wake of perennial disappointments in the search for a vaccine or cure for HIV, antiretroviral medications (ARV) first appeared as a beacon of hope for people living with the virus (see Section I for more information on the history and nature of ARV). Subsequently, ARV has brought longer and healthier lives to thousands of people living with HIV/AIDS (Palella et al. 1998). According to one estimate, at least three million years of life have been saved in the United States (U.S.) as a direct result of the significant advances made in HIV disease treatment (Walensky et al. 2006). Although access to the life-saving regimens was initially limited to the West, initiatives from international health activists and pharmaceutical companies eventually coalesced to make ARVs more accessible to the resource-constrained countries most devastated by the AIDS epidemic (Desvarieux et al. 2005).

However, ARV falls far short of a cure and several challenges to its full implementation and success still exist. Specifically, achieving optimum results requires near-perfect adherence to dosing schedules and strict attention to special instructions regarding dietary guidelines (Bangsberg et al. 2000; Garcia de Olalla et al. 2002). Few patients in the West have been able to achieve the strict adherence levels required. Indeed, poor adherence to medication regimens appears to be one of the primary reasons why the high degree of success with ARV in achieving undetectable HIV-1 RNA levels reported in clinical trials (i.e., 60–90 percent) has seldom been achieved in everyday practice, where, on average, 50 percent of patients achieve undetectable HIV-1 RNA (Curioso, Kurth, Blas, and Klausner, in press; Liu et al. 2001, Nieuwkerk et al. 2001; Rabkin and Chesney 1999). Early reports suggest that patients in sub-Saharan Africa have better adherence (Mills et al. 2006b), but maintenance of these levels may be difficult (Bangsberg, Ware, and Simoni 2006).

In this chapter, we overview the barriers to achieving optimal levels of ARV adherence, theoretical conceptualizations of these barriers and the factors facilitating ART (antiretroviral therapies) adherence, and, finally, research on the behavioral strategies evaluated to promote adherence.

BARRIERS TO ANTIRETROVIRAL THERAPY ADHERENCE

Many factors associated with non-adherence to prescribed medication regimens have been identified from cross-sectional studies across various illnesses. Ickovics and Meisler (1997) categorized these factors into five groups: patient variables, treatment regimen, disease characteristics, patient–provider relationship, and clinical setting. *Patient variables* include socio-demographic factors (which are generally not strongly related to non-adherence) and psychosocial factors such as active alcohol or other drug use, depression or psychiatric illness, degree of social support, concerns regarding body image, and self-efficacy. *Variables related to the treatment regimen* include the regimen's complexity (i.e., large number of medications, frequent doses, dietary restrictions, long-term duration, and various forms of administration) and the number and severity of side effects. However, given that medication adherence studies suggest that only 50 percent of the general population will follow much simpler prescribed regimens (DiMatteo 2004; Meichenbaum and Tuck 1987; O'Donohue and Levensky 2006), simplifying ARV regimens themselves may be important for many patients' adherence but is not anticipated to resolve the multiple and dynamic barriers to ARV adherence experienced by others. Also included in treatment regimen are patients' own perceptions of HIV and ARV, which may have important influences on adherence. Patients are less likely to adhere to medications at optimal rates when side effects are acute, although the relation between regimen complexity and adherence is less consistently supported. *Disease characteristics* include severity of symptomatology, reduced immune functioning, and opportunistic infections or complicating factors, which in other chronic conditions have been negatively associated with adherence. Interestingly, with positive beliefs towards the effectiveness of ARV, HIV acute symptoms may actually increase levels of adherence, perhaps because of increased motivation to adhere (Singh et al. 1996; Spire et al. 2002). It is likely that patients are less likely to adhere when their illness is chronic, has asymptomatic periods, or immediate effects of non-adherence are not experienced. *Aspects of the patient–provider relationship* include the patient's beliefs in the provider's competence; the provider's ability, knowledge, and time to implement interventions to help his or her patients; and the extent to which the patient–provider relationship is characterized by consistency, openness, friendliness, genuine interest, empathy, mutual trust, and respect. Aspects of the *clinical setting* that may influence adherence include access to ongoing primary care, involvement in a dedicated adherence program, availability of transportation and child care, pleasantness of the clinical environment, convenience in scheduling appointments, perceived confidentiality, and satisfaction with past experiences in the health care system.

With respect to non-adherence to ARV specifically, a number of empirical studies and reviews have found that several factors were often associated with non-adherence, including presence of adverse drug effects, neuropsychological dysfunction, psychological distress, substance use, lack of social or family support, low patient self-efficacy, inconvenience of treatment, and poor reading literacy skills (Ammassari et al. 2002). Several factors render the combination therapies an especially challenging treatment. These include the relative absence of significant symptoms related to HIV until later in the course of the disease; the often prophylactic nature of the treatment; indefinite duration of treatment; questionable treatment efficacy; and frequent and serious adverse effects.

Some of the important barriers to ARV adherence in resource-constrained countries are similar to those reported in the resource-rich countries. In a review of 72 studies (35 qualitative) conducted in resource-rich nations and 12 (two qualitative) conducted in resource-constrained nations, Mills et al. (2006a) noted that important barriers reported in both settings included fear of disclosure, concomitant substance abuse, forgetfulness, suspicions of treatment, regimens that are too complicated, number of pills required, decreased quality of life, work and family responsibilities, falling asleep, and access to medication.

Other prevalent barriers appear to be specific to sub-Saharan Africa, including: cost (Bangsberg et al. 2006; Crane et al. 2006; Laurent et al. 2004; Nachega et al. 2006); not disclosing HIV status to a loved one; and fear of being stigmatized (Nachega et al. 2004; Weiser et al. 2003). In China, fear, shame, and secrecy resulting from AIDS-related stigma and social disapproval were reported as major barriers to antiretroviral adherence (Starks et al. in press). Mills (2006a) underscored how suboptimal adherence levels among the poor in North America have mistakenly been interpreted as indicating that poverty itself is a barrier to adherence, thereby decreasing support for antiretroviral treatment in resource-constrained countries. However, non-adherence among impoverished individuals in North America appears to be related to ancillary factors such as poor patient–clinician relationships, untreated depression, and substance abuse, suggesting that poverty itself should not be considered a barrier to one's ability to adhere. In resource-limited settings, structural barriers such as shortages, cost, and inadequate health and transportation infrastructures may be the real "Achilles heel" to successful HIV treatment (Machtinger and Bangsberg 2005; Oyugi et al. 2007).

Research on barriers to antiretroviral adherence in pediatric populations is more limited. Pontali (2005) grouped factors that were capable of influencing adherence into those related to the prescribed medication, health care system, and patient and family/caregiver. Family/caregiver factors were crucial to pediatric adherence, because infants and younger children depend almost entirely on a caregiver to administer medications (Pontali 2005). Their adherence to treatment, therefore, is largely determined by the resources and efficacy of their caregivers. Caregivers who are biological parents of HIV-positive children often share their diagnosis and confront challenges associated with their own illness and its comorbidities. In these cases, treatment can become a reminder of the parents' guilt about their role in their child's acquisition of infection, which is yet another challenge to adherence (Simoni 2007; Wrubel et al. 2005).

THEORIES OF ARV ADHERENCE

Following a wave of research studies that identified correlates consistently identified as important to ARV adherence—and that produced some conflicting findings—comprehensive theoretical models of adherence began to appear as a way to organize and consolidate the findings. These models seek to identify the constellation of constructs that influence adherence and the manner in which these constructs coexist and influence one another. The development and evaluation of theoretical models has critical implications for intervention development and clinical practice.

In practice, many efforts to understand the dynamics of ARV adherence have involved the application of health behavior models developed outside of the domain of ARV adherence. These include the Health Beliefs Model (HBM), Social-Cognitive Theory (SCT), Theory of Reasoned Action (TRA), Theory of Planned Behavior (TPB), and Protective Motivation Theory (PMT). A common feature to all of these cognitive theories is their proposition that attitudes and beliefs about a behavior, as well as outcome expectancies, are critical determinants of a health behavior (Munro, Lewin, Swart, and Volmink 2007). This feature, however, is also the main source of criticism for these models in that the behavior in question may be assumed to be overly volitional or under the patient's immediate control and that these models do not fully address structural and social influences on health behavior choices (cf., Munro et al. 2007).

Several models have been proposed for, or applied specifically to, ARV adherence behavior. One of the more comprehensive and empirically supported models is the Information–Motivation–Behavioral Skills model of ARV adherence (Fisher, Fisher, Amico, and Harman 2006), which proposes that ARV adherence is a function of one's fund of accurate regimen-specific information, social and personal motivation, and adherence-related behavioral skills, which is further considered in relation to the relative presence of moderating factors, such as homelessness or severe depression.

Self-regulation theory's (SRT's) (Leventhal and Benyamini 1997; Leventhal et al. 1984) articulation to ARV adherence and HIV self-care behavior explicitly joins individuals' perceptions about their health with surrounding social, cultural, and environmental factors (Reynolds 2003; Reynolds et al. 2007). SRT assumes that individuals actively make health behavior decisions on the basis of their cognitive and emotional responses to their illness and more specifically to the health threats they perceive. As individuals attempt to make sense of their illness, understand it in the context of their surroundings, and manage perceived health threats, a cognitive representation of their illness and how to deal with it develops and influences self-care, including adherence behavior.

The importance of social factors in ARV adherence incorporated in the models previously discussed is highlighted more prominently in models using Social Action Theory (SAT) (Ewart 1991; Johnson et al. 2003; Remien et al. 2006) and recently evaluated social-cognitive models of adherence (Simoni, Frick, and Huang 2006). SAT models of ARV adherence assume that health protective behaviors, such as ARV adherence, are the interactive result of: a) the *environmental context* in which the patient exists and in which he or she must implement adherence behaviors; b) *responses to states of emotion*, which includes both positive and negative affect and can lead to changes in cognitive "action scripts" one has developed; and c) *self-regulatory capacities*, which include adherence self-efficacy, beliefs and attitudes towards treatment and adherence, and outcome expectancies, and other strategies that are used to maintain equilibrium between a behavior or "action script" and its consequences/outcomes.

Understanding the dynamics of ARV adherence for individuals living in limited-resource countries has involved modifications to models originally developed in the West (Ware, Wyatt, and Bangsberg 2006). Whereas models of adherence behavior in well-resourced settings appear to converge in the placement of information, social support, beliefs, self-efficacy, outcome expectancies, and behavioral strategies as key factors, preliminary models of ARV adherence in resource-limited settings emphasize information, social support, and, critically, structural barriers to adherence. One model for use in China, grounded in the IMB (information, motivation, and behavior) approach, suggests there are four components that are necessary for consistent medication adherence (Starks et al. in press). First, persons with HIV/AIDS must have *access to medications* and other supports to allow for ongoing monitoring of health and treatment regimens (a structural component). Second, they require correct *knowledge* (i.e., about dosing schedules, resistance, potential side effects) to take their medications (a cognitive component). Third, they must be *motivated* to take the medications (a psychological component). Fourth, they need to have the medication available and *remember* to take the medication at the appropriate time (an internal cue) or *be prompted* by a family member or an alarm (an external cue). These external cues represent a social/mechanical component.

In India, investigators applied a Social Cognitive Model of Health to adherence (Tarakeshwar et al. 2007). The model recognizes three broad domains that influence each other to produce health behaviors: the Personal Domain (self-concept, family-focused goals, and treatment optimism); the Environmental Domain (family-based support, treatment availability, access, and quality, HIV stigma and discrimination); and the Behavioral Domain (medication adherence and health habits, sexual behavior, and social relationships and emotional wellbeing).

BEHAVIORAL INTERVENTION STRATEGIES TO PROMOTE ARV ADHERENCE

The urgency of problems related to non-adherence to antiretroviral medications has sparked increasing work in the development of behavioral interventions to promote adherence. Several comprehensive reviews of this work have been published. Initial reviews focused on qualitative descriptions (Fogarty et al. 2002; Haddad et al. 2000; Ickovics and Meade 2002), and reported concerns over atheoretical intervention approaches, lack of methodological rigor, poor generalizability of results, and weak intervention outcomes. Ickovics and Meade's (2002) and Cote and Godin's (2005) reviews also clearly noted a dire need for improvements in methodology, although they did conclude that some interventions appeared to demonstrate efficacy (Cote and Godin 2005; Ickovics and Meade 2002).

Subsequent reviews incorporated more sophisticated approaches to research synthesis. Two recent meta-analyses summarizing intervention outcome studies published through December 2004 (Amico, Harman, and Johnson 2006) and September 2005 (Simoni, Pearson, Pantalone, Marks, and Crepaz 2006) suggested that intervention design, implementation, and evaluation has improved slightly in the field of ARV adherence, in terms of rigor and in the reporting of adequate detail, and that, generally, interventions do appear to improve ARV adherence. The authors concluded that various ARV adherence intervention strategies can be successful, but more research is needed to identify the most efficacious intervention components.

In terms of strategies, modified directly observed therapy has been a key feature in many of the presented or evaluated adherence interventions published over the last year (e.g., Ciambrone et al. 2006; Garland et al. 2007; Lucas et al. 2007; Mitchell, Freels, Creticos, Oltean, and Douglas 2007; Pearson et al. 2007; Smith-Rohrberg, Mezger, Walton, Bruce, and Altice 2006). Modified directly observed therapy (mDOT) or directly administered antiretroviral therapy (DAART) typically involves a program of intervention where research or clinic staff or trained peers observe patients ingesting a portion of their full ARV regimen. A recent mDOT RCT (randomized control trial) in the U.S. (Macalino et al. 2007) found mDOT participants were more likely to achieve PVL (plasma viral load) suppression (odds ratio, 2.16; 95 percent confidence interval, 1.0–4.7), and a significant treatment effect was also found in CD4 cell count change ($p < 0.05$). Likewise in Africa, Pearson et al. (2007) found mDOT participants, compared to those in standard care, showed significantly higher mean medication adherence at 6 months (92.7 percent versus 84.9, difference 7.8, 95 percent CI: .0.02, 13.0) and 12 months (94.4 percent versus 87.7 percent, difference 6.8 95 percent CI: 0.9, 12.9). There is growing sensitivity to the issue of overall cost-effectiveness of labor-intensive mDOT in resource-limited settings (Myung et al. 2007).

Recently, contingency management strategies have been highlighted as promising structural methods to support and improve adherence (Haug and Sorensen 2006). Contingency systems include voucher systems, rewards programs, or raffled prizes to perform a given behavior or meet a certain criteria (Javanbakht, Prosser, Grimes, Weinstein, and Farthing 2006; Rosen et al. 2007; Sorensen et al. 2007). When reinforced with prizes based on data collected from electronic pill caps, this type of intervention appeared to promote improved adherence in relation to standard of care, but improvements appear to dissipate after the removal of the incentive program (Rosen et al. 2007).

While mDOT and contingency management are based on Behavioral Theory, other interventions focus extensively on social support aspects of adherence. Intervention programs using tenets of Social Action Theory (e.g., Remien et al. 2006) and cognitive-affective models of social support (Simoni, Pantalone, Plummer, and Huang 2007) have received some degree of support for effectiveness in promoting adherence

An emerging area in ARV adherence interventions is the use of computer-supported technology to provide individually tailored education and support (Curioso et al. in press; Fisher, Amico, and Shuper 2007). In view of the sheer quantity of information available pertaining to HIV and ARV regimens, interactions, side effects, and the diversity in specific patient needs and barriers, computer technology may offer exceptionally comprehensive coverage of adherence-related issues and concerns. Additionally, despite high initial development costs, these types of interventions may ultimately be cost-effective and provide individually tailored interventions that can be sustained over time.

Research in adherence promotion strategies for pediatric HIV infection is much more limited. A review of the empirical literature through December 2005 located seven published studies, of which only one was a randomized controlled trial. These studies provided some support for the utility and efficacy of DOT, a 12-week educational program, gastrointestinal tube placement, and nursing home visits. However, most findings were based on pilot studies with very small samples, and adherence to the intervention itself often was problematic. The findings suggest that more intensive interventions are required to produce efficacious outcomes; one-time interventions in the absence of ongoing education and support may be insufficient.

In resource-constrained settings, strategies that are practical yet not costly are urgently needed. Barriers in terms of structural access to medications and clinics; costs associated with medications (e.g., Ivers, Kendrick, and Doucette 2005); acute HIV stigma; and instability of resources such as food and water are critical issues in adherence (e.g., Mukherjee et al. 2006; Nachega et al. 2006; Pearson et al. 2006). Coupled with often grossly understaffed clinics, adherence support must be both tailored and cost-effective. One cost-effective strategy is the use of media to assist in the widespread dissemination of accurate information (Wong et al. 2006). Recently, the straightforward provision of pill boxes and training on how to use them has been highlighted as an efficacious strategy that can be deployed and maintained with minimal resources (Mills and Cooper 2007; Petersen et al. 2007). The clear challenge to interventionists is to target the adherence needs of a given population carefully and always in relation to the sustainability of any intervention strategy over time, outside of the context of well-supported research.

CONCLUSION

Effective combination therapies are transforming HIV infection from an acute condition into a long-term chronic illness that is manageable and survivable. Regimens are becoming increasingly simple and tolerable, yet strict adherence is still required for optimal benefits for most regimens. Pharmacological improvements are introduced frequently, including ARV production on several continents, cost containment, and reductions in toxicities. However, the current formulary of available drugs is still in limited supply for those most in need, and even these formularies will soon be insufficient as drug resistance drives the need for new treatment options (Curran et al. 2005). Accessibility to several lines of ARVs and the use of the most adapted formulations are needed. In particular, future research must more specifically focus on ARV effects in chronically malnourished populations and under conditions of drug toxicities. Continued effort should be made to decrease the ARV drug prices as well as to ensure global production and accessibility (Curran et al. 2005). Finding the right balance is an important policy concern if scientific progress, technical innovation, and capital investment are not to be compromised.

Regimens should not only be accessible; they should also correspond to an individual's personal preferences and lifestyle to help ensure the high adherence that is required. Creativity and inventiveness in delivery approaches may include such strategies as an "ARV patch" that releases timely medications without requiring food and drink restrictions, chewable tablets, and non-refrigerated liquids and pills for all persons on ARVs (Ellis, Shumaker, Sieber, and Rand 2000).

In terms of both adherence theory development and intervention development, there is considerable need for further evaluation of which core determinants of ARV adherence are relevant for which patients at which time (Chesney 2006). Models of, and interventions targeting, adherence need to explicitly incorporate both structural and individual factors, including the role of stigma, access, cultural beliefs, economic constraints, complex histories with ARVs, non-adherence-related factors that could produce poor medical outcomes, climate and constraints in the provision of care, and the host of determinants of health behavior housed within a given individual (Dieckhaus and Odesina 2007; Herrmann et al. 2007). Our understanding of adherence must be inclusive and complex, but interventions to support adherence may be quite straightforward. Pill boxes, calendars, alarm clocks, pill splitters, and other inexpensive devices may adequately meet the adherence needs of some patients. Alternatively, it is likely that others will require a much larger compendium of strategies and resources to achieve and sustain optimal adherence. What may be the most critical factor in maximizing the potential benefit of an adherence promotion is careful preliminary study of the population at hand and the cultural, structural, and individual adherence barriers most pertinent to that population at that given time. Only with detailed understanding of that group's specific adherence barriers can models of adherence be fully articulated and interventions maximally effective.

REFERENCES AND FURTHER READING

Amico, K. R., J. J. Harman, and B. T. Johnson. "Efficacy of antiretroviral therapy adherence interventions: a research synthesis of trials, 1996 to 2004." *J Acquir Immune Defic Syndr* 41, no. 3 (2006): 285–97.

Ammassari, A., M. P. Trotta, R. Murri, F. Castelli, P. Narciso, P. Noto, S. Vecchiet, A.D. Monforte, A.W. Wu, A. Antinori, and ADICONA Study Group. "Correlates and predictors of adherence to highly active antiretroviral therapy: Overview of published literature." *J Acquir Immune Defic Syndr* 31 (2002): S123–S27.

Bangsberg, D. R., F. M. Hecht, E. D. Charlebois, A. R. Zolopa, M. Holodniy, L. Sheiner, J. D. Bamberger, M. A. Chesney, and A. Moss. "Adherence to protease inhibitors, HIV-1 viral load, and development of drug resistance in an indigent population." *AIDS* 14, no. 357–66 (2000).

Bangsberg, D. R., N. Ware, and J. M. Simoni. "Adherence without access to antiretroviral therapy in sub-Saharan Africa?" *AIDS* 20, no. 1 (2006): 140–141; author reply 41–2.

Chesney, M. A. "The elusive gold standard. Future perspectives for HIV adherence assessment and intervention." *J Acquir Immune Defic Syndr* 43, no. Suppl. 1 (2006): S149–S155.

Ciambrone, D., H. G. Loewenthal, L. B. Bazerman, C. Zorilla, B. Urbina, and J. A. Mitty. "Adherence among women with HIV infection in Puerto Rico: the potential use of modified directly observed therapy (MDOT) among pregnant and postpartum women." *Women's Health* 44, no. 4 (2006): 61–77.

Cote, J. K., and G. Godin. "Efficacy of interventions in improving adherence to antiretroviral therapy." *Int J STD AIDS* 16, no. 5 (2005): 335–43.

Crane, J. T., A. Kawuma, J. H. Oyugi, J. T. Byakika, A. Moss, P. Bourgois, and D. R. Bangsberg. "The price of adherence: qualitative findings from HIV positive individuals purchasing fixed-dose combination generic HIV antiretroviral therapy in Kampala, Uganda." *AIDS Behav* 10, no. 4 (2006): 437–42.

Curioso, W. H., A. E. Kurth, M. M. Blas, and J. D. Klausner. "Information and communication technologies for prevention and control of HIV infection and other STIs." edited by K. Holmes, in press.

Curran, J., H. Debas, M. Arya, P. Kelley, S. Knobler, and L. Pray. "Scaling up treatment for the global AIDS pandemic: challenges and opportunities." Edited by Committee on examining the probable consequences of alternative patterns of widespread antiretroviral drug use in resource-constrained settings: The National Academies Press, 2005.

Desvarieux, M., R. Landman, B. Liautaud, and P. M. Girard. "Antiretroviral therapy in resource-poor countries: illusions and realities." *Am J Public Health* 95, no. 7 (2005): 1117–22. Epub 2005, Jun 2.

Dieckhaus, K. D., and V. Odesina. "Outcomes of a multifaceted medication adherence intervention for HIV-positive patients." *AIDS Patient Care STDS* 21, no. 2 (2007): 81–91.

DiMatteo, M. R. "Variations in patients' adherence to medical recommendations: a quantitative review of 50 years of research." *Med Care* 42, no. 3 (2004): 200–209.

Ellis, S., S. Shumaker, W. Sieber, and C. Rand. "Adherence to pharmacological interventions. Current trends and future directions. The Pharmacological Intervention Working Group." *Control Clin Trials* 21, no. 5 Suppl. (2000): 218S–225S.

Ewart, C. K. "Social action theory for a public health psychology." *Am Psychologist* 46 (1991): 931–46.

Fisher, J. D., K. R. Amico, and P. A. Shuper. "Intervention demonstration: a CD-Rom delivered program to improve adherence in HIV-infected clinic patients." Paper presented at the NIMH/IAPAC International

Conference on HIV Treatment Adherence, Jersey City, NJ, 2007.

Fisher, J. D., W. A. Fisher, K. R. Amico, and J. J. Harman. "An information–motivation–behavioral skills model of adherence to antiretroviral therapy." *Health Psychol* 25, no. 4 (2006): 462–73.

Fogarty, L., D. Roter, S. Larson, J. Burke, J. Gillespie, and Richard Levy. "Patient adherence to HIV medication regimens: a review of published and abstract reports." *Patient Educ Couns* 46 (2002): 93–108.

Garcia de Olalla, P., H. Knobel, A. Carmona, A. Guelar, J. L. Lopez-Colomes, and J. A. Cayla. "Impact of adherence and highly active antiretroviral therapy on survival in HIV-infected patients." *J Acquir Immune Defic Syndr* 30 (2002): 105–10.

Garland, W. H., A. R. Wohl, R. Valencia, M. D. Witt, K. Squires, A. Kovacs, R. Larsen, N. Potterat, M. N. Anthony, S. Hader, and P. J. Weidle. "The acceptability of a directly-administered antiretroviral therapy (DAART) intervention among patients in public HIV clinics in Los Angeles, California." *AIDS Care* 19, no. 2 (2007): 159–67.

Haddad, M., C. Inch, R. H. Glazier, A. L. Wilkins, G. Urbshott, A. Bayoumi, and S. Rourke. "Patient support and education for promoting adherence to highly active antiretroviral therapy for HIV/AIDS." *Cochrane Database Syst Rev* 3 (2000).

Haug, N. A., and J. L. Sorensen. "Contingency management interventions for HIV-related behaviors." *Curr HIV/AIDS Rep* 3, no. 4 (2006): 154–9.

Herrmann, S., E. McKinnon, M. John, N. Hyland, O. P. Martinez, A. Cain, K. Turner, A. Coombs, C. Manolikos, and S. Mallal. "Evidence-based, multifactorial approach to addressing non-adherence to antiretroviral therapy and improving standards of care." *Intern Med J* Epub ahead of print, 2007.

Ickovics, J., and C. Meade. "Adherence to antiretroviral therapy among patients with HIV: a critical link between behavioral and biomedical sciences." *JAIDS* 31 (2002): S98–S102.

Ickovics, J. R., and A. W. Meisler. "Adherence in AIDS clinical trials: a framework for clinical research and clinical care." *J Clin Epidemiol* 50, no. 4 (1997): 385–91.

Ivers, I.C., D. Kendrick, and D. Doucette. "Efficacy of antiretroviral therapy programs in resource-poor settings: a meta-analysis of the published literature." *Clin Infect Dis* 41 (2005): 217–24.

Javanbakht, M., P. Prosser, T. Grimes, M. Weinstein, and C. Farthing. "Efficacy of an individualized adherence support program with contingent reinforcement among nonadherent HIV-positive patients: results from a randomized trial." *J Int Assoc Physicians AIDS Care* 5, no. 4 (2006): 143–50.

Johnson, M. O., S. L. Catz, R. H. Remien, M. J. Rotheram-Borus, S. F. Morin, E. Charlebois, C. Gore-Felton, R. B. Goldsten, H. Wolfe, M. Lightfoot, and M. A. Chesney. "Theory-guided, empirically supported avenues for intervention on HIV medication nonadherence: findings from the Healthy Living Project." *AIDS Patient Care STDS* 17, no. 12 (2003): 645–56.

Laniece, I., M. Ciss, A. Desclaux, K. Diop, F. Mbodj, B. Ndiaye, O. Sylla, E. Delaporte, and I. Ndoye. "Adherence to HAART and its principal determinants in a cohort of Senegalese adults." *AIDS* 17, Suppl. 3 (2003): S103–S108.

Laurent, C., C. Kouanfack, S. Koulla-Shiro, N. Nkoue, A. Bourgeois, A. Calmy, B. Lactuock, V. Nzeusseu, R. Mougnutou, G. Peytavin, F. Liegeois, E. Nerrienet, M. Tardy, M. Peeters, I. Andrieux-Meyer, L. Zekeng, M. Kazatchkine, E. Mpoudi-Ngole, and E. Delaporte. "Effectiveness and safety of a generic fixed-dose combination of nevirapine, stavudine, and lamivudine in HIV-1-infected adults in Cameroon: open-label multicentre trial." *Lancet* 364, no. 9428 (2004): 29–34.

Leventhal, H., and Y. Benyamini. "Illness representations: theoretical foundations." In *Perceptions of Health and Illness: Current Research and Applications*, edited by K. J. Petrie and J. A. Wieinman. Singapore: Hardwood Academic Publishers, 1997.

Leventhal, H., D. R. Nerenz, and D. J. Steele. "Illness representations and coping with health threats." In Baum, A., S. E. Taylor, and J. E. Singer (eds), *Handbook of Psychology and Health*. Hillsdale, NJ: Lawrence Erlbaum Associates vol. 4, 1984, pp. 219–252.

Liu, H., C. E. Golin, L. G. Miller, R. D. Hays, C. K. Beck, S. Sanandaji, J. Christian, T. Maldonado, D. Duran, A. H. Kaplan, and N. S. Wenger. "A comparison study of multiple measures of adherence to HIV protease inhibitors." *Ann Intern Med* 134, no. 10 (2001): 968–77.

Lucas, G. M., B. A. Mullen, M. E. McCaul, P. J. Weidle, S. Hader, and R. D. Moore. "Adherence, drug use, and treatment failure in a methadone-clinic-based program of directly administered antiretroviral therapy." *AIDS Patient Care STDS* 21, no. 8 (2007): 564–74.

Macalino, G. E., J. W. Hogan, J. A. Mitty, L. B. Bazerman, A. K. Delong, H. Loewenthal, A. M. Caliendo, and T. P. Flanigan. "A randomized clinical trial of community-based directly observed therapy as an adherence intervention for HAART among substance users." *AIDS* 21, no. 11 (2007): 1473–7.

Machtinger, E. L., and D. Bangsberg. *Adherence to HIV Antiretroviral Therapy* HIV InSite Knowledge Base Chapter, 2005. http://hivinsite.ucsf.edu/InSite?page=kb-03–02–09. Cited 2007.

Meichenbaum, D., and D.C. Tuck. *Facilitating Treatment Adherence: A Practitioner's Guidebook*. New York: Plenum Press, 1987.

Mills, E. J., and C. Cooper. "Simple, effective interventions are key to improving adherence in marginalized populations." *Clin Infect Dis* 45, no. 7 (2007): 916–17.

Mills, E. J., J. B. Nachega, D. R. Bangsberg, S. Singh, B. Rachlis, P. Wu, K. Wilson, I. Buchan, C. J. Gill, and C. Cooper. "Adherence to HAART: a systematic review of developed and developing nation patient-reported barriers and facilitators." *PLoS Med* 3, no. 11 (2006a): e438.

Mills, E. J., J. B. Nachega, I. Buchan, J. Orbinski, A. Attaran, S. Singh, B. Rachlis, P. Wu, C. Cooper, L.

Thabane, K. Wilson, G. H. Guyatt, and D. R. Bangsberg. "Adherence to antiretroviral therapy in sub-Saharan Africa and North America: a meta-analysis." *JAMA* 296, no. 6 (2006b): 679–90.

Mitchell, C. G., S. Freels, C. M. Creticos, A. Oltean, and R. Douglas. "Preliminary findings of an intervention integrating modified directly observed therapy and risk reduction counseling." *AIDS Care* 19, no. 4 (2007): 561–4.

Mukherjee, J. S., L. Ivers, F. Leandre, P. Farmer, and H. Behforouz. "Antiretroviral therapy in resource-poor settings. Decreasing barriers to access and promoting adherence." *J Acquir Immune Defic Syndr* 43, Suppl. 1 (2006): S123–S126.

Munro, S., S. Lewin, T. Swart, and J. Volmink. "A review of health behaviour theories: how useful are these for developing interventions to promote long-term medication adherence for TB and HIV/AIDS?" *BMC Public Health* 7 (2007): 104.

Myung, P., D. Pugatch, M. F. Brady, P. Many, J. I. Harwell, M. Lurie, and J. Tucker. "Directly observed highly active antiretroviral therapy for HIV-infected children in Cambodia." *Am J Public Health* 97, no. 6 (2007): 974–7.

Nachega, J. B., A. R. Knowlton, A. Deluca, J. H. Schoeman, L. Watkinson, A. Efron, R. E. Chaisson, and G. Maartens. "Treatment supporter to improve adherence to antiretroviral therapy in HIV-infected South African adults. A qualitative study." *J Acquir Immune Defic Syndr* 43, Suppl 1 (2006): S127–S133.

Nachega, J. B., D. M. Stein, D. A. Lehman, D. Hlatshwayo, R. Mothopeng, R. E. Chaisson, and A. S. Karstaedt. "Adherence to antiretroviral therapy in HIV-infected adults in Soweto, South Africa." *AIDS Res Hum Retroviruses* 20, no. 10 (2004): 1053–6.

Nieuwkerk, P. T., M. A. Sprangers, D. M. Burger, R. M. Hoetelmans, P. W. Hugen, S. A. Danner, M. E. van Der Ende, M. M. Schneider, G. Schrey, P. L. Meenhorst, H. G. Sprenger, R. H. Kauffmann, M. Jambroes, M. A. Chesney, F. de Wolf, and J. M. Lange. "Limited patient adherence to highly active antiretroviral therapy for HIV-1 infection in an observational cohort study." *Arch Intern Med* 161, no. 16 (2001): 1962–8.

O'Donohue, W. T., and E. R. Levensky. *Promoting Treatment Adherence: A Practical Handbook for Health Care Providers*. New York: Sage Publications, Inc., 2006.

Oyugi, J. H., J. Byakika-Tusiime, K. Ragland, O. Laeyendecker, R. Mugerwa, C. Kityo, P. Mugyenyi, T. C. Quinn, and D. R. Bangsberg. "Treatment interruptions predict resistance in HIV-positive individuals purchasing fixed-dose combination antiretroviral therapy in Kampala, Uganda." *AIDS* 21, no. 8 (2007): 965–71.

Palella, F. J., K. M. Delaney, A. C. Moorman, M. O. Loveless, J. Fuhrer, G. A. Satten, D. J. Aschman, S. D. Holmberg, and The HIV Outpatient Study Investigators. "Declining morbidity and mortality among patients with advanced human immunodeficiency virus infection." *N Engl J Med* 338 (1998): 853–60.

Parsons, J. T., E. Rosof, and B. Mustanski. "Patient-related factors predicting HIV medication adherence among men and women with alcohol problems." *Journ Health Psychol* 12, no. 2 (2007): 357–70.

Pearson, C. R., M. A. Micek, J. M. Simoni, P. D. Hoff, E. Matediana, D. P. Martin, and S. S. Gloyd. "Randomized control trial of peer-delivered, modified directly observed therapy for HAART in Mozambique." *J Acquir Immune Defic Syndr* 9 (2007).

Pearson, C. R., M. Micek, J. M. Simoni, E. Matediana, D. P. Martin, and S. Gloyd. "Modified directly observed therapy to facilitate highly active antiretroviral therapy adherence in Beira, Mozambique. Development and implementation." *J Acquir Immune Defic Syndr* 43, Suppl 1 (2006): S134–S141.

Petersen, M. L., Y. Wang, M. J. van der Laan, D. Guzman, E. Riley, and D. Bangsberg. "Pillbox organizers are associated with improved adherence to HIV antiretroviral therapy and viral suppression: a marginal structural model analysis." *Clin Infect Dis* 45, no. 7 (2007): 908–15.

Pontali, E. "Facilitating adherence to highly active antiretroviral therapy in children with HIV infection: what are the issues and what can be done?" *Paediatr Drugs* 7, no. 3 (2005): 137–49.

Rabkin, J. G., and M. A. Chesney. "Treatment adherence to HIV medications." In *Psychosocial and Public Health Impact of New HIV Therapies*, edited by S. C. Kalichman, 61–82. New York: Kluwer Academic/Plenum Publishers, 1999.

Remien, R. H., M. J. Stirratt, J. Dognin, E. Day, N. El-Bassel, and P. Warne. "Moving from theory to research to practice. Implementing an effective dyadic intervention to improve antiretroviral adherence for clinic patients." *J Acquir Immune Defic Syndr* 43, Suppl. 1 (2006): S69–S78.

Reynolds, N. R. "The problem of antiretroviral adherence: a self-regulatory model for intervention." *AIDS Care*, 15(1) (2003): 117–24.

Reynolds, N. R., L. Sanzero Eller, P. K. Nicholas, I. B. Corless, K. Kirksey, M. J. Hamilton, J. K. Kemppainen, E. Bunch, P. Dole, D. Wantland, E. Sefcik, K. M. Nokes, C. L. Coleman, M. Rivero, G. E. Canaval, Y. F. Tsai, and W. L. Holzemer. "HIV illness representation as a predictor of self-care management and health outcomes: a multi-site, cross-cultural study." *AIDS Behav* 18 (2007): 18.

Rosen, M. I., K. Dieckhaus, T. J. McMahon, B. Valdes, N. M. Petry, J. Cramer, and B. Rounsaville. "Improved adherence with contingency management." *AIDS Patient Care STDS* 21, no. 1 (2007): 30–40.

Simoni, J. M. "Adherence to antiretroviral therapy: state of the science." *The AIDS Reader* 17, no. 4 (2007): S5–S10.

Simoni, J. M., P. A. Frick, and B. Huang. "A longitudinal evaluation of a social support model of medication adherence among HIV-positive men and women on antiretroviral therapy." *Health Psychol* 25, no. 1 (2006): 74–81.

Simoni, J. M., D. W. Pantalone, M. D. Plummer, and B. Huang. "A randomized controlled trial of a peer support intervention targeting antiretroviral medication adherence and depressive symptomatology in HIV-positive men and women." *Health Psychol* 26, no. 4 (2007): 488–95.

Simoni, J. M., C. R. Pearson, D. W. Pantalone, G. Marks, and N. Crepaz. "Efficacy of interventions in improving highly active antiretroviral therapy adherence and HIV-1 RNA viral load. A meta-analytic review of randomized controlled trials." *J Acquir Immune Defic Syndr* 43, Suppl. 1 (2006): S23–S35.

Singh, N., C. Squier, C. Sivek, M. Wagener, M. Hong Nguyen, and V. L. Yu. "Determinants of compliance with antiretroviral therapy in patients with human immunodeficiency virus: prospective assessment with implications for enhancing compliance." *AIDS Care* 8 (1996): 261–9.

Smith-Rohrberg, D., J. Mezger, M. Walton, R. D. Bruce, and F. L. Altice. "Impact of enhanced services on virologic outcomes in a directly administered antiretroviral therapy trial for HIV-infected drug users." *J Acquir Immune Defic Syndr* 43, Suppl. 1 (2006): S48–S53.

Sorensen, J. L., N. A. Haug, K. L. Delucchi, V. Gruber, E. Kletter, S. L. Batki, J. P. Tulsky, P. Barnett, and S. Hall. "Voucher reinforcement improves medication adherence in HIV-positive methadone patients: a randomized trial." *Drug Alcohol Depend.* 88, no. 1 (2007): 54–63. Epub 2006, Oct 23.

Spire, B., S. Duran, M. Souville, C. Leport, F. Raffi, and J. P. Moatti. "Adherence to highly active antiretroviral therapies (HAART) in HIV-infected patients: from a predictive to a dynamic approach." *Soc Sci Med* 54, no. 10 (2002): 1481–96.

Starks, H., J. Simoni, H. Zhao, B. Huang, K. Fredriksen-Goldsen, C. Pearson, W. T. Chen, L. Lu, and F. Zhang. "Conceptualizing antiretroviral adherence in Beijing, China." *AIDS Care*, in press.

Tarakeshwar, N., A. K. Srikrishnan, S. Johnson, C. Vasu, S. Solomon, M. Merson, and K. Sikkema. "A social cognitive model of health for HIV-positive adults receiving care in India." *AIDS Behav* 11, no. 3 (2007): 491–504.

Walensky, R. P., A. D. Paltiel, E. Losina, L. M. Mercincavage, B. R. Schackman, P. E. Sax, M. C. Weinstein, and K. A. Freedberg. "The survival benefits of AIDS treatment in the United States." *J Infect Dis* 194, no. 1 (2006): 11–19. Epub 2006, Jun 1.

Ware, N. C., M. A. Wyatt, and D. R. Bangsberg. "Examining theoretic models of adherence for validity in resource-limited settings. A heuristic approach." *J Acquir Immune Defic Syndr* 43, Suppl. 1 (2006): S18–S22.

Weiser, S., W. Wolfe, D. Bangsberg, I. Thior, P. Gilbert, J. Makhema, P. Kebaabetswe, D. Dickenson, K. Mompati, M. Essex, and R. Marlink. "Barriers to antiretroviral adherence for patients living with HIV infection and AIDS in Botswana." *J Acquir Immune Defic Syndr* 34, no. 3 (2003): 281–8.

Wong, I. Y., N. V. Lawrence, H. Struthers, J. McIntyre, and G. H. Friedland. "Development and assessment of an innovative culturally sensitive educational videotape to improve adherence to highly active antiretroviral therapy in Soweto, South Africa." *J Acquir Immune Defic Syndr* 43, Suppl. 1 (2006): S142–S148.

Wrubel, J., J. T. Moskowitz, T. A. Richards, H. Prakke, M. Acree, and S. Folkman. "Pediatric adherence: perspectives of mothers of children with HIV." *Soc Sci Med* 61, no. 11 (2005): 2423–33. Epub 2005, Jun 3.

CHAPTER 13

Adherence Masters

Reaching for Perfection in ART Adherence

Jannette Berkley-Patton, Andrea Bradley-Ewing, Nikki Thomson, Tara Carruth, Mary M. Gerkovich, and Kathy Goggin

ABSTRACT

This chapter highlights the results of a study that demonstrated that the most frequently identified factors that facilitated mastery of taking medications included: understanding how to take medications, believing that HIV medications kept participants healthy, having a provider who was caring, keeping medical appointments, and having hope about the future. Identified barriers to overcome to maintain adherence included: being tired of taking medications, feeling overwhelmed, being stressed/worried or down, being around negative people, and not being able to afford medications. Factors identified for maintaining adherence despite challenges included being healthy, spiritual, knowledgeable, and in control. Participants suggested ART-naive individuals must be ready to start medications, be informed, and advocate for their quality care.

OVERVIEW

Significant advances in HIV disease management have been made since the first case of AIDS was identified over 25 years ago. Among the leading contributors to these advances has been the emergence of antiretroviral therapies (ART). ART medications have significantly reduced morbidity and mortality, transforming what was once a death sentence into an often controllable chronic disease (Jensen-Fangel et al. 2004; Hammer et al. 2006). The goal of ART is to attain maximum and long-lasting suppression of viral replication which leads to improved immunological functioning and better overall health (Lucas 2005; Shor-Posner et al. 2000). However, for these goals to be achieved, individuals must maintain near-perfect ART adherence.

Studies suggest that, to achieve viral load suppression and positive treatment outcomes, ≥95 percent adherence to ART may be necessary (e.g., Paterson et al. 2000). This is an incredible feat for compliance to any medication regimen. Adding to the difficulty of adherence is the degree of ART regimen complexity and dealing with ART-related side effects (Johnson et al. 2003; Sullivan et al. 2007). Understandably, many HIV-positive individuals are unable to adhere at optimal levels, and numerous studies have demonstrated average adherence rates that are far below this goal (33–88 percent; e.g., Chesney et al. 2000; Golin et al. 2006; Halkitis et al. 2003; Rosen et al. 2007). Unfortunately, suboptimal adherence not only negatively affects suppression of HIV—it also increases the risk of developing drug resistance to ART medications (Sethi et al. 2003), which has serious consequences for long-term HIV disease control.

A number of studies have identified individual, medical, and social factors that contribute to less than optimal adherence. Leading individual factors associated with nonadherence include substance abuse, depression, and younger age (e.g., Barclay et al. 2007; Sullivan et al. 2007). Also, individuals who are at increased risk for suboptimal adherence exhibit: limited knowledge about and belief in the efficacy of ART (Barclay et al. 2007; Beach et al. 2006; White et al. 2006), fewer supportive networks (Amico et al. 2007; Hamilton et al. 2007; Sunil and McGehee 2007), and less effective coping styles (Remien et al. 2006). Along with regimen complexity, other medical factors associated with suboptimal adherence include: nonengagement in routine medical appointments and poor patient–provider relationships (Beach et al. 2006; Gordillo et al. 1999; Johnson et al. 2006). Moreover, social factors—such as lack of access to adequate health insurance and medical services (Reif et al. 2006), chaotic living environments (Schönnesson et al. 2006; Sullivan et al. 2007), and HIV stigma (Rao et al. 2007; Rintamaki et al. 2006)—can also negatively impact ART adherence.

Findings from studies on factors associated with suboptimal adherence have guided the development of several theoretical models of adherence constructs and the design of adherence interventions. More recently, the Information–Motivation–Behavioral Skills (IMB) model has evolved as a theoretical framework for understanding the existing literature on adherence to ART (Fisher et al. 2006). As applied to ART adherence, the IMB model posits that adherence will more likely be achieved when an individual has: 1) accurate, comprehensible information on how to properly adhere to their ART regimen; 2) appropriate levels of motivation (personal and social) to adhere to ART; and 3) specific behavioral skills to take ART as prescribed (e.g., having designated dosing times and reminder strategies, following special instructions, adjusting daily activities to accommodate ART, reinforcing self for optimal adherence) (Amico et al. 2007; Fisher et al. 2006; Starace et al. 2006). In the IMB model, sufficient information and motivation each play independent critical roles in influencing adherence behavioral skills, which, in turn, are directly related to optimal adherence.

More recently, the IMB model has been employed in theory-based development of interventions for improving information, motivation, and behavioral skills to adhere to ART regimens (e.g., Gerkovich et al. 2005; Golin et al. 2006). Yet, one area of the IMB model that has not been fully explored is the qualitative aspects of the model's core constructs and their interrelated influence on ART adherence. Use of qualitative methods, such as focus groups, can provide a deeper understanding of the model's constructs and give new insights to inform the design of adherence interventions by identifying requisite knowledge, motivation, and behavioral skills for adherence. One strategy to better understand the qualitative aspects of the IMB model's influence on ART adherence is to elicit perspectives from HIV-positive individuals who have maintained optimal levels of adherence and have successfully managed their HIV disease. A few qualitative studies have reported on beliefs and behaviors related to ART adherence among successful adherers (Enriquez et al. 2004; Gray 2006; Lewis et al. 2006; Malcolm et al. 2003); however, these studies provide limited perspectives on information and motivation for adherence. This qualitative study sought to provide key insights on information and knowledge, personal and social motivation, and behavior skills for ART adherence as described by the IMB model and as reported by adherence masters in focus group discussions.

METHODS

Study Setting and Participants

Participants included 18 HIV-positive individuals who were recruited from two large infectious disease clinics in the metropolitan Kansas City area. Participants consisted of persons who were: a) HIV positive and taking ART medications; b) at least 18 years old; c) able to communicate proficiently in English; and d) able to provide informed consent. Medical records were also reviewed to determine eligibility based on whether participants: a) were on a stable ART regimen for at least nine months; b) showed engagement in medical care by keeping at least two medical appointment in the past nine months; and c) demonstrated stable clinical lab values as defined by viral loads ranging from undetectable to a low and stable viral load (less than 1,000 copies/mL). Patients with higher viral loads were eligible if the viral load was stable and the medical provider's chart notes indicated good reasons for not changing medications.

A pre-screening self-report measure of adherence was used as a final tool to determine eligibility. Adapted from measures used in other studies on adherence, the self-report adherence measure used a 30-day recall period for responding to three items: 1) number of days the patient missed any doses of his/her ART medications; 2) overall rating of how well he or she had taken HIV medications, using a six-point scale from "very poor" to "excellent"; and 3) ratings from "never" to "always" for three aspects of adherence (i.e., taking all HIV pills every day, taking medications on time, and following special instructions). To be eligible, participants had to report at least two of the following criterion: no more than three days of missed medications, at least "good" rating on taking medications, or report "often" or "always" on at least two of the adherence aspects.

Focus group participants received a meal and assistance with transportation. Each of the four group discussions lasted about two hours and were digitally audio-recorded. The focus group discussions were facilitated by a moderator and an assistant who recorded participants' comments on newsprint for the group to review for accuracy, took notes, and summarized the discussion at the close of each meeting. All aspects of this voluntary study were reviewed and approved by University of Missouri—Kansas City Institutional Review Board.

MEASURES

Focus Group Survey

A brief self-report survey was developed to collect information on participants': general knowledge about ART adherence; HIV ancillary service utilization (e.g., housing assistance, case management); and demographic data (age, gender, race/ethnicity, and education level). The survey was completed at the beginning of each focus group session.

Focus Group Questions

The focus group discussions were structured around nine questions, which addressed four primary topics: 1) expectations and ART information received prior to taking HIV medications (e.g., "When you first started taking meds, what did you expect? What were you told?"); 2) medication-taking behaviors (e.g., "Now think about times when you had a change in your normal routine. What did you do to continue taking your meds correctly?"); 3) personal values and motivators for taking medications (e.g., "In thinking about taking your meds, what motivates you to take your meds correctly?"; and 4) support systems that assist with taking medications (e.g., "What support systems have helped you take your meds?"). For question 3) above, participants were given a list of motivator/value items (e.g., in control, health, family) and were asked to mark each item that held great value or strongly motivated them. Participants then discussed their marked items, and the group ranked items in order of importance.

Data Analysis

Descriptive statistics were used to describe participant demographics, pill-taking knowledge and behaviors, and use of ancillary services. Audio recordings of focus group discussions were transcribed. Three of the studies' researchers (Berkley-Patton, Bradley-Ewing, Thomson) conducted a content analysis of the transcripts to identify themes on expectations and information, personal and social motivation, and behavioral skills related to ART adherence. Agreement between coders was noted, and thematic categories were named for descriptive purposes.

RESULTS

Participant Demographics

Of the 18 participants, 55 percent were female, and 44 percent were African American (28 percent Caucasian, 17 percent Hispanic, 11 percent other). The average age of participants was 45 years old (range 27–65 years). Educational levels ranged from having some high school (17 percent) to graduate degree (6 percent), with the majority having a high-school diploma (83 percent) or higher. Additionally, 83 percent had received case management services, and a portion of participants had received assistance with housing (39 percent), financial support (17 percent), and/or food (22 percent).

Focus Group Survey

On pill-taking behaviors, 78 percent of participants believed that ART should be taken within two hours (or sooner) of the designated target dosing time. Additionally, 64 percent reported that if they missed a dose they took it as long as it was not too close to the next dose; 12 percent took their missed doses no matter what time it was when they remembered; 12 percent took the missed dose with the next dose; and 12 percent never took missed doses.

Focus Group Discussion

In the focus group discussions, thematic issues relating to the IMB model were identified in the areas of: 1) ART information and expectations; 2) personal beliefs on motivation and supportive motivation; and 3) behavioral skills related to ART adherence. Samples of focus group participants' comments related to these IMB core constructs are provided below.

ART INFORMATION AND EXPECTATIONS

Provider-Delivered ART Information and HIV Care

All of the participants spoke of the importance of having an informed, caring provider who worked *with* the participant, as being critical to their positive expectation for survival and their commitment to adherence. Most of the participants expressed how they cared about and trusted their providers and felt that their providers respected them. Also, most of the participants had been informed by their providers about what to expect concerning drug resistance and side effects when they began taking their current ART regimen. In addition to their clinic appointments, it was important for participants to be able to get in touch with their providers by phone or email to discuss ART medication and other health issues.

> She didn't mind about answering as many questions as I had. She was in Boston a week or so ago, and I had a question. I e-mailed her, and she got right back to me—[she said], "I'll see you next week, but this is the answer." And if she doesn't know, we'll figure it out together. And I really feel comfortable in her care.

> I have stayed undetectable basically for the past 8 years being with this particular doctor, because she pays so close attention, and we're conversing with one another on a one-on-one basis. She expressed to me life—as opposed to death. This doc that I have is so wonderful. I called and left her a message and within a day's time [she says], "Let's talk about this." So with that type of relationship with the doctor, I mean, you can't help but do well.

Some of the participants stated that when they first started their medications their providers gave them "information overload" and that their ART regimen information was very difficult to understand. In addition, some of their providers overstated potential ART side effects and tried to reassure participants that medication and strategies were available to counteract the side effects. Most of the participants also expressed that they were initially afraid of ART-related side effects (e.g., nausea, diarrhea) and of the "toxicity" of the medications' overall effect on their bodies.

> You were inundated with so much information of all this stuff. It was overload. I was always just befuddled with all this stuff—to a point where you are thinking, "Okay, I should have written this down." I hope somebody is writing this down. I hope there's a list. You were just informed with so much that you didn't know what to follow.

> They prepared you for a lot of things in the beginning. See, you're going to have this problem and probably that. Then we've got a pill to counteract that and if that doesn't work.

> I thought it was going to be really bad. And it was bad for a little bit. I'd think I was delirious or something. I just had to go through the side effects.

Five participants had no memory of discussing drug resistance and optimal ART dosing intervals with their first providers in their initial use of ART, and most of these participants suffered suboptimal adherence during this period of lack of information. Some of these participants sought out new providers because they perceived their former providers were either not knowledgeable enough about HIV medications, did not provide enough information about how to take their medications, or did not communicate with them in a way that expressed concern about the participant's quality of life.

> He told me initially—"You need to take it. You need to take it on time." That was pretty much it. He didn't explain any of what he said, and you know it's always good to have a reason why you're doing what you're doing. And later on when I did get the education, I was glad I was adherent to it, because I learned about resistance and all of that other stuff.

Personal ART and HIV Information Seeking

Most of the participants conducted their own research to gain more information about HIV, their ART medications, other medication options, and ART-related side effects. Participants valued having multiple information sources and regularly sought out HIV and ART information from internet sources, HIV-positive friends, and from fellow support group members. This was particularly the case when participants felt that their providers had given them more information than they could comprehend during office visits or when participants did not trust provider-delivered information. They used the information they gathered to make medication decisions in partnership with their providers.

> Knowledge is always important. I mean I really need to know. The more I know, the more I can make good choices or [know] that I have a choice. Because without the knowledge, you're just going on what somebody says or you just accept it. But if I have the knowledge, I'm able to dispel ignorance, even if it's nothing but my own.

> I go to an HIV social group every Friday. It's been a blessing for me to sit and talk with [other HIV-positive persons] and find out some of . . . the meds they are going through. As a matter of fact, they started playing a part in the meds I was taking. They told me you don't want to start out with this. I opted to jump over my first [medication] choice. And that only left me with one more choice after that if the meds didn't work. I was willing to do that, because I didn't want to get sick like they were telling me how you could get sick.

MOTIVATION FOR ART ADHERENCE

Personal Beliefs and Attitudes

All of the participants expressed a strong desire to live and to stay healthy for as long as possible. They believed they would live longer if they took their ART medications and maintained a positive outlook on their ability to manage their HIV disease. Participants stated that exerting control over taking their medication was important to them and that they took pride in their consistent adherence. Most of the participants spoke of mentally preparing themselves to take ART medications and for taking medications for the rest of their lives. Also, almost all of the participants mentioned engaging in positive self-talk and using it to motivate themselves, which in turn helped them to renew their commitments to deal with side effects and daily hassles, be healthy, and attend to self-care.

> I'm the adherence king around here. Since I've been diagnosed and started on my medication, I have not missed a dose. I mean I just had a mindset, you know, when it came to that time when providers spoke to me about [adherence]. I was mentally prepared for that.

> I had to get to the point where I had to make a decision whether I was going to take medicine or not. I had to make the decision about it. That was one of the first of many decisions that I had to make for myself since I've been positive.

Additionally, most of the participants regularly had their CD4 and viral load lab work completed. They used their lab results to gauge their success with ART adherence and how well they were managing their HIV disease. Positive lab results were viewed as motivational and reinforcing elements in their commitment to adherence. Unfavorable lab results were used as a stimulus to make new commitments to ART adherence.

> [Taking my medications] . . . it reinforces it—when I have my blood work done, and my doctor says everything is fine. And even though I hate needles, to hear my doctor say, "Okay that your levels are still undetectable." You know. That's what reinforces me to keep taking it.

Personal Motivators for ART Adherence

Primary personal motivators for adhering to ART included the importance of being healthy and in control. Participants expressed a strong desire to live and to be as healthy as possible for as long as possible by taking HIV medications. They also discussed the importance of: being knowledgeable about HIV and ART medications in order to make informed decisions; being respected by their health care providers; and advocating for themselves and their HIV care. Many expressed the value of spirituality, prayer, and meditation in helping them to cope with living with HIV as a chronic disease and in giving them hope in living long enough to experience the benefits of a future HIV cure.

> That I am in control of my disease. My kids tell me all the time, "Mom, you are not the boss of everything." I say, "Well I beg to differ." So that gives me that little bit of being in control. So that's important. That's an important value for me.

> But my God and I had to have that one-on-one relationship. He was the only one I could share with—I knew he wouldn't tell anybody. So that's where I built my self up spiritually with where I was medically.

> And my spiritual life, that's first really. I trust God that the doctor will have some medicine that will work. That's really motivating for me.

Supportive Networks

All participants mentioned having a variety of support systems that kept them motivated. Many of the participants mentioned the motivational value of significant others, such as their children, spouses, friends, and support group members who cared about their adherence. Significant others supported participants by reminding them to take their medications and by providing a safe outlet to disclose/discuss their HIV status and related issues. Supportive others also provided companionship and participated with participants in positive social activities (e.g., camping, conferences, movies, exercise). Also, some of the participants mentioned that attending church gave them a positive outlook on life.

> Knowing that we can pick up the phone and call and say to this other person, "Hey, I feel lousy today," and this other person right away knows what you are feeling.

> My daughter will call and say, "Mom did you take your medicine?" I'll say, "Yes I did."

Most participants mentioned it was important to advocate for other HIV-positive people who may be experiencing difficulties with ART or accessing HIV services. Participants provided advice for others starting HIV medications, which included: wait until you are absolutely ready to start medications, find the right provider who you can trust, educate and advocate for yourself, get into adherence support groups, and dedicate yourself to excellent adherence.

BEHAVIORAL SKILLS RELATED TO TAKING ART

Reminder Strategies

All participants used reminder cues (e.g., favorite TV show, alarms, brushing teeth in the morning and at night) for taking ART at predetermined target dosing times. Participants reported experimenting with various strategies to identify one that worked best for their lifestyle. Also, participants had a back-up plan to assist with not missing doses, which primarily involved carrying an entire medication bottle or extra pills throughout the day. Because they always carried their medication, changes in lifestyle rarely interfered with taking medications. However, participants with significant lifestyle changes (e.g., new school, new work hours) pre-planned how to accommodate their new routines. Two of the participants reported borrowing medication from friends who were on the same HIV medication on the few rare occasions when they were away from home and had forgotten to take their medications.

> I just take the bottle with me all day long. If for some reason I didn't take it after brushing my teeth, I got the whole bottle with me. So I just basically take that around. It's convenient.

> There have been times when I didn't have my medicine with me. But I have a friend who takes the same medicine, and I'd hurry over to his place. But him and I fell out. Now I carry my medicine [with me], no matter what.

Side Effects

The primary strategy used to deal with HIV medication side effects was to make a commitment to continue taking medication and endure side effects in order to survive. Most of the participants expressed that they were very afraid of ART side effects prior to the start of taking ART, but resolved to take the medication no matter what happened. Many of the participants had talked with their providers about their side effects and had taken medications to reduce them. Participants spoke of being flexible in their daily habits in order to accommodate lifestyle changes that would help to circumvent side effects.

> I thought, "I hate those morning pills." You're supposed to take that [medication] with food—but I don't eat breakfast. Those things and whatever else would just make my stomach so nauseous. I would try eating toast, but I wanted my coffee and cigarette. Then I found out it works better with food. You learn to go buy a toaster and make toast.

> Every once in a while, I'll still have a bout with the diarrhea coming on me. There are certain foods that I can't eat anymore because of the medication. So I still have the bottle of what they gave me that's supposed to stop it—a brown pill. They told me to take one after every episode. And I just laughed. After an episode? I mean I done went all over myself. Anyway, it works.

Obstacles to Overcome

Most of the participants spoke of overcoming obstacles to improve their ability to effectively manage their HIV disease. These obstacles included finding new ART medications to improve health outcomes, finding new providers, and quitting substance use.

> I did crack, was in and out of prison, and just had a real destructive lifestyle. And when I became positive, I was faced with my demon that I was going to die. Subconsciously, when you do drugs and you're living that lifestyle—you're trying to kill yourself. I said I don't want to die, so all the risky behaviors stopped. I determined that I wanted to live. So I was going to do all that I could do within my power. I would tell people that HIV really saved my life. And people would be like, "Are you crazy?? She's crazy!!" I mean it really saved my life literally.

Participants reported that they surrounded themselves with positive people and tried to limit contact with negative people; nevertheless, they still had to deal with HIV stigma from family and friends who were ignorant about HIV. Several participants mentioned that they educated significant others about

HIV transmission and ART medication in order to help others understand the importance of ART adherence, enlist ART adherence support from others, and/or to reduce others' fear of contracting HIV from the participant, and thereby maintaining positive relationships.

> When I first got tested I was living with my daughter. She had her dishes and the kids' dishes. Mine were off to the side. As I learned more about the disease and what it could do and couldn't do, I told my kids there's no reason why we should be doing this. And she stopped. Today she doesn't care. She drinks out of my cup. That's when you can tell you've done your best.

> With the educational piece and knowledge piece I share that with my family, they have more information about the drugs and adherence. If my husband sees my medication sitting there, he'll say, "Okay what are you waiting on?" He'll hand me a glass of water and brings it to me.

DISCUSSION

Working from an IMB theoretical perspective, this qualitative study provides a deeper contextual understanding of interrelated information, motivation, and behavioral determinants of ART adherence among highly adherent HIV-positive individuals. Discussions with adherence masters revealed new strategies to address improvement of adherence for persons naive to ART, struggling with ART, or starting a new ART regimen. This study sheds light on the qualitative aspects of adherence mastery that complement quantitative studies' findings, and identifies issues for future research related to the design of IMB model-based interventions.

The literature on behavior change is replete with studies that demonstrate that information alone is not enough to influence uptake of behaviors. However, a minimal level of information is necessary to serve as basis for ART behavioral skills acquisition (Amico et al. 2007; Starace et al. 2006). Our findings indicated adherence information exchange in a caring patient–provider relationship was a critical component for adherence mastery. Participants mentioned the importance of providers providing accurate, up-to-date information and respecting their personal autonomy to make informed health care decisions. Conversely, participants were concerned about their providers delivering an excessive amount of information and information that was difficult to comprehend, especially when initiating use of ART. These findings are particularly important to note, and may suggest why 36 percent of our adherence masters were unclear on what they should do if they missed their ART target dose time. This speaks to the need for ongoing booster sessions on adherence-related information and assessments of adherence behaviors (Stirratt and Gordon 2007).

To become better informed, participants initiated contacts with providers outside of regular medical visits via phone and email and gathered information from Internet sources. Some of the participants relied on their HIV-positive friends' experiential knowledge—even more so than provider-delivered information—to make ART medication decisions. Studies have shown that the more HIV-positive patients are involved in decision-making, the more information sources they tend to seek (e.g., Kremer and Ironson 2007). Our findings give context to quantitative studies that have demonstrated an association between perceived support for autonomous decision-making and better ART adherence (Kennedy et al. 2007) and suggest the need for ongoing autonomous support to maintain adherence. Moreover, given that participants highly valued HIV-positive friends' opinions about ART, consideration could be given to exploring provider- or support group-delivered health communication tools, such as role model stories (Liston et al. 2006), that provide health information in an engaging, comprehensible, and timely manner. By design, role model stories depict experiences of individuals with good ART adherence behaviors, provide pertinent information (e.g., dosing intervals, handling missed doses), and link readers to resources that provide ongoing, accurate updated information and support services.

In our focus group discussions, we used a values clarification process to prompt participants for statements about adherence-related motivators that was similar to the values clarification strategies used by Walters, Ogle, and Martin (2002). This elicitation process resulted in participants stating that their primary motivational beliefs were staying healthy, having faith that their ART medications will keep them healthy, and having a strong desire to live. These findings are consistent with findings from studies demonstrating that health beliefs are strongly associated with adherence (e.g., Barclay et al. 2007). Unique to this study are the comments participants provided which illuminate the connection between these motivating beliefs and their commitment to adherence. Participants reported that they saw themselves as having control over, and responsibility for, their HIV disease management and that this view of themselves was a strong motivator for ART adherence. Other studies (e.g., Berg et al. 2005; Remien et al. 2003) have noted the strong association between taking personal responsibility for medical care and better adherence. Our work here suggests that a structured values clarification approach may be a successful strategy for assisting individuals in making the link between their personal values and adherence behavior. Other highly valued personal characteristics that provided motivation included being a spiritual person, being an advocate for other HIV-positive individuals, and being a positive person. More research is needed on approaches that increase motivation for ART adherence by focusing on the link to personal values (e.g., desire to live, spirituality, positive outlook, advocacy for others) in an autonomy-supportive environment. Recent studies using motivational interviewing as an adherence counseling technique employ such motivational enhancement strategies and may have promise of increasing personal autonomy for adherence (Golin et al. 2006; Gerkovich et al. 2005). However, little is known about how to translate these counseling strategies for use by HIV providers in real-world clinical settings.

In addition to possessing high motivation, participants' comments revealed strong behavioral skills for adherence. Many had struggled with how to fit adherence into their already chaotic lives, but because they had the requisite knowledge and motivation they persevered to develop the necessary adherence behavioral skills. Many comments revealed strong problem-solving skills and a willingness to keep adapting to make ART adherence work. For example, participants reported learning to carry extra doses, making lifestyle changes, and actively engaging others to ensure ART success. Overall, our findings were interestingly reminiscent of the key attributes of social action theory (i.e., self-regulation, personal change mechanisms, social contexts on adherence—Ewart 1991), which, together with the IMB model, may assist in providing important insights for adherence interventions that particularly focus on sustained personal autonomy and empowerment.

This study's results may be limited by the small sample of adherence masters. However, our sample of adherence masters was representative of a wide range of ages, educational levels, and ethnicities. Only a few studies have been conducted on this population whose perspectives and experiences can shed light on critical aspects of successful ART adherence (e.g., Lewis et al. 2006; Malcolm et al. 2003). Also, this study was largely focused on data collection through qualitative procedures in an urban Midwestern population, which may limit the generalization of findings to other regions and populations. The design also precluded exploration of causality. However, our intent was to explore adherence masters' rich descriptive perspectives on ART adherence related to their experiences, knowledge, beliefs and behaviors, and motivation, and to map their responses to the IMB model. Additionally, our study did not track our adherence masters' adherence levels beyond their focus group participation. Studies have shown that ART adherence can be a moving target and tends to wane for long-time adherers (e.g., Gardner et al. 2006). Our adherence masters weren't perfect, yet they strived to maintain their adherence despite their encountered challenges and refused to give up hope of long-term survival.

HIV is a chronic disease for which there is no cure. However, new ART options continue to emerge that reduce regimen complexity and improve health outcomes for HIV-positive individuals. Further understanding of how to improve adherence to these medications is critical for assisting HIV-positive individuals in disease management. Studies based on the IMB model with adherence masters may provide invaluable insights and new discoveries of adherence intervention strategies that could facilitate excellent adherence and decreased mortality for HIV-positive individuals.

REFERENCES AND FURTHER READING

Amico, K. R., Barta, W., Konkle-Parker, D. J., Fisher, J. D., Cornman, D. H., Shuper, P. A., and Fisher, W. A. (2007). The Information–Motivation–Behavioral Skills Model of ART adherence in a Deep South HIV+ clinic sample. *AIDS Behavior*. Advance copy.

Barclay, T. R., Hinkin, C. H., Castellon, S. A., Mason, K. I., Reinhard, M. J., Marion, S. D. Levine, A. J., and Durvasula, R. S. (2007). Age-associated predictors of medication adherence in HIV-positive adults: health beliefs, self-efficacy, and neurocognitive status. *Health Psychology, 26*(1), 40–49.

Beach, M. C., Keruly, J., and Moore, R. D. (2006). Is the quality of the patient–provider relationship associated with better adherence and health outcomes for patients with HIV? *Journal of General Internal Medicine, 21*(6), 661–665.

Berg, M. B., Safren, S. A., Mimiaga, M. J., Grasso, C., Boswell, S., and Mayer, K. H. (2005). Nonadherence to medical appointments is associated with increased plasma HIV RNA and decreased CD4 cell counts in a community-based HIV primary care clinic. *AIDS Care, 17*(7), 902–907.

Chesney, M. A., Morin, M., and Sherr, L. (2000). Adherence to HIV combination therapy. *Soc Sci Med, 50*, 1599–1605.

Enriquez, M., Lackey, N. R., O'Connor, M. C., and McKinsey, D. S. (2004). Successful adherence after multiple HIV treatment failures. *Journal of Advanced Nursing, 45*(4), 438–446.

Ewart, C. K. (1991). Social action theory for a public health psychology. *American Psychol, 46*(9), 931–946.

Fisher, J., Fisher, W., Amico, K. R., and Harmon, J. J. (2006). An information–motivation–behavioral skills model of adherence to antiretroviral therapy. *Health Psychology, 25*, 463–473.

Gardner, E., Burman, W. J., Maravi, M. E., and Davidson, A. J. (2006). Durability of adherence to antiretroviral therapy on initial and subsequent regimens. *AIDS Patient Care STDS, 20*(9), 628–636.

Gerkovich, M. M., Goggin, K. J., Wright, J., Catley, D., Williams, K., Bradley, A. et al. (2005). Design and implementation of a multi-modal adherence trial. Poster presented at the Enhancing Adherence: A State of the Science Meeting on Intervention Research to Improve Anti-Retroviral Adherence, New Haven, CT, November.

Golin, C. E., Earp, J., Tien, H. C., Stewart, P., Porter, C., and Howie, L. (2006). A 2-arm, randomized, controlled trial of a motivational interviewing-based intervention to improve adherence to antiretroviral therapy (ART) among patients failing or initiating ART. *Journal of Acquired Immune Deficiency Syndromes, 42*(1), 42–51.

Gordillo, V., del Amo, J., Soriano, V., and Gonzalez-Lahoz, J. (1999). Sociodemographic and psychological variables influencing adherence to antiretroviral therapy. *AIDS, 13*, 1763–1769.

Gray, J. (2006). Becoming adherent: experiences of persons living with HIV/AIDS. *Journal of the Association of Nurses in AIDS Care, 17*(3), 47–54.

Halkitis, P. N., Parsons, J. T., Wolitski, R. J., and Remien, R. H. (2003). Characteristics of HIV antiretroviral treatments, access and adherence in an ethnically diverse sample of men who have sex with men. *AIDS Care, 15*, 89–102.

Hamilton, M. M., Razzano, L. A., and Martin, N. B. (2007). The relationship between type and quality of social support and HIV medication adherence. *Journal of HIV/AIDS and Social Services, 6*(1–2), 39–63.

Hammer, S., Saag, M., Schechter, M., et al. (2006). Treatment for adult HIV infection. 2006 recommendations of the International AIDS Society-U.S.A. panel. *JAMA*, 296(7), 827–843.

Jensen-Fangel, A., Pedersen, L., Pedersen, C., Larsen, C. S., Tauris, P., Moller, A., et al. (2004). Low mortality in HIV-infected patients starting highly active antiretroviral therapy: a comparison with the general population. *AIDS, 18*, 89–97.

Johnson, M. O., Catz, S. L., Remien, R. H., Rotheram-Borus, M. J., Morin, S. F., Charlebois, E., et al. (2003). Theory-guided, empirically supported avenues for intervention on HIV medication nonadherence: findings from the Healthy Living Project. *AIDS Patient Care STDs, 17*, 645–656.

Johnson, M. O., Chesney, M. A., Goldstein, R. B., Remien, R. H., Catz, S., Gore-Felton, C., et al. (2006). Positive provider interactions, adherence self-efficacy, and adherence to antiretroviral medications among HIV-infected adults: a mediation model. *AIDS Patient Care STDS, 20*(4), 258–268.

Kennedy, S., Goggin, K., and Nollen, N. (2007). *Adherence to HIV medications: utility of Self-Determination Theory*. Manuscript in progress.

Kremer, H., and Ironson, G. (2007). People living with HIV: sources of information on antiretroviral treatment and preferences for involvement in treatment decision-making. *Eur J Med Res, 31, 12*(1), 34–42.

Lewis, M. P., Colbert, A., Erlen, J., and Meyers, M. (2006). A qualitative study of persons who are 100% adherent to antiretroviral therapy. *AIDS Care, 18*(2), 140–148.

Liston, R. J., Berkley-Patton, J., and Goggin, K. (2006) *Tell me a story: using role model stories to promote use of HIV/AIDS prevention and care services.* Poster presentation at the American Public Health Association 134th Annual Meeting, Boston, MA.

Lucas, G. M., (2005). Antiretroviral adherence, drug resistance, viral fitness, and HIV disease progress. A triangle web is woven. *Journal of Antimicrobial Chemotherapy, 55*, 413–416.

Malcolm, S. E., Ng, J. J., Rosen, R. K., and Stone, V. E. (2003). An examination of HIV/AIDS patients who have excellent adherence to HAART. *AIDS Care, 15*(2), 251–261.

Palella, F. J., Deloria-Knoll, M., Chmiel, J. S., Moorman, A. C., Wood, K. C., Greenberg, A. E., et al. (2003). Survival benefit of initiating antiretroviral therapy in HIV-infected persons in different CD4+ cell strata. *Ann Intern Med, 138,* 620–626.

Paterson, D. L., Swindells, S., Mohr, J., Brester, M., Vergis, E. N., Squier, C., et al. (2000). Adherence to protease inhibitor therapy and outcomes in patients with HIV infection. *Ann of Intern Med, 133*, 21–30.

Rao, D., Kekwaletswe, T. C., Hosek, S., Martinez, J., and Rodriguez, F. (2007). Stigma and social barriers to medication adherence with urban youth living with HIV. *AIDS Care, 19*(1), 28–33.

Reif, S., Whetten, K., Lowe, K., and Ostermann, J. (2006). Association of unmet needs for support services with medication use and adherence among HIV-infected individuals in the southeastern United States. *AIDS Care, 18*(4), 277–283.

Remien, R. H., Hirky, A. E., Johnson, M. O., Weinhardt, L. S., Whittier, D., and Le, G. M. (2003). Adherence to medication treatment: a qualitative study of facilitators and barriers among a diverse sample of HIV+ men and women in four U.S. cities. *AIDS Behav, 7*, 61–72.

Remien, R. H., Stirratt, M. J., Dognin, J., Day, E., El-Bassel, N., and Warne, P. (2006). Moving from theory to research to practice: implementing an effective dyadic intervention to improve antiretroviral adherence for clinic patients. *Journal of Acquired Immune Deficiency Syndromes, 43* (Suppl. 1), S69–S78.

Rintamaki, L. S., Davis, T. C., Skripkauskas, S., Bennett, C. L., and Wolf, M. S. (2006). Social stigma concerns and HIV medication adherence. *AIDS Patient Care STDs, 20*(5), 359–368.

Rosen, M. I., Dieckhaus, K., McMahon, T. J., Valdes, B., Petry, N. M., Cramer, J., and Rounsaville, B. (2007). Improved adherence with contingency management. *AIDS Patient Care STDS*, 21(1), 30–40.

Schönnesson, L. N., Diamond, P. M., Ross, M. W., Williams. M., and Bratt., G. (2006). Baseline predictors of three types of antiretroviral therapy (ART) adherence: a 2-year follow-up. *AIDS Care, 18*(3), 246–253.

Sethi, A. K., Celentano, D. D., Gange, S. J., Moore, R. D., and Gallant, J. E. (2003). Association between adherence to antiretroviral therapy and human immunodeficiency virus drug resistance. *Clin Infect Dis*, 37, 1112–1118.

Shor-Posner, G., Lecusay, R., Miguez-Burbano, M. J., Quesada, J., Rodriguez, A., Ruiz, P., et al. (2000). Quality of life measures in the Miami HIV-1 infected drug users cohort: relationship to gender and disease status. *J Subst Abuse, 11*, 395–404.

Starace, F., Massa, A., Amico, K. R., and Fisher, J. D. (2006). Adherence to antiretroviral therapy: an empirical test of the Information–Motivation–Behavioral Skills Model. *Health Psychology, 25*(2), 153–162.

Stirratt, M. J., and Gordon, C. M. (2007). HIV treatment adherence research and intervention: current advances and future challenges. *Journal of HIV/AIDS and Social Services, 6*, 9–22.

Sullivan, P., Campsmith, M. L., Nakamura, G. V., Begley, E. B., Schulden, J., and Nakashima, A. K. (2007). Patient and regimen characteristics associated with self-reported nonadherence to antiretroviral therapy. *PLoS ONE, 2*(6), e552.

Sunil, T. S., and McGehee, M. A. (2007). Social and religious support on treatment adherence among HIV/AIDS patients by race/ethnicity. *Journal of HIV/AIDS and Social Services, 6* (1–2), 83–99.

Walters, S. T., Ogle, R., and Martin, J. E. (2002). Perils and possibilities of group-based motivational interviewing. In M. Miller and S. Rollnick (eds.), *Motivational Interviewing: Preparing People for Change*, 2nd edition (pp. 377–390). New York: Guilford Press.

White, B. L., Wohl, D. A., Hays, R. D., Golin, C. E., Liu, H., Kiziah, C. N., et al. (2006). A pilot study of health beliefs and attitudes concerning measures of antiretroviral adherence among prisoners receiving directly observed antiretroviral therapy. *AIDS Patient Care STDs. 20*(6), 408–417.

SECTION 4

Explorations in New Forms of Intervention and Prevention

FRAMING ESSAY

A Social Contextual Perspective to Optimize the Prevention and Control of STIs/HIV among Adolescents

Ralph J. DiClemente, Colleen P. Crittenden, Eve S. Rose, and Jessica M. Sales

OVERVIEW

The threat of acquiring a sexually transmitted infection (STI) is one of the most significant public health risks facing adolescents today (Blum and Nelson-Mmari 2004). From an economic and social perspective, these infections continue to exact a significant toll on adolescents and society, in general, worldwide (Barnett et al. 2001). The real concern, however, is that in an era where a sexually transmitted infection, human immunodeficiency virus (HIV), can result in a fatal illness, the acquired immunodeficiency syndrome (AIDS), we have begun to measure the impact in terms of deaths of adolescents and young adults from AIDS. As HIV-related morbidity increases in salience, the need for more effective measures to prevent disease transmission must become a high public health priority (WHO 2007a).

ADOLESCENTS' RISK FOR STI/HIV INFECTION: A GLOBAL ASSESSMENT

Globally, adolescents are disproportionately affected by a wide range of STIs, including bacterial, viral, and parasitic infections. More than 340 million new STIs occur annually, with at least one third occurring in young people under 25 years (WHO 2007a). Each year, it is estimated that 1 in 20 adolescents worldwide will contract an STI (WHO 2007b). Although many STIs can be effectively treated with medication (e.g., chlamydia), others such as viral STIs (e.g., genital herpes) remain impervious to cure. Although there is effective suppressive treatment for HSV-2, this viral STI and many others are a significant source of morbidity for adolescents as they transition to adulthood. Notably, females are much more likely than males to be diagnosed with STIs and, if left untreated, experience adverse sequelae, including reproductive abnormalities such as infertility and ectopic pregnancy.

HIV has emerged as a major source of morbidity and mortality among adolescents, riveting international attention from prevention researchers and clinicians. Twenty-five percent of all global HIV infections occur among young people between the ages of 15 and 24 years, with new infections among some subgroups reaching epidemic proportions (UNAIDS 2006). In sub-Saharan Africa, HIV is the leading cause of mortality among adolescents/young adults of 15–29 years and the second major cause of mortality worldwide (Kiragu 2001), with over 60 million new infections over the last two decades (Blum and Nelson-Mmari 2004). It has been estimated that in some areas of sub-Saharan Africa, which contains roughly 75 percent of all youth living with HIV/AIDS (Kiragu 2001), over 10 percent of female adolescents aged 15–19 years and 25–33 percent of young women aged 20–24 years are infected with HIV (UNAIDS 2005).

At highest risk for STI/HIV acquisition are several discrete, but related groups: 1) sex workers, 2) injection drug users, 3) men who have sex with men, 4) incarcerated or institutionalized youth, and 5) those living in extreme poverty (Hoffman et al. 2006). Disease prevalence rates within these high-risk groups vary by country. For example, in Southeast Asia it is estimated that females under the age of 25 years represent between 41–71 percent of women working in high-risk sex environments such as brothels (Family Health International 2003; Indonesia Ministry of Health 2002), whereas in African regions such as Zambia and Tanzania it is more common for women working in high-risk environments to be younger females, under the age of 20 years (Vandepitte et al. 2006). Across each high-risk group, one trend remains constant: young people ages 15–24 years are at substantial risk for HIV acquisition (Monasch and Mahy 2006).

In addition, minority adolescents in industrialized countries experience a disproportionate burden of STIs. Results from a survey of U.S. adolescents aged 14–21 years indicated that African Americans were more than three and a half times more likely to report ever contracting an STI relative to same-age adolescents of different ethnicity; a finding not attributable to differential sexual risk behavior or demographic factors (Hallfors et al. 2007). In industrialized countries the majority of new HIV infections occur as a result of heterosexual contact as opposed to other routes of acquisition (e.g., injection drug use) (Rosenberg and Biggar 1998).

THERE IS AN URGENT NEED TO DEVELOP AND DISSEMINATE INTERVENTIONS FOR ADOLESCENTS

Despite the large proportion of adolescents in jeopardy of contracting HIV, targeted preventive interventions are extremely limited based on geographic region. There is a critical need to increase the number of effective prevention programs worldwide, as adolescents represent the subgroup at greatest risk for HIV acquisition and also signify the group perhaps most amenable to change (Aggleton and Rivers 1997). In a recent WHO review, Monasch and Mahy (2006) reported that, globally, relatively little is known about the specific needs of young people. Further, while existing prevention programs are genuinely concerned with reducing the incidence of STI/HIV among adolescents, many of these programs are deficient in effectively evaluating whether preventive measures actually achieve their goals (Grassly et al. 2001).

With the possible exception of hepatitis B and more recently, Human Papillomavirus (HPV), two vaccine-preventable STIs, behavioral interventions are the most promising strategy for preventing STIs/HIV among adolescents. STI/HIV behavioral interventions have evolved markedly over the course of the epidemic—from predominantly knowledge-based approaches to sexual communication skills-based approaches, with more recent studies investigating the usefulness of life-skills approaches (e.g., youth development programs). The primary goal of behavioral interventions is to impact the antecedents associated with STI/HIV-associated sexual risk behaviors and, as a consequence, reduce the likelihood of disease acquisition.

Few behavioral interventions conducted in the developing world provide sufficient data in terms of outcome or impact (Kirby et al. 2005), thus making it difficult to gauge the efficacy of behavior change interventions. On the other hand, interventions conducted in higher resource areas, such as the United States, have produced some of the most promising findings (Lyles et al. 2007). Further, many interventions implemented globally are often adapted from or patterned after prevention approaches in the United States (Smith and Katner 1995). As an in-depth review of global STI/HIV interventions is beyond the scope of this chapter, prevention and intervention efficacy within the United States (U.S.) will serve as the foundation for our discussion. After highlighting the design and evaluation of adolescent prevention programs in the U.S., the sections that follow will address the importance of shifting prevention efforts from an individualized paradigm to encompass a broader risk environment utilizing a socio-contextual perspective and how this perspective can be applied to future prevention efforts on a global scale.

STI/HIV PREVENTIVE INTERVENTIONS FOR ADOLESCENTS IN THE U.S.

Behavioral interventions have been successfully delivered through diverse venues, the most common being community settings (Jemmott and Jemmott 2000), schools (Kirby 2000), clinical venues (DiClemente et al. 2005a), and locations targeting particularly high-risk adolescents such as prisons (Magura et al. 1994), detention centers (St. Lawrence et al. 1999), and in-patient substance abuse treatment facilities (St. Lawrence et al. 2002). Several recent reviews have summarized the effects of STI/HIV interventions for adolescents in the United States (Robin et al. 2004; Pedlow and Carey 2003; Sales et al. 2006).

Regardless of the intervention venue (community settings, schools, clinics, incarceration/treatment facilities), some degree of reduction in STI/HIV-associated risk behaviors as a result of participation in the intervention is typically observed (Robin et al. 2004). The most frequently reported behavioral outcome is the reduction in frequency of unprotected sexual intercourse or increased condom use (Sales et al. 2006). Less common, however, are intervention effects that result in a delay in initiation of intercourse (Downs et al. 2004), a decrease in the frequency of intercourse (Rotheram-Borus et al. 1998), or a reduction in the number of sexual partners (Orr et al. 1996).

Characteristically, STI/HIV behavioral intervention programs for adolescents are most effective when they employ: 1) a theoretical framework to guide the design and implementation of the program; 2) diverse learning techniques that emphasize interactive learning; 3) developmentally appropriate skills-based instruction; 4) strategies to foster peer norms supportive of safer sex practices; 5) gender-specific methodologies; 6) culturally specific methodologies; and 7) trained peer facilitators (Janz et al. 1996; Wingood and DiClemente 1996). Specifically, the use of a theoretical framework in intervention development and implementation has been associated with improved STI/HIV risk reduction outcomes. Social learning theory and social cognitive theory are the frameworks most consistently used in successful programs (Jemmott et al. 1999; Fisher et al. 2002). These programs incorporate modeling, and skills building, and attempt to increase self-efficacy with regard to safer sexual behavior. Additionally, interventions that provide adolescents with a broad base of skills may be highly effective for the prevention of STI/HIV-associated risk behaviors. For example, programs that include broader content, such as problem solving, capacity building, social skill building, and that enhance gender and ethnic pride, have been shown to impact STI/HIV-associated sexual behavior (DiClemente et al. 2004; Pedlow and Carey 2004).

While empirical evidence suggests that behavioral interventions can be effective, estimating the true magnitude of intervention efficacy has been difficult. Historically, the field of HIV research has been dominated by an individual-level perspective, one that primarily focuses solely on the adolescent. While such interventions are successful at reducing HIV-associated sexual behavior, individual-level interventions may not be sufficient to promote the adoption and maintenance of HIV-preventive behaviors over time. To truly optimize the development and evaluation of future STI/HIV prevention interventions for adolescents on a larger scale, prevention must move beyond the individual to address the larger circumstantial context of risk.

MOVING BEYOND THE INDIVIDUAL TO ADDRESS THE BROADER RISK CONTEXT

Traditionally, biomedical trials inclusive of vaccines and the use of daily antiretrovirals have been viewed as some of the most effective HIV prevention strategies in the highest-risk countries (McQueen and Karim 2007; Stover et al. 2006). However, expanding intervention development and implementation to incorporate a broader spectrum of determinants of adolescents' sexual risk for STI/HIV acquisition may provide an opportunity to more effectively confront disease acquisition and transmission (Blum and Nelson-Mmari 2004). Within the last decade health researchers have gone beyond focusing just on treatment and have begun to recognize the value of adopting a socio-ecological approach to examine individual risk behavior (Bronfenbrenner 1979). A socio-ecological approach involves examining individuals' behavior within the context of their social and physical environment, inclusive of family context, social relationships, peer, and societal influences (Boyer et al. 2000). Psychosocial influences reciprocally shape one another and collectively impact the balance of risk for STI/HIV infection while ultimately influencing behavior change.

UNDERSTANDING ADOLESCENT RISK BEHAVIOR: A SOCIAL CONTEXTUAL APPROACH

Emerging evidence indicates that a spectrum of contextual factors and exposures are prominent and interact with each other in promoting or preventing adolescents' HIV/STI-associated sexual behavior, including psychological, social, relational, familial, developmental, structural, environmental, and cultural factors. By utilizing a social contextual perspective, HIV/STI intervention research can generate new kinds of data, formulate innovative hypotheses regarding adolescents and their risk of HIV, and, most important, produce novel approaches for primary prevention of HIV/STI infection among adolescents.

The Individual

Although adolescents typically perceive STI/HIV as a severe disease, a great deal of variability exists regarding individual perception of susceptibility. Studies suggest that adolescents who perceive that they are at risk for STI/HIV tend to engage in less risky sexual behavior than those who do not have these perceptions (Zimet et al. 1992). Furthermore, adolescents who feel confident in using condoms (Rosenthal et al. 1991), in their ability to negotiate condom use with their partners (Sionean et al. 2002), in their ability to refuse sexual intercourse without condom use (Crosby et al. 2001), and in their ability to openly communicate about their sexual history (Crosby et al. 2002a), tend to use condoms more often and have lower rates of STIs (DiClemente et al. 2001). Conversely, adolescents who engage in unprotected sexual intercourse tend to perceive more barriers toward condom use (Crosby et al. 2000), believe that condom use is less pleasurable (Jemmott et al. 1999), hold more negative attitudes toward condom use (Fisher et al. 1992), and perceive susceptibility to STI/HIV infection to be low (Bandura 1994).

Individual characteristics such as low self-esteem, depression, and psychological distress also place many adolescents at risk for engaging in STI/HIV-associated sexual behaviors (Spencer et al. 2002). Adolescents' STI/HIV risk behavior appears to cluster with other risk-taking behaviors (e.g., substance use) (Donohew et al. 2000), antisocial behavior and delinquency (Millstein and Moscicki 1995), and pregnancy (Crosby et al. 2002b), making it relatively easy to identify subgroups at highest risk. Moreover, adolescents with high levels of impulsivity or who are prone toward sensation-seeking behaviors may place themselves at greater risk for contracting an STI/HIV (Khan et al. 2002).

The Family Context

Adolescent sexual risk behavior has been frequently associated with the family structure (Romer et al. 1999; Li et al. 2000a). Protective factors such as perceived family support, family cohesiveness, parental monitoring, and parent–adolescent communication about sex mitigate adolescents' risky sexual behavior (DiClemente et al. 2001; DiIorio et al. 1999). Of particular importance is parental monitoring and parental communication. Evidence suggests that adolescents who perceive that their parents (or parental figure) know where they are and who they are with outside of the home are substantially less likely to engage in STI/HIV sexual risk behaviors (Whitaker and Miller 2000). Likewise, adolescents who engage in conversations about sexual issues with their mothers are generally less experienced sexually (Jaccard et al. 1996), report fewer lifetime sex partners (Dutra et al. 1999), report engaging in sex less frequently (Miller et al. 2000), and, if sexually active, use contraception methods (including condoms) more often (Dutra et al. 1999) in comparison to those not having open conversations.

Social Relationships

Outside of the family environment, relationship characteristics play an important role in influencing adolescents' risk behavior and likelihood of contracting STIs/HIV. This form of social influence may be especially strong when one partner has more power and control in the romantic relationship. Although similarities occur across gender, some differences do exist. Primary limitations among females are that they often lack control in the relationship (Fortenberry et al. 2002), engage in longer relationships (Catania et al. 1989), fear condom negotiation with their male partner (Crosby et al. 2002a), communicate less frequently with their partner about sex (Sionean et al. 2002), and have older sexual partners (DiClemente et al. 2002)—all of which have been associated with greater likelihood of engaging in STI/HIV sexual risk behavior. Extensive research on partner control (Weisman et al. 1991) and perceived partner support (Lindberg et al. 1998) as relational risk factors have likewise been documented. For males, partner communication about sex (Wilson et al. 1994), belief in contraception responsibility (Ku et al. 1994), being in the early stages of a relationship (Brown et al. 1986), and perceptions of partners' sexual inexperience have been associated with increased condom use (Tremblay et al. 1995), thus acting more as protective factors to prevent risky sexual behavior. However, perceived partners' negative attitude toward condom use has been related to unprotected intercourse and an increased number of sexual partners (Bachanas et al. 2002).

Peer Influence

Perhaps one of the most dominant influences on adolescents' sexual risk behavior is the perception about the behavior of their peers. Although it has been established that parents and sexual partners have considerable influence on adolescents' decisions to engage in risk behaviors in comparison to peers (Bachanas et al. 2002), perceived peer norms surrounding sexual behavior and condom use have been shown to also be key influencers of risky sexual behavior. As group norms frequently dictate sexual scripts, conformity to these prescribed roles is rewarded with peer approval (Fisher et al. 1992). If adolescents and young adults perceive that their friends are having unprotected sex or engage in risky sex, they may be more likely to adopt their friends' behaviors (Fortenberry et al. 2002). Similarly, perceptions of low levels of social support among peers have also been associated with the likelihood of participating in risky sexual behavior (Fullilove 1998). In contrast, perceived peer norms supportive of STI/HIV-protective behaviors can have a significant influence on the adoption and maintenance of protective behaviors over time (Millstein and Moscicki 1995).

Societal Influence

Societal factors play an integral role in shaping cultural norms and influencing behavior. Surveillance data indicate African-American adolescent females are disproportionately affected by STIs/HIV relative to other racial/ethnic groups and males (DiClemente et al. 2005b). The apparent influences of race/ethnicity may be confounded by a variety of environmental factors (Small and Luster 1994). Societal influences such as neighborhoods devoid of adequate community resources (Aral and Wasserheit 1995), poor community supervision, and extreme poverty (Ennett et al. 1999) are each likely to foster STI/HIV risk behavior. Adolescents living in stressful environments are generally more likely to take sexual risks (Lown et al. 1993).

More recently, in an era bombarded by technology and entertainment, the media has moved to the forefront as a key influence on the sexual health of adolescents. Overt sexual imagery coupled with situations depicting unprotected sexual intercourse, violence, aggression, and subordination of women is ubiquitous (Peter and Valkenburg 2006). There is emerging empirical evidence for an association between both exposure to rap music videos (Peterson et al. 2007; Wingood et al. 2003) and pornographic movies (Wingood et al. 2001) with greater levels of problem behavior and increased sexual risk-taking. Unfortunately, little is known about the psychosocial mechanism that might explain the observed associations between the media and adolescent risk behavior. Existing studies suggest that one potentially important society-level predictor of adolescents' sexual risk behavior may be their association with organized social groups (Crosby 2002c).

Optimizing Prevention Programs From A Social Contextual Perspective

Future interventions with sexually active adolescents should target behaviors like condom use that have been empirically demonstrated across a variety of adolescent subgroups and venues to be amenable to change. By incorporating a more focused approach and targeting only specific areas of behavioral change that are realistic for adolescents to accomplish, STI/HIV prevention programs may prove more efficacious and sustainable over protracted time periods. For example, the SiHLE (Sisters Informing, Healing, Living, and Empowering) intervention, a gender and culturally appropriate HIV risk-reduction intervention for African-American adolescent females, was able to significantly increase condom use, while reducing the number of chlamydia infections by targeting condom skills, frequency of condom use, and partner communication techniques (DiClemente et al. 2004).

Moving Beyond the Individual-Level Perspective

Contemporary thinking in public health practice has shifted focus from the adolescent alone to the adolescent embedded in a complex network of family, social relationships, peers, and cultural factors that constantly shape their STI/HIV-associated risk and protective behaviors (DiClemente and Wingood 2000; DiClemente et al. 2007). It is possible that the next generation of STI/HIV risk-reduction interventions will be developed using a multi-tier intervention framework. Such an intervention would be designed to reinforce and amplify the preventive message initially delivered to the adolescent using group-formatted or social network intervention strategies that create an atmosphere conducive to and supportive of adolescents' adoption and maintenance of STI/HIV-preventive practices. For example, we are currently engaged in a multi-site trial (iMPPACS) designed to assess the relative efficacy of an evidence-based face-to-face risk-reduction intervention alone, paired with electronic mass media intervention messages, versus a control condition, in terms of initial behavior change and sustaining or amplifying behavior change over an 18-month follow-up period. The underlying assumption is that targeting adolescents through multiple levels of intervention may have a synergistic effect on STI/HIV preventive behaviors that exceeds that of a single-level intervention. From this perspective, adolescents' STI/HIV risk behavior should not be conceptualized as "individual deficits," but rather more appropriately and favorably viewed as a reflection of their socio-contextual environment (DiClemente and Crosby 2006; DiClemente et al. 2005b).

Tailor Interventions to the Needs of the Population

Tailored interventions are generally more effective relative to general or broad-based interventions in terms of reducing STI/HIV-associated behaviors. Tailored interventions reflect the recognition that adolescents are not a homogeneous group, but rather a heterogeneous mosaic of subgroups, comprising different ethnicities/cultures, behavioral risk characteristics, developmental levels, sexual preferences, and gender differences. Because of the myriad differences between adolescent subgroups, customizing interventions specifically for a subgroup of adolescents may produce more favorable results in terms of reducing risk-associated behavior. Thus, acknowledging that adolescents are not a monolithic group, and tailoring messages and intervention strategies to specific subgroups, is a critical step in providing an impetus toward positive behavior change (DiClemente et al. 2003).

Developing a Long-Term Maintenance Strategy

For behavior change to be meaningful, it must be durable. Given the scope and complexity of factors that can affect adolescents' sexual behavior, it is unclear whether short-term STI/HIV preventive changes, observed as a result of intervention participation, can be sustained over protracted periods of time. Therefore, it is necessary to develop and incorporate innovative maintenance strategies to sustain and, if possible, increase STI program efficacy. For example, below we describe a multi-level intervention designed to reinforce prevention messages that may enhance sustainability by intervening with adolescents' families.

Utilize the Family Structure as a Vehicle for Behavior Change

Given the fundamental role the family plays in many developmental processes, utilizing adolescents' families as a behavioral change agent could be particularly beneficial. Involving parents may be an especially important strategy to help delay adolescents' sexual debut, reduce frequency of intercourse, limit number of sexual partners, or support health-promoting behaviors, such as using condoms during intercourse. These goals may be achieved by fostering improved communication between parents and adolescents and intensified parental monitoring (Li et al. 2000b). We are currently collaborating on a multi-site trial (Project STYLE) designed to evaluate the efficacy of a parent–adolescent intervention relative to an adolescent-only intervention and a control condition in enhancing STI/HIV-preventive behaviors. Again, as previously noted, the key assumption is that multi-leveled interventions may yield greater efficacy and sustainability of intervention effects.

Incorporate Biological Outcomes as an Assessment of Program Efficacy

Historically, interventions have relied almost exclusively on adolescents' self-reported behavior change to assess program efficacy. Self-reported data has been criticized as subject to potential reporting biases, inaccurate recall, and social desirability bias (Zenilman et al. 1995). Recently, the use of newly developed DNA assays (PCR) to detect prevalent STIs has been advocated as a complementary measure for evaluating program efficacy (DiClemente 2000). Thus, future STI/HIV intervention studies, when applicable and feasible, should consider the utility of including biological markers as an objective and quantifiable outcome measure of program efficacy.

Translate and Disseminate Effective STI/HIV Interventions

It is unlikely that any single STI/HIV intervention would be appropriate and equally effective for all adolescents given the heterogeneity of this population. The true challenge concerns moving beyond the rigorously controlled intervention trial and taking the necessary steps towards translating those interventions that have demonstrated programmatic efficacy in a particular venue (Sales et al. 2006), and with a particular group (O'Donnell et al. 1999) into sustainable programs that can be widely disseminated among similar venues and populations. Ultimately, preventing STI/HIV infections in adolescents does not only depend on the development and evaluation of innovative behavior change approaches, but on how effectively these interventions can be translated and integrated into self-sustaining components of clinic practice, school curricula, or community programs, particularly among populations most adversely impacted by STIs/HIV (DiClemente and Wingood 2003).

A Look Ahead: STI/HIV Intervention on A Global Level

Globally, the intersecting STI and HIV epidemics continue to exact a heavy toll on the health and wellbeing of adolescents and the resources of many countries to address the prevention and treatment needs of youth. While great strides have been made in advancing our understanding of social and behavioral strategies to reduce STI/HIV infection, much more needs to be accomplished if we are to control these epidemics.

We have addressed a number of issues integral to STI/HIV prevention research in the sections above. Many of these issues have focused on optimal research designs to evaluate programmatic efficacy. However, perhaps the central theme from our examination of research pertaining to the prevention and control of STI/HIV suggests that the majority of prevention efforts have been dedicated to identifying individual-level risk and protective factors. The disregard for the importance of a social-ecological perspective delimits our ability not only to motivate youth to adopt STI/HIV-preventive behaviors but also to sustain newly acquired behaviors over extended periods of time. In the face of pervasive countervailing influences (e.g., peer networks, media), we need to transcend our focus on the individual, to rethink prevention, and reconceptualize interventions to focus on the adolescent-within-social-context.

Integrated interventions, which traverse multiple levels of causation in the socio-ecological model, can marshal new kinds of data, ask new and broader questions regarding the range of influences that affect risk of STI/HIV, and, most important, create new and promising options for STI/HIV prevention. If we are to confront the challenge of STI/HIV among adolescents, then prevention programs targeting social change will play a major role. For the science of STI/HIV prevention to progress more rapidly, a comprehensive and coordinated infrastructure to conceptualize, stimulate, and support STI/HIV intervention research that focuses on the social ecology of risk and prevention is of critical importance.

REFERENCES AND FURTHER READING

Aggleton, Peter, and Kim Rivers. 1997. "Preventing HIV: behavioral interventions with young people." Retrieved on August 27, 2007 from http://www.id21.org/insights/insights22/insights-iss22art05.html.

Aral, Sevgi O., and Judith N. Wasserheit. 1995. "Interactions among HIV, other sexually transmitted diseases, socioeconomic status, and poverty in women." In *Women at risk: issues in the primary prevention of AIDS*, ed. Anne O'Leary and Loretta S. Jemmott, 13–42. New York, NY: Plenum Press.

Bachanas, Pamela J., Mary K. Morris, Jennifer K. Lewis-Gess, Eileen J. Sarett-Cuasay, Adriana L. Flores, Kimberly S. Sirl, and Mary K. Sawyer. 2002. "Psychological adjustment, substance use, HIV knowledge, and risky sexual behavior in at-risk minority females: developmental differences during adolescence." *Journal of Pediatric Psychology* 27: 373–84.

Bandura, Albert. 1994. "Social cognitive theory and exercise control over HIV infection." In *Preventing AIDS: theories and methods of behavioral intervention*, ed. Ralph J. DiClemente and John L. Peterson, 25–60. New York, NY: Plenum Press.

Barnett, Tony, Alan Whiteside, and Chris Desmond. 2001. "The social and economic impact of HIV/AIDS in poor countries: a review of studies and lessons." *Progress in Development Studies* 2: 151–70.

Blum, Robert W., and Kristin Nelson-Mmari. 2004. "The health of young people in a global context." *Journal of Adolescent Health* 35: 402–18.

Boyer, Cherrie B., Mary-Ann B. Shafer, Charles J. Wibbelsman, Donald Seeberg, Eileen Teitle, and Nydia Lovell. 2000. "Associations of sociodemographic, psychosocial, and behavioral factors with sexual risk and sexually transmitted diseases in teen clinic patients." *Journal of Adolescent Health* 27: 102–11.

Bronfenbrenner, Urie. 1979. *The ecology of human development*. Cambridge, MA: Harvard University Press.

Brown, B. Bradford, Donna R. Clasen, and Sue A. Eicher. 1986. "Perceptions of peer pressure, peer conformity dispositions, and self reported behavior among adolescents." *Developmental Psychology* 22: 521–30.

Catania, Joseph A., Thomas J. Coates, Ruth M. Greenblatt, and Margaret Dolcini. 1989. "Predictors of condom use and multiple partnered sex among sexually-active adolescent women: implications for AIDS related health interventions." *Journal of Sex Research* 26: 514–24.

Crosby, Richard A., Ralph J. DiClemente, Gina M. Wingood, Catlainn Sionean, Brenda K. Cobb, and Kathy Harrington. 2000. "Correlates of unprotected vaginal sex among African American female teens: the importance of relationship dynamics." *Archives of Pediatrics and Adolescent Medicine* 154: 893–9.

Crosby, Richard A., Ralph J. DiClemente, Gina M. Wingood, Catlainn Sionean, Brenda K. Cobb, Kathy Harrington, Susan L. Davies, Edward W. Hook, and M. Kim Oh. 2001. "Correct condom application among African American adolescent females: the relationship to perceived self-efficacy and the association to confirmed STDs." *Journal of Adolescent Health* 29: 194–9.

Crosby, Richard A., Ralph J. DiClemente, Gina M. Wingood, Brenda K. Cobb, Kathy Harrington, Susan L. Davies, Edward W. Hook III, and M. Kim Oh. 2002a. "Condom use and correlates of African American adolescent females' infrequent communication with sex partners about preventing sexually transmitted diseases and pregnancy." *Health Education and Behavior* 29: 219–31.

Crosby, Richard A., Ralph J. DiClemente, Gina M. Wingood, Kathy Harrington, Susan L. Davies, and Robert Malow. 2002b. "African American adolescent females' membership in social organizations is associated with protective behavior against HIV infection." *Ethnicity and Disease* 12: 186–92.

Crosby, Richard A., Ralph J. DiClemente, Gina M. Wingood, Catlainn Sionean, Kathy Harrington, Susan L. Davies, and M. Kim Oh. 2002c. "Pregnant African American adolescent females are less likely to use condoms than their non-pregnant peers." *Preventive Medicine* 34: 524–52.

DiClemente, Ralph J. 2000. "Looking forward: future directions for HIV prevention research." In *The handbook of HIV prevention*, ed. John L. Peterson and Ralph J. DiClemente, 311–24. New York, NY: Plenum Press.

DiClemente, Ralph J., and Richard A. Crosby. 2006. "Preventing STIs in adolescents: the glass is half full." *Current Opinion in Infectious Diseases* 19: 39–43.

DiClemente, Ralph J., and Gina M. Wingood. 2000. "Expanding the scope of HIV prevention for adolescents: beyond individual-level interventions." *Journal of Adolescent Health* 26: 377–8.

DiClemente, Ralph J., and Gina M. Wingood. 2003. "HIV prevention for adolescents: windows of opportunity for optimizing intervention effectiveness." *Archives of Pediatrics and Adolescent Medicine* 157: 319–20.

DiClemente, Ralph J., Gina M. Wingood, and Richard A. Crosby. 2003. "A contextual perspective for understanding and preventing STD/HIV among adolescents." In *Reducing adolescent risk: toward an integrated approach*, ed. Daniel Romer, 366–73. Thousand Oaks, CA: Sage Publications.

DiClemente, Ralph J., Gina M. Wingood, Richard A. Crosby, Catlainn Sionean, Brenda K. Cobb, Kathy Harrington, Susan L. Davies, Edward W. Hook III, and M. Kim Oh. 2001. "Parental monitoring and its association with a spectrum of adolescent health risk behaviors." *Pediatrics* 107: 1363–8.

DiClemente, Ralph J., Gina M. Wingood, Richard A. Crosby, Catlainn Sionean, Brenda K. Cobb, Kathy Harrington, Susan L. Davies, Edward W. Hook, and M. Kim Oh. 2002. "Sexual risk behaviors associated with having older sex partners: a study of African American female adolescents." *Sexually Transmitted Diseases* 29: 20–24.

DiClemente, Ralph J., Gina M. Wingood, Kathy Harrington, Delia L. Lang, Susan L. Davies, Edward W. Hook, M. Kim Oh, Richard A. Crosby, Victoria S. Hertzberg, Angelita B. Gordon, James W. Hardin, Shan Parker, and Alyssa Robillard. 2004. "Efficacy of an HIV prevention intervention for African American adolescent girls: a randomized controlled trial." *Journal of the American Medical Association* 292: 171–9.

DiClemente, Ralph J., Robin Milhausen, Jessica M. Sales, Laura F. Salazar, and Richard A. Crosby. 2005a. "Programmatic and methodologic review and synthesis of clinic-based sexually transmitted infection risk reduction interventions: research and practice implications." *Seminars in Pediatric Infectious Diseases* 16: 199–218.

DiClemente, Ralph J., Laura F. Salazar, Richard A. Crosby, and Susan L. Rosenthal. 2005b. "Prevention and control of sexually transmitted infections among adolescents: the importance of a socio-ecological perspective—a commentary." *Public Health* 119: 825–36.

DiClemente, Ralph J., Laura F. Salazar, and Richard A. Crosby. 2007. "STD/HIV preventive interventions for adolescents: sustaining effects using an ecological approach." *Journal of Pediatric Psychology* 32(8): 888–906.

DiIorio, Colleen, Maureen Kelley, and Marilyn Hockenberry-Eaton. 1999. "Communication about sexual issues: mothers, fathers, and friends." *Journal of Adolescent Health* 24: 181–9.

Donohew, Lewis, Rick Zimmerman, Pamela S. Cupp, Scott Novak, Susan Colon, and Ritta Abell. 2000. "Sensation seeking, impulsive decision-making, and risky sex: implications for risk-taking and design of interventions." *Personality and Individual Differences* 28: 1079–91.

Downs, Julie S., Pamela J. Murray, Wandi Bruine de Bruina, Joyce Penrose, Claire Palmgren, and Barunch Fischhoff. 2004. "Interactive video behavioral intervention to reduce adolescent females' STD risk: a randomized controlled trial." *Social Science and Medicine* 59: 1561–72.

Dutra, Robin, Kim S. Miller, and Rex Forehand. 1999. "The process and content of sexual communication with adolescents in two-parent families: associations with sexual risk-taking behavior." *AIDS and Behavior* 3: 59–66.

Ennett, Susan T., Belle E. Federman, Susan L. Bailey, Christopher L. Ringwalt, and Michael L. Hubbard. 1999. "HIV-risk behaviors associated with homelessness characteristics in youth." *Journal of Adolescent Health* 25: 344–53.

Family Health International. 2003. *Behavioural surveillance survey in Lao People's Democratic Republic, 2000–2001*. Lao PDR: National Committee for the Control of AIDS Bureau.

Fisher, Jeffrey D., Stephen J. Misovich, and William A. Fisher. 1992. "Impact of perceived social norms on adolescents' AIDS-risk behavior and prevention." In *Adolescents and AIDS: A generation in jeopardy*, ed. Ralph J. DiClemente, 117–36. Thousand Oaks, CA: Sage Publications.

Fisher, Jeffrey D., William A. Fisher, Angela D. Bryan, and Stephen J. Misovich. 2002. "Information–motivation–behavioral skills model-based HIV risk behavior change intervention for inner-city high school youth." *Health Psychology* 21: 177–86.

Fortenberry, J. Dennis, Wanzhu Tu, Jaroslaw Harezlak, Barry P. Katz, and Donald P. Orr. 2002. "Condom use as a function of time in new and established adolescent sexual relationships." *American Journal of Public Health* 92: 211–13.

Fullilove, Robert E. 1998. "Race and sexually transmitted diseases." *Sexually Transmitted Diseases* 25: 130–31.

Grassly, Nicholas C., Geoff P. Garnett, Bernhard Schwartlander, Simon Gregson, and Roy M. Anderson. 2001. "The effectiveness of HIV prevention and the epidemiological context." *Bulletin of the World Health Organization* 79: 1121–32.

Hallfors, Denise D., Bonita J. Iritani, William C. Miller, and Daniel J. Bauer. 2007. "Sexual and drug behavior patterns and HIV and STD racial disparities: the need for new directions." *American Journal of Public Health* 97: 125–32.

Hoffmann, Oliver, Tania Boler, and Bruce Dick. 2006. "Achieving the global goals on HIV among young people most at risk in developing countries: young sex workers, injecting drug users and men who have sex with men." *World Health Organization Technical Report Series*, 938: 287–515.

Indonesia Ministry of Health. 2002. *Behavioural surveillance among populations at risk for HIV*. Jakarta, Indonesia: Directorate of Communicable Disease Control and Environmental Health, Ministry of Health and Central Bureau of Statistics.

Jaccard, James, Patricia J. Dittus, and Vivian V. Gordon. 1996. "Maternal correlates of adolescent sexual and contraceptive behavior." *Family Planning Perspectives* 28: 159–65, 185.

Janz, Nancy K., Marc A. Zimmerman, Patricia A. Wren, Barbara A. Israel, Nicholas Freudenberg, and Rosalind J. Carter. 1996. "Evaluation of 37 AIDS prevention projects: successful approaches and barriers to program effectiveness." *Health Education Quarterly* 23: 80–97.

Jemmott, John B., and Loretta S. Jemmott. 2000. "HIV behavioral interventions for adolescents in community settings." In *The handbook of HIV prevention*, ed. John L. Peterson and Ralph J. DiClemente, 103–28. New York, NY: Plenum Press.

Jemmott, John B., Loretta S. Jemmott, Geoffery T. Fong, and Konstance McCaffree. 1999. "Reducing HIV risk-associated sexual behavior among African American adolescents: testing the generality of intervention effects." *American Journal of Community Psychology* 27: 161–87.

Kahn, Jessica A., Rebekah A. Kaplowitz, Elizabeth Goodman, and Jean S. Emans. 2002. "The association between impulsiveness and sexual risk behaviors in adolescent and young adult women." *Journal of Adolescent Health* 30: 229–32.

Kiragu, Karungari. 2001. "Youth and HIV/AIDS: can we avoid a catastrophe?" *Population Reports, Series L. No. 12*. Baltimore, MD: Johns Hopkins University Bloomberg School of Public Health, Population Information Program.

Kirby, Douglas. 2000. "School-based interventions to prevent unprotected sex and HIV among adolescents." In *The handbook of HIV prevention*, ed. John L. Peterson and Ralph J. DiClemente, 83–102. New York, NY: Plenum Press.

Kirby, Douglas, B. A. Laris, and Lori A. Rolleri. 2005. *Impact of sex and HIV education programs on sexual behavior in developed and developing countries. Youth Research Working Paper No. 2*. Research Triangle Park, NC: Family Health International Youth Net Program.

Ku, Leighton C., Freya L. Sonenstein, and Joseph H. Pleck. 1994. "The dynamics of young men's condom use during and across relationships." *Family Planning Perspectives* 26: 246–51.

Li, Xioaming, Susan Feigelman, and Bonita Stanton. 2000a. "Perceived parental monitoring and health risk behaviors among urban low-income African American children and adolescents." *Journal of Adolescent Health* 43: 43–8.

Li, Xioaming, Bonita Stanton, and Susan Feigelman. 2000b. "Impact of perceived parental monitoring on adolescent risk behavior over 4 years." *Journal of Adolescent Health* 27: 49–56.

Lindberg, Laura D., Leighton Ku, and Freya L. Sonenstein. 1998. "Adolescent males' combined use of condoms with partners' use of female contraceptive methods." *Maternal and Child Health Journal* 2: 201–209.

Lown, Anne E., Karen Winkler, Robert E. Fullilove, and Mindy T. Fullilove. 1993. "Tossin' and tweakin': women's consciousness in the crack culture." In *Women and AIDS: psychological perspectives*, ed. Corinne Squire, 90–106. Thousand Oaks, CA: Sage Publications.

Lyles, Cynthia M., Linda S. Kay, Nicole Crepaz, Jeffrey H. Herbst, Warren F. Passin, Angela S. Kim, Sima M. Rama, Sekhar Thadiparthi, Julia B. DeLuca, and Mary M. Mullins. 2007. "Best-evidence interventions: findings from a systematic review of HIV behavioral interventions for U.S. populations at high risk, 2000–2004." *American Journal of Public Health* 97: 133–43.

McQueen, Kathleen M., and Quarraisha Abdool Karim. 2007. "Practice brief: adolescents and HIV clinical trials: ethics, culture, and context." *Journal of the Association of Nurses in AIDS Care* 18: 78–82.

Magura, Stephen, Sung-Yeon Kang, and Janet L. Shapiro. 1994. "Outcomes of intensive AIDS education for male adolescent drug users in jail." *Journal of Adolescent Health* 15: 457–63.

Miller, Kim S., Rex Forehand, and Beth A. Kotchick. 2000. "Adolescent sexual behavior in two ethnic minority samples: a multi-system perspective delineating targets for prevention." *Adolescence* 35: 313–33.

Millstein, Susan G., and Anna-Barbara Moscicki. 1995. "Sexually transmitted disease in female adolescents: effects of psychosocial factors and high risk behaviors." *Journal of Adolescent Health* 17: 83–90.

Monasch, Roeland, and Mary Mahy. 2006. "Young people: the centre of the HIV epidemic." *World Health Organization Technical Report Series* 938: 15–41.

O'Donnell, Lydia, Ann Stueve, Alexi San Doval, Richard Duran, Deborah Haber, Rebecca Atnafon, Norma Johnson, Uda Grant, Helen Murray, Greg Junn, Julia Tang, and Patricia Piessens. 1999. "The effectiveness of the reach for health community service learning program in reducing early and unprotected sex among urban middle school students." *American Journal of Public Health* 89: 176–81.

Orr, Donald P., Carl D. Langefeld, Barry P. Katz, and Virginia A. Caine. 1996. "Behavioral intervention to increase condom use among high-risk female adolescents." *Journal of Pediatrics* 128: 288–95.

Pedlow, C. Teal, and Michael P. Carey. 2003. "HIV sexual risk-reduction interventions for youth: a review and methodological critique of randomized controlled trials." *Behavior Modification* 27: 135–90.

Pedlow, C. Teal, and Michael P. Carey. 2004. "Developmentally appropriate sexual risk reduction interventions for adolescents: rationale, review of interventions, and recommendations for research and practice." *Annals of Behavioral Medicine* 27: 172–84.

Peter, Jochen, and Patti M. Valkenburg. 2006. "Adolescents' exposure to sexually explicit online material and recreational attitudes toward sex." *Journal of Communication* 56: 639–60.

Peterson, Shani H., Gina M. Wingood, Ralph J. DiClemente, Kathy Harrington, and Susan Davies. 2007. "Images of sexual stereotypes in rap videos and the health of African American female adolescents." *Journal of Women's Health* 16: 1157–64.

Robin, Leah, Patricia Dittus, Daniel Whitaker, Richard A. Crosby, Kathleen Ethier, Jane Mezoff, Kim Miller, and Katina Pappas-Deluca. 2004. "Behavioral interventions to reduce incidence of HIV, STD, and pregnancy among adolescents: a decade in review." *Journal of Adolescent Health* 34: 3–26.

Romer, Daniel, Bonita Stanton, Jennifer Galbraith, Susan Feigelman, Maureen Black, and Xiaoming Li. 1999. "Parental influence on adolescent sexual behavior in high-poverty settings." *Archives of Pediatrics and Adolescent Medicine* 153: 1055–62.

Rosenberg, Philip S., and Robert J. Biggar. 1998. "Trends in HIV incidence among young adults in the United States." *Journal of the American Medical Association* 279: 1894–9.

Rosenthal, Dan, Susan Moore, and Irene Flynn. 1991. "Adolescent self-efficacy, self-esteem and sexual risk-taking." *Journal of Community and Applied Social Psychology* 1: 77–88.

Rotheram-Borus, Mary Jane, Marya Gwadz, Isa Fernandez, and Shobha Srinivasan. 1998. "Timing of HIV interventions on reductions in sexual risk among adolescents." *American Journal of Community Psychology* 26: 73–96.

Sales, Jessica M., Robin Milhausen, and Ralph J. DiClemente. 2006. "A decade in review: building on the experiences of past adolescent STI/HIV interventions to optimize future prevention efforts." *Sexually Transmitted Infections* 82: 431–6.

Sionean, Catlainn, Ralph J. DiClemente, Gina M. Wingood, Richard A. Crosby, Brenda K. Cobb, Kathy Harrington, Susan L. Davies, Edward W. Hook, and M. Kim Oh. 2002. "Psychosocial and behavioral correlates of refusing unwanted intercourse among African American female adolescents." *Journal of Adolescent Health* 55: 55–63.

Small, Stephen A., and Tom Luster. 1994. "Adolescent sexual activity: an ecological, risk-factor approach." *Journal of Marriage and the Family* 56: 181–92.

Smith, Mike U., and Harold P. Katner. 1995. "Quasi-experimental evaluation of three AIDS prevention activities for maintaining knowledge, improving attitudes, and changing risk behaviors of high school seniors." *AIDS Education and Prevention* 7: 391–402.

Spencer, Jennifer M., Gregory D. Zimet, Matthew C. Aalsma, and Donald P. Orr. 2002. "Self-esteem as a predictor of initiation of coitus in early adolescents." *Pediatrics* 109: 581–4.

St. Lawrence, Janet, Richard A. Crosby, Lisa Belcher, Nanolla Yazdani, and Ted L. Brasfield. 1999. "Sexual risk reduction and anger management interventions for incarcerated male adolescents: a randomized controlled trial of two interventions." *Journal of Sex Education and Therapy* 24: 9–17.

St. Lawrence, Janet, Richard A. Crosby, Ted L. Brasfield, and Robert E. O'Bannon. 2002. "Reducing STD and HIV risk behavior of substance-dependent adolescents: a randomized controlled trial." *Journal of Consulting and Clinical Psychology* 70: 1010–21.

Stover, John, Stefano Bertozzi, Juan-Pablo Gutierrez, Neff Walker, Karen A. Stanecki, Robert Greener, Eleanor Gouws, Catherine Hankins, Geoff P. Garnett, Joshua A. Salomon, Ties J. Boerma, Paul De Lay, and Peter D. Ghys. 2006. "The global impact of scaling up HIV/AIDS prevention programs in low-and middle-income countries." *Science* 311: 1474–6.

Tremblay, Richard E., Louis C. Masse, Frank Vitaro, and Patricia L. Dobkin. 1995. "The impact of friends' deviant behavior on early onset of delinquency: longitudinal data from 6 to 13 years of age." *Developmental Psychopathology* 7: 649–67.

UNAIDS. 2005. *AIDS epidemic update: December 2005*. Geneva, Switzerland: UNAIDS/WHO.

UNAIDS. 2006. *Report on the global AIDS epidemic: a UNAIDS 10th anniversary special edition*. Geneva, Switzerland: UNAIDS.

Vandepitte, Jan, Rob Lyerla, Gina Dallabetta, Frederick Crabbé, Michel Alary, and Anne Buve. 2006. "Estimates of the number of female sex workers in different regions of the world." *Sexually Transmitted Infections* 82, supplement 3. Retrieved on September 1, 2007 from http://sti.bmj.com/cgi/content/abstract/82/suppl_3/iii18.

Weisman, Carol S., Stacy Plichta, Constance A. Nathanson, Margaret Ensminger, and J. Courtland Robinson. 1991. "Consistency of condom use for disease prevention among adolescent users of oral contraceptives." *Family Planning Perspectives* 23: 71–4.

Whitaker, Daniel J., and Kim S. Miller. 2000. "Parent–adolescent discussions about sex and condoms: impact on peer influences of sexual risk behavior." *Journal of Adolescent Research* 15: 251–73.

Wilson, Michelle D., Mariana Kastrinakis, Lawrence D'Angelo, and Pamela Getson. 1994. "Attitudes, knowledge, and behavior regarding condom use in urban black adolescent males." *Adolescence* 29: 13–26.

Wingood, Gina M., and Ralph J. DiClemente. 1996. "HIV sexual risk reduction interventions for women: a review." *American Journal of Preventive Medicine* 12: 209–17.

Wingood, Gina M., Ralph J. DiClemente, Jay M. Bernhardt, Kathy Harrington, Susan L. Davies, Alyssa A. Robillard, and Edward W. Hook III. 2003. "A prospective study of exposure to rap music videos and African American female adolescents' health." *American Journal of Public Health* 93: 437–9.

Wingood, Gina M., Ralph J. DiClemente, Kathy Harrington, Susan L. Davies, Edward W. Hook III, and M. Kim Oh. 2001. "Exposure to X-rated movies and adolescents' sexual and contraceptive-related attitudes and behaviors." *Pediatrics* 107: 1116–19.

World Health Organization (WHO). 2007a. *Global strategy for the prevention and control of sexually transmitted infections: 2006–2015*. Geneva: Switzerland: WHO Press.

World Health Organization (WHO). 2007b. *Towards universal access: scaling up priority HIV/AIDS interventions in the health sector: progress report, April 2007*. Geneva, Switzerland: WHO Press.

Zenilman, Jonathan M., Carol S. Weisman, Anne M. Rampalo, Nancy J. Ellish, Dawn M. Upchurch, Edward W. Hook, and David Celentano. 1995. "Condom use to prevent incident STD: the validity of self-reported condom use." *Sexually Transmitted Diseases* 22: 15–21.

Zimet, Gregory D., Debra L. Bunch, Trina M. Anglin, Rina Lazebnik, Paul Williams, and Daniel P. Krowchuk. 1992. "Relationship of AIDS-related attitudes to sexual behavior changes in adolescents." *Journal of Adolescent Health* 13: 493–8.

CHAPTER 14

Evidence-Based Community Interventions

The Community Readiness Model

H. Virginia McCoy, Robert Malow, Ruth W. Edwards, Anne Thurland, and Rhonda Rosenberg

ABSTRACT

Translational research has been prioritized by funders of HIV/AIDS behavioral risk prevention research in ongoing efforts to bring efficacious interventions to culturally diverse and underserved populations and communities. Adaptation of evidence-based interventions to population and community context is an important part of this work, and the Community Readiness Model is one strategy for informing and facilitating this process. This chapter discusses the history, methods, and significance of this model and presents an application of its use in the U.S. Virgin Islands, a U.S. territory in the Caribbean.

OVERVIEW

Just as the basic sciences of HIV prevention are increasingly allowing a clearer view of individual variation in biological risk and susceptibility (Ames and McBride 2006), so too are the sociobehavioral sciences demonstrating that there is *community* variation in how HIV risk—in all its complicated variations—will be acknowledged and met (Foster-Fishman, Cantillon, Pierce, and Egeren 2007). A long, hard lesson of the AIDS epidemic is the complexity of community as well as individual sensibility and capacity in responding to the risk from HIV (Jumper-Thurman, Vernon, and Plested 2007). This has meant that the development of evidence-based prevention interventions has been a necessary but not sufficient condition for making progress in reducing individual behavioral risk reduction. Consequently, translational research has been prioritized in recent years, emphasizing participatory designs, techniques of cultural adaptation, and community capacity building (Solomon, Card and Malow 2006).

Foster-Fishman, Cantillon, Pierce, and Egeren (2007: 103) have recently noted that "[d]espite significant interest in community capacity and readiness across many disciplines and by foundations and federal funders, the measurement of these two constructs is still in its infancy." Before the contributions by researchers at the Tri-Ethnic Center for Prevention and Research at Colorado State University, no methodology or tools existed for empirically studying the phenomenon of community readiness, except for partial theoretical antecedents such as community development theory (Jumper-Thurman 2000).

The Community Readiness Model offers one solution for responding to this issue of translating research to practice. As a public health approach for intervention design, Community Readiness (CR) directly links people, places, and time—core elements of epidemiological science—on the basis of a community's capacity to make use of available prevention strategies. Moreover, it links the psychological with the structural because its theoretical, evaluative, and intercessional features are rooted in the research tradition of individual psychological readiness for treatment and the field of community development for effective social action. In the most basic sense, Community Readiness reinforces the importance of taking a case history in planning a prevention response. It combines objective and participatory elements by integrating the observations of researchers with those of community members and government representatives and providing a framework for collaboration between academic institutions, community organizations, and all levels of government.

International research has demonstrated the potential of structural interventions for reducing HIV risk. For example, in Thailand, there was an 80 percent increase in condom use among commercial sex workers following implementation of a policy requiring the use of condoms in brothels (Sumartojo, Doll, Holtgrave, Gayle, and Merson 2000). HIV prevention interventions at the community level, such as the Population Opinion Leader, have already demonstrated their usefulness in increasing condom use among gay men (Kelly, St. Lawrence, Diaz, Stevenson, Hauth, Brasfield, Kalichman, Smith, and Andrew 1991; Kelly, St. Lawrence, Stevenson, Hauth, Kalichman, Diaz, Brasfield, Koob, and Morgan 1992; Kelly 2004). In addition, they show encouraging signs of being able to reduce risk behaviors among female commercial sex workers and the female sexual partners of injection drug users (Lauby, Smith, Stark, Person, and Adams 2000). Recent work by Morisky et al. (Morisky, Ang, Coly, and Tiglao 2004; Morisky, Chiao, Stein, and Malow 2005; Morisky and Ebin 2000) underscore how participatory and peer components aimed at the social organizational level can have dramatic effects on not only individual risk behavior, but also social norms—even among commercial sex workers and the managers of bar and entertainment establishments.

The development of participatory approaches may greatly benefit HIV/AIDS prevention. Over the past two decades the use of collaboration has escalated, in part because opportunities for partnerships of mutual benefit are created through joining different sectors of the community (DiClemente, Crosby, and Kegler 2002). They cite the National Heart, Lung and Blood Institute's community advisory boards to plan and implement cardiovascular disease prevention programs in the Stanford Three Community and Five City Projects and the Minnesota and Pawtucket Heart Health community (DiClemente, Crosby, and Kegler 2002). Feinberg, Greenberg, and Osgood (2004) researched factors associated with effectiveness of 21 community coalitions in Pennsylvania which were focusing on implementation of the Communities that Care (CTC) prevention program addressing substance use. They found a strong link between Community Readiness and the perceived effectiveness of a coalition with readiness being mediated by internal coalition functioning. In addition, success of a community-based participatory research partnership was demonstrated in the Detroit community—Academic Urban Research Center (URC) (Lantz et al. 2001). These projects brought together diverse sectors of the community which otherwise might not have a chance to communicate or use a community base with academic research advisors or community advisors.

It is important to note here the argument by Castro and Farmer (2005) that HIV/AIDS-related stigma is more a function of ineffective or poor-quality treatment and intervention than the influence of adverse sociocultural norms. Typically, the effectiveness of interventions is viewed more as a scientific or cost-saving value rather than as directly tied to perceptions of a disease and a community's readiness to cope with it. In fact, community sources of knowledge often do not have credible, evidentiary standing within public health models, except as a preparatory or adjunct component. Legitimizing frameworks are needed, according to Castro and Farmer (2005), which can integrate academic and community knowledge so that the voices of the community are heard. The Community Readiness Model provides this bridge and resource for documentation that can be accessible to both academic researchers and community leaders and health workers. The basic premise is that all partners in HIV/AIDS prevention need a translational tool for turning community and participatory sources into usable knowledge that can be applied to improving the effectiveness of intervention and treatment.

BACKGROUND

Like most of the Caribbean region, the U.S. Virgin Islands has witnessed alarming increases in AIDS and HIV. Among U.S. territories, U.S. Virgin Islands ranks second to Puerto Rico in AIDS cases (15.6/100,000) (CDC 2005a); however, the AIDS rates among women adults and adolescents (19.4/100,000) is higher than in Puerto Rico (19.4/100,000) (CDC 2005b). The CDC's 2005 HIV/AIDS Surveillance Report estimates that the prevalence of adults and adolescents living with HIV infection declined between 2003 (285.2/100,000) and 2005 (274.5/100,000), and living with AIDS declined from 345.4 to 343.0 (CDC 2003, 2005a).

The U.S. Virgin Islands, a U.S. territory, has a population of 108,612 and consists of four main islands—St. Croix, St. Thomas, St. John, and Water Island, situated east of Puerto Rico in the Caribbean. Each island is distinctly different from the other in population composition, size, and economy. Water Island has the smallest population (161) and is primarily residential; St. John is the next largest, more than half of which is national park and with a population of just over 4,000; St. Thomas has the strongest tourism economy and cruise ship traffic; St. Croix is the largest island, where the local residents call themselves Crucians and the island accommodates one of the world's largest petroleum refineries (U.S. Central Intelligence Agency 2005). The population is 76.19 percent black, 13.09 percent white, and 13.99 percent Hispanic (U.S. Census Bureau 2000); 74 percent are West Indian, most of whom were born in the U.S. Virgin Islands, 13 percent from the U.S. mainland, and 5 percent from Puerto Rico. Virgin Islanders form a close-knit society, with constant interaction on both the social and professional levels. A Community Advisory Board (CAB),[1] composed of representatives from all three islands who were community leaders with expertise HIV/AIDS, was assembled to collaborate with researchers to provide the essential community perspective in applying the CR Model. The CAB comprises both the systemic and individual stakeholders who have sufficient influence to promote needed interventions. They are local HIV/AIDS advocates, health department officials, substance abuse treatment agency staff, and other community leaders.

HISTORY OF THE COMMUNITY READINESS MODEL

The CR Model is based on two research traditions: psychological readiness for treatment and community development. The Colorado State University (CSU) research team that developed the model in 1995 has continued to refine it as they have conducted over 5,000 key informant interviews in over 1,500 communities throughout the U.S., addressing a wide variety of social, health, and environmental issues over the past 20 years.

The development of the model followed standard procedures for the development of anchored rating scales, working directly with communities on problems from substance abuse to violence (Dickinson and Tice 1977; Edwards et al. 2000; Oetting et al. 1995). The team has applied the model to HIV/AIDS prevention and conducted interviews in 30 rural communities throughout the U.S. (from 3 to 5 per community) including African-American, Mexican-American and white, non-Hispanic communities (Plested, Edwards, and Jumper-Thurman 2007). Findings of that study showed relatively low levels of readiness in rural communities to address HIV/AIDS prevention, with Mexican-American communities even somewhat lower than white, non-Hispanic or African-American communities (Plested, Edwards, and Jumper-Thurman 2007). Community knowledge of the issue—the need for HIV/AIDS prevention efforts—was a key dimension which was particularly low, indicating the importance of focusing on culturally appropriate and targeted education about HIV/AIDS infection and what can be done to prevent it.

The CSU team has since conducted over 200 workshops to train community members and professionals in how to use the model to develop efficient, effective, and economical local solutions to local problems including youth drug use, intimate partner violence, methamphetamine use, HIV/AIDS prevention, cultural competency of organizations, traffic and highway issues, prevention of head injuries, etc. Many community groups have used the CR Model as integral parts of applications for funding and to guide design and implementation of community interventions. Studies utilizing the model conducted by its CSU authors suggest a high level of success in supporting the development of community-wide prevention efforts, success measured as moving communities to higher levels of community prevention readiness in whatever the topic of interest (Edwards, Jumper-Thurman, and Plested 2000; Kelly, Edwards, Comello, Plested, Jumper-Thurman, and Slater 2003; Slater, Edwards, Plested, Jumper-Thurman, Kelly, Comello, and Keefe 2005).

COMMUNITY READINESS METHODS

Community Readiness is assessed by conducting semi-structured interviews with key members of the community, asking a set of questions on each of six dimensions about what is occurring in that community. Key respondents are selected for their knowledge of community affairs, not necessarily for formal leadership positions or status. An example of the questions used to assess the dimension of community climate for HIV/AIDS can be found in Appendix 1. Responses to the questions are then used by two trained raters (coming to agreement) to rate the community on each of the six dimensions of readiness using anchored rating scales (Plested, Edwards, and Jumper-Thurman 2006). The scores on the dimensions are averaged to achieve an overall score of community readiness, but primary attention is paid to the scores on the individual dimensions for guiding development of prevention strategies.

Reliability of the method was determined by interviews of key respondents by a number of different interviewers and scoring of the transcripts by independent scorers, which resulted in very close agreement on each dimension and stage. Results of interviews with more than three key informants (four, five, or six) proved generally consistent with the first three interviews. Consequently, in small communities especially, reliable data can be obtained from as few as three key respondents (Oetting, Jumper-Thurman, Plested, and Edwards 2001). The use of key respondent interviews is an acceptable method in ethnographic research (Agar 1996).

The CR Model describes nine stages of community readiness (see Exhibit 14.1) based on six dimensions: Community Efforts (programs, activities, policies, etc.); Community Knowledge of the Efforts; Leadership (formal and informal); Community Climate; Community Knowledge About the Issue; and Resources Related to the Issue (people, time, money, space, etc.). There are six processes involved in application of the CR Model: identifying the issue, defining the "community," conducting key interviews, scoring to determine the readiness level, developing strategies (conducting workshops), and implementing action plans which result in community change (Plested, Edwards, and Jumper-Thurman 2004). From a sound theoretical basis, the CR Model offers a respectful, step-by step methodology for involving communities in finding solutions to local problems utilizing local resources.

The CR Model suggests appropriate types of interventions for each level of readiness that will lead to changing community norms, behaviors, and attitudes. It sets the stage for community acceptance and understanding of HIV and involves community members in creating efforts that result in community ownership.

Effective community prevention must be based on involvement of multiple sys-

Exhibit 14.1 Stages of Community Readiness

Stages	*Brief description*	*Goal*
Stage 1: No Awareness	Issue is not generally recognized by the community or leaders as a problem.	Raise awareness of issue.
Stage 2: Denial/Resistance	At least some community members recognize that it is a problem, but there is little or no recognition that it might be a local problem or resistance to addressing it.	Raise awareness that problem exists in community.
Stage 3: Vague Awareness	Some may feel that there is a local problem, but there is no immediate motivation to do anything about it.	Raise awareness that community can do something.
Stage 4: Preplanning	There is clear recognition that something must be done, and there may even be a committee. However, efforts are not focused or detailed.	Raise awareness with concrete ideas to address problem.
Stage 5: Preparation	Active leaders begin planning in earnest. Community offers modest support of efforts.	Gather information with which to plan efforts and/or programs.
Stage 6: Initiation	Enough information is available to justify efforts, and activities are underway.	Provide community-specific information.
Stage 7: Stabilization	Activities are supported by administrators or community decision makers. Staff are trained and experienced.	Stabilize efforts/programs.
Stage 8: Confirmation/Expansion	Standard efforts are in place. Community members feel comfortable in using services and support expansions. Local data regularly obtained and utilized to evaluate effectiveness of efforts and guide expansion.	Evaluate, expand and enhance services.
Stage 9: High Level of Community Ownership	Detailed and sophisticated knowledge exists about prevalence, risk factors and causes. Staff members are highly trained. Effective evaluation is in place and utilized routinely to monitor effectiveness and need for change.	Maintain momentum and continue growth.

tems and utilization of within-community resources and strengths. Efforts must be culturally relevant and accepted as long term in nature. The CR Model takes these factors into account and provides a research-based tool that focuses and directs community efforts (Edwards, Jumper-Thurman, and Plested 2000). The six dimensions on which determination of readiness level is based address levels of *acceptance* and *awareness* of HIV/AIDS as a community problem that needs to be addressed among members of the community and their leadership.

In summary, the CR Model has been found useful in program development and evaluation, research, community-based prevention, and organizational analysis. The Model is useful in identifying resources, identifying obstacles, providing to a community an assessment of how ready it is to address a specific issue, and identifying appropriate intervention strategies appropriate for the community's stage of readiness. The procedures include identifying the issue, defining community, conducting key respondent interviews, scoring to determine readiness level, and developing strategies. The CR Model facilitates community ownership, utilizes existing resources—deemphasizing money, provides an evaluation tool, requires no "outside experts," creates a community vision translatable into a sustainable effort, and guides development of culturally appropriate strategies.

FINDINGS FROM APPLICATION OF THE CR MODEL IN THE U.S. VIRGIN ISLANDS

In order to assess readiness of residents of the U.S. Virgin Islands to address HIV/AIDS, key interviews (see Appendix 1) were conducted on the islands of St. Thomas, St. Croix, and St. John with 12 respondents (5 in St. Thomas, 5 in St. Croix, and 2 in St. John) including police officers, senators, educators, social and health service providers, and other community members. Each island was assumed to be a separate community, following the CR Model that community is defined as it relates to a targeted issue. Respondents, recruited by community residents and Advisory Board members, were asked questions addressing each of the six dimensions (see Appendix 1 for sample questions) and each dimension was scored using an anchored rating scale based on the nine levels of readiness identified in the CR Model. The interviews were conducted by a Master's-level interviewer from the West Indies and then were scored independently by three scorers using an anchored rating scale. Scores were averaged across scorers, with high reliability among scorers, and interviews for each island, producing the dimension scores and an overall score for each island (see Exhibit 14.2).

All three communities (islands) scored highest in Knowledge of Community Efforts (programs, activities, policies). Although the number of such efforts was small, this indicated that respondents recognized these activities as having been planned and/or implemented.

Representative comments included, "local ads on the radio, ranging from condom use to abstinence" and "workshops, AIDS Awareness Day." All three communities scored lowest in Community Climate, indicating a sense of hopelessness or general lack of knowledge that HIV is a local problem and affects them. Representative comments included, "they are aware and sometimes they are scared; religion, culture, and stigma act as barriers" and "there is a stigma. People think AIDS is a curse, a sin from God; people think that it won't happen to them. I think we are in denial about the impact of AIDS."

Overall, the island of St. John, the smallest, most ethnically homogeneous, wealthiest population of all three islands, and in the same health service district as St. Thomas, scored at Stage 3—Vague Awareness. As described by the authors of the model, in this stage, "there is a general feeling among some in the community that there is a local problem and that something ought to be done about it, but there is no immediate motivation to do anything. There may be stories or anecdotes about a problem, but ideas about why the problem occurs and who has the problem tend to be stereotyped and/or vague. Few identifiable leaders exist. Community climate does not serve to motivate leaders" (Edwards, Jumper-Thurman, Plested, Oetting, and Swanson 2000: 298). The CR Model suggests that communities at Stage 3 need to raise awareness that the issue can, in fact, be dealt with by the community. Efforts need to be fairly low intensity at this stage in order to begin raising awareness. Rather than attempt to have community informational meetings at this stage, efforts such as distributing flyers at local events and putting up posters pertaining to local HIV/AIDS issues in public places have been found by communities to be more effective. If they show local relevance, newspaper editorials and articles presenting general information about HIV/AIDS and its implications to local communities can be effective at this stage.

The findings show that, overall, St. Thomas and St. Croix scored at the Stage 4 of Prevention Readiness: Preplanning. The

Exhibit 14.2 Community Readiness dimensions and scores by Island

Dimension area	*Typical comments*	*St. Thomas*	*St. Croix*	*St. John*
Community Efforts	"AIDS Awareness Day" "condoms during Carnival"	6.80	5.45	6.75
Knowledge of Community Efforts	"we are slowly progressing in awareness and involvement"	3.85	4.55	3.00
Leadership	"concerned . . . most are reactive" "not involved enough"	3.50	4.75	3.75
Community Climate	"there is a stigma" "we are in denial"	2.00	3.65	2.00
Knowledge About Community Issues	"there are still misconceptions" "they know the difference between HIV and AIDS"	4.70	5.50	3.37
Resources Related to the Issue	"first turn to a private physician" "turn to a family member"	4.50	4.25	3.87
Overall		**4.20**	**4.69**	**3.79**

description of this stage states that "there is clear recognition on the part of at least some that there is a local problem and that something should be done about it. There are identifiable leaders, and there may even be a committee, but efforts are not focused or detailed. There is discussion, but no real planning of actions to address the problem. Community climate is beginning to acknowledge the necessity of dealing with the problem" (Edwards, Jumper-Thurman, Plested, Oetting, and Swanson 2000: 299).

DEVELOPMENT OF APPROPRIATE INTERVENTION STRATEGIES

According to the Community Readiness Model, the goal of efforts in communities at this stage is to present concrete ideas for action to address HIV/AIDS. Appropriate activities might include visiting community leaders to gain their support for addressing the problem locally. At this stage it may be useful to conduct focus groups with local residents to discuss local issues. Increasing media exposure to HIV/AIDS issues through public service announcements on television and radio are likely to be effective.

The real key to effective prevention efforts lies in paying attention to the scores on each of the dimensions. By examining each dimension score in Exhibit 14.2, it is clear that, although overall readiness levels are in the Vague Awareness to Preplanning range for the islands, the Community Climate score for all three islands lags behind scores on the other dimensions. Without raising this readiness level, community-wide efforts for prevention will not be effective. Stigma and judgmental beliefs about HIV/AIDS infection prevalent on all three islands needs to be addressed first in order to provide a sound foundation for HIV/AIDS prevention efforts to go forward. In the process of addressing community attitudes giving rise to stigma, the community must acknowledge and address the pervasiveness of the perception that nothing can really be done, which is reflected in the low scores on the dimension of Community Climate and which likely is a large part of why previous efforts at prevention of HIV/AIDS have not been effective.

While addressing stigma and judgmental beliefs is only a part of the answer to HIV in the U.S. Virgin Islands, the CR Model suggests that raising Community Climate will help prepare the communities to have more success with future interventions. Better-quality services and interventions are expected to arise out of the community problem-solving efforts underway. Using the suggested strategies, such as media advocacy in St. John and modeling of local

HIV-infected persons in St. Croix, to address stigma and discrimination should move community readiness along the stages of change and not allow stigma to become "markers for failure" (Castro and Farmer 2005: 57).

The findings of the Community Readiness assessment validated the informal assessments of community members. Prior to viewing the findings of the CR survey and scores, the members "guessed" the scores. This demonstrates that the community members are aware of their community's attitude and knowledge in respect to HIV/AIDS. Following the scientific method in the CR Model merely confirmed their assessments and heightened their sense of knowledge and power about addressing HIV in their community. The assessment helped empower them to confront the issues of prevention using community action. Guided by the discussion of stage-appropriate strategies set forth in the CR Model, the community members brainstormed strategies to move the communities along the stages of prevention readiness. Their recommendations included media campaigns with spokespersons, faith community involvement, outreach, and engagement of community leaders. While these are not unusual strategies, they work because they begin at the stage where the community is "ready" for prevention. The ideas provided by the community members are valuable to guide prevention efforts in the U.S. Virgin Islands because they know their communities and their recommendations are culturally appropriate to reach the population, validating the CR Model. For example, previous campaigns which used "off islanders" as role models failed miserably, while local celebrities would more likely personalize the risks for HIV. Their input on tailoring prevention efforts specifically for their communities will greatly aid the creation of effective HIV/AIDS prevention programs.

CONCLUSION

The CR Model provides a participatory tool for empirical measurement of Community Readiness. It can be utilized by the communities to provide guidance in selecting intervention efforts likely to have the most impact based on the stage of readiness as programs are implemented. The integral role that the community participation brings is a collective history and ownership. Community partners are the best equipped to identify the "HIV risk environment" in their communities (Rhodes et al. 2005), the interplay of social, structural, and political-economic factors, that will lead to the development of effective HIV prevention interventions. The CR Model requires respect for cultural differences and response from various community power structures.

In conclusion, the adaptation and use of evidence-based intervention strategies derived from the CR Model may impact how various intervention efforts will contribute to successful community change outcomes. Probably the most important measure of success is the level of health change to be effected by the translation process (Roussos and Fawcett 2000; Zakocs and Edwards 2006). Communities that follow standard frameworks of adaptation may, in fact, experience unintended outcomes of empowerment through enhancing their capabilities for decision-making, consensus-building strategies, priority-setting and other related skills (Zakocs and Edwards 2006; Soloman, Card, and Malow 2006).

Appendix 1 Example of Community Readiness Model Interview Questions on Community Climate Dimension

D. COMMUNITY CLIMATE

19. Describe____ (name of your community).
20. Are there ever any circumstances in which members of your community might think that this issue should be tolerated? Please explain.
21. How does the community support the efforts to address this issue?
22. What are the primary obstacles to efforts addressing this issue in your community?
23. Based on the answers that you have provided so far, what do you think is the

overall feeling among community members regarding this issue?

Source: Barbara A. Plested, Ruth W. Edwards, and Pamela Jumper-Thurman. *Community Readiness: A Handbook for Successful Change*. Ft. Collins, CO: Tri-Ethnic Center for Prevention Research, Colorado State University, 2004.

ACKNOWLEDGMENT

Barbara Plested; Pamela Jumper-Thurman of CASAE, Colorado State University; Brenda Luna of Florida International University; USVI Community Advisory Board Members (Anne Thurland, Chanie Lang, Marjorie Williams, Donna Walcott-Kelly MPH, Lois Sanders, Dr. Frank Mills, Maren Roebuck, Pat Odoms, Josephine Shim, Fran Jacobson, Dr. Gayann Hall).

NOTE

1. A Community Planning Board (CPB), funded by CDC, acts in an official capacity to advise the Health Department and other government officials on HIV/AIDS. The Community Advisory Board supports the research project's aims of HIV prevention among substance users. A few of the members overlap the CPB and the CAB.

REFERENCES AND FURTHER READING

Agar, Michael. C (1996). *The Professional Stranger: An Informal Introduction to Ethnography*, 2nd edition, Academic Press.

Ames, Susan and McBride, C (2006). "Translating Genetics, Cognitive Science, and Other Basic Science Research Findings into Applications for Pevention." *Evaluation and the Health Professions*, 29(3), 277–301.

Castro, A. and Farmer, P. (2005). "Understanding and Addressing AIDS-Related Stigma: From Anthropological Theory to Clinical Practice in Haiti." *American Journal of Public Health*, 95(1), 53–59.

Centers for Disease Control and Prevention (CDC). (2003). *HIV/AIDS Surveillance Report*. Centers for Disease Control, 15(1): 1–46. Retrieved on December 6, 2004, from http://www.cdc.gov/hiv/stats/2003 surveillanceReport.pdf.

Centers for Disease Control and Prevention (CDC). (2005a). *HIV/AIDS Surveillance Report*. Centers for Disease Control, 15(1): 1–46. Retrieved on October 12, 2007 from http:/0-www.cdc.gov.mill1.sjlibrary .org/hiv/topics/surveillance/resources/slides/epidemiol ogy/slides/EPI-AIDS.pdf and http://0-www.cdc.gov .mill1.sjlibrary.org/hiv/topics/surveillance/resources/ reports/2005report/map1.htm.

Centers for Disease Control and Prevention (CDC). (2005b). *HIV/AIDS Surveillance Report*. Centers for Disease Control, 15(1): 1–46. Retrieved on October 12, 2007 from www.cdc.gov/hiv/topics/surveillance/ resources/slides/women/slides/Women.pdf.

Dickinson, T.L. and Tice, T.E. (1977). "The Discriminant Validity of Scales Developed by Retranslation." *Personnel Psychology*, 30, 217–228.

DiClemente, R.J., Crosby, R.A. and Kegler, M.C.C. (2002). *Emerging Theories in Health Promotion Practice and Research: Strategies for Improving Public Health*, San Francisco, Jossey-Bass.

Edwards, R.W., Jumper-Thurman, P., Plested, B.A., Oetting, E.R. and Swanson, L. (2000). "Community Readiness: Research to Practice." *Journal of Community Psychology*, 28(3), 291–307.

Feinberg, M.E., Greenberg, M.T. and Osgood, D.W. (2004). "Readiness, Functioning and Perceived Effectiveness in Community Prevention Coalitions: A Study of Communities That Care." *American Journal of Community Psychology*, 33(3/4), 163–176.

Foster-Fishman, P.G., Cantillon, D., Pierce, S.J. and Van Egeren, L.A. (2007). "Building an Active Citizenry: The Role of Neighborhood Problems, Readiness, and Capacity for Change." *American Journal of Community Psychology* (2007), 39, 91–106.

Jumper-Thurman, P. (2000). In Bigfoot D, (ed.) *Community Readiness: A promising model for community healing (Native American topic specific mongraph series)*. Oklahoma: University of Oklahoma Health Sciences Center, US Department of Justice. http:// www.triethniccenter.colostate.edu/docs/Article3.pdf

Jumper-Thurman, P., Plested, B.A., Edwards, R.W., Helm, H.M., Oetting, E.R. (2001). "Using the Community Readiness Model in Native Communities." In J. E. Trimble and F. Beauvais (eds.), *Health promotion and substance abuse prevention among American Indian and Alaska Native communities. Issues in cultural competence* (DHHS Publication No. SMA 99-3440), pp. 129–158. Rockville, MD: U.S. Department of Health and Human Services.

Jumper-Thurman, P., Vernon, I.S. and Plested, B. (2007). "Advancing HIV/AIDS Prevention among American Indians through Capacity Building and the Community Readiness Model." *Journal of Public Health Management and Practice*, January (Suppl.), S49–S54.

Kelly, J.A. (2004). "Popular Opinion Leaders and HIV Prevention Peer Education: Resolving Discrepant Findings, and Implications for the Development of Effective Community Programmes." *AIDS Care*, 16(2), 139–150.

Kelly, J.A., St. Lawrence, J.S., Diaz, Y.E., Stevenson, L.Y., Hauth, A.C., Brasfield, T.L., Kalichman, S.C., Smith, J.E. and Andrew, M.E. (1991). "HIV Risk Behavior Reduction Following Intervention with Key Opinion Leaders of Population: An Experimental Analysis." *American Journal of Public Health*, 81(2), 168–171.

Kelly, J.A., St. Lawrence, J.S., Stevenson, L.Y., Hauth, A.C., Kalichman, S.C., Diaz, Y.E., Brasfield, T.L., Koob, J.J., and Morgan, M.G. (1992). "Community

AIDS/HIV Risk Reduction: The Effects of Endorsements by Popular People in Three Cities." *American Journal of Public Health*, 82(11), 1483–1489.

Kelly, K., Edwards, R.W., Comello, M.L.G., Plested, B.A., Jumper-Thurman, P.J., and Slater, M.D. (2003). "The Community Readiness Model: A Complementary Approach to Social Marketing." *Marketing Theory*, 3(4), 411–426.

Lantz, P.M., Viruell-Fuentes E., Israel, B.A., Softley, D. and Guzman, R. (2001). "Can Communities and Academia Work Together on Public Health Research? Evaluation Results from a Community-Based Participatory Research Partnership in Detroit." *Journal of Urban Health*, 78(3), 495–507.

Lauby, J.L., Smith, P.J., Stark, M., Person, B. and Adams, J. (2000). "A Community-Level HIV Prevention Intervention for Inner-City Women: Results of the Women and Infants Demonstration Projects." *American Journal of Public Health*, 90(2), 216–222.

Morisky, D.E., Ang, A., Coly, A. and Tiglao, T.V. (2004). "A model HIV/AIDS Risk Reduction Program in the Philippines: A Comprehensive Community-Based Approach through Participatory Action Research." *Health Promotion International*, 19(1), 69–76.

Morisky D.E., Chiao, C., Stein, J.A., Malow, R. (2005) "Impact of Social and Structural Influence Interventions on Condom Use and Sexually Transmitted Infections among Establishment-Based Female Bar Workers in the Philippines." *Journal of Psychology and Human Sexuality* 17(1/2), 45–63.

Morisky, D.E. and Ebin, V.J. (2000). "The Effectiveness of Peer Education in HIV/STD Education." In S.B. Kar, R. Alcalay and S.J. Alex (eds.), *Health Communication: A Multicultural Perspective*. Sage Publications, Inc.

Oetting, E.R., Donnermeyer, J.F., Plested, B.A., Edwards, R.W., Kelly, K. and Beauvais, F. (1995). "Assessing Community Readiness for Prevention." *International Journal of the Addictions* 30(6), 659–683.

Oetting, E.R., Jumper-Thurman, P., Plested, B.A. and Edwards, R.W. (2001). "Community Readiness and Health Services." *Substance Use and Misuse* 36 (6/7), 825–843.

Plested, B.A., Edwards, R.W. and Jumper-Thurman, P. (2004). *Community Readiness: A Handbook for Successful Change*. Fort Collins, CO: Tri-Ethnic Center for Prevention Research, Colorado State University.

Plested, B.A., Edwards, R.W. and Jumper-Thurman, P. (2007) "Disparities in Community Readiness for HIV/AIDS prevention." *Substance Use and Misuse* 42, 729–739.

Rhodes, T., Singer, M., Bourgois, P., Friedman, S.R. and Strathdee, S.A. (2005). "The Social Structural Production of HIV Risk Among Injecting Drug Users." *Social Science and Medicine*, 61, 1026–1044.

Roussos S.T. and Fawcett, S.B. (2000). "A Review of Collaborative Partnerships as a Strategy for Improving Community Health." *Annual Review of Public Health*, 21, 369–402.

Slater, M.D., Edwards, R.W., Plested, B.A., Jumper-Thurman, P.J., Kelly, K.J., Comello, M.L.G. and Keefe, T.J. (2005). "Using Community Readiness Key Informant Assessments in a Randomized Group Prevention Trial: Impact of a Participatory Community Media Intervention." *Journal of Community Health*, 30(1), 39–53.

Solomon, J., Card, J.J. and Malow, R.M. (2006). "Adapting Efficacious Interventions: Advancing Translational Research in HIV Prevention." *Evaluation and the Health Professions*, 29(2), 162–194.

Sumartojo, E., Doll, L., Holtgrave, D., Gayle, H. and Merson, M. (2000). "Structural Factors in HIV Prevention: Concepts, Examples, and Implications for Research." *AIDS*, 14 (Suppl. 1), S3–S10.

U.S. Census Bureau. (2003). *2000 Census of Population and Housing, Social, Economic, and Housing Characteristics, PHC-4-VI, U.S. Virgin Islands*. U.S. Census Bureau, U.S. Department of Commerce, Washington DC. Retrieved on December 4, 2006 from http://www.census.gov/prod/cen2000/phc-4-vi.pdf.

U.S. Central Intelligence Agency (2005). "The World Factbook—U.S. Virgin Islands." Retrieved on December 4, 2006 from http://www.cia.gov/cia/publications/ factbook/geos/vq.html.

Zakocs, R.C. and Edwards, E.M. (2006). "What Explains Community Coalition Effectiveness? A Review of the Literature." *American Journal of Preventive Medicine*, 30(4), 351–361.

Latex gloves being washed for reuse in a Haitian hospital

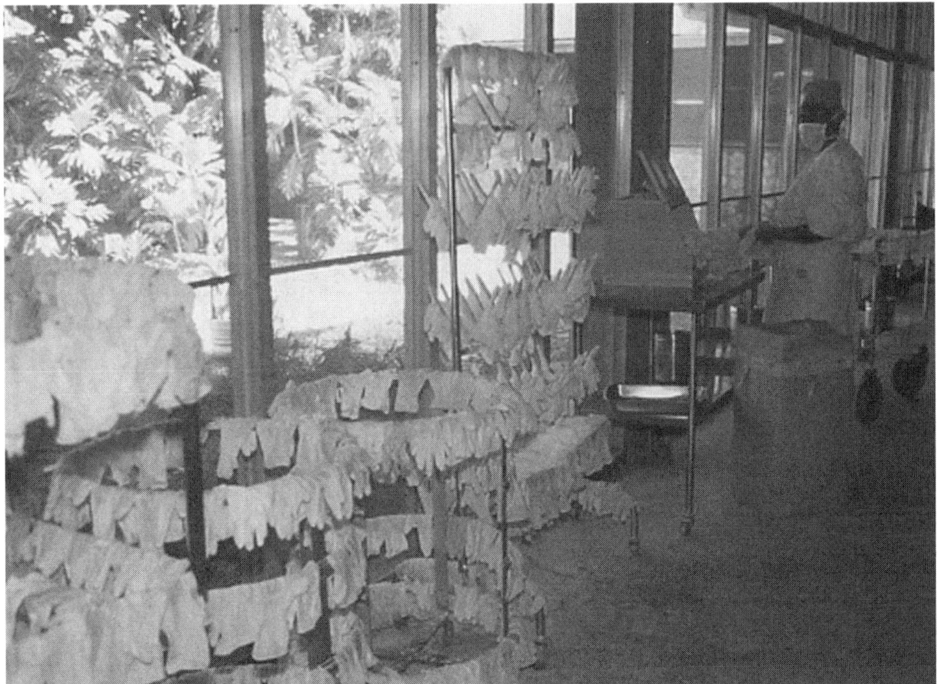

Source: Photo courtesy of Alyx Kellington

CHAPTER 15

Barriers to Care among HIV-positive Haitians

An Examination of Sociocultural Factors

Jessy G. Dévieux, Marie-Marcelle Deschamps, Robert Malow, Jean W. Pape, Rhonda Rosenberg, Michèle Jean-Gilles, Gilbert Saint-Jean, and Lisa Metsch

ABSTRACT

This chapter examines the personal, sociocultural, and structural barriers associated with receiving timely medical care for HIV-positive individuals in Haiti. Results of a pilot study involving 356 patients receiving antiretroviral treatment at the GHESKIO Centers in Port-au-Prince indicated that personal barriers such as economic dependence on a partner, sociocultural barriers such as stigma and secrecy associated with the disease, and structural barriers such as costly transportation continued to pose significant obstacles, keeping patients in need of services from receiving early treatment.

OVERVIEW

Haiti has the highest documented rate of HIV outside of sub-Saharan Africa; an estimated 180,000 adults (15 years and older) and 17,000 children (0–14 years) live with HIV/AIDS (UNAIDS, 2006). The latest HIV data for Haiti estimates national adult HIV prevalence at 2.2 percent. In 2001, 30,000 Haitians died from AIDS: twice the number who succumbed to the disease in the U.S. (Guly 2004). HIV transmission is predominantly heterosexual, with a male/female ratio of 1.2:1 in 2001 (PAHO/WHO 2001). Multiple factors have contributed to the generalized level of the epidemic, including poverty, gender inequality, limited access to health care, and lack of coordination among the various entities doing work to address HIV/AIDS in Haiti (Hempstone, Diop-Sidibe, Ahanda, Lauredent, and Heery 2004; Magee, Small, Frederic, Joseph, and Kershaw 2006). Furthermore, sociopolitical instability and lack of access and availability of services create challenges to receiving proper care. As of 1998, there were an estimated 2.7 physicians per 10,000 population; only 60 percent of the Haitian population had access to health services (UNAIDS/WHO 2004), and estimates are that only approximately 2,800 Haitians were receiving antiretroviral therapy, though the actual need was closer to 40,000 (Pape et al. 2004; UNAIDS/WHO 2004).

These disparities in access to care also affect the rate of progression of AIDS. A pilot study in Haiti showed that time to AIDS (5.2 years) and time to death (7.4 years) was almost twice as fast in the Haitian sample compared to the progression of the disease in developed countries (Deschamps, Fitzgerald, Pape, and Johnson 2000).

Early in the HIV/AIDS epidemic, the inclusion of Haitians in the Centers for Disease Control's list of HIV risk groups and the FDA's (Food and Drug Administration) regulation excluding Haitians from donating blood[1] contributed to the high levels of denial surrounding HIV/AIDS issues in Haiti (St. Cyr-Delpe 1995). While efforts to assign blame are largely absent from peer-reviewed literature, efforts to find the "last common ancestor" to pinpoint the origin of HIV are still ongoing (e.g., Korber et al. 2000). These efforts may contribute to continuing levels of stigma associated with the disease.

The high levels of denial exhibited by Haitians led to a great reluctance to receive testing for the disease while also contributing to the high levels of stigma and discrimination surrounding those who admit to having HIV. As one of the poorest countries in the Western Hemisphere, and one with low levels of infrastructure from which to provide treatment services, researchers and clinicians in Haiti have had to be creative in addressing service delivery needs in the country. Review of an *accompagnateur* program in rural Haiti, which included providing community assistance to HIV-positive individuals, noted a reduction in social stigma attached to HIV due to the involvement of community members in the daily lives of the participants (Behforouz, Farmer, and Mukherjee 2004). Additionally, research in rural areas suggests that with the provision of quality HIV care there is an increase in testing (Castro and Farmer 2005), which may lead to further reductions in stigma. These facts highlight the vital need to provide timely access to care by reducing potential barriers.

This chapter will discuss issues surrounding barriers to HIV medical treatment in Haiti. It will draw on historical and sociocultural research and provide data from a pilot study conducted at the Groupe Haitien d'Etude du Sarcome de Kaposi et des Infections Opportunistes (GHESKIO), the largest voluntary, counseling, testing (VCT), and treatment center on the island nation.

BACKGROUND

Early efforts at preventing the spread of HIV worldwide focused on the ABC mantra: Abstinence, Be faithful to one partner and Condom use. However, in Haiti's social context, where formal marriage is not the norm and men have multiple sexual relations, cultural adaptations had to be made in message delivery. In addition, the role of Voodoo and the widespread belief that HIV could be spread by supernatural causes was a further complicating factor.

There are existing cultural barriers to using condoms in many developing countries, including Haiti; however, the widespread effects of the epidemic led to collaborative efforts by non-governmental organizations (NGOs) and government agencies to reduce the impact of the disease by increasing commercial and social marketing techniques, increasing the number of outlets where condoms were available, and reducing prices of condoms (Dadian 1997a, 1997b). Early studies showed that there was a significant negative relationship between prices and the number of condoms sold (Harvey 1994) and that a one-year supply of condoms should cost much less than 1 percent of per capita gross national product in order to have an effect on family planning or HIV prevention. In Haiti, specifically, the most heavily marketed condom, Pantè, from 1991 to 1995 saw an increase in sales from 3,000 to more than 400,000 per month due to widespread efforts to publicize preventive measures (Dadian 1997b). While this significant increase in condom sales suggested a broader acceptance by Haitians of the need for prevention, many sociocultural and structural factors complicate the marketing and receipt of testing for HIV and the delivery of HIV treatment services in the country.

STIGMA AS A BARRIER TO CARE

Historically, stigma has been associated with diseases of undefined origin, coupled with the lack of effective treatments (Sontag 1978). Because HIV is primarily associated with the sex act and, by implication, morality, attention and conversation focusing on issues surrounding prevention and transmission are often difficult to broach. Furthermore, the fact that sexual acts are more often than not perceived as voluntary further appears to validate the appropriateness of negatively labeling those with the disease.

In the literature, stigma and knowledge are often negatively correlated. For example, a study in Haiti among expectant fathers revealed that high stigma and low HIV knowledge was found to be related to having multiple sexual partners (Magee et al. 2006). These data suggested a statistically significant link between stigma and knowledge and engagement in risky sexual practices, and underline the importance of improving knowledge among the general populace.

Stigma and the fear of repercussions associated with potential discrimination appear to be serious barriers to care in Haiti. For example, one study showed that HIV-positive individuals with signs of depression often do not return for medical care (Fitzgerald, Maxi, Marcelin, Johnson, and Pape 2004). In the case of HIV, depression may be linked to the perception that stigmatization and discrimination will follow a positive HIV diagnosis. In addition, women who are afraid of domestic violence or the withdrawal of economic support from their partners may not notify their sexual partners, thus perpetuating a cycle initiated by fears of discrimination. Denial and lack of disclosure of HIV status, which is also indirectly related to the presence of stigma, has also been significantly related to not seeking medical care (Fitzgerald et al. 2004). These issues may have less salience with the reduction of stigma in the country.

KNOWLEDGE AND SUPERSTITION

The practice of Voodoo and the power ascribed to it in the transmission of HIV has complicated the delivery of HIV testing and treatment services in Haiti. Several years ago, Pierre and colleagues noted, that although information about HIV transmission was widely known, surveys still revealed deficits in HIV knowledge and education (Pierre and Fournier 1999). More recently, in a national survey, even though almost all individuals knew about the existence of HIV/AIDS, 24 percent of women and 14 percent of men believed that HIV could not be prevented (Cayemittes, Placide, Barrere, Mariko, and Severe 2001). More importantly, 35 percent of the women and 19 percent of the men surveyed knew that HIV could be prevented, but could not name any method of prevention (Cayemittes et al. 2001), suggesting the continuing need for widespread knowledge dissemination on this topic.

As further evidence of this need, more than 50 percent of females and 43 percent of males in a national survey believed definitely, or are unsure about whether transmission can occur by supernatural means (Cayemittes et al. 2001). Previous research has shown that believing that HIV can be transmitted by supernatural means is a significant predictor that an HIV-positive individual will not seek medical care (Fitzgerald et al. 2004), highlighting the vital need for education.

LOGISTICAL BARRIERS TO CARE

More than stigma, however, some research points to logistic and economic barriers as greater factors in accessing testing and HIV treatment services in Haiti (Castro and Farmer 2005). Qualitative data from the GHESKIO centers in Haiti strongly suggest that the costs associated with transportation, and sociopolitical violence, which often prevents travel and may result in the interruption of the distribution of medication supplies, were common challenges to the delivery of service in the country (Dévieux et al. in press). Researchers have shown that poverty may be the primary reason that people living with HIV suffer from greater AIDS-related stigma (Castro and Farmer 2005), and being poor has been shown to predict refusal to notify one's sexual partner of one's HIV status (Fitzgerald et al. 2004).

THE EFFECTS OF GENDER ON BARRIERS

In Haiti, women are at high risk for contracting HIV due to the serial nature of heterosexual relationships in the country and the common male practice of having concurrent multiple partners. Magee and colleagues (2006) note that the patriarchal system, which leads to power imbalances within relationships, has increased women's vulnerability to HIV. Their study among expectant fathers showed that high decision-making power was associated with having multiple female partners—leading to the increased chances of contracting HIV among women. In addition, due to high levels of unemployment and underemployment in the country, women often are economically dependent on their male partners.

This power imbalance and economic dependence has implications for engaging and maintaining ongoing use of HIV primary care. For example, Fitzgerald and colleagues (2004) found that being poor and female were significant predictors of people refusing to disclose to their sexual partners about their HIV status. This is a significant barrier to care for not only the infected woman, but also for her partner (who may not know his HIV status) and any additional sex partners that he may have.

Researchers have hypothesized that women are increasingly entering sexual relationships due to economic vulnerability and that this factor is a contributor to the HIV epidemic in Haiti (Fitzgerald et al. 2000). Results of an exploratory study showed that almost 30 percent of the women in the study entered into a sexual relationship due to economic necessity, which resulted in a sixfold increase in the odds of contracting HIV. Approximately 40 percent of the women in this study had at least one sexually transmitted infection. Other studies have shown that gender and power factors accounted for 18 percent and 25 percent of the variance, above and beyond HIV knowledge and demographic covariates, in terms of condom use and intention to use condoms (Kershaw et al. 2006). Additional research has also shown that forced sex, another unfortunate behavior that has been linked to HIV transmission, has been significantly associated with economic vulnerability (Smith Fawzi et al. 2005). There may be some hopeful signs, however, specifically among the younger populations, where research has revealed that having fewer lifetime sexual partners was significantly associated with lower traditional gender norms among Haitian adolescents (Holschneider and Alexander 2003).

CULTURAL ADAPTATION

In the early stages of the HIV epidemic in Haiti, researchers from developed nations attempted to deliver interventions in a cultural context very different from their own. They soon learned about the importance of cultural adaptation and of integrating cultural beliefs into their intervention practices. For example, in an effort to integrate these beliefs into prevention programs, organizations have utilized Voodoo priests in order to influence and educate Haitians about HIV transmission (Fitzgerald and Simon 2001; Barker 2004).

Researchers have also learned the importance of addressing the individual needs of the people they are working with; for example, if money is needed for transportation or encouragement to utilize the medical systems by offering free services, then efforts will be made to do so. For example, a program to reduce the incidence of fungiasis, a disease common to poor communities in Haiti, provided shoes to individuals to prevent further transmission of the disease. This simple intervention importantly acknowledged the context of extreme poverty and successfully reduced the incidence of the disease (Joseph et al. 2006). This program provides a good model for effective interventions.

PRELIMINARY STUDY

In an effort to further understand the potential barriers to care among a sample of HIV-positive individuals, an exploratory study was conducted at the GHESKIO centers. GHESKIO serves as a model for determining the feasibility of introducing HIV care in urban Haiti. The clinic programs integrate VCT for HIV and syphilis services with reproductive health services (family planning, antenatal services, and care for rape victims), treatment for sexually transmitted infections, screening, treatment and prophylaxis for tuberculosis (TB).

In this current study, 356 HIV-positive patients who received antiretroviral treatment at GHESKIO were administered a questionnaire on barriers to care. Seventy-one percent of the sample was female. The mean age of men was 41.5 years, and 34.1 years for women. The majority of the patients consulted with medical personnel within six months after finding out their diagnosis; however, approximately 30 percent waited more than six months.

Fifty percent of those who waited more than six months to seek HIV care did not seek treatment earlier because they did not believe that the medical staff were telling them the truth about their diagnosis. Sixty-seven percent of those who were afraid their partners would leave them after learning their HIV diagnosis waited more than six months, compared to only 51 percent of those who were not afraid of this ($p = 0.004$). Sixty-six percent delayed seeking care because of lack of finances. Results from our qualitative data revealed that, even when care is free, the costs associated with transportation to the clinic and sustenance can be significant barriers to accessing the free health services. Many of the patients reported that, when they are too weak to travel long distances alone, they are accompanied to the clinic by a trusted relative or friend and must purchase food for themselves as well as their companions due to the long waits associated with receiving services. Finally, 97 percent of the sample, regardless of when they sought care, thought that HIV was a punishment for past mistakes. These preliminary results suggest that distance, denial, fear of partner repercussions, and finances were major reasons for delay in accessing medical care for HIV.

In addition to this exploratory study, qualitative research was conducted to clarify persistent barriers to access and utilization of HIV/AIDS-related services. Three focus groups—two client groups and one provider group—were conducted with 20 HIV-positive individuals and 11 health providers. The participants were recruited from community-based organizations providing HIV prevention and treatment services.

Both the client and provider focus groups independently identified and agreed on a number of major sociocultural, structural, and personal barriers. These included stigma and secrecy that prevent disclosure to loved ones, partners, and employers for fear of violence or loss of support; traditional health beliefs that cause misconceptions and denial of HIV; lack of confidentiality and/or comfort with conditions at health facilities; negative attitudes of health care personnel; low level of literacy and education about HIV and other sexually transmitted infections (STIs); prohibitive transportation costs; lack of information about available treatments and services; and insufficient HIV care within primary health services. This study revealed a high degree of agreement among providers and patients on persistent barriers to access and utilization. Results from both groups suggest that access must now become as important as HIV sociobehavioral prevention interventions.

DISCUSSION

These data confirm that there are barriers to care that include personal, sociocultural, and environmental factors. These factors have an impact on access and utilization of treatment services for HIV-positive individuals in Haiti and indicate the need for multilevel approaches in addressing these challenges. Previous research in Haiti has shown that demographic factors—being male and older; sociocultural factors such as the belief that HIV symptoms were not due to natural causes; and structural factors such as distance from medical clinic, lack of access to effective care, inability to pay, and previous negative experiences with the medical system—have all played a causative role in delaying presentation for care (Louis et al. 2007). Also overriding these issues is the existence of extreme poverty which itself acts as an almost insurmountable barrier to care (Louis et al. 2007).

Past studies also suggest that the provision of available HIV care may lead to the reduction of stigma, which may also result in increased levels of HIV testing. Castro and Farmer (2005) have conducted research in rural Haiti suggesting that the introduction of effective HIV treatment may lead to a reduction of stigma and increased testing. These researchers have piloted a program in which HIV-positive individuals participate in a program in which they have directly observed therapy and *accompagnateurs* (community health providers), who provide psychosocial support and also act to connect patients with medical staff and resources (Behforouz et al. 2004). These programs have proven effective in increasing the numbers of persons who access care.

Reducing stigma may also involve normalizing the issues surrounding HIV, for example, by incorporating HIV care into the basic provision of primary care services. Peck and colleagues (2003) suggested that integrating primary care—e.g., services for communicable diseases and reproductive services—with voluntary counseling and testing services may attract more persons to services. Walton and colleagues (2004) made similar findings, noting that integrated HIV prevention and care may also have a positive impact on primary health care goals, for example on family planning and TB case finding and cure. Therefore addressing issues of stigma and discrimination, by integrating HIV services with existing medical care, may be an important component of reducing barriers to care.

As further evidence of the importance of providing effective and integrated services in reducing stigma, the results of a mother-to-child transmission program in the Dominican Republic suggested that effective therapies for pregnant mothers have helped in reducing the stigma associated with patients. The researchers indicated that this change may have occurred partially due to the fact that health professionals focused on preventing transmission to unborn children, rather than on the status of the mother (Cáceres Ureña et al. 1998).

Some have argued that, in resource poor-nations, service delivery and adherence will be hampered due to lack of sufficient infrastructure. However, researchers have proven that effective interventions in rural Haiti are possible. For example, in one rural district, over 8,000 HIV-positive patients were followed, and adherence to medication was very high (Koenig, Leandre, and Farmer 2004). These interventions involved activities that may not be the norm in developed nations, for example, the renovation of medical clinics and the hiring of additional staff (Koenig et al. 2004). The successful model also included the provision of *accompagnateurs*, community health workers (CHWs) who supervised the delivery of antiretroviral therapy (ART) and provided community outreach to marginalized populations (Mukherjee and Eustache 2007). This model of community workers, along with the inclusion of directly observed therapies which keeps medication adherence rates high, may also have a synergistic effect in reducing the impact of other diseases, e.g., TB-related mortality (Jacquet et al. 2006).

Increasing levels of service access among HIV-positive individuals in Haiti have led to higher levels of testing, reductions in incidence rates, and measured reductions in mother-to-child transmission (MTCT) of HIV. For example, studies conducted at GHESKIO suggest that MTCT of HIV was as high as 27 percent prior to the availability of a mother/infant targeted program (Jean et al. 1999), compared to the current overall rate of 9.2 percent (Deschamps et al. in press).

Recent studies have shown that there have been increases in condom use with occasional partners at last contact, increases in abstinence and fidelity, and a decrease in the number of occasional partners (Gaillard et al. 2006). Researchers strongly suggest that the recent reductions in HIV prevalence found in Kenya, Zimbabwe, and Haiti, are due to reductions in risky sexual behaviors (Hallett et al. 2006), highlighting the growing impact of education interventions on these populations.

Though reductions in stigma may lead to increased testing and access to medical services, logistical and structural challenges may still represent insurmountable barriers to care in Haiti. A study in Uganda, for example, found that one of the primary reasons for non-adherence to medication was the inability of patients to pay for their medication (Byakika-Tusiime et al. 2005). In addition to these barriers, depression and denial may represent further challenges for HIV-positive individuals in terms of access to care and medication adherence (Fitzgerald et al. 2004).

Pettit (2000) notes that, especially in marginalized rural areas, by allowing people to participate in the process, by defining priorities and finding solutions that fit their realities, interventions have a greater chance of being perpetuated. For these reasons, working with the cultural realities, acknowledging the structural and personal barriers to care, and providing services to address these realities, may provide the best chances of reducing the impact of HIV on the Haitian population.

ACKNOWLEDGMENT

Preparation of this chapter was supported in part by grants from the NIH: DA13802 and 5UZRTW 006896.

NOTE

1. This was later repealed.

REFERENCES AND FURTHER READING

Barker, K. (2004). "Diffusion of innovations: A world tour." *Journal of Health Communication, 9, Suppl. 1*, 131–137.

Behforouz, H.L., Farmer, P.E., and Mukherjee, J.S. (2004). "From directly observed therapy to accompagnateurs: Enhancing AIDS treatment outcomes in Haiti and in Boston." *Clinical Infectious Diseases, 38*, S429–S436.

Byakika-Tusiime, J., Oyugi, J.H., Tumwikirize, W.A., Katabira, E.T., Mugyenyi, P.N., and Bangsberg, D.R. (2005). "Adherence to HIV antiretroviral therapy in HIV+ Ugandan patients purchasing therapy." *International Journal of STD and AIDS, 16*, 38–41.

Cáceres Ureña, F.I., Duarte, I., Moya, E.A., Pérez-Then, E., Hasbún, M.J., and Tapia, M. (1998). *Análisis de la situación y la respuesta al VIH/SIDA en República Dominicana*. Instituto de Estudios de Población y Desarrollos (IEPD) and Asociación Dominicana Pro-Bienestar de la Familia (PROFAMILIA). Santo Domingo, Dominican Republic.

Castro, A., and Farmer, P. (2005). "Understanding and addressing AIDS-related stigma: From anthropological theory to clinical practice in Haiti." *American Journal of Public Health, 95*, 53–59.

Cayemittes, M., Placide, M.F., Barrere, B., Mariko, S., and Severe, B. (2001). *Enquête mortalité, morbidité, et utilisation des services*, Haiti 2000 (Demographic and Health Survey). Ministère de la Santé Publique et de la Population, Institut Haitien de l'Enfance et ORC Macro. Calverton, MD.

Dadian, M.J. (1997a). "Condom sales boom as Rwanda and Haiti struggle to rebuild." *Aidscaptions, 4*, 4–8.

Dadian, M.J. (1997b). "NGO participation boosts condom sales in Haiti." *AIDSlink, 43*, 10–11.

Deschamps, M., Fitzgerald, D.W., Pape, J.W., Johnson, W.D., Jr. (2000). "HIV infection in Haiti: Natural history and disease progression." *AIDS, 14*, 2515–2521.

Deschamps, M., Noel, F., Bonhomme, J., Dévieux, J.G., Samuels, D., Saint-Jean, G., Zhu, Y., Wright, P., Pape, J.W., and Malow, R.M. (in press). "Prevention of mother to child transmission of HIV in Haiti." *Pan American Journal of Public Health*.

Dévieux, J.G., Deschamps, M.M., Malow, R.M., Jean-Gilles, M., Saint-Jean, G., Samuels, D., Marcelin, A., and Pape, J.W. (in press). "Knowledge, attitudes and behaviors among a sample of HIV-positive and HIV-negative females visiting an urban voluntary counselling and testing VCT center in Haiti." *Journal of Health Care for the Poor and Underserved*.

Fitzgerald, D.W., and Simon, T.S. (2001). "Telling stories of people with AIDS in rural Haiti." *AIDS Patient Care, 15*, 301–309.

Fitzgerald, D.W., Behets, F., Caliendo, A., Roberfroid, D., Lucet, C., Fitzgerald, J.W., and Kuykens, L. (2000). "Economic hardship and sexually transmitted diseases in Haiti's rural Artibonite Valley." *American Journal of Tropical Medicine and Hygiene, 62*, 496–501.

Fitzgerald, D.W., Maxi, A., Marcelin, A., Johnson, W.D., and Pape, J.W. (2004). "Notification of positive HIV test results in Haiti: Can we better intervene at this critical crossroads in the life of HIV-infected patients in a resource-poor country?" *AIDS Patient Care and STDs, 18*, 658–664.

Gaillard, E.M., Boulos, L.M., Andre Cayemittes, M.P., Eustache, L., Van Onacker, J.D., Duval, N., Louis-saint, E., and Thimote, G. (2006). "Understanding the reasons for decline of HIV prevalence in Haiti." *Sexually Transmitted Infections, 82, Suppl. 1*, i14–i20.

Guly, C. (2004). "Haiti emerging from chaos to face health care crisis." *Canadian Medical Association Journal, 170*(9), 1379.

Hallett, T.B., Aberle-Grasse, J., Bello, G., Boulos, L.M., Cayemittes, M.P., Cheluget, B., Chipeta, J., Dorrington, R., Dube, S., Ekra, A.K., Garcia-Calleja, J.M., Garnett, G.P., Greby, S., Gregson, S., Grove, J.T., Hader, S., Hanson, J., Hladik, W., Ismail, S., Kassim, S., Kirungi, W., Kouassi, L., Mahomva, A., Marum, L., Maurice, C., Nolan, M., Rehle, T., Stover, J., and Walker, N. (2006). "Declines in HIV prevalence can be associated with changing sexual behaviour in Uganda, urban Kenya, Zimbabwe, and urban Haiti." *Sexually Transmitted Infections, 82, Suppl. 1*, i1–i8.

Harvey, P.D. (1994). The impact of condom prices on sales in social marketing programs. *Studies in Family Planning, 25*, 52–58.

Hempstone, H., Diop-Sidibe, N., Ahanda, K.S., Lauredent, E., and Heery, M. (2004). "HIV/AIDS in Haiti: A literature review." USAID/Health Communication. Retrieved October 24, 2004, from http://www.jhuccp.org/africa/haiti/LitreviewAIDS_en.pdf.

Holschneider, S.O., and Alexander, C.S. (2003). "Social and psychological influences on HIV preventive behaviors of youth in Haiti." *Journal of Adolescent Health, 33*, 31–40.

Institut Haitien de l'Enfance et Centres GHEISKIO (2001). "Etude de Serosurveillance par Methode Sentinelle de la Prevalence de VIH, de la Syphilis, et de l'Hepatite B chez les Femmes Enceintes en Haiti 1999–2000." Port au Prince, Haiti: Pan American Health Organization (PAHO).

Jacquet, V., Morose, W., Schwartzman, K., Oxlade, O., Barr, G., Grimard, F., and Menzies, D. (2006). "Impact of DOTS expansion on tuberculosis related outcomes and costs in Haiti." *BMC Public Health, 156*, 209.

Jean, S.S., Pape, J.W., Verdier, R.I., Reed, G.W., Hutto, C., Johnson, W.D., and Wright, P.F. (1999). "The natural history of human immunodeficiency virus 1 infection in Haitian infants." *Pediatric Infectious Disease Journal, 18*, 58–63.

Joseph, J.K., Bazile, J., Mutter, J., Shin, S., Ruddle, A., Ivers, L., Lyon, E., and Farmer, P. (2006). "Tungiasis in rural Haiti: A community-based response." *Transactions of the Royal Society of Tropical Medicine and Hygiene, 100*, 970–974.

Kershaw, T.S., Small, M., Joseph, G., Theodore, M., Bateau, R., and Frederic, R. (2006). "The influence of power on HIV risk among pregnant women in rural Haiti." *AIDS and Behavior, 10*, 309–318.

Koenig, S.P., Leandre, F., and Farmer, P.E. (2004). "Scaling-up HIV treatment programmes in resource-limited settings: The rural Haiti experience." *AIDS, 18, Suppl. 3*, S21–S25.

Korber, B., Muldoon, M., Theiler, J., Gao, F., Gupta, R., Lapedes, A., Hahn, B.H., Wolinsky, S., and Bhattacharya, T. (2000). "Timing the ancestor of the HIV-1 pandemic strains." *Science, 288*, 1789–1796.

Louis, C., Ivers, L.C., Smith Fawzi, M.C., Freedberg, K.A., and Castro, A. (2007). "Late presentation for HIV care in central Haiti: Factors limiting access to care." *AIDS Care, 19*, 487–491.

Magee, E.M., Small, M., Frederic, R., Joseph, G., and Kershaw, T. (2006). "Determinants of HIV/AIDS risk behaviors in expectant fathers in Haiti." *Journal of Urban Health, 83*, 625–636.

Mukherjee, J.S., and Eustache, F.E. (2007). "Community health workers as a cornerstone for integrating HIV and primary healthcare." *AIDS Care, 19, Suppl. 1*, S73–S82.

PAHO/WHO, Institut Haitien de l'Enfance Centres GHEISKIO. (2001) *Etude de Serosurveillance par Methode Sentinelle de la Prevalence de VIH, de la Syphilis, et de l'Hepatite B chez les Femmes Enceintes en Haiti 1999-2000.* Port au Prince, Haiti: Pan American Health Organization (PAHO/WHO).

Pape, J.W., Deas Van Onacker, J.D., Cayemittes, M., Deschamps, M.M., Verdier, R.I., Severe, P.D., et al. (2004, July). "Haiti's response to the AIDS epidemic: A success story." Poster session presented at the annual meeting of the International AIDS Conference, Bangkok, Thailand.

Peck, R., Fitzgerald, D.W., Liautaud, B., Deschamps, M.M., Verdier, R.I., Beaulieu, M.E., GrandPierre, R., Joseph, P., Severe, P., Noel, F., Wright, P., Johnson Jr, W.D., and Pape, J.W. (2003). "The feasibility, demand, and effect of integrating primary care services with HIV voluntary counseling and testing: Evaluation of a 15-year experience in Haiti 1985–2000." *AIDS, 33*, 470–475.

Pettit, Jethro. (2000). "Strengthening local organization: 'Where the rubber hits the road.'" *IDS Bulletin, 31*, 57–67.

Pierre, J.A., and Fournier, A.M. (1999). "Human immunodeficiency virus infection in Haiti." *Journal of the National Medical Association, 91*, 165–170.

St. Cyr-Delpe, M. (1995). "On the eve of destruction." In E. Reid (ed.), *HIV and AIDS: The Global Interconnection.* West Hartford, CT: Kumarian Press. Retrieved on November 4, 2004, from http://www.undp.org/hiv/publications/book/bkchap06.htm.

Smith Fawzi, M.C., Lambert, W., Singler, J.M., Tanagho, Y., Leandre, F., Nevil, P., Bertrand, D., Claude, M.S., Bertrand, J., Louissaint, M., Jeannis, L., Mukherjee, J.S., Goldie, S., Salazar, J.J., and Farmer, P.E. (2005). "Factors associated with forced sex among women accessing health services in rural Haiti: Implications for the prevention of HIV infection and other sexually transmitted diseases." *Social Science and Medicine, 60*, 679–689.

Sontag, S. (1978). *Illness as Metaphor.* New York, NY: Farrar, Straus and Giroux.

UNAIDS. (2006). "Country report: Haiti, 2006." Retrieved June 14, 2007, from: http://www.unaids.org/en/Regions_Countries/Countries/haiti.asp.

UNAIDS/WHO. (2004). "*Haiti: Epidemiological fact sheets on HIV/AIDS and sexually transmitted infections.*" Retrieved October 23, 2004, from http://www.who.int/GlobalAtlas/PDFFactory/HIV/EFS_PDFs/EFS2004_HT.pdf.

Walton, D.A., Farmer, P.E., Lambert, W., Leandre, F., Koenig, S.P., and Mukherjee, J.S. (2004). "Integrated HIV prevention and care strengthens primary health care: Lessons from rural Haiti." *Journal of Public Health Policy, 25*, 137–158.

CHAPTER 16

The Evolution of the ABC Strategy for HIV Prevention in Uganda

Domestic and International Implications

Peter Ibembe

ABSTRACT

Uganda has been deemed as a success story in the fight against HIV/AIDS. In a relatively short time, HIV infection rates fell dramatically. It is all the more remarkable, given the prevailing environment over the last few years, a situation severely constrained by lack of resources, poverty and mass illiteracy, and the presence of war over the last two decades. This chapter traces the evolution of the much-lauded ABC strategy in Uganda, and how state and international support for the strategy has impacted on public health. It examines the influence of varying approaches of the strategy and whether it is still relevant in a changing environment.

OVERVIEW

The ABC approach is a strategy to prevent HIV/AIDS espoused by the Ugandan government and quickly adopted by United States funding programs. "A" stands for **A**bstaining from sex or a delay of sexual debut. "B" stands for **B**eing faithful or reducing the number of one's sexual partners," while "C" refers to the correct and consistent use of **C**ondoms. Uganda has been much lauded as a success story in the fight against HIV/AIDS; in a relatively short time, HIV infection rates fell dramatically in that country. This success is all the more remarkable, given a lack of resources, the prevalence of poverty and mass illiteracy, and the presence of war over the last two decades.

This chapter traces the evolution of the much-lauded ABC strategy, and how state and international support for the strategy has affected public health in Uganda. This chapter is an insider's view of the varying dynamics of the pandemic and the varying responses to the condition over time. To better understand the sociopolitical context in which the ABC strategy operates, it is essential to examine the general context in which HIV developed and flourished. To that end, I have divided the conceptual framework into three distinct time periods. International interventions, and more specifically U.S. government support, are analyzed to help decipher the popularity of the ABC programs with international funding portfolios.

THE CONTEXT

Uganda is still largely a patriarchal society, where disadvantage for the female gender is rife. There are inequalities in educational opportunity, access to resources, and political participation, and polygamy is common (Parikh 2007). Virtually no insurance mech-

Exhibit 16.1 The ABC prevention strategy—Uganda

Je... UNAJUA YA KWAMBA...

SALAMA CONDOMS NI SALAMA KWELI ???
Salama Condoms hutengenezwa katika hali ya usafi wa hali ya juu inayozingatia afya yako. Utengenazaji wake hulingana na masharti ya Shirika la Afya Duniani (WHO), na hivyo kuhakikisha ya kwamba hazibebi magonjwa au uchafu wa aina yoyote. Kuanzia mwaka 1993 hadi sasa, *Salama* Condoms zaidi ya **milioni 50** zimeuzwa hapa Tanzania, na wote wanaozitumia wana furaha na wana afya nzuri. Uthibitisho tosha kuwa *Salama* Condoms ni kinga thabiti dhidhi ya virusi vya UKIMWI na magonjwa ya zinaa, na pia ni njia safi ya kupanga uzazi. **Jikinge. Tumia *Salama* Condoms ipasavyo kwa kila tendo.**
ZINGATIA: UNAPOVAA KONDOM, SHIKA CHUCHU ILI KUONDOA HEWA NA HAKIKISHA KWAMBA UPANDE UTAKAOUKUNJUA UKO KWA NJE.
KUMBUKA KUWA UNAWEZA KUEPUKANA NA UKIMWI NA MAGONJWA YA ZINAA KWA:
A) Kutofanya kabisa mapenzi B) Kuwa na mpenzi mmoja ambae hajaambukizwa C) Kutumia Kondom ipasavyo na kila mara

NEW
Salama
CONDOMS
Chaguo la Kisasa

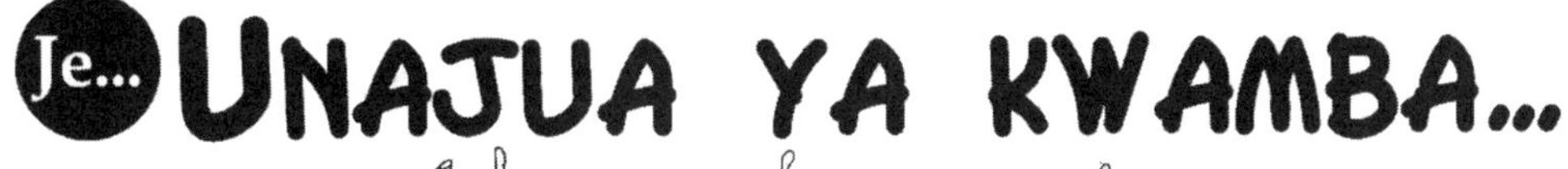

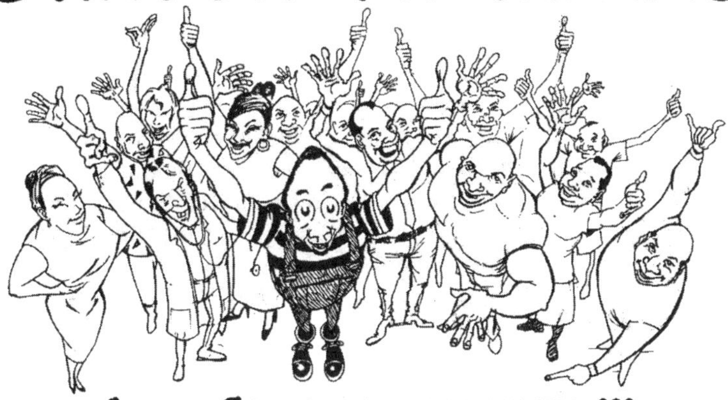

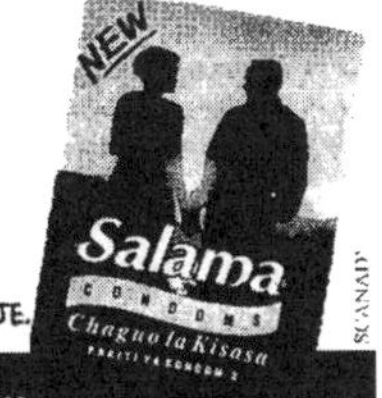

anism exists, and the main form of insurance in one's old age is still one's children or close relatives. Marriage at an early age, especially in the rural areas, is still widespread. The current society is a mix of traditional practices, modern influences, and religious interaction. In the traditional setup, women were largely expected to be chaste at marriage, though at the same time men were largely anticipated to have a degree of sexual experience. This ambivalent and contradictory position concerning abstinence was difficult to interpret or enforce, and instances of premarital sex were quite common, though the levels of this at the time, and the source of prior sexual experience, have not been systematically studied. It nevertheless points to cultural norms that lead to an unequal distribution of power and decision-making authority in the country.

In Uganda AIDS is a predominantly heterosexual condition, with preponderance in urban locations. The prevalence of HIV among the sexes is evenly balanced, with preponderance among younger women and older men (Ministry of Health 2006). It also has one of the highest rates of population growth in the world and one of the highest teenage pregnancy rates in the world, which reflects the levels of unprotected sex. In recent years there has been a reduction in the rates of teenage pregnancy, though population growth rates remain high.

1978–1990

Genesis and Evolution of the Pandemic: War, Poverty, and Pestilence

There is evidence that the AIDS epidemic in Central Africa has its origin in the late 1950s, although the condition became most noticeable in Uganda only in the early 1980s (Berry and Noble 2007). The epidemic first manifested itself on the back of two wars that took place in a relatively short time. The first war, from 1978 to 1979, had resulted in the overthrow of Idi Amin by armed opposition from Tanzania. The other was a protracted civil war in the center of the country from 1981 to 1986 that swept Yoweri Museveni into power. The main outbreaks of the condition were first noticed among people living or working in the far west of the country, in the area neighboring Tanzania. These were relatively wealthy people who were involved in fishing or trading along the common border, and in this area transactional sex was common. The earliest local interpretations of this inexplicable and lethal disease were that the condition was caused by witchcraft or retribution for business deals gone sour. The linkages to sex were made only later. There was no structured response to the spreading condition, and in a situation of war, displacement, and disorder the spread of the disease was intensified. Social services had by and large broken down due to war and there were no ways of making science-based diagnoses. Anyone losing weight could arbitrarily be pronounced to be suffering from "Slim Disease," as AIDS was then known (PANOS 1990). The main "victims" of the condition were from along the Great North Road, running from Rwanda in the West to Mombasa in Kenya. In Uganda the greatest impact was felt in the western areas of Rakai, and Masaka. Later, when it was realized that the condition was linked to sexual intercourse, the local response was to avoid such persons or their sexual contacts.

Uganda's nationwide anti-AIDS awareness campaign began in March 1986, with the main priority being information and education (PANOS 1990), although it also included screening and protection of the blood supply, epidemiological surveillance, and the improvement of laboratory facilities. Seminars were held to promote less risky sexual behavior, and brochures and leaflets were developed urging people to "Love Carefully," or "Love Faithfully," and were broadcast over radio in most of Uganda's major languages. These imply a focus on abstinence and the promotion of fidelity. A mixture of fear and morality was employed to convince or cajole people into more "responsible" behavior. The most popular messages were chastity before marriage, and fidelity within marriage (PANOS 1990). Key members of the community, such as tribal chiefs, traditional midwives, and local political and church leaders, were involved in reaching different constituencies. Popular entertainers were actively employed to help reduce stigma against AIDS and give the disease a "human face."

The international response to the evolving pandemic at the time was mainly to channel additional funding to diagnostic facilities, and to grassroots anti-AIDS organizations such as The AIDS Support Organization (TASO), which has a close interaction with those directly affected. By the time HIV testing became more available in Uganda in 1986, the condition had already reached epidemic proportions.

1991–2000

Information, Education, Communication

By 1991, the overall HIV prevalence in Uganda stood at 21 percent (Low-Beer and Stoneburner 2003). By 2001, the levels had fallen to 6 percent. The government was faced with two stark options: either deny that the epidemic actually existed, or make informed inroads into it with a concerted and focused campaign to inform and educate people about it. The critical components of Uganda's prevention program was a combination, to various degrees, of strong political support, especially from President Yoweri Museveni, interventions such as affirmative action to empower women and girls, a strong emphasis on behavior change in youths such as adoption of safer sex behaviors, active efforts to give AIDS a human face and to fight stigma and discrimination, with emphasis on more open communication about the condition, an involvement and engagement of the religious leadership and faith-based organizations such as the Protestant, Catholic and Muslim community, the introduction of confidential counseling and testing facilities for HIV, and the emphasis on STI prevention and management. Additionally, drama and song are still a popular way of passing on messages to the local communities, and almost all songs developed have a moral or educational message. The use of radio as a means of communication, common in Uganda, helped to spread the messages across the different communities. Commercial sex and "promiscuous" behavior was frowned upon, and many messages were words of warning or admonition (author's personal observation).

Aside from this, the different communities were adapting various coping mechanisms to help them survive. The youth were advised to avoid sexual activity before marriage and, if this were not possible, to get married as soon as possible. Instances where a wife was inherited by the husband's close male relative, a practice which hitherto had been quite common, declined precipitously. During this time period, there was a reversal in the age-old tendency for the young to look after the old. With the death or ailment of younger members of the community, the elder uncles, aunts, and grandparents took on a greater role to protect and look after their blood. In some situations, children who had belonged to the deceased were "distributed" among one's brothers and other relations to look after and to educate. Widows were in some instances apportioned clan land to cultivate and produce food for the children.

In the 1990s HIV was detected mainly among the 20–24 age group. This segment of the population constituted more than half of the new infection (Uganda Bureau of Statistics 2002). The ABC approach was then developed to help fight the pandemic in the country, with the Ministry of Health taking a leading role in this (Okware et al. 2005). Another crucial proponent in the changing picture of HIV/AIDS at the time was President Yoweri Museveni. Although it is widely assumed that he had been a champion of condom use from the onset, the following observation discounts this assertion:

> President Yoweri K. Museveni of Uganda recently reviewed findings from an AIDSTECH computer modeling project which demonstrated that consistent condom use could help reduce future HIV infection. Two days later, President Museveni expressed public support for condom use, reversing a long-held position against their use. (Lamptey 2002)

Therefore, it seems that President Museveni was not an early proponent of condom use, but only took up the message in the early 1990s. His main focus before was to advocate for early marriage and to avoid multiple sex partners. However, once he came out in support of condom use, he embraced the idea wholeheartedly. While it was important to elucidate components of ABC, there was a need to communicate the message as clearly and as simply as possible. Uganda used the media and the President himself, who personally toured the country educating people about AIDS (Berry and Noble 2007). Besides coming out openly in support of condoms, the President broke many age-old taboos in the country. He was willing to discuss sex openly, a situation deemed unacceptable in the past. He openly supported people living with HIV/AIDS as normal human beings and also gave hope to many, by asserting that managing AIDS was easy, because, "unlike most other conditions like malaria or cancer which come looking for you, it is you who goes looking for AIDS. So stop looking for it, and you will be fine." He was willing to speak openly at funeral services concerning what had caused the death of the deceased (author's personal observations).

The country almost completely embraced the President's messages. The main strategies Uganda adopted at the same time included reducing stigma, bringing discussions on sex more into the open, promoting the need for counseling and testing, mainstreaming AIDS in society and integrating more participants in the AIDS prevention campaigns, such as religious leaders and traditional healers (Cohen 2003). Additionally, these measures were complemented with other broader holistic structural aims, such as the empowerment of women (Population Secretariat 2004), education, and interventions aimed at reducing poverty. Gender relationships were redefined through affirmative action, which included increased parliamentary representation and the passing of laws supporting patients' rights in the workplace.

International interventions at the time were focused mainly on developing and rolling out diagnostic facilities and prompting HIV education about the ABC strategy through non-government organizations. Most importantly, there was greater leeway to sponsor home-grown interventions that had already proven their worth.

Uganda's subsequent decline in HIV prevalence has been linked to change in all three ABC behaviors. These interventions are heralded as the main causes of the remarkable decline in HIV prevalence at the time, which resulted from increased abstinence and delay in sexual debut (decreased teenage pregnancy rate, STI), increased faithfulness and a reduction in sexual partners, and an increase in condom use between casual partners (USAID 2003).

2001–PRESENT

The Current HIV and ABC Situation in Uganda

To help understand the impact of the ABC intervention in Uganda, it is necessary to unravel the package of interventions in the light of statistical evidence. The following results were mainly obtained from a sero-behavioral survey carried out in the country. HIV prevalence rates, after falling precipitously from 18.5 percent from the early 1990s, have stagnated at 6.4 percent, or even risen in some parts of the country (Population Secretariat 2004). There are other factors that have had an impact on HIV prevalence levels. It is possible that the rise in AIDS-related deaths beginning in the 1990s could partly explain some of the decline in HIV prevalence in the country. The condition could have disproportionately removed those affected from the population through opportunistic infections and subsequent death. Another factor that could also partly explain this is the high population growth rate. The average Ugandan woman gives birth to six to seven children in her lifetime (UBOS 2007), and the population doubles every 25 years. This has implications for the prevalence rate, especially if the rate of population increase far outnumbers the rate of spread of HIV. In the context of high population growth, prevalence rates could fall. The stagnating prevalence rate in the country, then, must have dire consequences for a fast-growing population.

Regarding the outcomes of the ABC strategy, from 1995 to 2005 the proportion of women aged 15–19 who have never had sex increased from 38 to 54 percent, and from 52 percent to 58 percent among men of similar age in the same period (Ministry of Health 2006). More recent data (UBOS 2007) indicates that the percentage of men aged 15–19 has increased from 58 percent to 65 percent, and those remaining faithful to their partners from 45 percent to 53 percent. More than 50 percent of young women have had sex by the age of 17, and by 19 years among young men. However, the percentage of people who have had sex before the age of 18 had reduced from 74 percent to 58 percent of women, and from 64 percent to 42 percent of men, between 1995 and 2006. Moreover, in the preceding 12 months, only 4 percent of women reported having sex with more than one partner, compared to 29 percent of men. Polygamy is relatively common in Uganda. Just over one fourth of married women (28 percent) and 17 percent of married men are in polygamous unions (Uganda Bureau of Statistics 2007).

Regarding condom use, generally speaking it is the younger people aged 15–19 who are more likely to have used a condom at last intercourse, and this percentage decreases substantially with age. Fifteen percent of women and 37 percent of men aged 15–49 who were sexually active in the 12 months preceding the survey had engaged in sex with a non-marital, non-cohabiting partner; of these, 47 percent of women and 53 percent of men had reported using condoms. However, in the 15–19 age group 27 percent of women reported condom use at their last sexual encounter, compared to only 5.7 percent in the 35–39 age group. This implies that condom use in Uganda varies greatly with age, and that the older members of society are less likely to be using them. Another survey has shown that among men aged 20–24 who have one partner, the proportion who did not use a condom at last sex increased more than the proportion who use a condom, but the percentage of men in the same age group who had multiple partners in the last 12 months and did not use a condom decreased from 14 percent to 9 percent (Uganda Bureau of Statistics 2007).

Generally speaking, then, condom use in the country has increased, but is the level of use sufficient to make an appreciable impact on the spread of HIV? At present, HIV prevalence is now highest among those aged 30–34, and lowest in the 15–19 age group (Population Secretariat 2007). This would imply that the age group that is using condoms more often is safer than others, but this is also the group that is generally abstaining from sex.

There has been a recorded rise in the number of discordant couples; 5 percent of those who are HIV positive have an HIV-negative spouse (Ministry of Health 2006). This necessarily opens up a situation of constant exposure and risk to infection, with added implications on the possibility of "being faithful" leading to exposure to HIV. A pattern of decline in condom use is also seen when relations become more emotional or intimate, even in higher-risk categories (Parikh 2007).

Regarding gender, there are still glaring disparities concerning HIV in Uganda. Only 31 percent of women have comprehensive knowledge of HIV/AIDS, compared to 42 percent of men, and only 35 percent of sexually active women report condom use at last intercourse, compared to 57 percent of men (Uganda Bureau of Statistics 2007). Four in ten women in the 15–49 age group have experienced sexual violence.

Concerning voluntary counseling and testing for HIV, a key component in countering the condition, only 13 percent of women and 11 percent of men in the 15–49 age group had ever tested for HIV and received the results. For the overwhelming majority of the population, therefore, HIV transmission is still a question of "Russian roulette."

In Uganda, HIV has been crowding out patients who suffer from conditions that are deemed to be less severe than HIV. It is a drain on the meager resources and disproportionately eats into the health budget (Population Secretariat 2007). Treatment using antiretroviral therapy (ART) has usually hitherto been unaffordable, but access has increased as a result of increased donor support.

MONEY, POLITICS, AND IDEOLOGY

In the dynamic context of more and more people living with HIV, and with the development of antiretroviral therapy, more resources are needed for HIV management reduction to address the challenge of inadequate financial and technical resources and help bridge the gap between available resources and the needs of the people living with HIV. This has resulted in increased funding for the condition in the form of resources for antiretroviral therapy (Okware et al. 2005). However, additional investment circumvents the glaring fact that other health conditions—such as malaria, malnutrition, and unsafe pregnancies—are the primary causes of mortality in the country and affect a disproportionately higher number of people (Population Secretariat 2007).

The international response to the AIDS pandemic in Uganda has been spearheaded by the United States and Britain. The following quotation bears testament to added American investment:

> The Bush Administration is basing its AIDS initiative on the success of Uganda which has experienced the greatest decline in HIV prevalence of any country in the world. Studies show that from 1991 to 2001, HIV infection rates in Uganda declined from about 15 percent to 5 percent. Among pregnant women in Kampala, the capital of Uganda, HIV prevalence dropped from a high of approximately 30 percent to 10 percent over the same period. (Laconte 2003)

This added international response, especially from the U.S., resulted in increased investments in HIV management programs. However, these came with strings attached. The U.S. required emphasis on abstinence as a key strategy to prevent the spread of HIV in recipient countries (Sussman 2006). The related leadership response in Uganda has been a championing of the use of abstinence. One of the key proponents of the abstinence until marriage campaign has been the first lady, Janet Museveni, an evangelical Christian. Even President Museveni, who had been a major champion of condom use in the past, made an abrupt shift to emphasize abstinence. At the 15th International AIDS Conference in 2004 in Bangkok, Museveni made a highly public policy shift, denouncing the use of condoms at the expense of abstinence (Chan 2004; Sanders 2005). National and international ire at this position resulted in a denial that he changed positions. The official government position was that the first statement had been misunderstood, though it was reported that, in Ugandan schools supported by U.S. funds, contractors instructed teachers not to discuss condoms in schools (Mbogo 2007).

The change in strategic focus in the anti-AIDS drive by the Musevenis has been tied to U.S. funding for the pro-abstinence campaigns (Sussman 2006). However, the U.S. continues to provide substantial support for President Museveni's Presidential Initiative for AIDS Strategy for Communication to Youth (PIASCY), which champions abstinence among youth (United States Presidential Emergency Plan for AIDS Relief 2007). These funds are channeled to Uganda despite the fact that abstinence-only programmes have not been found to be very effective in the U.S. (Human Rights Watch 2007). This continued funding, based on ideology, has raised grave moral and ethical questions about funding an intervention that is of doubtful scientific value and infringes the human rights of the individual concerning access to comprehensive and quality services, including accurate and all-inclusive sex education.

However, it has also been argued that this debate around condoms has developed ideological undertones, and has led to the integration of other hitherto peripheral bodies, such as faith-based organizations (Planned Parenthood 2006). The public health lobby in the West, using the rights-based approach, has placed too much emphasis on condom use as an AIDS intervention, and political conservatives have placed too little (Epstein 2007). This debate has crowded out indigenous interventions to the crisis and moved the focus of attention away from epidemiology to ideology (Wilson 2004).

The Uganda AIDS programs, as supported by the international community, belie a more fundamental question. In a country where the main health priorities are death from malaria, malnutrition, and stunted growth among children, and poor sexual and reproductive health indices, such as high maternal mortality, abortion and runaway population growth (Population Secretariat 2004), was the accelerated U.S. support for this intervention aimed primarily at the local communities in question—with their needs in acute focus, and grounded in humanitarian reality—or was it for another audience, a political intervention for the consumption of Western ears? An effect of the intervention has been that much-needed funding has been channeled to HIV at the expense of other more cost-effective and proven public health interventions. There have also been concerns raised about the capacity of governments to absorb and manage donor funding. There is uneasiness about the replacement of community responses with exotic interventions in areas where there is limited absorptive or infrastructural capacity to cope with added capital investment (Halmshaw and Hawkins 2004).

ISSUES AND CHALLENGES

There have been different key actors and differing strategic responses to Uganda's ABC approach. The fight against HIV has the formative picture of one trying to hit a moving target. As the pandemic evolves in time to reflect changing patterns of at-risk groups, the strategies and focus against it must necessarily be dynamic. To piece together whether the ABC approach has affected public health is to appreciate the highly complex interrelations that impact upon and affect sexuality. Have the varying points of emphasis concerning the ABC approach succeeded in reducing the incidence and prevalence of HIV in Uganda, thus contributing to public health and general welfare? Why has the prevalence of HIV stabilized at 6.4 percent of the population, and what added interventions can further catalyze its reduction? Has the relative shift towards abstinence-only campaigns led to stagnation or an increase in the HIV rates?

The changing face of HIV/AIDS in Uganda is evident in the changing age cohorts most affected. HIV/AIDS in Uganda is now an aging disease. HIV prevalence levels are rising fastest in married people in the thirties age group. How relevant is abstinence or being faithful in preventing HIV, where most cases are now occurring among married people in their thirties? How will the ABC campaign play out in such an older age group usually more set in their ways, and where levels of sexual fidelity vary?

Abstinence becomes irrelevant once one gets married. Being faithful is only absolutely safe once both partners remain faithful to each other. However, condom use in Uganda has never been appreciably high, though the actual levels of use are not known. Why did the HIV prevalence decrease, even in the absence of widespread condom use? This picture is further complicated by the fact that usage varies by age group, and also according to whether one is in a monogamous or higher-risk relationship. Additionally, there are implications concerning people who are surviving longer as a result of ART. The long-term sexual behavior of this group in the Ugandan context warrants further study.

It is evident that state support for the comprehensive ABC policy has not always been consistent or steadfast. National support has evolved over the years, either in support of or against different sections of its components, as a result of scientific fact, ideology, or political expediency. The continuing adaptation of public sexual behavior in response to leadership inclinations, especially in age groups that are less impressionable, is food for thought.

Another challenge to the ABC strategy is to ask about the effects of the feminization of HIV/AIDS through gender inequalities, increasing levels of transactional sex, and an ingrained structure of patriarchy. What is the impact of the ABC strategy in communities where the female gender has a low level of social and economic empowerment, and where polygamy and gender and sex-based violence are commonplace?

There has been a recent preponderance of vertical funding for HIV, while relatively little goes to address the overarching challenge of improving people's sexual and reproductive health (SRH). As it were, HIV is the "rich nephew" of impoverished SRH. To what extent can HIV continue being compartmentalized without addressing SRH in its entirety is a question still open to debate. What is the influence and effect of one of the highest population growth rates in the world on the picture of HIV/AIDS prevalence in contemporary Uganda?

Is the emphasis on HIV at the expense of broader SRH or other graver public health concerns in the country, as well as an emphasis on abstinence at the expense of the other components of ABC, a deliberate strategy? Or is it a result of the foreign mindset that focuses on an interventionist "project" approach to development? Has the Uganda anti-AIDS agenda has been hijacked by foreign interests, or was it a marriage of like minds in the U.S. and Uganda leaderships? And what are the implications of this on other public health donor funding? It is obvious that cost-effective and proven interventions are necessary to continually improve and fine-tune interventions tailored to the local context. The history of donor support and the decisions and thought processes that informed its implementation will need further analysis. Nevertheless, it would seem that the current international support for the intervention promoting abstinence at the expense of condom use was fatally flawed from the outset. HIV had become an intensely political condition, crowding out malaria and other conditions of greater public health concern to the country.

CONCLUSION

The ABC strategy has proved its resilience for more than 20 years. The ABC approach is a vital ingredient in preventing HIV transmission, and it will remain the cornerstone of Uganda's anti-HIV drive for some time to come. However, given the changing dynamics of HIV, it will be necessary to devise new strategies developed from evolving insights and perceptions. It is necessary to continually revisit this prevention strategy in light of the changing social dynamics of the condition. Intervention measures and messages have to be seen within the context of the country's reality and developed from the foundation of the community's social context. For example, HIV needs to be tackled within the framework of the overall picture of sexual and reproductive health, which includes maternal health and family planning.

In recent years, the greater international response to the epidemic in Uganda has served to help mitigate the effects of the condition. However, the impact of these interventions is still subject to debate. Without international support for the preventive measures, it is difficult to see how the country could have coped any better, especially regarding care and support of people living with HIV/AIDS. However, these interventions, all with their different agendas, written or unwritten, should be seen as learning experiences upon which better and more refined strategies can be developed.

At the end of the day it is the balance and experience from different interventions that will cause the most impact on public health. With the chorus of voices at the national and international level, it is possible to drown out the small voice of community interventions and priorities. Proven interventions are those that allow broad coverage and are most cost-effective to apply. They are better understood by the population and more socially relevant. It must take into account the fact that there are many partners in health care and that we all need our differing contributions, insights, and perceptions, because if we do not hang together we will surely be hanged separately.

REFERENCES AND FURTHER READING

Berry, Steve and Rob Noble. July 30 2007. "HIV and AIDS in Uganda: Why is Uganda Interesting?" www.avert.org/aidsuganda.htm, July 30 (accessed 8/3/2007).

Chan, Kenneth. 2004. "Experts Debate Over Abstinence, Condom Controversy at AIDS Conference." *The Christian Post*. http://www.christianpost.com/article/20040720/1159, July 20 (accessed 9/27/2007).

Cohen, Susan A. 2003. "Beyond Slogans: Lessons from Uganda's Experience with ABC and HIV/AIDS." *The Guttmacher Report on Public Policy* (December 2003) 6:5.

Epstein, Helen. 2007. *The Invisible Cure: Africa, the West and the Fight Against AIDS*. New York: Viking Press.

Halmshaw C. and K. Hawkins. 2004. "Capitalising on Global HIV/AIDS Funding: The Challenge for Civil Society and Government." *Reproductive Health Matters* (2004) 12: 24.

Human Rights Watch. 2007. "The Less They Know, the Better: Abstinence Only HIV/AIDS Programs in Uganda—Arguments for and Against Abstinence-Only Programs in Uganda." http://hrw.org/reports/2005/Uganda0305/8.htm (accessed 9/27/2007).

Laconte, Joseph. 2003. "The White House Initiative to Combat AIDS: Learning from Uganda," The Heritage Foundation. Backgrounder #1692, www.Heritage.org/Research/Africa/BG1692, September 29 (accessed 8/3/2007).

Lamptey, Peter. 2002. "Reducing Heterosexual Transmission of HIV in Poor Countries." *British Medical Journal* (2002) 324(7331): 207–211.

Low-Beer, D and R.L. Stoneburner. 2003. "Behaviour and Communication Change in Reducing HIV: Is Uganda Unique?" *African Journal of AIDS Research* (2003) 2(1): 9–21.

Mbogo, Stephen. 2007. *Uganda Denies Claims That Focusing on Abstinence Harms Anti-AIDS Efforts*. http://www.crosswalk.com/1322513 (accessed 9/27/2007).

Ministry of Health. 2006. *Uganda HIV/AIDS Sero-behavioural Survey 2004–2005, Kampala*. Uganda Ministry of Health and Calverton, MD, U.S.A.

Okware, S., J. Kinsman, S. Onyango, A. Opio, and P. Kaggwa. (2005). "Revisiting the ABC Strategy: HIV Prevention in Uganda in the Era of Antiretroviral Therapy." *Postgraduate Medical Journal* (2005) 81: 625–628. pmj.bmj.com (accessed 8/3/2007).

PANOS Dossier No. 2, 1990. *The 3rd Epidemic: Repercussions of the fear of AIDS*. London: Panos Inst.

Parikh, Shanti A. 2007. "The Political Economy of Marriage and HIV: The ABC Approach, 'Safe' Infidelity, and Managing Moral Risk in Uganda." *American Journal of Public Health* (July 2007) 97: 7.

Planned Parenthood. 2006. "Global HIV/AIDS: The Politics of Prevention Issue Brief." http://www.plannedparenthood.org/news-articles-press/politics-policy-issues/international-issues/aids-prevention-9657.htm (accessed 9/11/2007).

Population Secretariat. 2004. *The State of Uganda Population Report 2004: Promises, Performances and Opportunities*. Ministry of Finance, Planning and Economic Development, Kampala, 2004. www.popsec.org.

Population Secretariat. 2007. *The State of Uganda's Population Report 2007: Planned Urbanization for*

Uganda's Growing Population. Ministry of Finance, Planning and Economic Development, Kampala, 2007. www.popsec.org.

Sanders, Edmund. 2005. "Uganda Takes Up Abstinence Campaign." *Los Angeles Times*, October 31, A8, http://www.ph.ucla.edu/epi/seaids/ugandaabstinence.html (accessed 9/27/2007).

Sussman, Anna Louie. 2006. Uganda's Shift in AIDS Policy Tied to U.S. www.womensenews.org/article.cfm=aid=2645, February (accessed 9/27/2007).

Uganda Bureau of Statistics (UBOS) and Macro International Inc. 2002. *Uganda Demographic and Health Survey 2001–2002*. Calverton, MD: UBOS and Macro International Inc.

Uganda Bureau of Statistics (UBOS) and Macro International Inc. 2007. *Uganda Demographic and Health Survey 2006*. Calverton, MD: UBOS and Macro International Inc.

United States Agency for International Development (USAID). 2003. *The "ABCs" of HIV Prevention: Report of a USAID Technical Meeting on Behaviour Change Approaches to Primary Prevention of HIV/AIDS*. Washington DC: Population, Health and Nutrition Information Project.

United States Presidential Emergency Plan for AIDS Relief (PEPFAR). 2007. *Uganda Fiscal Year 2007 Country Operational Plan (COP)*. Washington, DC, 2007. www.pepfar.gov/about/82442.htm (accessed 9/28/2007).

Wilson, David. 2004. "Partner Reduction and the Prevention of HIV/AIDS: The Most Effective Strategies Come from Within Communities." *British Medical Journal* (April 2004) 328: 848–849.

CHAPTER 17

The Role of South African Traditional Health Practitioners in HIV/AIDS Prevention and Treatment

Kathy Goggin, Megan Pinkston, Nceba Gqaleni, Thandi Puoane, Douglas Wilson, Jannette Berkley-Patton, and David A. Martinez

ABSTRACT

This chapter provides findings from a study of herbal interventions for HIV disease management used by Traditional Health Practitioners (THPs) in in Kwa-Zulu Natal, which has the highest incidence of HIV in South Africa. THPs provide health care for many who do not have access to or wish to use allopathic health care. It is estimated that the majority of South Africans seek the services of THPs at some point. Despite a long history of marginalization, many in South Africa, including the government, have begun to recognize this and view THPs as a valuable health resource. However, their inclusion in the mainstream public health care system is only beginning due to the long-standing distrust between THPs and allopathic health care providers.

> *"Why must it be the doctor or the traditional healer? I find some things work from both, but you can never tell one about the other. If they worked together, it would benefit the patients. As it is, I've had to work out the balance for myself but it's really helping. Herbs counteract the side-effects of some of the drugs."*
>
> Priscilla, Zimbabwe (from *A Positive Woman's Survival Kit*, The International Community of Women Living with HIV/AIDS)

HIV/AIDS IN SOUTH AFRICA

By the end of 2005, 38.6 million people were living with the human immunodeficiency virus (HIV) worldwide. Sub-Saharan Africa is home to three-quarters of all HIV-positive (HIV+) women and 90 percent of all HIV+ children (UNAIDS/WHO 2006). HIV+ adult women (59 percent) outnumber men in this region and female youth (15–24 years old) account for 90 percent of all new HIV infections (Rehle et al. 2007; Human Science Research Council 2005). By the end of 2006, 2.1 million sub-Saharan individuals had died of AIDS. In the sub-Saharan country of South Africa, the number of deaths is so overwhelming that in some parts of the country the cemeteries are running out of space and the dead are being buried on top of other bodies (Wines 2004).

Currently, there are an estimated 5.4 million HIV+ South Africans (Dorrington et al. 2004b). Estimated at 22 percent among adults and 18 percent among 15- to 24-year-olds, HIV/AIDS prevalence in South Africa is one of the highest in the world. HIV has extracted a huge toll on the health of the country, driving life expectancy down from 62 years in 1990 to 47 years in 2005 (United Nations Population Fund 2007). As HIV incidence continues to climb, South African life expectancy is predicted to be as low as 40 years by 2010 (UNFPA).

Rates of HIV in South Africa are highest in the province of KwaZulu-Natal, where the prevalence is estimated to be as high as 40 percent (Dorrington et al. 2004b; Dorrington et al. 2004a). Additionally, four out of every ten pregnant women in KwaZulu-Natal are HIV+ (Anderson and Phillips 2006). According to a recent South African survey, more than twice as many people had been to a funeral in the past year than had been to a wedding (South African Advertising Research Foundation 2004). Sadly, the AIDS epidemic in South Africa shows no evidence of decline (UNAIDS/WHO 2006).

UNIQUE BARRIERS TO HIV PREVENTION AND ACCESS TO CARE IN SOUTH AFRICA

Indigenous beliefs about HIV prevail in South Africa and unfortunately often hinder prevention and treatment activities. For instance, Simbayi et al. (2005) have demonstrated that, despite prevalence of appropriate AIDS knowledge and education, 29 percent of young adult respondents believe that cleansing one's genitals after sexual intercourse will prevent HIV infection. Further, one in five men reported that having sexual intercourse with a virgin would cleanse their bodies of HIV (Meel 2003). Research in KwaZulu-Natal indicated that such indigenous beliefs are more prevalent among older individuals (Liddell et al. 2006); however, sexually active youth who reported being more accepting of modern prevention methods also reported never using condoms (Eaton et al. 2003). Lack of access to condoms is also a commonly cited barrier, but clearly misconceptions are also contributing to the problem (Karim et al. 1995).

One of the most publicized barriers to effective treatment is lack of access to antiretroviral medication therapy (ART). Despite a large push by the South African government to facilitate a medication rollout program to increase access, only one in six individuals (i.e., 17 percent) in need of treatment were able to receive it in 2005 (UNAIDS/WHO 2006). For instance, in the Western Cape and Gauteng, only 60 percent of qualified HIV+ patients have received ART (Baleta 2004). Worse yet, only a small portion of South Africa's HIV+ population, those with advanced disease (CD4 < 200 cells/mm^3), qualify for the rollout. South Africa based its qualification criteria on the 2002 World Health Organization (WHO) guidelines for initiating and prescribing ART medications, which instruct clinicians to initiate treatment once individual's CD4 cell counts are < 200 cells/mm^3 (WHO 2003a). However, in developed countries individuals are typically started on ART well before this point (CD4 < 350 cells/mm^3; United States Department of Health and Human Services 2007), as delaying treatment beyond this point has demonstrated negative health effects (Badri et al. 2006; Holmes et al. 2006). Recognizing these grim facts, WHO revised their 2002 guidelines, encouraging initiation of ART between 200 and 350 CD4 cells/mm^3 (WHO 2006). Unfortunately, the South African government has yet to adopt these new guidelines.

Further complicating ART access issues is the overall lack of an adequate health care infrastructure in rural South Africa (Busgeeth and Rivett 2004). The vast majority of rural HIV+ individuals are referred to tertiary hospitals and then to district hospitals, requiring individuals to travel great distances (Bateman 2006). Unfortunately, the lack of sufficient medical infrastructure means that many HIV+ people who need ART never make it to care (Buor 2003; Wilson and Blower 2007). In peri-urban and rural areas where resources are scarce and travel distances extensive, the Department of Health estimated that 70 percent of South Africans consult the country's 200,000 Traditional Health Providers (THPs) for health-related issues (Watson 2005).

Patients see THPs for a variety of reasons; however, one of the most common is symptoms of sexually transmitted infections, including HIV/AIDS (e.g., Ndulo et al. 2001; Peltzer 1998, 2001, 2003; Peltzer et al. 2006; Wilkinson and Wilkinson 1998; Zachariah et al. 2002). In fact, so many make this decision that most experts now believe that this "second system" of traditional medicine is actually bearing the brunt of HIV/AIDS care and support (Morris 2001). How South Africa has arrived at this point of having a "second system" is intractably linked to the historical legacy of apartheid.

HISTORICAL CONTEXT OF THPs' ROLE IN THE HIV EPIDEMIC

Racial strife between the White minority and the Black majority of South Africa culminated in the segregationist movement of the National Party in 1948, better known as apartheid (i.e., meaning "apart-ness" in Afrikaans). Between 1948 and 1993, the laws that defined apartheid provided advantages to the White minority and oppressed the Black South African majority. Blacks were disadvantaged by almost every standard including income, education, medical care, housing, and life expectancy.[1] Apartheid rules dictated the classification of people into separate racial groups. Restrictions delegated where one could live and work based on one's assigned race. Blacks were segregated to specific areas of South Africa and were only allowed to travel outside of their designated "homeland" areas to work in another area (Cornell et al. 2004).

The end of apartheid in 1990 was marked by several important historical events, including: the resignation of the National Party and the lifting of the ban on the African National Congress (ANC), the release of Nelson Mandela after 27 years in prison, and the slow repeal of apartheid laws and formal segregation. The first multi-race elections were held in 1994 and the ANC, led by Nelson Mandela, won with an overwhelming majority of votes (Sampson 1999). While these historic elections marked the end of apartheid and lifted the spirits of a people who had suffered greatly under years of oppression, these events could do little to address decades of neglect. With no immediate relief in sight, the majority of South Africans continue to live in impoverished settings with limited access to the most basic of human needs, including limited access to health care. Worse yet, during the years leading up to the end of apartheid a new and deadly epidemic was silently making its way into the lives of far too many South Africans.[2]

The first case of AIDS was confirmed in South Africa in 1982. In 1990, the South African case count of HIV had increased to 500. Incidence rates of HIV dramatically increased between 1993 and 2000, during which time the country's focus was consumed by the political changes noted above. Sadly, after the political change and the new awareness of the HIV epidemic, the once prosperous Republic of South Africa fell by 35 places in the Human Development Index, a global directory that ranks countries by their level of development (UNAIDS/WHO 2006).

The legacy of the apartheid era would make it nearly impossible to control the spread of HIV. Despite the end of formal laws requiring segregation, hospitals continued to be segregated. By apartheid design, White hospitals were better equipped, staffed and supported. Black hospitals, which continue to provide care for the majority of the population, were the least prepared to deal with the magnitude of the epidemic (Oppenheimer and Bayer 2007: 12). For example, in the 1980s a Black hospital named King Edward VII was so overcrowded that many patients were forced to sleep under the beds of other patients (Oppenheimer and Bayer 2007: 12). The apartheid medical system, much of it based on Nazi doctrine (Oppenheimer and Bayer 2007: 8), reflected the theorized differential worth of Blacks and Whites. A fee-for-service private market was available to Whites with health insurance-sponsored voluntarily by their employers. The majority of the Black population never had access to such employment and necessarily had to depend on publicly supported hospitals and clinics. The medical care offered to Whites was comparable to that found in developed countries (van Rensburg 1992:

80–83), but the average Black South African was not as lucky. In the mid-1980s, the hospital bed ration for Blacks was one quarter of that for Whites in South Africa (van Rensburg 1992). In an attempt to draw attention to the plight of their patients, physicians at Chris Hani Baragwanath Hospital banded together and sent a letter detailing the overcrowding and inhumane conditions. The government responded by firing the physicians (Oppenheimer and Bayer 2007: 13). "It is not the least of the ironies of AIDS in South Africa that, in its death throes, the apartheid regime fueled an epidemic that would so mark the first decade of freedoms" (Oppenheimer and Bayer 2007: 20). After suffering decades of oppression during apartheid and then facing a new and deadly epidemic, the country looked to their leader for assistance. However, Nelson Mandela's successor, the newly elected Thabo Mbeki, chose to place AIDS low on his priority list.

Thabo Mbeki, known for his commitment to fighting apartheid, more recently has become known for his unfounded statements that HIV is not the cause of AIDS (Gellman 2000; Achmat and Simcock 2007). President Mbeki's Health Minister, Manto Tshabalala-Msimang, has publicly encouraged the use of garlic, olive oil, beetroot, and the African potato rather than ART to treat HIV. Tshabalala-Msimang was quoted as saying, "Raw garlic and a skin of the lemon—not only do they give you a beautiful face and skin but they also protect you from disease" (Tshabalala-Msimang 2005). The Mbeki administration has repeatedly stated that the leading causes of death in South Africa are malnutrition and poverty, not HIV. In the summer of 2007, Deputy Health Minister, Nozizwe Madlala-Routledge, was fired for questioning the administration's stance and for her efforts to revitalize anti-AIDS campaigns in South Africa (Nullis 2007).

IMPACT OF STIGMA AND DISCRIMINATION

Fueled by the political battle surrounding HIV, stigma has played a significant role in the development and maintenance of South Africa's epidemic. A wealth of research exists establishing the negative impact of stigma. For example, HIV+ women often do not seek care for their illness because of the stigma and discrimination they fear they will face (Kilewo et al. 2001). Stigma is a real barrier to HIV prevention efforts as individuals often do not want to know their status and will avoid testing and further accessing treatment to avoid being seen as an HIV+ person (Daftary et al. 2007; Kalichman and Simbayi 2003; Skinner and Mfecane 2004; Petros et al. 2006). Fear of discrimination also often prevents HIV+ individuals from disclosing their status to their sexual partners (Simbayi et al. 2007). Despite efforts to reduce AIDS stigma in South Africa, recent studies reveal that: 29 percent of South African respondents would not buy food from a vendor who has HIV (Shisana et al. 2005); 20 percent believe that HIV+ children should be isolated to prevent infection (Shisana et al. 2005); 43 percent believe that HIV+ people should not be allowed to work with children; and 41 percent felt that HIV+ people should expect to have restrictions placed on their freedom (Kalichman et al. 2005).

Studies in South Africa have demonstrated the negative impact of AIDS stigma. For example, in Cape Town, 25 percent of HIV+ individuals queried have never spoken with friends or family members about their status and 33 percent of those who have disclosed their HIV status report being treated differently after telling others (Shisana et al. 2005; Simbayi et al. 2007). One in five HIV+ individuals report losing their jobs or housing subsequent to disclosing their HIV status (Shisana et al. 2005, Simbayi et al. 2007). In addition, qualitative research has revealed that HIV+ individuals prefer to tell others that they have tuberculosis (TB) rather than deal with the stigma of being HIV+ (Daftary et al. 2007). Not surprisingly, many struggle to cope with the many challenges of having HIV, and studies have demonstrated that 30–42 percent of HIV+ South Africans report symptoms of depression (Shisana et al. 2005, Simbayi et al. 2007). It is against this backdrop that many HIV+ South Africans seek the care of THPs.

TRADITIONAL MEDICINE IN SOUTH AFRICA

The World Health Organization defines traditional medicine as: "health practices, approaches, knowledge and beliefs incorporating plant, animal and mineral-based medicines, spiritual therapies, manual techniques and exercises, applied singularly or in combination to treat, diagnose and prevent illnesses or maintain well-being" (WHO 2003b). For thousands of years, traditional medicine has been practiced by THPs, who have provided services for the majority of people in Africa (Nyika 2007). During colonialism, traditional medicine was portrayed as primitive superstition based on witchcraft (Tolsi 2007; Nyika 2007). Efforts to suppress traditional medicine and the perceived political threat of non-colonial ideas that it represented led to a series of Witchcraft Acts that outlawed its practice (Gordon 2003; Andrews and Sutphen 2003). Despite attempts to suppress its practice, the availability of allopathic health care and valid concerns about the lack of safety and efficacy data for traditional methods, traditional medicine still remains the first choice option for the majority of South Africans (Nyika 2007). Estimates are that 80 percent of all South Africans will consult with a THP during their lifetime (Puckree et al. 2002). A recent study of 300 patients of THPs in Durban revealed that 70 percent consulted THPs as their first choice health care provider (Puckree et al. 2002).

Many South Africans choose traditional over allopathic health care, as the existing government-run health care system is overstressed and cannot meet the needs of all who currently need it (e.g., Wilson and Blower 2007). The legacy of institutionalized inequality in health facilities, infrastructure and staffing has left the majority of South Africans with a system that simply was not built to accommodate them (Oppenheimer and Bayer 2007). Despite local clinics in urban and peri-urban settings, most South Africans have to travel great distances, with little or no existing public transportation, on dangerous roads, to visit a government-run health care facility. Once there, they often face long lines, required fees, and an overwhelmed bureaucracy that is buckling under the weight of caring for all who need it. In contrast, there are often more than a few THPs' practices within walking distance of individuals' homes and THPs often make house calls. While there are often other patients to be seen and fees for the services rendered, patients of THPs are warmly welcomed and assured a cure for what ails them. Not surprisingly, many choose the ease and familiarity of their local THP over a trip to the allopathic health care clinic.

Recognizing this reality, in 2004 the South African government passed the THP Act, which formally acknowledged the contributions of THPs. It established a "regulatory framework to ensure the efficacy, safety and quality of TH care services" and "for control over the registration, training and conduct" of traditional health practitioners and students" (Traditional Health Practitioners Act 2004: Preface). The act established the national Interim THP Council, which is charged with establishing and instituting professional standards while maintaining the dignity and integrity of traditional healing and promoting public health (Traditional Health Practitioners Act 2004: Chapter 2, Clause 5).

TRADITIONAL HEALTH PROVIDERS IN KWAZULU-NATAL

In the South African province of KwaZulu-Natal, there are a number of different types of THPs including: *sangomas* (*izangoma*), who are diviners; *inyangas* (*izinyanga*), who are herbalists; *abathandazi*, who are faith healers; and others (e.g., traditional birth attendants, traditional surgeons, and *muthi* (medicine) traders) (Devenish 2005).

Sangomas divine the cause of illnesses in several ways, including communicating with ancestral spirits through dreams, visions, and "throwing of the bones." Depending on the presumed cause of the symptoms/illness, *sangomas* prescribe rituals and/or natural remedies. *Inyangas* prescribe traditional medicines to treat patients after consulting with them about their symptoms. Both *sangomas* and *inyangas* employ rituals and/or symbolic offerings to address illness and maintain health. While there is overlap between the techniques used in diagnosis and treatment offered by different types of THPs, in general *inyangas* do not use divination as a diagnostic technique. Also, *sangomas* are usually female and *inyangas* mostly male (Ngubane 1981); however, there are many exceptions to this general pattern in modern South Africa.

Medicine provided by *sangomas* and *inyangas* is called *muthi* (*umuthi*). In isiZulu, *muthi* literally translates as "tree" or "shrub," but it is widely used throughout South Africa to describe any type of medicine. *Muthis* prescribed by THPs typically consist of herbal, bark, and animal products that are specially prepared to address a particular symptom or illness. Formulas for *muthis*, including where exactly the ingredients are collected, are often closely guarded secrets handed down from healer to apprentice.

While a thorough discussion of THPs' extremely complex belief system of the etiology of disease is beyond the scope of this chapter (see Ngubane 1977), we offer a concise summary here. Most illnesses from the common cold to serious outbreaks of disease are believed to be caused by biological factors and are referred to as *umkhuhlane*. The causes of these illnesses are linked to the body's natural tendency to break down as it ages and are believed to "just happen" (Ngubane 1977). Diagnosis and effective medicines to treat these illnesses can come from allopathic and/or traditional health traditions. In contrast, *ukufa kwabantu* or "disease of the African peoples," are inextricably linked to traditional African beliefs regarding health and disease, and require the attention of a THP. The cause of these diseases is seen as a problem in the interaction of the individual and their environment or due to sorcery, ancestral possession, or evil spirits. Diagnosis and treatment for these disorders is attainable only from THPs, as allopathically trained professionals do not share an understanding of the presumed etiology or treatment of these traditional ailments.

TRADITIONAL HEALTH PROVIDERS' IMPACT ON HEALTH CARE

Many South Africans are familiar with traditional beliefs regarding health and disease (Oppenheimer and Bayer 2007: 106) and choose between allopathic or traditional medicine based on what they believe to be the cause of their symptoms. If they believe that their symptoms are caused by traditional causes, then they seek traditional treatment approaches rather than allopathic health care (Kayombo et al. 2007; Oppenheimer and Bayer 2007: 106).

Despite the ease with which patients move between the allopathic and traditional worlds of health care, many do not share their use of both, approached with either type of provider. This is not surprising, as many allopathic providers and THPs are not pleased with their patients seeking services from other types of providers. Allopathic providers are often quite hostile towards the use of traditional medicine, which they view as unscientific and potentially harmful. Likewise, some THPs discourage their patients from seeking allopathic health care, as they believe that the ancestors do not want to be mixed with White people's medicine because it will weaken the effect of their treatments (Bradley and Puoane 2007). Needless to say, many patients avoid this potential conflict by not disclosing their use of both forms of health care. Unfortunately, utilizing services from both systems without the full awareness of all providers can lead to negative consequences for patients. For example, there may be interactions, some quite serious in nature, between the different medications provided by the allopathic providers and THPs. One of us (Puoane) reports on the case of a 54-year-old man who had been in the hospital for one week suffering from heart problems. His condition had improved considerably since being admitted, until one afternoon, when his visitors gave him a Coke to drink. Thirty minutes after taking the Coke, he experienced palpitations and unfortunately died. The Coke in the bottle was actually traditional medicine brought by the relatives. The combination of the traditional medicine and the medicines provided to him in the hospital proved to be fatal.

Another common pattern is for patients to start and stop medications just before seeing the different types of providers, which can have serious implications for proper assessment, treatment, and disease management. Our own work (Puoane) illustrates this pattern, as explained by one patient, who did not share his use of traditional health care with his allopathic provider.

> When I came from the hospital, I went to my traditional healer, who gave me a mixture for control of my disease. I used this until a few weeks before I went for checkup. After my [allopathic] doctor checked me he said, "Your health is good. Continue with the way in which you have been taking your treatment."

Delays in obtaining effective treatment for disorders can also occur when patients are going back and forth between the two systems. One of us (Puoane) provides the following example to illustrate how delays in treatment can affect patient outcomes.

> A traditional healer reported that she had been diagnosed with high blood pressure and prescribed tablets by her allopathically trained provider; however, she had stopped taking them. "I use snuff everyday to relieve the stress. I was told that I have the HI-HI. I don't use the tablets that they gave me, I don't like them. I use the snuff and medicine that I make from bark of a certain tree. A few minutes after sniffing it, I feel dizzy, then I feel relieved of the stress."

Finally, some individuals suffer severe and sometimes life-threatening effects from traditional medicines. These adverse effects include bradycardia, brain damage, cardiogenic shock, diabetic coma, encephalopathy, heart rupture, intravascular hemolysis, liver failure, respiratory failure, toxic hepatitis, and even death (Ernst 2003). Many believe that the lack of regulation of traditional *muthis* means that they may unknowingly contain toxic plant material, be contaminated with heavy metals, or tainted with synthetic drugs (Ernst 2003). Unfortunately, it is not uncommon to see infants in the emergency department of hospitals die from herbal intoxication (Steenkamp et al. 2003) and/or dehydration (Moore and Moore 1998) after receiving *muthi*, especially in the form of enemas. This condition is unfortunately so common that it has actually been named "paediatric enema syndrome" (Moore and Moore 1998). Despite the potential for iatrogenic results, the convenience and presumed efficacy of traditional medicine leads many individuals to seek care from a THP.

CURRENT EFFORTS TO WORK WITH THPs

Despite their popularity, few properly designed trials have been conducted to establish the safety and efficacy of traditional medicines for HIV (Food and Agriculture Organization of the United Nations 2006). Unfortunately, this has not prevented some THPs from making claims that their treatments can cure HIV infection (Abdulbaqi 2002). Despite the intense media attention to these most extreme cases of false claims, the vast majority of THPs provide what many believe is effective treatment for the symptoms of HIV disease and side effects of the ART medications. There are presently several efforts underway to determine the veracity of these claims of safety and efficacy in formal randomized clinical trials (e.g., Goggin et al. 2007; Tolsi 2007). For example, several of us (Goggin, Gqaleni, Wilson) are working together on a study funded by the National Center for Complementary and Alternative Medicine to conduct a randomized clinical trial to test the safety of a particular herb used by THPs (i.e., Sutherlandia or *unwele*) in a sample of HIV+ adults with ≥350 CD4 cells. To our knowledge, this is the first clinical trial of Sutherlandia (*unwele*) in HIV+ individuals and the first trial to utilize a fully integrated team of allopathic providers and THPs. We are hopeful that our efforts will be a model for how allopathic providers and THPs can work together.

Our ability to establish this groundbreaking study is a direct result of the longstanding collaborative relationship among leaders at the Nelson R. Mandela School of Medicine, eThekwini Traditional Health Practitioners Council, eThekwini Municipality Health Unit, and eThekwini District Office of the KwaZulu-Natal Department of Health. There have been many successful efforts that have grown out of this historic partnership. For example, one of us (Gqaleni) has been central in the development and implementation of a President's Emergency Plan for AIDS Relief (PEPFAR)-funded project to establish a district/local government level collaboration between allopathic health care clinics and THPs. This novel partnership has led to the development of an HIV prevention and integration in-care program that has reached 221 THPs from all 11 sub-districts of eThekwini thus far. Each of these THPs have completed a one-week workshop covering: HIV awareness, prevention, voluntary counseling and testing, clinical guideline for care, monitoring and evaluation, and potential interactions between traditional and allopathic medications. A comparable course which introduces allopathic health care providers to traditional medicine has also been developed. A piloted test of this curriculum with 20 allopathic health care workers has been completed with the goal of implementing the full program with 200 health care workers in 2007 and 2008 (Gqaleni 2007).

In addition to the cross-training curriculums, this project also includes a data collection component where THPs were asked to use co-jointly developed monitoring forms to track the patients seen in their practice for HIV-related issues and treatments provided. Results from the first wave of data collection in October of 2006 indicated that 82 percent of THPs (126 of 154) had completed the monitoring forms. Results indicate that a total of 2,067 patients were seen in the preceding month, with slightly more women (58 percent) than men (39 percent) receiving care. THPs reported treating 150 HIV+ patients who were not currently on ARVs (antiretrovirals). Nearly a third of these patients (32 percent) had blood work done by an allopathic health care provider, which was being used by their THP to track treatment progress. The majority of patients with blood work (76 percent) reportedly had CD4 cell counts of ≥ 200, making them ineligible for the rollout under current guidelines. THPs reported providing care for 84 patients with < 200 CD4 cells who were not on ARVs and were receiving only prophylactic or palliative care. A third of THPs (60 percent) had referred patients (n = 112) to volunteer HIV counseling and testing. An additional 396 patients received treatment for STIs other than HIV/AIDS.

In terms of HIV prevention, THPs reported providing patients with advice on abstinence (n = 54) and being faithful (n = 1816). They also provided education on condom use to 1,889 patients and advice on nutrition to 1,917 patients. They reportedly provided prevention advice (e.g., other STIs, general health) to 1,967 of their patients.

These are the first published data of this type and, while provisional, clearly demonstrate that THPs are providing prevention and treatment services to HIV and at-risk individuals, using hematology reports in their practices, and are willing to make referrals to allopathic health care. While further refinement to the monitoring system is needed, this is also a first look at what THPs are willing to do in terms of record-keeping and integration with allopathic health care systems. This revolutionary program also demonstrates that a respectful exchange of information between the traditional and allopathic worlds can lead to better communication and treatment for Black South Africans.

SUMMARY

South Africans are dying from HIV in record-breaking numbers. Given the complex historical and political context of HIV in South Africa, any successful response to this epidemic will need to involve every sector of the government, as well as the formal and informal health care systems. In short, any successful response will have to include Traditional Health Providers.

THPs have historically played and continue to play an important role in HIV prevention and treatment in South Africa. Minimizing their contributions or ignoring their status within society is a mistake that we cannot afford to make. Luckily, serious strategic efforts to build bridges between the allopathic and traditional health worlds have already demonstrated some success; however, sustained coordinated efforts are needed to build on these successes. Carefully conceived strategies to facilitate enhanced communication and infrastructure systems between the traditional and allopathic health care worlds can only benefit public health in South Africa.

NOTES

1. The act of segregation by race was not new and had been occurring in South Africa since the seventeenth century.
2. The full complexity of the relationship between the fall of apartheid and the rising of HIV is beyond the scope of this chapter. See Achmat and Simcock (2007).

REFERENCES AND FURTHER READING

Abdulbaqi, A. (2002). HIV cure gives folk medicine the upper hand, trans. I. Alayoubi. Retrieved September 18, 2007, from Doha: Islam Online, http://www.islamonline.net/English/science/2002/11/article07.shtml.

Achmat, Z., and Simcock, J. (2007). Combining prevention, treatment and care: Lessons from South Africa. *AIDS*, *21*, S11–S20.

Anderson, B. A., and Phillips, H. E. (2006). *Adult mortality (age 15–64) based on death notification data in South Africa: 1977–2004* (Report No. 03–09–05). Pretoria Statistics South Africa, 15.

Andrews, B., and Sutphen, M. (2003). Introduction. In B. Andrews and M. Sutphen (eds.), *Medicine and Colonial Identity* (pp. 1–13). London: Routledge.

Badri, M., Lawn, S. D., and Wood, R. (2006). Short-term risk of AIDS or death in people infected with HIV-1 before antiretroviral therapy in South Africa: A longitudinal study. *Lancet*, *368*, 1254–1259.

Baleta, A. (2004). Antiretroviral rollout in South Africa fails to meet demands. *Lancet Infectious Diseases*, *44*(11), 652.

Bateman, C. (2006). Inspiring rural health—a fierce and distant light. *South African Medical Journal*, *96*, 576–577.

Bradley, H.A., and Puoane, T. (2007). Prevention of hypertension and diabetes in an urban setting in South Africa: Participatory action research with community health workers. *Ethnicity and Disease*, *17*, 49–54.

Buor, D. (2003). Analysing primacy of distance in utilization of health care services in Ahafo-ano south district, Ghana. *International Journal of Health Planning and Management*, *18*, 298–311.

Busgeeth, K., and Rivett, U. (2004). The use of a spatial information system in the management of HIV/AIDS in South Africa. *International Journal of Health Geographics*, 7(1), 13.

Cornell, M., Reid, G., and Walker, L. (2004). *Waiting to happen: HIV/AIDS in South Africa: The bigger picture.* Boulder, CO: Lynne Rienner.

Daftary, A., Padayatchi, N., and Padilla, M. (2007). HIV testing and disclosure: A qualitative analysis of TB patients in South Africa. *AIDS Care*, *19*(4), 572–577.

Devenish, A. (2005). Negotiating healing: Understanding the dynamics amongst traditional healers in Kwazulu-Natal as they engage with professionalisation. *Social Dynamics*, *31*(2), 243–284.

Dorrington, R. E., Bradshaw, D., Johnson, L., and Budlender, D. (2004a). *The demographic impact of HIV/AIDS in South Africa: National indicators for 2004.* Cape Town: Centre for Actuarial Research, South African Medical Research Council and Actuarial Society of South Africa.

Dorrington, R. E., Johnson, L. F., Bradshaw, D., and Daniel, T. (2004b). *The demographic impact of HIV/AIDS in South Africa. National and provincial indicators for 2006.* Cape Town: Centre for Actuarial Research, South African Medical Research Council and Actuarial Society of South Africa.

Eaton, L., Flisher, A. J., and Aarø. L.E. (2003). Unsafe sexual behaviour in South African youth. *Social Science and Medicine*, *56*(1), 149–165.

Ernst, E. (2003). Serious adverse effects of unconventional therapies for children and adolescents: A systematic review of recent evidence. *European Journal of Pediatrics*, *162*, 72–80.

Food and Agriculture Organization of the United Nations (FAO). (2006). *Living well with HIV/AIDS.* Retrieved September 18, 2007, from ftp://ftp.fao.org/docrep/fao/005/y4168/y4168 E00.pdf.

Gellman (2000). South African president escalates AIDS feud. *Washington Post.*

Goggin, K., Mbhele, A. L., Makhathini, M. E., Buthelezi, T. D., Ndlovu, S. W., Shange, V. F., Thabethe, M. A., Mkhwanazi, D. A., Nkomo-Gwala, B. L., Hlongwane, T., Mdlalose, T., Ngubane, L., Gqaleni, N., Wilson, D., Wu, A. W., Bartman, P., Gerkovich, M., Williams, K., Berkley-Patton, J., Johnson, Q., and Folk, W. (2007). The translation and cultural adaptation of patient-reported outcome measures: A report from the field. Manuscript submitted for publication.

Gordon, D. (2003). A sword empire? Medicine and colonialism at King William's Town, Xhosaland, 1856–91. In B. Andrews and M. Sutphen (eds.), *Medicine and Colonial Identity* (pp. 41–60). London: Routledge.

Gqaleni, N. (2007). Leadership in HIV/AIDS magazine, July.

Holmes, C. B., Wood, R., Badri, M., Zilber, S., Wang, B., Maartens, G., Zhena, H., Lu, Z., Freedberg, K.A., and Losina, E. (2006). CD4 decline and incidence of opportunistic infections in Cape Town, South Africa: Implications for prophylaxis and treatment. *Journal of Acquired Immune Deficiency Syndromes, 42*, 464–469.

Human Science Research Council (2005). *South African national HIV prevalence, HIV incidence, behavior, and communication survey*. Cape Town: HSRC Press.

Kalichman, S., and Simbayi, L. (2003). HIV testing attitudes, AIDS stigmas, and voluntary HIV counseling and testing in the Western Cape, South Africa. *Sexually Transmitted Infections, 79*, 442–447.

Kalichman, S. C., Simbayi, L., Jooste, S., Toefy, Y., Cain, D., Cherry, C., and Kagee, A. (2005). Development of a brief scale to measure AIDS-related stigmas in South Africa. *AIDS and Behavior, 9*, 135–143.

Karim, Q. A., Karim, S. S., Soldan, K., and Zondi, M. (1995). Reducing the risk of HIV infection among South African sex workers: Socioeconomic and gender barriers. *American Journal of Public Health, 85*(11), 1521–1525.

Kayombo, E. J., Uiso, F. C., Mbwambo, Z. H., Mahunnah, R. L., Mosh, M. J., and Mgonda, Y. H. (2007). Experience of initiating collaboration of traditional healers in managing HIV and AIDS in Tanzania. *Journal of Ethnobiology and Ethnomedicine, 3*(6), 1–9.

Kilewo, C., Massawe, A., Lyamuya, E., Semali, I., Kalokola, F., Urassa, E., et al. (2001). HIV counseling and testing of pregnant women in sub-Saharan Africa: Experiences from a study on prevention of mother-to-child HIV-1 transmission in Dar es Salaam, Tanzania. *Journal of Acquired Immune Deficiency Syndrome, 28*(5), 458–462.

Liddell, C., Barrett, L., and Bydawell, M. (2006). Indigenous beliefs and attitudes to AIDS precautions in a rural South African community: An empirical study. *Annals of Behavioral Medicine, 32*(3), 226.

Meel, B. L. (2003). The myth of child rape as a cure for HIV/AIDS in Transkei: A case report. *Medical Science Law, 43*, 53–88.

Moore, D. A., and Moore, N. L. (1998). Paediatric enema syndrome in a rural African setting. *Annals of Topical Paediatrics, 18*(2), 139–144.

Morris, K. (2001). Treating HIV in South Africa—a tale of two systems. *The Lancet, 357*, 1190.

Ndulo, J., Faxelid, E., and Krantz, I. (2001). Traditional healers in Zambia and their care for patients with urethral/vaginal discharge. *Journal of Alternative and Complementary Medicine, 7*(5), 529–536.

Ngubane, H. (1977). *Body and mind in Zulu medicine: An ethnography of health disease in Nyuswa-Zulu thought and practice*. London: Academic Press Inc.

Ngubane, H. (1981). Aspects of clinical practice and traditional organisation of indigenous healers in South Africa. *Social Science and Medicine, 15B*, 361–365.

Nullis (2007). Mbeki hits back on AIDS. *Washington Post*.

Nyika, A. (2007). Ethical and regulatory issues surrounding African traditional medicine in the context of HIV/AIDS. *Developing World Bioethics, 7*(1), 25–34.

Oppenheimer, G. M., and Bayer, R. (2007). *Shattered dreams? An oral history of the South African AIDS epidemic*. New York, NY: Oxford University Press.

Peltzer, K. (1998). A community survey of traditional healers in rural South Africa. *South African Journal of Ethnology, 21*, 191–197.

Peltzer, K. (2001). An investigation into the practices of traditional and faith healers in an urban setting in South Africa. *Health SA Gesondheid, 6*, 3–11.

Peltzer, K. (2003). HIV/AIDS/STD knowledge, attitudes, beliefs and behaviours in a rural South African adult population. *South African Journal of Psychology, 33*, 250–260.

Peltzer, K., Mngqundaniso, N., and Petros, G. (2006). HIV/AIDS/STI/TB knowledge, beliefs and practices of traditional healers in KwaZulu-Natal, South Africa. *AIDS Care, 18*(6), 608–613.

Petros, G., Airbihenbuwa, C. O., Simbayi, L., Ramlagan, S., and Brown, B. (2006). HIV/AIDS and "othering" in South Africa: The blame goes on. *Culture, Health, and Sexuality, 8*(1), 67–77.

Puckree, T., Mkhize, M., Mgobhozi, Z., and Lin, J. (2002). African traditional healers: What health care professionals need to know. *International Journal of Rehabilitation Research, 25*(4), 247–251.

Rehle, T., Shisana, O., Pillay, V., Zuma, K., Puren, A., and Parker, W. (2007). National HIV incidence measures—new insights into the South African epidemic. *South African Medical Journal, 97*(3), 194–199.

Sampson, A. (1999). *Mandela: The authorized biography*. New York: Knopf.

Shisana, O., Rehle, T., Simbayi, L., Parker, W., Bhana, A., Zuma, K., Connolly, C., Jooste, S., and Pillay, V. (2005). *South African national HIV prevalence, incidence, behaviour and communication survey*. Cape Town: Human Science Research Council Press.

Simbayi, L. C., Kalichman, S. C., Jooste, S., Cherry, C., Mfecane, S., and Cain, D. (2005). Risk factors for HIV-AIDS among youth in Cape Town, South Africa. *AIDS and Behavior, 9*(1), 53–61.

Simbayi, L. C., Kalichman, S., Strebel, A., Cloete, A., Henda, N., and Mqeketo, A. (2007). Internalized stigma, discrimination, and depression among men and women living with HIV/AIDS in Cape Town, South Africa. *Social Science and Medicine, 64*, 1823–1831.

Skinner, D., and Mfecane, S. (2004). Stigma, discrimination and the implications for people living with HIV/AIDS in South Africa. *Journal of Social Aspects of HIV/AIDS Research, 1*(3), 157–164.

South African Advertising Research Foundation. (2004). All Media Products Survey March 2004.

Steenkamp, V., Stewart, M. J., and Zuckerman, M. (2003). Death due to use of traditional medicine in Africa: A preventable cause of neonatal and infant mortality. *Journal of Pediatric Gastroenterology and Nutrition, 36*(2), 294–295.

Tolsi, N. (2007). Sowing the seeds of HIV hope. Mail

and Guardian Online, August. Retrieved September 4, 2007, from http://www.mg.co.za/articlePage.aspx?area=/insight/insight_national/&articleid=317928.

Traditional Health Practitioners Act. (2004). South Africa.

Tshabalala-Msimang, M. (2005). Natural products and molecular therapy. Closing remarks. *Annals of the New York Academy of Science*, *1056*, 494–496.

UNAIDS/WHO (2006). *2006 Report on the Global AIDS Epidemic*, Chapter 4, The impact of AIDS on people and societies. Joint United Nations Programme on HIV/AIDS.

United Nations Population Fund (2007). Overview: South Africa. Retrieved August 20, 2007, from http://www.unfpa.org/profile/southafrica.cfm?Section=1.

United States Department of Health and Human Services (2007). AIDS Information: Offering information on HIV/AIDS treatment, prevention and research. Retrieved September 28, 2007, from: http://www.aidsinfo.nih.gov/.

Van Rensburg, H.C.J. (1992). *Health care in South Africa*, pp. 80–83.

Watson (2005). Traditional healers fight for recognition in South African AIDS crisis. *Nature Medicine*, *11*, 6.

Wilkinson, D., and Wilkinson, N. (1998). HIV infection among patients with sexually transmitted diseases in rural South Africa. *International Journal of AIDS*, *9*, 736–739.

Wilson, D. P., and Blower, S. (2007). How far will we need to go reach HIV-infected people in rural South Africa? *BMC Med*, *5*, 16.

Wines (2004). South Africa "recycles" graves for AIDS victims. *New York Times*.

World Health Organization (2003a). Scaling up anti-retroviral therapy in resource-limited settings: Treatment guidelines for a public health approach. Geneva: WHO. Retrieved September 28, 2007, from http://www.who.int/3by5/publications/documents/arv_guidelines/en/index.html.

World Health Organization (2003b). Traditional medicine. Geneva: WHO. Retrieved September 28, 2007, from: http://www.who.int/mediacentre/factsheets/2003/fs134/en/.

World Health Organization (2006). HIV/AIDS anti-retroviral newsletter. Geneva: WHO. Retrieved September 28, 2007, from http://www.wpro.who.int/NR/rdonlyres/BBC0070D-FD29-4871-B269-432B63A3160E/0/ARV_Newsletter_Issue_13.pdf.

Zachariah, R., Nkhoma, W., Harries, D., Arendt, V., and Chantulo, A. (2002). Health seeking and sexual behavior in patients with transmitted infections. The importance of traditional healers in Thyolo, Malawi. *Sexually Transmitted Infections*, *78*, 127–129.

SECTION 5

Policies of (In)Justice: Structural Responses to HIV

FRAMING ESSAY

HIV, Public Health, and Social Justice

Reflections on the Ethics and Politics of Health Care

Renée T. White, Cynthia Pope, and Robert Malow

The AIDS pandemic has laid bare a deceptively simple reality—that economically and socially vulnerable populations cannot sustain what is necessary to improve their quality of life without viable institutional and structural changes both within and outside of their countries. With increased economic polarization, sexual and gender exploitation, political instability, shifting global economies, and the like, it is no wonder that "questions of health can never be separated from broader struggles for responsibility, fairness, and social justice" (Parker 2002, 345).

Throughout the history of the HIV/AIDS pandemic, epidemiologists, public health experts, activists, non-governmental organizations (NGOs) and some policymakers have confronted a bio-behavioral approach to disease which posits that disease can be halted by targeting the individual or the risk group. This approach frequently converges with the rational choice paradigm, which posits that transmission rates will decrease once an individual is given incentives and made accountable for his or her choice to engage in risk behavior and understands the availability of alternatives. However, public health has generally been the responsibility of the government, and individual rights historically have been subject to limitation if there is a communicable risk or a severe public risk, such as in the case of drug-resistant tuberculosis. The maintenance and improvement of the public's health requires collective or social action, involves governmental, non-governmental, and professional actors, and must operate from the local to the international level (Breslow et al. 2002; Gandy 2005). Further, many decades of social epidemiological research have established that social context is a serious component of disease risk, and that choice is mediated by what is available to the individual actor, or to the community in which he or she lives.

Thus, a more useful analytical strategy is to place the individual actor within a larger social environment in which external variables affecting life chances (whether HIV-specific or not) can be understood. For example, utilizing a social epidemiological approach to HIV allows for the identification of social determinants that affect susceptibility and vulnerability at the population level. By using this approach, one can identify the complex web of intersecting factors that affect HIV/AIDS (Poundstone, Strathdee, and Celentano 2004). Some of these factors are at the social level: cultural context, social networks, neighborhood, and social capital. Cultural beliefs and practices can be reinforced by social networks and result in the continued stigmatization of people living with HIV/AIDS (PLHA) and the stigmatization of certain risk behaviors (see Faubion this volume). Naturally, stigma and fear of discrimination can result in many barriers for people seeking information or health services.

Structural factors affecting HIV/AIDS, such as the interaction of poorly functioning social institutions (government, education, and media, for example) and a lack of will, can result in what Paul Farmer (2003) has termed "structural violence." Structural violence occurs when harmful or untenable structural conditions persist and result in the undue suffering of groups of people who often are already vulnerable to marginalization due to their race, ethnicity, religion, citizenship status, gender, economic status, or sexuality. Structure refers to phenomena that are "embedded in the political and economic organization of [the] social world: they are violent because they cause injury to people (typically not those responsible for perpetuating such inequalities)" (Farmer, Nizeye, Stulac, and Keshavjee 2006, 1686). Therefore, structural violence may be caused by institutional forces, such as forced migration, unequal law and criminal justice processes, and war/militarization. For example, armed conflict and stagnant economies are linked with health crises in developing countries (Epstein 2003) and an absence of political will and rule of law in nations like Ethiopia and Zambia (Mohiddin and Johnston 2006). It is clear that the most vulnerable to disease, whether in the global North (northern hemisphere) or global South (southern hemisphere), are the economically and socially marginalized. Those who are the most vulnerable require structural supports in order to survive. Therefore, the eradication of diseases presumes government effectiveness, the absence of violence, the rule of law, lack of corruption, and civil engagement or the ability to select a government and influence domestic policy (Menon-Johansson 2005; Irwin and Scali 2007). All of these social and structural impacts on HIV/AIDS are systemic rather than merely individual and behavioral, in that social and structural factors feed off of each other and shape the lived context of the populations affected by them. Furthermore, other actors such as NGOs, multinationals, and the governments of developed nations have influenced the development of responses to the social and structural challenges faced by the governments of developing nations and their citizens.

Engaging in a social epidemiological analysis or structural analysis of the impact of HIV in resource-poor nations requires multiple lenses, such as understanding the social and structural variables within a particular nation while recognizing the impact of systems outside of the country. For example,

> As poverty increases so usually do income and class inequality. Mobility increases as people seek to escape poverty and work away from their homes. Increased poverty, inequality and mobility weaken or break up the social framework in which people live—a framework that may have disciplined sexual relations in ways that reduce disease transmission. This framework may be thought of, in part, as "social capital." Finally, rapid change and insecurity often increase the incidence of transactional sex as part of women's livelihoods. When, against this background, a government cuts back spending on health and education, it creates an environment conducive to HIV transmission (Barnett and Blackwell 2004, 4).

Social epidemiological analyses also necessitate recognizing that there are moral and ethical concerns that intersect society and structures. Key stakeholders have made decisions which both directly and indirectly affect the development of many nations' infrastructures. A person's inability to afford life-saving health care obstructs his or her ability to act as an autonomous being and thus becomes a human rights problem (Hein and Kohlmorgen 2005). As such, it is important to address the ways in which such decisions constrain a nation's ability to respond to the needs of its citizenry and to what extent multiple actors are culpable in the building of nations' infrastructures (Henry Kaiser Family Foundation 2007). The physical health of citizens is directly predicated upon the social health of the nation. The social health of a nation depends upon many factors—political, cultural, and economic. All of these factors shape and are shaped by the AIDS pandemic. Political structures impact the development of public health policy, fiscal decision-making, the building of infrastructures which facilitate health, and the decentralization of power within systems required to provide aid to citizens. Cultural factors such as the influence of gendered and sexual stigma, social norms concerning caregiving, and reliance on indigenous spiritual and health-seeking practices are influential as well. Movement of capital and labor within and between countries, trends in worker employability, and wage stagnation, are some of the viable economic factors associated with HIV/AIDS in developing countries. While developing such an extensive analysis is outside of the scope of this framing essay, what is feasible is to provide an introductory sketch of how one of these mechanisms is connected to HIV/AIDS—namely, economic influences.

STRUCTURAL FACTORS AND POWERFUL STAKEHOLDERS

Global gaps in income and investment have been growing over the past 20 years to 86:1 between the richest and poorest 20 percent of the global population. While poor state-level economic and political management are implicated in this trend, the influence of bilateral and multilateral financial support cannot be denied. For example, foreign direct investment (FDI) involves the influx of overseas foreign funds into a country to be used in manufacturing or services. The foreign investor retains at least partial control and ownership of this investment (e.g., the increasing trend among U.S.-based multinationals to outsource information technologies). FDI in the global South targeted 10 countries, including China, Indonesia, Colombia, Malaysia, and Taiwan.

> At the other extreme, the 48 Less Developed Countries (LDCs) received around $800 million in FDI in 1999—roughly the same size as flows into Brazil, and less than 1 percent of the total transfer to developing countries . . . This uneven distribution of global investment patterns with its associated selectivity and polarization of societies has given rise to: a growing gap between the rich and poor within and between nations (Commission on HIV/AIDS and Governance in Africa 2004: 5; see also BBC 2005).

Arguably, macroeconomic policy has had a profound impact on the economic viability of developing nations. Macroeconomic policies affect health and development because they alter absolute poverty and the distribution of wealth. As a result, both households and health systems are affected (Federici 2002; Gostin 2004; Poundstone, Strathdee, and Celentano 2004). Since the 1980s, the overarching macroeconomic policy that has generated substantial debate concerning its impact on health care provision and on national responses to HIV has been structural adjustment programs (SAP). The World Bank and the International Monetary Fund were the two key architects of SAPs in the 1980s. SAPs are vehicles for economic stabilization, sustained economic growth, and poverty reduction in developing countries. Eligible countries that receive low interest rate loans agree to satisfy certain conditions, including trade liberalization and reductions in state budgets (Abouharb and Cingranelli 2003; Muuka 1998). This economic model and the resulting conditions were predicated on a neoliberal political-economic premise emphasizing the power of the free market to dictate resource mobilization and patterns of consumption.[1] With a reduction in state controls on production and export of goods, economic growth was to be stimulated and all resources needed for the public good would be more efficiently distributed. Stimulating economic growth might necessitate a reduction in investments for the social good, including health care provision, but would promise long-term benefits. Within this framework, responsibility for health care would shift from the state as provider to the individual as consumer (Irwin and Scali 2007).

Under SAP guidelines, countries with a high debt burden would garner restructuring of debt as long as they satisfy certain requirements. These included the reorganization of their economic system and social policy initiatives to focus on privatization of goods and services, reduction of price controls on goods, a focus on exporting goods, and the use of fees for social goods such as education and health care (Irwin, Millen, and Fallows 2003; Barnett and Blackwell 2004; Heimer 2007). An unintended outcome was the reduction of spending in the social sector at the same time that the HIV pandemic was emerging (Irwin and Scali 2007). Ironically, alongside the expansion and popularization of neoliberalism there was an increase in available medical technologies to wealthy nations, liberalization of trade, increased economic vulnerability and marginalization of the already vulnerable, and increased intervention by non-state actors as problem solvers (Hein and Kohlmorgen 2005). All of the societal tools needed to confront the pandemic were weakened exactly when they were most needed by the governments of developing countries to launch effective, strategic, and long-term responses to HIV. There were limited resources for AIDS education through traditional and non-traditional outlets, infrastructures for health provision had been stripped, and thus developing nations faced the reality of borrowing more to offset the cost of care. While the SAPs and related neoliberal policies did not cause the rapid transmission of HIV in developing countries, particularly in sub-Saharan Africa, they inadvertently diverted resources that could have been used by poor nations in response to the pandemic. It would be problematic to argue that poor nations would have been equipped to contain the prevalence of HIV but it is possible that such macroeconomic policies weakened those nations with some modicum of infrastructure (Federici 2002; London 2007).

The economic destabilization of developing nations was so profound that by the end of the 1990s the debt to foreign aid ratio reached a high of 1.5:1 in sub-Saharan Africa, where expenditures on debt service outpaced health care 2:1 (Harris and Siplon 2001). Among the many outcomes of this debt load is that the provision of proven treatments such as antiretroviral drug therapies (ARVs) were too costly for countries to afford (Krieger 2001). Access to ARVs is literally a life-and-death issue, since taking these drug cocktails makes the difference between HIV being a chronic disease and a fatal one. Along with the increasing demand for ARVs is the need for health care providers, educators, and other health workers necessary to the provision of care: "This increased demand is putting pressure on the limited health resources in many developing countries . . . As more and more people turn to the public sector to help pay for health services after their own resources are depleted, governments will be faced with important choices regarding responses to HIV/AIDS" (Henry Kaiser Family Foundation 2007, 5).

A lack of infrastructural support has also been linked to an increased likelihood of structural violence within societies. Such violence is defined as the impact of both intentional and unintentional processes of institutional forces that constrain agency. Some scholars, such as Farmer (2003) and Poundstone, Strathdee, and Celentano (2004), have viewed the impact of SAPs and other institutional forces on the provision of care to individuals in resource-poor countries as a form of structural violence. One of the outcomes of this structural violence and public health debate is a new human rights and health discourse which calls for a renewed commitment to providing for the sustainability of health care and the reduction of rates of HIV transmission. Within this discourse, what comes to the fore is that developing nations may be resource-poor but asset-rich (Mohiddin and Johnston 2006). This shifts the health-as-social-problem debate from a pathologizing discourse to a collaborative problem-solving approach.

International law and human rights law have provided useful guideposts to this asset-rich, collective problem-solving strategy. What is especially instructive is that the application of a human rights orientation facilitates the leadership of developing nations to confront their HIV/AIDS crises with the help of both wealthy nations, NGOs, and other international actors. Responding to structural violence and the legacy of neoliberal economic policy demands the integration of human rights law in a way that addresses the importance of socioeconomic rights (Ammann 2002; Patterson and London 2002). Some scholars argue that the right to health is a binding component of international law extending to essential medicines,[2] a system of health protection and various other goods, services, and facilities allowing for the enjoyment of the highest possible level of health (Blaylock 2006; Hein and Kohlmorgen 2005). One of the most visible applications of the human rights discourse has concerned access to affordable ARVs. Even the most affordable ARVs are prohibitively expensive for the average person in a developing country, where the average daily wage might be no more than U.S.$1. Attempts to address questions of access within the World Trade Organization (WTO) illustrated the ongoing institutional conflicts between nations. Debates over the manufacture and distribution of pharmaceuticals highlighted the persistent tensions among stakeholders concerning the intersection of human rights, multinationals, and poverty. In 1995, the WTO drafted the agreement on Trade Related Aspects of Intellectual Property Rights (TRIPS), which was intended to protect the intellectual property of corporations (e.g., the patent rights of pharmaceuticals) to promote further incentives to advance ARV therapies for those pharmaceuticals operating in market-based economies. All WTO member nations, including developing ones, were obligated to alter their state laws so they paralleled the TRIPS agreement. But paying full price for medicines protected by patent law is untenable for most developing nations (see Craddock this volume for an expansion of this point). A logical alternative would be the production or import of generics or a pricing structure that would relieve poorer nations of this untenable economic burden (Perry 2002; Blaylock 2006).

Despite the aggressive resistance to these affordable alternatives launched by some pharmaceuticals and the United States government in particular, poorer nations could employ other options. There was a clause in TRIPS that granted countries a grace period before full application of intellectual property protections was expected. Initially, this grace period was slated to expire in 2005. Also, since the 2001 Doha Declaration on the TRIPS Agreement and Public Health, there is some authority for developing nations to suspend patent protection due to national emergencies (Calfee and Bate 2004). Further, a number of state actors, with the support of the World Health Organization and other United Nations organizations and activists, have explored the definition of "national emergency" with reference to the AIDS pandemic. In response to the overwhelming global public criticism, the TRIPS council has extended the transition period to 2016, during which less developed nations do not need to guarantee patent protection. Developing nations can utilize either parallel imports (drugs purchased in countries where manufacturing costs are low and resold in countries where costs would have been too high) or the manufacture of generics for domestic use but not imports. This means that countries with the technological capacity to manufacture generics can do so; both Brazil and South Africa took advantage of the grace period and produced generic versions of ARVs. However, many other poor nations are not able to do the same and are also unable to afford the cost of the imported drugs.

IMPLICATIONS FOR FUTURE COLLABORATIVE EFFORTS

SAP and neoliberal social and economic policies have contributed to the destabilization of developing nations (Avafia and Narasimhan 2006; Epstein 2003; Gandy 2005). These are coupled with the impact of the AIDS pandemic, which has contributed to the reduced life-expectancy rate in many developing nations, weakened the economic viability of nations, and become a national security risk (Parker 2002). It is important to recognize that some research indicates no causal relationship between SAP and the growth of HIV/AIDS, but rather a correlation (Barnett and Blackwell 2004). Even so, SAP and other policies created before the advent of HIV/AIDS could be modified to become more responsive to the ways in which HIV and structural factors *are* related.

The evolution of international policies allowing for the manufacture of affordable ARVs makes clear the relevance of structural human rights-oriented approaches to health care access (Beyrer 2007; Gandy 2005). It also highlights the importance of collaborative initiatives that use a multi-sectoral approach which is both vertical (focused on disease control) and horizontal (capacity building) (Henry Kaiser Family Foundation 2007; Poundstone, Strathdee, and Celentano 2004). NGOs and other international actors do have an important role to play in devising useful strategies to confront the AIDS pandemic—both vertical and horizontal (Dickinson 2006; Menon-Johansson 2005; Mohiddin and Johnston 2006). In 2006, international AIDS assistance totaled U.S.$5.6 billion (Kates, Izazola, and Lief 2007). The United States contributes 47 percent of all donor nation funds committed to HIV/AIDS programs. They are followed by the Netherlands (16.7 percent) and the United Kingdom at (14 percent). When based on the proportion of national wealth, The Netherlands, Sweden and Ireland are the three leading government donors for global programs.

The most successful collaborations between NGOs, international interests, and state actors include strong state-level leadership and political will, a national health care regulatory strategy, the incorporation of indigenous health provision—all of these encourage the capacity-building support of NGOs, private donors, and other international funds.

> [S]olutions and measures—money, expertise, technology—are readily available in countries with the ability to supply them (most often the world's wealthy countries). Moreover, doing so does not significantly harm those providing the aid (and may indeed benefit them materially in the long term, for example when those aided become trading partners). Therefore, those with the ability to provide the necessary aid ought to administer it even if they are not directly complicit in causing the problem—but the obligation is much more profound if they are (Harris and Siplon 2001, 9).

The Global Fund to Fight AIDS, Tuberculosis and Malaria was developed as a multilateral funding mechanism in 2002 and thus far has received financial commitments exceeding U.S.$4 billion from over 50 countries and numerous foundations such as the Bill and Melinda Gates Foundation (Feachem and Sabot 2007; Global Fund 2007; Hein and Kohlmorgen 2005). Its governance structure consists of 14 nation states (seven each from the North and South), NGOs foundations, and companies. The WHO, World Bank, and UNAIDS are non-voting members. Any country applying for programmatic funds must establish a nationwide coordinating structure that enables the participation of public and private partners. When compared with other stakeholders, the Global Fund represents a multi-sectoral partnership with tangible global power and influence, plus an effective strategic approach to prevention (Wornham 2005). For example, funds have been dedicated to voluntary counseling and testing (VCT) for over three million people and ARV provision to over 300,000 individuals globally. While the United States has been recognized as a leading contributor to the Global Fund, much of these dedicated funds have now been earmarked for the President's Emergency Plan for AIDS Relief (PEPFAR). In 2003, President Bush introduced PEPFAR as a mechanism to distribute U.S.$15 billion dollars over five years to existing bilateral programs, the Global Fund, and 14 target nations in the Caribbean and Africa. There is a debate among scholars (Pope and White 2007; see also Blankenship et al. 2006 for a review of the impact of other contingent funding on international reproductive health programs) regarding the extent to which PEPFAR will engender innovative programs or whether it is merely an ideological policy to promote a singular prevention and treatment agenda. In the meantime, the United States remains the biggest contributor to the Global Fund program, comprising 28 percent of its funds from donor nations, even with the PEPFAR mechanism (Global Fund 2007).

There are other innovative strategies which have been developed in response to the stated structural barriers faced by developing nations. The Essential Drugs Program of the World Health Organization, adopted in 1978, is one example that may enhance access to ARVs. International clinical research is another vehicle for the distribution of drugs in developing nations (Heimer 2007). The Clinton Foundation and the Bill and Melinda Gates Foundation have been instrumental in brokering tiered pricing of drugs (where cost is adjusted to reflect the financial viability of the recipient nations) and bulk purchases at reduced cost. NGOs such as the Treatment Action Campaign (TAC) in South Africa have actively engaged in public debates about policies concerning access (London 2007; Treatment Action Campaign 2007). TAC coordinates a treatment literacy campaign that provides accurate information—at various reading skill levels—about access to and use of ARVs. They have utilized mobilizing strategies to demand transparency and accountability from the South African Minister of Health and to encourage voluntary counseling and testing at the national level. On May 2, 2007, they issued a press release describing their "National Strategic Plan on HIV/AIDS:

A New Opportunity for a Fairer South Africa," in which they commit to advocating for human rights protection, widespread access to ARVs, increased voluntary testing, and endorsing policies mitigating the impact of HIV on the citizens of South Africa. They call upon state actors to work in collaboration with other national and international interests in their realization of their vision.

As explorations of effective ways to develop new alliances continue, the continuing impact of the AIDS pandemic on developing nations remains unchanged. Given the possible ways that some wealthy nations may have benefited materially from these policies, the ensuing focus of public health policy researchers and ethicists is likely to be whether wealthier nations have a moral and structural obligation to facilitate both vertical and horizontal forms of prevention (Wornham 2005): "History shows the vulnerability of social determinants policies [policies addressing the social roots of health inequality and disease] to resistance mounted by national and global actors concerned with maintaining existing distributions of economic and social power" (Irwin, Millen, and Fallows 2003, 251). Strategic structural interventions will need to be more explicitly linked with the goal of HIV treatment and prevention. Such interventions include innovations in research and technology, structural policy reform, public–private partnerships, and (above all), recognition that the social and political will must be embraced by all if such change is to become a reality (Feachem 2001; Myer, Ehrlich, and Susser 2004). It has been demonstrated that there is some ideological incompatibility between governments, NGOs, and global actors that embrace a structural or social epidemiological approach to HIV and those focused on international financial and development (Blankenship, Friedman, Dworkin, and Mantell 2006; London 2007). Perhaps the divide can be breached by recognizing that moral, ethical, human rights, and fiscal goals can be simultaneously achieved. There is an implicit profit for all actors involved, whether based on humanitarian and human rights discourse or human and labor capital investment. Employing strategies that encourage economic growth in developing nations without causing undue burdens on social goods and services may result in economic stability and profit for foreign investors, and enhance the life chances of the citizens (Gruskin, Mills, and Tarantola 2007; Lee 1988). Ultimately, responding to the chronic and institutional impact of HIV/AIDS will continue to require navigation through the rough waters of ideology, geopolitics, transnational economies, and social justice.

NOTES

1. Neoliberalism is a policy geared to the expansion of global economies. It presumes that free private enterprise should be encouraged (allowing for the flow of capital, goods, and services), that reduction of public expenditures frees up revenue to be invested in production of goods, government deregulation of policies that might obstruct profits, privatization of enterprises and infrastructures (like water, highways, telecommunications, and electricity), and focuses on individual responsibility for solving societal problems (Martinez and Garcia 2000).
2. Essential medicines are defined by the WHO as "[T]hose that satisfy the priority health care needs of the population. They are selected with due regard to public health relevance, evidence on efficacy and safety, and comparative cost-effectiveness. Essential medicines are intended to be available within the context of functioning health systems at all times in adequate amounts, in the appropriate dosage forms, with assured quality and adequate information, and at a price the individual and the community can afford" (World Health Organization 2007).

REFERENCES AND FURTHER READING

Abouharb M. Rodwan, and David L. Cingranelli. "When the World Bank Says Yes: Determinants of Structural Adjustment Lending." Paper prepared for presentation at The Impact of Globalization on the Nation State From Above: The International Monetary Fund and The World Bank, Yale University, April 2003.

Ammann, Arthur J. "Governments as Facilitators or Obstacles in the HIV Epidemic." *BMJ* (2002): 184–185.

Avafia, Tenu, and Savita Mallapudi Narasimhan. *The TRIPS Agreement and Access to ARVs*. Background Paper, New York: United Nations Development Program, 2006.

Barnett, Tony, and Michael Blackwell. *Structural Adjustment and the Spread of HIV/AIDS*. Working Paper, London: Christian Aid, 2004.

BBC. "Foreign Investment Rises, Says UN." *BBC News*. September 29, 2005. http://news.bbc.co.uk/1/hi/business/4295022.stm (retrieved November 3, 2007).

Beyrer, Chris. "HIV Epidemiology Update and Transmission Factors: Risks and Risk Contexts—16th International AIDS Conference Epidemiology Plenary." *Clinical Infectious Diseases* 44 (2007): 981–987.

Blankenship, Kim, Sam Friedman, Shari Dworkin, and Joanne E. Mantell. "Structural Interventions: Concepts, Challenges and Opportunities for Research." *Journal of Urban Health* 83, no. 1 (2006): 59–72.

Blaylock, Jean. *Access to Medicines: A Briefing Paper for the Trade Campaign and the HIV and AIDS campaign*. Working Paper, Geneva: Ecumenical Advisory Alliance, 2006.

Breslow, Lester, Bernard D. Goldstein, Lawrence W. Green, C. William Keck, John M. Last, and Michael McGinnis. *Gale Encyclopedia of Public Health*. New York: Macmillan Reference U.S.A., 2002.

Calfee, John E., and Roger Bate. "Pharmaceuticals and the Worldwide HIV Epidemic: Can a Stakeholder Model Work?" *Journal of Public Policy and Marketing* 23, no. 2 (2004): 140–152.

Commission on HIV/AIDS and Governance in Africa. *Globalized Inequalities and HIV/AIDS*. Working Paper, Addis Ababa: Commission on HIV/AIDS and Governance in Africa, 2004.

Dickinson, Clare. *The Politics of National HIV/AIDS Responses: A Synthesis of Literature*. Working Paper, London: HLSP Institute, 2006.

Epstein, Helen. "The Global Health Crisis." In *Biological Security and Public Health: In Search of a Global Treatment*, edited by Kurt M. Campbell and Philip Zelikow. Queenstown: The Aspen Institute, 2003.

Farmer, Paul. *Pathologies of Power: Health, Human Rights, and the New War on the Poor*. Berkeley and Los Angeles: University of California Press, 2003.

Farmer, Paul, Bruce Nizeye, Sara Stulac, and Salmaan Keshavjee. Structural Violence and Clinical Medicine." *PLoS Medicine* 3, no. 10 (2006): 1686–1691.

Feachem, Richard G.A. "Globalization: From Rhetoric to Evidence." *Bulletin of the World Health Organization* 79, no. 9 (2001): 804.

Feachem, Richard, and Oliver Sabot. "The Global Fund 2001–2001: A Review of the Evidence." *Global Public Health* 2, no. 4 (2007): 325–341.

Federici, Silvia. "War, Globalization and Reproduction." *Alternatives: Turkish Journal of International Relations* 1, no. 4 (2002): 254–267.

Gandy, Matthew. "Deadly Alliances: Death, Disease and the Global Politics of Public Health." *PLoS Medicine* 2, no. 1 (2005): e4.

Global Fund. *How the Fund Works*. 2007. http://www.theglobalfund.org/en/about/how/ (retrieved November 3, 2007).

Gostin, Lawrence O. *The AIDS Pandemic: Complacency, Injustice, and Unfulfilled Expectations*. Chapel Hill: University of North Carolina Press, 2004.

Grusin, Sofia, Edward J. Mills, and Daniel Tarantola. "History, Principles, and Practice of Health and Human Rights." *The Lancet* 370 (2007): 449–455.

Harris, Paul G., and Patricia Siplon. "International Obligation and Human Health: Evolving Policy Responses to HIV/AIDS." *Ethics and International Affairs* 15, no. 1 (2001): 29–52.

Heimer, Carol A. "Old Inequalities, New Disease: HIV/AIDS in Sub-Saharan Africa." *Annual Review of Sociology* 33 (2007): 551–577.

Hein, Wolfgang, and Lars Kohlmorgen. *Global Health Governance: Conflicts on Global Social Rights*. Working Paper, Hamburg: German Overseas Institute, 2005.

Henry Kaiser Family Foundation. *The Multisectoral Impact of the HIV/AIDS Epidemic—A Primer*. Washington DC: Kaiser Family Foundation, 2007.

Irwin, Alec, and Elena Scali. "Action on the Social Determinants of Health: A Historical Perspective." *Global Public Health* 2, no. 3 (2007): 235–256.

Irwin, Alexander, Joyce Millen, and Dorothy Fallows. *Global AIDS: Myths and Facts*. Cambridge: South End Press, 2003.

Kates, Jennifer, José-Antonio Izazola, and Eric Lief. "Financing the Response to AIDS in Low- and Middle-Income Countries: International Assistance from the G8, European Commission and Other Donor Governments, 2006." The Henry H. Kaiser Family Foundation and UNAIDS, June 2007. http://www.kff.org/hivaids/upload/7347_03.pdf (retrieved November 30, 2007).

Krieger, Nancy. "Theories for Social Epidemiology in the 21st Century: An Ecosocial Perspective." *International Journal of Epidemiology* 30 (2001): 668–677.

Lee, Kelley. "Shaping the Future of Global Health Cooperation: Where Can We Go From Here?" *The Lancet* 351 (1998): 899–902.

London, Leslie. "Issues of Equity are also Issues of Rights: Lessons from Experiences in South Africa." *BMC Public Health* 7 (2007): 14–24.

Martinez, Elizabeth, and Arnoldo Garcia. "What is Neo-Liberalism?" *Global Exchange*. February 26, 2000. http://www.globalexchange.org/campaigns/econ101/neoliberalDefined.html (retrieved November 4, 2007).

Menon-Johansson, Anatole S. "Good Governance and Good Health: The Role of Societal Structures in the Human Immunodeficiency Virus Pandemic." *BMC International Health and Human Rights* 5 (2005): 4–13.

Mohiddin, Abdu, and Deborah Johnston. "HIV/AIDS Mitigation Strategies and the State in Sub-Saharan Africa—The Missing Link?" *Globalization and Health* 2 (2006): 1–5.

Muuka, Gerry Nkombo. "In Defense of World Bank and IMF Conditionality in Structural Adjustment Programs." *The Journal of Business in Developing Nations*, 1998. http://www.ewp.rpi.edu/jbdn/jbdnv202.htm (retrieved November 30, 2007).

Myer, Landon, Rodney I. Ehrlich, and Ezra Susser. "Social Epidemiology in South Africa." *Epidemiologic Reviews* 26 (2004): 112–123.

Parker, Richard. "The Global HIV/AIDS Pandemic, Structural Inequalities, and the Politics of International Health." *American Journal of Public Health* 92, no. 3 (2002): 343–346.

Patterson, David, and Leslie London. "International Law, Human Rights and HIV/AIDS." *Bulletin of the World Health Organization* 80, no. 12 (2002): 964–969.

Perry, David. "The Global Distribution of AIDS Pharmaceuticals." *Markkula Center for Applied Ethics*. 2002. http://www.scu.edu/ethics/publications/submitted/Perry/aids.html (retrieved November 3, 2007).

Pope, Cynthia, and Renée T. White. "Global Impact: U.S. Sexual Health and Reproductive Policy." *21st Century Sexualities: Contemporary Issues in Health, Education, and Rights*, edited by G. Herdt and C. Howe, London and New York: Routledge, 2007.

Poundstone, Katharine E., Steffanie A. Strathdee, and David D. Celentano. "The Social Epidemiology of Human Immunodeficiency Virus/Acquired Immonodeficiency Syndrome." *Epidemiologic Reviews* 26, (2004): 22–35.

Treatment Action Campaign. "National Strategic Plan." *Treatment Action Campaign*. May 4, 2007. http://www.tac.org.za/index.html (retrieved November 5, 2007).

World Health Organization. "Essential Medicines." 2007. http://www.who.int/topics/essential_medicines/en/ (retrieved November 4, 2007).

Wornham, David. "The AIDS Epidemic and Pharmaceutical Companies: Ethics, Stakeholders, and Obligations." *Bristol Business School Teaching and Research Review* Summer (2005): 1–15.

"You can't get HIV/AIDS by sharing mate." Public service announcement to combat stereotypes about HIV transmission in Argentina.

NO SE CONTRAE
POR
COMPARTIR EL
La verdad sobre el VIH/SIDA.

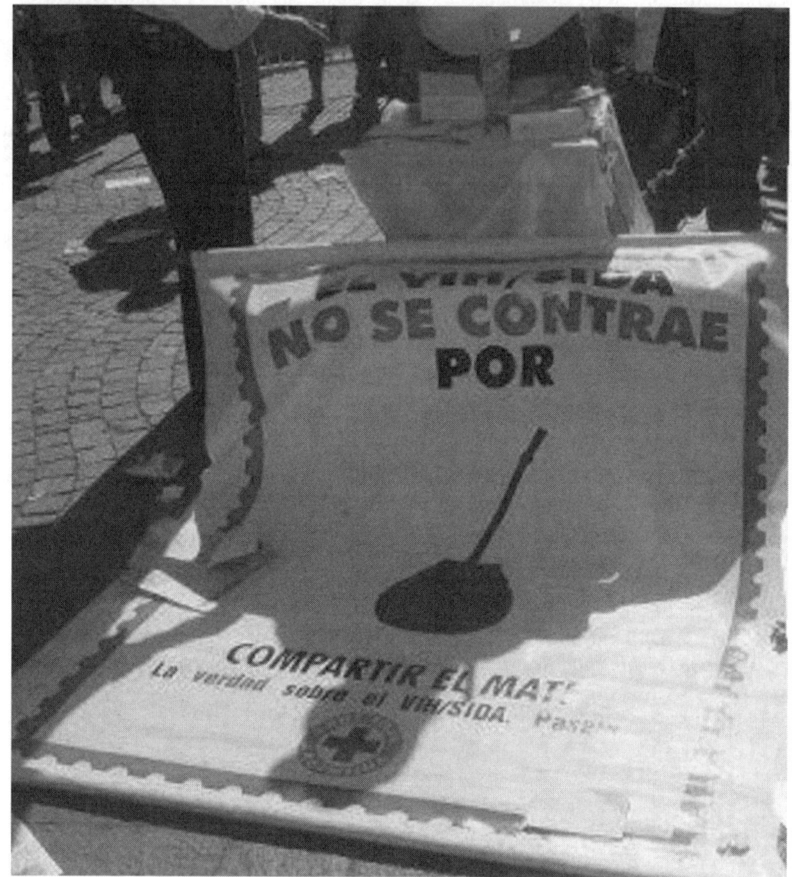

Source: Photo courtesy of Ashley Toombs

CHAPTER 18

AIDS and the Politics of Violence

Susan Craddock

ABSTRACT

This chapter investigates a specific juncture that points towards the inseparability—at least in particular regions of the globe—of market relations, scientific technologies, social ideologies, and transnational institutional assemblages in shaping biological and therapeutic citizenship. It focuses on this juncture as it relates to AIDS in Africa because this region remains a primary locus of therapeutic debate and denial. While well-organized transnational movements have succeeded in raising the visibility of antiretroviral access as a human rights issue, forged regional pockets of drug availability, and underscored the moral bankruptcy of government and corporate regulatory practices, they have arguably not succeeded yet in altering the fundamental coordinates of biological citizenship underlying unconscionable levels of preventable death and suffering.

The 1990s saw the convergence of two phenomena bearing equally critical impact on what Nicholas Rose has termed "the politics of life itself" (Rose 2001). The first is the advent of antiretrovirals designed to prolong the lives of people living with AIDS by intervening in viral replication and destruction of the immune system; and the second is the simultaneous development of global intellectual property regulations largely preventing those same drugs from reaching the vast majority of those who need them. What makes this politics of life more than just another blip on the radar screen of contested practices of economic globalization are the massive number of lives at stake: in 2005 alone, somewhere in the vicinity of three million people died of AIDS, two million of them in Africa (UNAIDS 2005).

Epidemics that kill millions are not unprecedented, and neither is the reality of preventable deaths from a variety of infectious and chronic diseases (cf. Farmer 2001, 2004). What marks this juncture as a critical chapter in recent discussions of health and citizenship is the existence of an effective therapy capable of preventing deaths from AIDS that has been proactively confined in circulation by governments, pharmaceutical companies, and high-level international policy organizations as exemplified by the passage of the 2001 World Trade Organization's Trade Related Aspects of Intellectual Property, or TRIPS. The Doha agreement, as it is sometimes called, ostensibly generates conditions for easier transfer of technologies to lower income countries, and it pays lip service to protecting a country's public health in the course of such transfers. Yet the essential purpose of this global "agreement" is to ensure that countries recognize patents on all forms of intellectual property, including essential medicines such as antiretrovirals, a move with profound reverberations because it effectively changes pharmaceutical drugs' occupation of a more variable zone of government subsidization and citizen's rights of access to one of global restriction and regulation. Essential medications and designer jeans thus now occupy similar trade-regulated terrain in an exemplification of what Rose and Novas characterize as the increasing intrusion of market relations into new areas of biomedicine and the "vital life processes of the citizenry" (2005, 457).

Under the terms of TRIPS, pharmaceutical companies have latitude to charge what they want for patented drugs and all countries, no matter what their income level, will be obliged to pay those prices by 2016 or earlier in order to supply their populations with necessary medicines. Perhaps not surprisingly, then, it is commonly understood that TRIPS was pushed through by western governments such as the US under pressure from strong pharmaceutical industry lobbies to ensure global patent recognition, and thus increased profits, on new and existing pharmaceutical products; as suggested by a 2001 United Nations report on TRIPS and human rights, "the overall thrust of the TRIPS Agreement is the promotion of innovation through the provision of commercial incentives." Subsequently, "the various links with . . . the promotion of public health, nutrition, environment and development are generally expressed in terms of exceptions to the rule" (article 22,7). In effect, the political landscape of preventable deaths from AIDS points to a particularly violent juncture where an array of global assemblages (Ong and Collier 2005) including pharmaceutical companies, international trade organizations, government trade representatives, scientists, and social movements both collide and collude.

My intention in this chapter is to examine this collision/collusion as a way of extending conversations on the new modes of citizenship that have emerged within the nexus of medical research, biotechnological innovations, bioethics, and global mechanisms of governance. Though the term "biological citizenship" has been variously defined (Petryna 2002; Rose and Novas 2005), discussions have so far focused on the ways in which individuals negotiate access to state resources through biological definitions of incapacity (Petryna 2002), form methods of activism revolving around understandings of disease, or negotiate novel methods of governance through genetic and biomedical knowledge (Rose 2001; Rose and Novas 2005). As Rose and Novas recognize, however, these discussions primarily describe networks, relationships, and technological access more characteristic of western Europe and the United States and suggest "no visible presence in whole geographic regions" (2005, 451). The kinds of governance and its contestation that has revolved around access to antiretrovirals, or ARVs, suggest new dimensions to these discussions of how biological citizenship is defined and the players involved in shaping that definition and its experience. As I suggest, a restricted circulation of effective biotherapies in low-income regions in the heart of a pandemic certainly points towards more ominous formulations of citizenship and its corollary, bare life (Agamben 1998).

More specifically, I raise the question of what representational practices, contradictions, and ideologies underlie formulations of biological citizenship that are at the heart of responses to AIDS in hard hit regions such as Africa. Global regulations governing access to antiretrovirals and similar responses to the AIDS epidemic are never neutral apparatuses but rather rest upon ideological and symbolic foundations produced from multiple histories, geopolitical relations, and unequal global economic coordinates. At one level, these ideologies constituting particular geographic regions such as Africa as zones of exception to global economic and social progress circulate through high-level governmental, trade, and funding policies regarding AIDS. These policies in turn constitute the two million Africans who died of AIDS last year and the twenty-eight million more infected with HIV (UNAIDS 2005) as noncitizens and thus expendable people, an exemplification of what Agamben (1998), Bauman (1989), and others have suggested is at the heart of modern biopolitics: the ability of governments to administer death as well as life.

Contesting these policies at another level are grassroots, national, and transnational organizations, which have gone far in procuring antiretrovirals in low-income regions while also making visible the continuing paucity of options for most poor people living with AIDS in Africa and worldwide. Organizations such as South Africa's Treatment Action Campaign have had considerable success in making the devastating effects of pharmaceutical industry and governmental practices visible, and in achieving greater access to ARVs.[1] The networks and skilled negotiations for treatment options among those facing limited resources—what Nguyen calls therapeutic citizenship (2005)—have been critically important in forging alternative models of biological citizenship based on universal inclusion rather than exception and pivoting around population- rather than market-centered allocations of therapeutic resources. In tracing a few of these deployments of biopolitics, one of my intentions is to highlight some of the frictions (Tsing 2005) between new scientific technologies, the array of individuals involved in the larger field of antiretroviral treatment, and the complex political context in which drug access is playing out.

I also want to extend the UN reports' interrogation of links between TRIPS and human rights, to posit the question of whether it makes sense ethically and strategically to call current global political responses to AIDS genocide. This is not the first time that a charge of genocide has been raised in the context of governmental responses to AIDS. As Epstein notes in his account of early AIDS activism in the US (1997), charging scientists and government with genocide early in the epidemic arguably resulted in better governmental responsiveness and accountability, as well as productive partnerships between scientists and activists. The question now is whether similar charges aimed not at one government but at multiple governmental and international political apparatuses would have similar productive effect in galvanizing more, and more appropriate, responses from US and European governments, and less punitive global regulatory policies. Intentionality is often termed the bottom line in designating acts of genocide, and this is something I will outline in the following pages, not only to decide the more legal question of genocide but to bring attention to the proactive rather than passive nature of current coordinates of drug access. Contrary to a common impression of global economic policies as somehow reflective of collective interests as well as beyond human control, it has taken an inordinate amount of time, work, and money to implement global intellectual property regulations and to maintain the primacy of patents over the protests of nations, NGOs, and social movements worldwide.

Before moving on to an investigation of the representational practices underlying responses to AIDS in Africa, I need to make clear here that this chapter does not attempt a comprehensive overview of treatment issues. The larger picture encompassing access to AIDS drugs involves questions of infrastructure, tariffs, stigma, distribution, testing and storage technologies, as well as delayed, inappropriate, or inadequate responses to the epidemic by some African heads of state. A comprehensive overview also would raise important questions, as does Bastos (1999), of why particular technologies such as antiretrovirals gain biomedical primacy to the detriment of other, more comprehensive treatment approaches. Finally, more recent work is recognizing the problematic politics of intervention underlying expanded drug access, focusing in particular on the controversial contingencies and language of biosecurity attached to ramped-up ARV funding from sources such as the US's PEPFAR (Craddock forthcoming; Ingram 2005).

What I am trying to do here is a much more constrained investigation of a specific juncture that points towards the inseparability—at least in particular regions of the globe—of market relations, scientific technologies, social ideologies, and transnational institutional assemblages in shaping biological and therapeutic citizenship. In the next section, I focus on this juncture as it relates to AIDS in Africa, because this region remains a primary locus of therapeutic debate and denial. In particular, I want to draw out the imbrication of ideological formations with regulatory restrictions as these have played out over the course of a decade. While well organized social movements have succeeded in raising the visibility of antiretroviral access as a human rights issue, negotiated increased drug availability, and questioned the ethics of government and corporate regulatory practices maintaining high drug prices, they have arguably not succeeded yet in altering the fundamental coordinates of biological citizenship underlying unconscionable levels of preventable death and suffering.

REPRESENTATIONS AND CIRCULATIONS

The first step in examining this interrelation of ideology and policy—that is, the first step in investigating what forces are producing Africans as expendable in the AIDS equation—is to extend the argument made by medical anthropologists such as Paul Farmer (2001) and Charles and Clara Briggs (2003) that culturalist explanations about people and their practices predominate in interpreting disproportionate burdens of disease. Assumptions of ignorance or indifference have gained more attention from many social scientists, in other words, than have the structures of violence including poverty that drive patterns of disease and suffering (Farmer 2001). Similarly, Jarosz (1992), Jones (2004), and Machungo (2004) have separately argued that among other factors, representations of Africa and Africans are in both implicit and explicit ways informing transnational responses to AIDS.

An early and continuing target of AIDS analysts for example is the African sex worker. This is relatively predictable given the historical tendency to attribute blame for sexually transmitted infections on women exhibiting behaviors outside historically-bounded norms of sexual exchange (Brandt 1987; Adams and Pigg 2005). In the context of AIDS in Africa, however, iconographies of sex workers remain problematic for their narratives of viral danger devoid of socio-economic context or male agency. Early in the epidemic, for example, the term "reservoirs of infection" was applied by medical and epidemiological researchers uncovering high rates of HIV among particularly urban sex workers. Though the intent of these researchers was to find a focal point for intervention, the term is significant both for what it broadcasts and what it effectively elides. Rather than a neutral phrase designating heightened risk, "reservoirs of infection" clearly signals sex workers as the locus of unidirectional viral flow outward from themselves to clients. It thus designates blame, if not intentionality, rather than recognizing the variable and negotiated dynamic of transactional sex. Other than leaving the question of male agency out, the continued use of the term "reservoirs of infection" also makes invisible the often inequitable power relations within which most sex workers undertake their trade and that often places them at greater risk of HIV infection from their male clients.

The moral opprobrium implicit in linguistic designations of sex workers also underlies policies such as the US government's 2003 Global AIDS Act prohibiting the allocation of any US government funds to organizations that promote or advocate legalization and practice of prostitution, even if these organizations are attempting to intervene in higher levels of HIV infection among sex workers. Though the impacts of this law have received inadequate attention so far, at least one study has traced its negative effects on the ability to provide HIV prevention to migrant sex workers in Cambodia (Busza 2006). Less visible but nonetheless significant in contesting such ideological signals are the increasing number of sex worker organizations and programs highlighting sex work as a locus for safe sex, educational outreach, and supportive community. In the 2004 International AIDS conference held in Bangkok, for example, was a photojournal display chronicling the words and approaches of Nairobi sex workers in introducing condom use to their clientele.

Media coverage of AIDS in Africa over twenty years into the epidemic, however, shows little sign of moving away from its reliance upon colonial stereotypes of a primitive continent unable to address its problems and reliant upon—or intractably resistant to—western knowledge. In one 2003 example from *Newsweek* titled "Witchcraft, vengeful spirits, and the plague," Mercedes Sayagues suggests that "Most Africans know what to say when asked about AIDS. HIV causes AIDS. Western-style advertising campaigns have accomplished that much. So why aren't prevalence rates plummeting? [Because] they might hold to one belief system by day, and another by night" (2003). Not only does Sayagues' language evoke images of the devious African, but her stark opposition of a "real" western biomedical knowledge of AIDS against a primitive spirit-based belief system illustrates Farmer's insight that such wildly inaccurate culturalist interpretations of phenomena like AIDS disguise complex structural and historical antecedents to disease (Farmer 2001).

Sayagues' approach is by no means unique. In his compilation of recent US-based newspaper articles covering AIDS in Africa, Francis Machungo effectively shows the repetitive quality of tropes used to depict a continent and its populations. "Death Stalks a Continent" (*Time* February, 2001), "AIDS: The Agony of Africa" (*Village Voice* November, 1999), "Dark Continent Still Dark" (*Village Voice* May, 2000), "AIDS and the African: A Continent's Crisis" (*Boston Globe* October, 1999), and "Africa's Lost Generation" (CNN 2003) are remarkable for their Conradian invocation of Africa as the Dark Continent (Machungo 2004) and their geographical essentializations that assume what happens in one region can be extrapolated to the whole. Nowhere in these titles is there any indication of the highly disparate rates of HIV across Africa, nor the regional variations in negotiation, successful response to, and containment of disease.

The point here is not for the media to avoid covering AIDS in Africa, but that its coverage is consistently one-sided and tediously reliant upon historical iconographies that should have been soundly unpacked decades ago rather than revivified under the pretense of "news" coverage. As Beverly Hawk notes in her book on images of Africa (1992, 7), events in Africa seem to require a different vocabulary than violent events in places like Northern Ireland or the former Yugoslavia—a vocabulary that connotes a primitiveness and brutality that is somehow special to Africa. As Paul Gilroy puts it, the "torrent of images of casual death and conflict . . . transmitted instantaneously from all over the African continent . . . make savagery something that occurs exclusively beyond the fortified borders of the new Europe" (2000, 26). In his analysis of the verisimilar distance between African colonialism and the "postcolony," Achille Mbembe in turn comments that western typification of Africa is still based on "a grotesque dramatization . . ., [where] what political imagination is in Africa is held incomprehensible, pathological, and abnormal . . . [and where] human action there is seen as stupid and mad, always proceeding from anything but rational calculation" (2001, 8).

Taking Mbembe's point further, these images of death and conflict also produce perceptions of Africa's problems as internally produced because they ignore international factors such as the multiple legacies of colonialism, IMF structural adjustment policies, overwhelming debt burdens, trade constraints, and the legions of failed western development efforts—all of which have not only left many regions of Africa in greater poverty over the last few decades, but have by most accounts left millions of newly or more profoundly impoverished Africans more vulnerable to HIV.

One of the most explicit and thorough illustrations of journalistic deployment of African Otherness is Robert Kaplan's article and subsequent book "The Coming Anarchy" (1994, 1996). With the subtitle of "how scarcity, crime, overpopulation, tribalism, and disease are rapidly destroying the social fabric of our planet," Kaplan focuses attention on West Africa as the locus where these ominous forces merge to disastrous effect. Written as an informed travel narrative, he roams across physical and imagined landscapes where lawlessness, withered government capacity, and crime predominate with no signs of optimism to vary the universally desultory scene. In this surficial iteration, Kaplan contends that "West Africa is becoming *the* symbol of worldwide demographic, environmental, and societal stress" and where, among other things, "loose family structures are largely responsible for the world's highest birth rates and the explosion of the HIV virus on the continent" (1994, 46). As Kevin Dunn suggests, Kaplan's representation of Africans is not only a colonizing act that reemploys tropes from an earlier era to produce visions of extreme insecurity, it also signals a profound western anxiety over the definitions and boundaries of modernity as well as "Africans' refusal to accept . . . exclusive Western authorship" of those definitions (2004, 485).[2]

More disturbing than the erroneous simplicity of narratives such as Kaplan's, however, is the impact that they have. As noted by Dunn, the message conveyed by Kaplan is that "Western modernity has failed to take hold in the backward Third World" and thus poses a direct security threat to the First World. Indications that the US government took this message seriously lay in its directives to fax a copy of "The Coming Anarchy" to every US embassy around the world, while placing Kaplan himself in the role of "expert" on post-9/11 security issues (Dunn 2004, 293). Another illustration is found in high-level US policy statements on responses to AIDS in Africa that incorporate the kinds of colonial and colonizing tropes employed by Kaplan and other reporters. In a paper linking discourses of overpopulation with responses to AIDS, Lisa Richey points out that the continued spotlight on African "exceptionalism" in demographic transitions to lower fertility levels has generated opinions among some policy makers that AIDS in Africa actually has a positive angle as a "Malthusian check" on the rate of population growth in the continent. A 1992 World Bank Report, for example, contained a statement by an economist suggesting that "If the only effect of the AIDS epidemic were to reduce the population growth rate [in Africa], it would increase the growth rate of per capita income in any plausible economic model" (cited in Richey, 7). A USAID administrator similarly was quoted in 2001 as stating that antiretrovirals were too costly and inappropriate for Africans because they "don't know what Western time is" (Donnelly, *Boston Globe* June 7, 2001).

Though the question of adherence is obviously important given the specter of drug-resistant forms of HIV, the point here is that narratives of African backwardness serve as an apparently convincing rationale for withholding effective therapies, a maneuver with direct links to colonial tactics of othering and deprivation (Said 1979). Incidentally, studies reported in the *Bulletin of the WHO* (Farmer 2001), and an issue of the journal *AIDS* (2003) have found adherence rates among populations in South Africa, Côte D'Ivoire, Senegal, and Uganda averaging twenty percent higher than rates for the United States (see also Severe et al. 2005). Nonetheless the rationalization of nonaccess through myths of nonadherence goes far to disguise the reality that many Africans do not have to worry about their drug regimens because European and US government lobbying and intellectual property regulations until very recently have ensured their scarcity. It also overlooks the potential of restricted access itself to generate drug resistance because more tenuous means of gaining supplies of ARVs appear in the wake of more standard, and more stable, channels of procurement (Nguyen 2005).

PROMISES AND POLITICS

The impact of othering techniques does not stop at the blundering of high level policy officials, however. It informs as well the strenuous work performed by the former US Trade Representative Robert Zoellick at various rounds of WTO meetings, congressional discussions concerning international aid and trade regulations, pronouncements made by former US Global AIDS coordinator Randall Tobias, and the Bush administration's initiatives on AIDS and free trade agreements. The combined work of these individuals and institutions has effectively restricted access to antiretrovirals and other essential on-patent medications to low-income regions while veiling the inhumanitarian nature of these restrictions through more visible initiatives boosting "science" and earmarking new funds towards AIDS prevention and treatment in several African and Caribbean countries. It is the contradictions of these policies and the various locations within which "science" and politics get done that I want to focus on in this section.

Within the larger economic climate of deregulation, privatization, and corporate preeminence it should not be so surprising that the pharmaceutical industry lobbied vehemently and paid large sums of money to political parties in order to achieve global recognition of intellectual property as stipulated in the TRIPS agreement. Given increasing difficulties producing blockbuster new drugs, mergers and global patent enforcement are two ways for the pharmaceutical industry to maintain higher profits and industry ranking (Wallace, personal communication; Goozner 2005).

With pharmaceutical backing and under the rubric of free trade, it was then-US Trade Representative Robert Zoellick who "developed a strategy to launch new global trade negotiations at the WTO meeting in Doha and to press the negotiations forward" (www.whitehouse.gov/government/zoellick-bio.html). That strategy involved not only the global enforcement of patent regulations on pharmaceutical drugs, but the extension of patent licenses to twenty years, both measures pushed through despite vehement protests from representatives of low income countries who could foresee their humanitarian implications. Only through sustained negotiations on the part of affected countries and despite US opposition were two measures passed that somewhat softened the punitive nature of TRIPS: the extension by ten years, until 2016, of when lowest income countries are required to recognize patents, and in 2003 the Cancun agreement's amendment that in the meantime, generically-produced antiretrovirals can be exported to countries lacking capacity either to produce or otherwise purchase generic ARVs. The inflexibility with which Zoellick and his US team of trade representatives confronted these negotiations, however, generated what one negotiator from Medécins Sans Frontières said was the most tension-filled round of WTO negotiations she had ever witnessed (T'Hoen 2003, personal communication).[3] Though a partial political gain for low-income countries, the 2003 agreement in particular passed with so many added stipulations dictating when and how countries could import generic ARVs that Raymond Offenheiser, president of Oxfam America, called it a "gift wrapped in red tape" (Offenheiser 2004).

Despite the limited flexibilities of the latest TRIPS amendments, however, the Bush administration has been tireless in undermining its terms by pursuing bilateral free trade agreements that among other things require countries to recognize intellectual property rights immediately despite WTO guidelines. With eleven[4] of these "agreements" solidified, often under threat of trade sanctions and other punitive measures on the part of the US (Heywood 2002), and five more under negotiation,[5] Bush is making steady progress in eroding whatever public health protections are afforded under current TRIPS stipulations. As boldly suggested on the government's FTA website, these free trade agreements are overwhelmingly geared to helping US commercial interests as they "provide new market access for US consumer and industrial products . . . provide unprecedented access to government procurement in the partner countries . . . protect US investments in the region, and strengthen protections for US patents, trademarks, and trade secrets" (www.export.gov/fta/complete/CAFTA). Buried within the optimistic rhetoric of new markets and patent protections, however, are the human rights abuses generated by the automatic escalation of drug prices as generically produced medications become illegal under the terms of free trade agreements and average costs for yearly triple antiretroviral therapy go from two hundred dollars to at least three times that amount because governments and individuals will be obligated to pay for patented antiretrovirals, the lowest-cost versions of which are still much more expensive than generics. The inevitable result is that thousands will end up without access to drugs at all.

Coupled with its desultory funding pledge of $200 million to the UN-based Global Fund to Fight AIDS, Malaria, and Tuberculosis for 2005 and beyond, it is not surprising that the United States took a public relations beating during the 2004 International AIDS conference in Bangkok. Daily protests outside the main conference building demanded more Global Fund money and access to antiretrovirals, while Thai protestors targeted their president with pleas to stand firm against US demands for patent recognition as part of free trade negotiations still ongoing between Thailand and the United States. Former French President Jacques Chirac went so far as to accuse the US of blackmailing low-income countries in free trade negotiations where "favourable trade deals [are] being dangled before poor nations in return for those countries halting production of life-saving generic drugs" (Boseley 2004).[6]

At the same time that the US was working strenuously to erode the meager protections afforded by TRIPS, President Bush announced in 2003 his $15 billion President's Emergency Plan for AIDS Relief (PEPFAR), an initiative to earmark AIDS prevention and treatment money for fifteen countries in Africa and the Caribbean. Designed in part to respond to accusations that Bush was not doing anything to combat global AIDS, PEPFAR quickly came under global fire among other things for its insistence on funding abstinence programs, for naming Randall Tobias, the former head of the pharmaceutical giant Eli Lilly, as the head of the new US Global AIDS initiative, and for backing off the original promise to support generic antiretrovirals as part of PEPFAR grants (Klein 2003). Claiming concerns about the safety of generic combination antiretroviral pills even though they were preapproved by the World Health Organization's safety qualification program, Bush gave pharmaceutical manufacturers a boost by insisting that PEPFAR recipients purchase name-brand antiretrovirals until a new FDA generic drug qualification program could be implemented. This only happened in mid-2005. Despite the fact that fixed-dose combination pills (a pill combining all three antiretrovirals in one pill, taken twice a day) have made drug regimens cheaper and far easier to manage, Tobias in his testimony before Congress stuck to the argument that "We need to have principles—standards by which the purchase decisions can be made" (Langley 2004).

Behind this blatant privileging of corporate profit over people's lives is the resounding silence of many scientists who are strategically positioned to make a difference in access. Of course there are huge exceptions to this statement, most visibly exemplified in the organization Médecins Sans Frontières, or Doctors Without Borders, an international agency that among other things has mobilized the media, medical expertise, and "witnessing" to make access to antiretrovirals more visible as a human rights issue, while galvanizing efforts in hard-hit regions to import generic antiretrovirals and make them available to local populations (Redfield 2006). I am referring here to scientists located in research or high-level funding institutions whose work on biotechnologies places them in a unique position to highlight the critical importance of issues such as access once new products move beyond the laboratory and into a larger social setting.

The majority of antiretrovirals on the market today were developed and patented at research universities using NIH funds, then licensed to pharmaceutical companies who had the money and production capacity to market the new drugs. Since the passage of the Bayh-Dole Act in 1980 allowing NIH-funded products to be licensed commercially, the number of patents has risen sharply, as have the relationships between universities, biotech firms, and pharmaceutical companies (Krimsky 2004). Among the scientists whom I have interviewed, increased patenting has the obvious rewards of getting new discoveries out more quickly, though some scientists bemoaned the trend in "upstream" patenting of initial discoveries and delivery models, making some forms of biotechnical research more problematic. When questioned about restrictions on access to products, the most frequent reply was that it was the government's responsibility to ensure widespread dissemination of intellectual property.[7]

Scientists at the NIH, however, have been forced to divest themselves of any such political blinders in recognizing the contradictions between government-supported scientific development and dissemination. The 2004 Office of AIDS Research Fiscal Year

2005 Budget Report states that "the overarching priorities that continue to frame the NIH AIDS research agenda are: . . . therapeutics research to develop simpler, less toxic, and cheaper drugs and drug regimens to treat HIV infection . . .; [and] international research, particularly to address the critical needs in developing countries" (Whitescarver 2004). By the next year, the report had changed its priorities to ". . . research to develop better therapies for those who are already infected; [and] international research, particularly to address the pandemic in developing countries" (OAR 2005). The omission of both the word "cheaper" and the phrase "critical needs" from the 2005 statement speaks volumes about NIH's apparent turn away from ethical considerations in AIDS research, and its disciplined subscription to Bush administration policies. Though the reasons for scientists' collusion with inequitable regulation and commercialization of biotechnology varies between laboratory blinders, financial incentive, and political survival, it is nevertheless troubling that there has been no significant protest coming from the scientific arena on an issue that speaks so directly to the impossibility of doing science outside of complex political terrains.[8] Indeed as Adam Sitze asks, "how are we to understand [the relation between deregulated capital and the replication of HIV globally] given that the striated disciplines that today remain in charge of the study of the virus (macroeconomics, epidemiology, and virology, not to mention actuarial science, business management, and demography) are incapable of posing the question of their immanence?" (2004, 777).[9] This determined incapacity is what in part allows Bush to triumphantly claim on World AIDS Day in 2005 that "after two years of sustained effort [of PEPFAR], approximately 400,000 sub-Saharan Africans are receiving the treatment they need" (PEPFAR 2005, 2) without demanding to know why that number is so remarkably low in the face of US economic, political, and biotechnical capabilities. Meanwhile, a WHO plan to get three million people on antiretroviral treatment by 2005 collapsed in part because the US withheld funding in opposition to UN plans to use generic low cost three-in-one combination pills (Langley 2004).

Returning to one of the main themes of this chapter, however, it is critical to point to the geographic contours defining the boundaries of administrative efforts at enforcing patent regulations. During the post-9/11 anthrax scare, the Bush administration threatened to override Bayer's patent on the antibiotic Cipro after the deaths of five American individuals. The override became unnecessary when Bayer drastically dropped the price of Cipro and donated two million pills to the US, but the threat nevertheless signaled an acknowledgment on the part of the Bush administration that under some circumstances, placing lives in front of free market ideals when the two contradict is not out of the question; the only question remains as to which lives are worth the intervention, and here it is clear where the boundaries of biological citizenship have been drawn.[10]

A QUESTION OF GENOCIDE

When the technological means exist to prevent deaths from AIDS but when pharmaceutical companies, elected officials, and government administrations take unprecedented steps to block access to those means, do the resulting deaths constitute genocide? Clearly this is a fraught question on a number of fronts, not least of which is the fact that applying the term "genocide" to current responses to AIDS threatens to dilute and therefore disempower Lemkin's original definition centering on ethnic or religious-based extermination. If the current definition of genocide as written in 1948 and utilized by the United Nations is altered to encompass new situations unforeseen in the original, does this intervene in the power of genocide as a political tool to mobilize international responses to drastic situations of human rights abuses?

Possibly. On the other hand, however, concepts developed in one historical era and maintaining definitional stasis risk diminished impact if they no longer adequately encompass new ways of supporting life and administering death. Part of the point of this chapter is to show that new forms of scientific research and biomedical technologies coupled with particular coordinates of global economic privatization map onto existing social faultlines of region, race, class, colonial history, or gender to create widespread and devastating possibilities for human rights abuses. Though new scientific knowledge has also created positive forms of biological citizenship for some (Rose and Novas 2005), in other words, for others it has created situations of expendability that are no less violent for having distant institutional and regulatory perpetration. As several scholars have argued (Peluso and Watts 2001; Scheper-Hughes and Bourgois 2004; Farmer 2001), our conceptualizations of violence must be expanded to encompass its possibilities in everyday life, as "a continuum comprised of a multitude of 'small wars and invisible genocides' conducted in . . . normative social spaces" and "encompassing all forms of 'controlling processes' (Nader 1997b) that assault basic human freedoms and individual or collective survival" (Scheper-Hughes and Bourgois 2004, 19 and 22). Rather than signalling exceptional breakdowns in the "norm" of national and global governance, genocide instead needs to be recognized as part and product of current regulatory structures and the normative inequality of their deployment. The three million preventable deaths from AIDS in 2005 is only one, albeit powerful, example.

A subsequent question would be whether a designation of genocide would be strategically helpful for activists and affected countries in galvanizing more appropriate responses to global AIDS. There is no guarantee that it would, particularly given the United States' track record in refusing to recognize even more conventional forms of genocide as they unfold around the world (Powers 2002) not to mention their role in shaping current coordinates of genocide. Yet it is not just a question of United States recognition. A United Nations designation of genocide has the potential to mobilize international action among governments and activists in ways that otherwise might not happen, or happen as quickly. On the part of governments, a designation of genocide might be the impetus needed to provide desperately needed money to the Global Fund and the World Health Organization, both of which have failed thus far to convince high-income countries to provide adequate resources for treatment and prevention programs. Similarly, for treatment activists at all levels from regional grassroots to international NGOs, a designation of genocide could potentially shift the defensive terms under which much campaigning has been conducted so far, to a more cooperative context in which access to antiretrovirals becomes a given and it is the logistics of regional access that become the focus of collaborative negotiation.

A recognition that current responses to global AIDS constitute genocide clearly will not in itself solve the problem of access to antiretrovirals. Yet it holds the possibility, as in the 1980s, for generating greater visibility to a situation that exists in part because of egregiously inappropriate government response; for holding scientists in the public and private sectors accountable to the downstream implications of their research; and for raising questions about the humanitarian contradictions of intellectual property regulation. As Edwin Cameron, a South African High Court justice living with HIV, poignantly stated at the 2000 International AIDS Conference in Durban:

> Those of us who live affluent lives, well-attended by medical care and treatment, should not ask how Germans or white South Africans could tolerate living in proximity to moral evil. We do so ourselves today, in proximity to the impending illness and death of many millions of people with AIDS . . . No more than Germans in the Nazi era . . . can we . . . say that we bear no responsibility for more than 30 million people in resource-poor countries who face death from AIDS unless treatment is made accessible and available to them. (2000, 9)

Not recognizing millions of preventable deaths as a form of genocide, on the other hand, maintains the status quo of global governance and condones through collective silence the primacy of corporate over human capital. The question is whether millions dead from AIDS is enough to galvanize not the capacity, but the willingness, to concede fundamental changes in trade regulations and the implicit construction of biological noncitizenship upon which they rest. Until that happens, forty million lives and more remain precarious.

ACKNOWLEDGMENTS

I would like to thank Jennifer Pierce, Jeff Crump, Joanna O'Connell, George Henderson, Rachel Schurman, Sam Bullington, Doreen Montag, participants of the International Population Geography Conference, St. Andrews University, 2004, and the Feminist Geography Colloquium Series, University of Minnesota, Fall 2004 for comments on previous iterations of this chapter.

NOTES

1. In fact, in the few years between writing this chapter and this volume going to press, the number of individuals on ARV regimes has increased considerably. Though universal access has yet to be achieved, ARVs are more affordable and accessible now largely through the efforts of grassroots and transnational campaigns and increased funding from countries like the US.
2. Also see Peluso and Watts (2001) for a similar critique of Kaplan and his functionalist equation of population, environment, and violence.
3. Such unflinching inflexibility on the part of the US ensured, however, that the 2003 Cancun agreement was so mired in qualifications and contingencies as to be commended by Harvey Bale, the president of the Federation of Pharmaceutical Manufacturers Associations.
4. Australia, Bahrain, Central America-Dominican Republic, Chile, Israel, Jordan, Morocco, NAFTA, Oman, Peru, and Singapore (www.export.gov/fta).
5. Andes, Panama, Thailand, South African Customs Union, United Arab Emirates (ibid).
6. Though France came out as favoring free access to antiretrovirals for low-income nations (Boseley 2004), and Europe in general has taken a more moderate line on patent regulations, the EU nevertheless has several large pharmaceutical companies within its rubric, placing it in a somewhat more ambivalent position between industry protection and essential medicine access (T'Hoen 2003).
7. These interviews of biologists, biochemists, physicians, and pharmacology researchers were conducted between October 2003 and May 2004. They are by no means construed to be representative of all scientists either in the private or public sectors, but rather indicate a variety of different perspectives on patents which scientists are likely to hold given the nature of their research and their desire to have new discoveries gain visibility and marketability.
8. One exception to this is an organization called Universities Allied for Essential Medicines, a largely medical and law school student-run campaign to get research universities to incorporate humanitarian licensing clauses in contracts with biotech and pharmaceutical companies, thereby ensuring broad global access of new technologies.
9. The media also share in this collusion, as evidenced by an article in the *Washington Post* earlier this year announcing the imminent marketing of a fixed-dose pill that combines antiretrovirals from Bristol Myers Squibb and Gilead, the first time major pharmaceutical companies have managed to surmount their rivalry to come up with the simpler drug regimen. While understandably touting the significance of this move, nowhere in the *Post*'s suggestion that this "would be a milestone in the development of treatments for the human immunodeficiency virus" (Gillis 2006) is there any acknowledgment that Indian pharmaceutical companies have been manufacturing a low-cost generic three-in-one combination pill for years now. Claims by both pharmaceutical companies that they "are committed to providing the treatment to poor people overseas" also goes unchallenged by the *Post*, despite evidence putting such a claim in doubt. Three weeks after the *Post* announcement, an Associated Press article outlined a Doctors Without Borders accusation that Gilead's supposed Access Program making its antiretrovirals available to low-income countries at no profit was a sham, stating that Gilead had yet to submit regulatory approval to 91 of the 97 countries it claimed to be targeting (Elias 2006).
10. Similarly, and ironically, facing the possibility of a flu pandemic nine congressional representatives urged the Bush administration to invoke a clause in the TRIPS agreement allowing override of patents in the face of an emergency in order to enable the US to manufacture Tamiflu despite Roche's patent (*USA Today*, December 7, 2005).

REFERENCES AND FURTHER READING

Adams, Vincanne, and Stacey Pigg. 2005, *Sex in Development: Science, Sexuality, and Morality in Global Perspective*. Raleigh: Duke University Press.

Agamben, Giorgio. 1998, *Homo Sacer: Sovereign Power and Bare Life*, trans. D. Heller-Roazen. Stanford: Stanford University Press.

AIDS 2003, 17 (Supplement 13), July.

Bastos, Cristiana. 1999, *Global Responses to AIDS: Science in Emergency*. Bloomington: Indiana University Press.

Bauman, Zygmunt. 1989, *Modernity and the Holocaust*. Cambridge: Polity Press.

Boseley, Sarah. 2004, "France Accuses US of AIDS Blackmail." *Guardian*, July 14.

Boston Globe, 1999, "AIDS and the African: A Continent's Crisis," October.

Boston Globe, 2001, "Prevention Urged in AIDS Fight; Natsios Says Fund Should Spend Less on HIV Treatment," June 7.

Brandt, Allan. 1987, *No Magic Bullet: A Social History of Venereal Disease in the United States Since 1880*. Oxford: Oxford University Press.

Briggs, Charles, with Clara Mantini-Briggs. 2003, *Stories in the Time of Cholera: Racial Profiling During a Medical Nightmare*. Berkeley: University of California Press.

Busza, J. 2006, "Having the Rug Pulled From Under Your Feet: One Project's Experience of the US Policy Reversal on Sex Work." *Health Policy and Planning* 21(4): 329–332.

Cameron, Edwin. 2000, "The Deafening Silence of AIDS." *Health and Human Rights* 5(1): 7–24.

CNN, 2003, "Africa's Lost Generation."

Craddock, Susan. Forthcoming, "The Politics of HIV/AIDS in Africa." In *Reframing Contemporary Africa: Politics, Economics, and Society in a Global Era*, Peyi Soyinka-Airewele and Rita Kiki Edozie (eds.), Washington, DC: CQ Press.

Donnelly, John. 2001, "Prevention Urged in AIDS Fight; Natsios Says Fund Should Spend Less on HIV Treatment." *Boston Globe*, June 7.

Dunn, Kevin. 2004, "Fear of a Black Planet: Anarchy Anxieties and Postcolonial Travel to Africa." *Third World Quarterly* 25(3): 483–499.

Elias, Paul. 2006, "Biotech Company Gilead Criticized for AIDS Drug Supply." *Associated Press*, February 8.

Epstein, Steven. 1997, "AIDS Activism and the Retreat from the Genocide Frame." *Social Identities* 3(3): 415–438.

Farmer, Paul. 2001, *Infections and Inequalities: The Modern Plagues*. Berkeley: University of California Press.

Farmer, Paul. 2004, *Pathologies of Power: Health, Human Rights, and the New War on the Poor*. Berkeley: University of California Press.

Gillis, Justin. 2006, "Once-a-Day AIDS Pill Could Be Ready Soon." *Washington Post*, January 19.

Gilroy, Paul. 2000, *Against Race: Imagining Political Culture Beyond the Color Line*. Cambridge: Harvard University Press.

Goozner, Merrill. 2005, *The $800 Million Pill: The Truth Behind the Cost of New Drugs*. Berkeley: University of California Press.

Hawk, Beverly. 1992, *Africa's Media Image*. New York: Praeger Press.

Heywood, Mark. 2002, "Drug Access, Patents and Global Health: 'Chaffed and Waxed Sufficient.'" *Third World Quarterly* 32(2): 217–231.

Ingram, Alan. 2005, "The New Geopolitics of Disease: Between Global Health and Global Security." *Geopolitics* 10: 522–545.

Jarosz, Lucy. 1992, "Constructing the Dark Continent: Metaphor as Geographic Representation of Africa." *Geografiska Annaler* 74B: 105–115.

Jones, Peris. 2004, "When Development Devastates: Donor Discourses, Access to HIV/AIDS Treatment in Africa and Rethinking the Landscape of Development." *Third World Quarterly* 25(2): 385–404.

Kaplan, Robert. 1994, "The Coming Anarchy: How Scarcity, Crime, Overpopulation, and Disease Are Rapidly Destroying the Social Fabric of Our Planet," *Atlantic Monthly*, February: 44–76.

Kaplan, Robert. 1996, *The Ends of the Earth: A Journey at the Dawn of the 21st Century*. New York: Random House.

Klein, Naomi. 2003, "Bush's AIDS 'Gift' Has Been Seized by Industry Giants." *Guardian*, October 13.

Krimsky, Sheldon. 2004, *Science in the Private Interest: Has the Lure of Profits Corrupted Biomedical Research?* New York: Rowman and Littlefield Publishing.

Langley, Alison, 2004. "African AIDS Drug Plan Faces Collapse." *Observer*, March 14.

Machungo, Francis Gatua. 2004, "The Representation of the AIDS Epidemic in Africa by the US Media: A Critical Analysis." Presented at the Gender and Empowerment: AIDS in Africa conference, University of Illinois, Champaign-Urbana, April 14.

Mbembe, Achille. 2001, *On the Postcolony*. Berkeley: University of California Press.

Nader, Laura. 1997, "Controlling Processes: Tracing the Dynamic Components of Power," *Current Anthropology* 38(5): 711–737.

Nguyen, Vinh-kim. 2005, "Antiretroviral Globalism, Biopolitics, and Therapeutic Citizenship." In *Global Assemblages: Technology, Politics, and Ethics as Anthropological Problems*, Aihwa Ong and Stephen J. Collier (eds.), Boston: Blackwell Publishing.

Offenheiser, Raymond. 2004, Speech given at the Global Business and Global Poverty Conference, Stanford Graduate School of Business, May 19.

Office of AIDS Research (OAR). 2005. *Fiscal Year 2006 Budget*. Washington DC: Department of Health and Human Services, National Institutes of Health.

Ong, Aihwa and Stephen J. Collier (eds.), 2005, *Global Assemblages: Technology, Politics, and Ethics as Anthropological Problems*. Boston: Blackwell Publishing.

Orrell, C. 2003, "Adherence is Not a Barrier to Successful Antiretroviral Therapy in South Africa." *AIDS* 17(9): 1997–1997.

Peluso, Nancy and Michael Watts, (eds.), 2001, *Violent Environments*. Ithaca: Cornell University Press.

Petryna, Adriana. 2002, *Life Exposed: Biological Citizens after Chernobyl*. Princeton: Princeton University Press.

Piot, Peter. 2004, Presentation given at the International Conference on AIDS, Bangkok, July 16.

Powers, Samantha. 2002, *"A Problem from Hell:" America and the Age of Genocide*. New York: Perennial Press.

President's Emergency Plan for AIDS Relief (PEPFAR), 2005, "Annual Report." Washington DC.

Redfield, Peter. 2006, "A Less Modest Witness: Collective Advocacy and Motivated Truth in a Medical

Humanitarian Movement," *American Ethnologist* 33(1): 3–26.

Richey, Lisa. 2002, "Is Overpopulation Still the Problem? Global Discourse and Reproductive Health Challenges in the Time of HIV/AIDS." *Centre for Development Research Working Paper* 2, 1.

Rose, Nicholas. 2001, "The Politics of Life Itself." *Theory, Culture and Society* 18(6): 1–30.

Rose, Nicholas and Carlos Novas. 2005, "Biological Citizenship." In *Global Assemblages: Technology, Politics, and Ethics as Anthropological Problems*, Aihwa Ong and Stephen J. Collier (eds.), Boston: Blackwell Publishing.

Said, Edward. 1979, *Orientalism*. New York: Vintage Press.

Sayagues, Mercedes. 2003, "Witchcraft, Vengeful Spirits, and the Plague: The AIDS battle needs new approach." *Newsweek*, December, www.newsweek.com/id/60874.

Scheper-Hughes, Nancy, and Philippe Bourgois. 2004, *Violence in War and Peace*, Boston: Blackwell Press.

Second Annual Report to Congress. 2005, "Action Today, A Foundation for Tomorrow: The President's Emergency Plan for AIDS Relief." Washington DC: Office of US Global AIDS.

Severe, Patrice et al. 2005, "Antiretroviral Therapy in a Thousand Patients with AIDS in Haiti." *New England Journal of Medicine* 353(22): 2325–2334.

Sitze, Adam. 2004, "Denialism." *South Atlantic Quarterly* 103(4): 769–811.

T'Hoen, Ellen. 2003, Personal communication. April 10.

Time magazine. 2001, "Death Stalks a Continent." February 4.

Tsing, Anna Haupt. 2005, *Friction: An Ethnography of Global Connection*. Princeton: Princeton University Press.

UNAIDS. 2005, "Epidemic Update." Geneva: World Health Organization and United Nations.

USA Today. 2005, "Tamiflu Maker Treads Minefield." December 7.

Village Voice, 1999, "AIDS: The agony of Africa." November.

Village Voice, 2000, "Dark Continent Still Dark." May.

Wallace, Roger. 2002, Personal communication, October 9.

Whitescarver, Jack. 2004, *Fiscal Year 2005 Budget Request*. Washington DC: Office of AIDS Research, Department of Health and Human Services, National Institutes of Health.

CHAPTER 19

Lessons from the Latin American AIDS Epidemic

Tim Frasca

ABSTRACT

Despite improved access to AIDS drugs, clinical services for most people with HIV in Latin America are limited. Advocacy groups demand that governments act to "save lives now" by ensuring access to medicines, but backers of good sexuality education for future generations fight a rearguard action against powerful forces of social conservatism. Governments are weak in promoting condom use, while large segments of the population ignore the message. The region's predominantly homosexual pattern of HIV transmission has prevented seroprevalence from reaching the frightening levels seen in Africa and appearing in Asia, but mostly as a result of luck, not sound public policy.

Is the AIDS glass in Latin America half-full or half-empty? There is often evidence for both observations, even within a single country. The main actors—governments, health providers, social organizations, gay men, churches, people with HIV—have accomplished remarkable things, sometimes in spite of themselves. There have been heroic efforts interspersed with a great deal of negligence, sometimes nefarious, more often indifferent. Overall, help has reached some people, while others are barely touched by the scientific advances, drug treatments, improved services, and enlightened social attitudes. The 20-year period that has elapsed since the epidemic gathered steam around the continent provides an opportunity to stand back and take stock of these efforts.

The question is not merely of historical interest. The sharp influx of new resources to Latin America—since its inception in 2002 the Global Fund To Combat AIDS, Malaria and Tuberculosis alone has granted over a half-billion dollars to the region[1]—has sparked an uneven, continent-wide process of "scaling up" of HIV/AIDS-related efforts based on the assumption that what is being done is effective and needs to be expanded or at least that "best practices" can be identified even if they are not yet universally applied (Family Health International/UNAIDS 2001; World Bank et al. 2003; Institute of Medicine 2004; WHO/UNAIDS/UNICEF 2007). Whether or not these assumptions are entirely justified, the full-fledged industry that has emerged around HIV needs to channel its increased resources wisely while they last.

The record so far is a mixed bag: as conditions evolve and shift, current wisdom about the proper mix of tactics and programs suffers from excessive consensus. In addition, an atomization of beneficiary populations has occurred that tends to favor prevention interventions over prevention and interest groups over interests. A look at the role of each set of actors may shed valuable light on the historical roots of present trends.

GOVERNMENTS

AIDS reached the continent at a unique historical moment. After the dominance of military dictatorships throughout the region during the 1970s, democratic rule slowly came back to most countries just as the first HIV infections were appearing.[2] Although the regimes were highly unpopular, the attitudes and habits that they installed among the populace often survived the formal end of authoritarian rule. The dictatorships were inspired to varying degrees by the Doctrine of National Security fomented by Washington consistent with U.S. global strategy (Lernoux 1980; Dinges 2004): rather than external enemies, said the Argentine, Chilean and Salvadoran generals, the nation must ward off the internal threat represented by Marxist subversion. Even though this internal "enemy" was comprised of the country's own citizens, the de facto regimes saw them as vehicles of foreign (i.e., Soviet or Cuban) intervention, by which they justified the widespread use of torture and political murder.

Even after the thug regimes were discredited in country after country, their purported defense of the "essence" of the nation or the body politic from corrosive internal dangers retained a substantial and sometimes subliminal appeal. Revolutionary politics or urban guerrilla movements no longer represented a real threat in most cases, but new alarms fitting the same psychosocial pattern were raised regularly by the political and economic elites about rising crime rates, immigrants or unhealthy foreign influences, such as pornography, abortion, and sexual libertinism. In this dangerous environment a scary disease like HIV could easily have stimulated far more repressive measures in the name of "protecting the majority" than actually occurred, and it is a credit to the social movements that defended people affected by HIV that, despite some ugly outbursts, worse repression did not occur. By contrast, the record of the countries of the former Soviet Union, which faced similar conditions a few years later, often was much more punitive (Atlani et al. 2000; Atlani-Duault 2005).

Activists, sometimes including Catholic clergy, quickly reframed the discussion from a human rights or Christian charity focus, and this discourse easily resonated in political and intellectual circles in Latin America, where many people understood its importance from their recent experience with state impunity (Gilmore and Somerville 1994; Orlov 2006). The more astute government AIDS programs quickly picked up the cue (Rico et al. 1995).[3] So, despite the foot-dragging that characterized governmental response in most countries, the coincidence of AIDS and the restoration of democracy sometimes worked in favor of a coherent, humane public health approach to the epidemic in Latin America, which gradually would filter into policymaking circles (Uribe et al. 1998; del Río and Sepúlveda 2002; Galvão 2005).[4]

However, Latin America also experienced AIDS in a slightly different way from the rest of the developing world and thus remained somewhat off the global AIDS map. There are no countries in the region with anywhere near the prevalence rates of 10, 15, or even 30 percent seen in Africa, and heterosexual transmission—a key factor in creating those rates—was not the primary route of dissemination in South America in the first decades of the epidemic (PAHO 2005), notwithstanding the frequent attempts to make the epidemiological data say so.[5] AIDS in Latin America emerged as heavily concentrated among men engaged in homosexual relations, enabling opinion leaders and officials to act as though only marginalized populations were involved even while confining their public expressions of concern to the heterosexual majority (McKenna 1996; Parker, et al. 1998; Frasca 2003). This contradictory attitude often resulted in rather tepid official AIDS programs that emphasized tolerance, humanitarian concern, and sensitivity along with some discreet support to narrowly targeted interventions well off the radar of society at large. Given the possible alternatives, this result is far from the worst possible scenario.

But as long as AIDS was viewed as a phenomenon limited to sex workers, gay men and injecting drug users, no radical rethinking of sexual mores and practices would be required, either by the state or by the broader society. Nor would Latin American societies have to prepare children and teens to manage their sexual lives during the increasingly extended adolescence that was installed in the region along with the economic modernity that Latin America could no longer avoid (Altman 1999). And it was exactly this confrontation with human sexuality that Catholic, patriarchal Latin America found impossibly discomfiting, just as the Vatican under Pope John Paul II systematically shifted toward militant obscurantism about sex (Shepard 2006).

Now, heterosexual HIV transmission rates are indeed edging up, and male/female sero-prevalence ratios steadily shrink; but most of the region's governments continue to flounder when tasked to come up with a credible strategy for this shifting scenario. When they have tried to introduce massive sexuality education for youth, for example, Catholic hard-liners eagerly mobilize to block them and extract a high political price for daring to acknowledge the widespread reality of sexual practices that stray from traditional standards (Shepard 2006). An important exception is Brazil (Berkman et al. 2005).

Nonetheless, it is now much harder for governments to deny that HIV/AIDS is a long-term public health concern likely to affect many thousands of people and to require considerable resources. In addition, leaders face a test of moral credibility as growing numbers of their citizens acquire HIV infection and realize that the modern treatments that can save their lives remain out of reach. For the most part—and unlike the situation in Malawi or the Ivory Coast—the region's governments cannot wriggle free from this claim with the excuse that their countries are too poor or too unstable or too lacking in modern infrastructure to provide the treatments.

Another important contrast with the situation in Africa was that AIDS hit Latin America along with the rising tide of neo-liberalism. Under the so-called Washington Consensus fomented by the International Monetary Fund and the U.S. government (Williamson 1990; Gore 2000), the private sector driven by market forces is presumed to be the prime motor of economic efficiency, prosperity, and development, and inherently superior to the centralized state. Neo-liberal boosters—who continue to dominate policy formulation in Latin America despite recent developments in Venezuela and Bolivia—tend to view government as an inherent obstacle, an innately inefficient user of resources, which should cede the field to private entrepreneurs, perhaps even in the provision of social services. Although the final outcome of these trends remains to be seen, the Washington Consensus has been ascendant until recently with nominal "socialists" throughout the region signing on to extreme versions of neo-liberal dogma, including business-friendly free-trade pacts and other long-term explorations of private sector hegemony.

By contrast, the African experiments in structural adjustment pushed by the World Bank and others in the 1980s are now discredited after already weak state-run services in Africa were dismantled with nothing to replace them. AIDS showed the short-sightedness of that experiment in wholesale re-engineering by overconfident theoreticians. But Latin America is just prosperous and modern enough that privatized social services of considerable quality can be offered to the privileged, and in many countries there is a large enough middle class to pay for them. The probability that this model will not work in any remotely fair way for the majority is less obvious, and the experiment therefore can still be vigorously defended all across the political spectrum, while the only resistance of any weight comes from easily caricatured mavericks like Venezuela's Hugo Chávez.

This triumph of the neo-liberal will was so pervasive that the movement for universal access to HIV treatments might have floundered in Latin America had it not been for the example of Brazil, which gradually cleared away the considerable obstacles and established full and open access for its citizens (Berkman et al. 2005; Galvão 2005). Given the now general acceptance of this demand, it is easy to forget that the movement to treat all HIV cases is anomalous in the neo-liberal context of pushing health care further into the marketplace and away from established entitlements. One might even wonder if the long-term governmental commitment to universal treatment as a centerpiece of national AIDS strategies automatically must survive if external funding for dealing with AIDS ever were to plunge from its present generous levels.[6] Had AIDS been merely an endemic, rather than an epidemic, problem, there is no reason to think that it would have been treated any differently from chronic diabetes, Dengue fever or, for that matter, malnutrition—as just another health disparity in the immutable landscape of social inequity.

THE CATHOLIC CHURCH

Catholicism also defined the AIDS epidemic in Latin America through its permanent political role, as a major cultural influence and through its many charities. In the 1970s and 1980s Latin American Catholicism was a thorn in the side of ruling elites due to its announced "preferential option for the poor," that is, the radical implications of liberation theology and its cautious support for social and economic transformations to alleviate poverty. Furthermore, Catholic bishops often backed civilian democratic reformers eager to be rid of military rule, and many priests and lay activists were among the generals' victims (Lernoux 1982; Klaiber 1998; Goldman 2007).

But by the mid-1990s the Polish pope had shifted to a preferential option for the chaste: instead of justice on earth, Catholicism had come to represent conformity—or at least obeisance—to traditional concepts of sexual propriety (Wills 2001; Steinfels 2003). This would have profound implications for the HIV/AIDS epidemic as soon as the issue of sexuality moved away from the doctor's office or low-profile peer education projects and dared to enter the public sphere. Meanwhile, the new civilian governments were often beholden or at least sympathetic to the Catholic hierarchy, which in some cases had boosted their cause and protected them personally during the grim days of dictatorship.

Not surprisingly given its size and internal diversity, the Catholic role in the HIV/AIDS epidemic sometimes was ambiguous. Despite its retrograde posture on sex, Catholic institutions often defended those afflicted especially in the context of charitable works under church auspices. Their paternalistic attitude toward the sick could be irritating, but their call for Christian charity was an important buffer against further victimization and partially reinforced the human rights discourse about the epidemic. Occasionally, Catholic priests would avoid ideological confrontation and look the other way or discreetly support AIDS projects, even while going to the mat over official condom-promotion campaigns or government-sponsored sex education in schools.[7]

But notwithstanding this ever-shrinking gray area, Latin American Catholicism eventually aligned itself against sexual autonomy or any official loosening of community standards around sex. The result was a permanent softening of governmental determination to promote sexual health with the required vigor once its attempts were demonized by Catholic hierarchs. John Paul II encouraged this posture with his steady promotion of the most rigid and uncompromising bishops, some of whom were openly sympathetic to the ousted generals (such as Chile's Cardinal Medina, who announced the election of John Paul's successor from a Vatican balcony).

One frequent outcome of Catholic intransigence was that AIDS prevention campaigns eventually fell into a crude binary, a battle between the cloth and the lab coat, a mass-media set-piece controversy in which priests would condemn immorality as symbolized by condom promotion and medical professionals would defend disease prevention—also symbolized by condom promotion. The sterile superficiality of this condom-centered debate, as it dragged on repetitively year after year, confused citizens and reinforced many individuals' deep-seated ambivalence about their public sexual roles and their private sexual acts—not to mention condom use itself.

Although the political and religious conservatives' strict objection to condom use was a minority position, their dogged persistence succeeded in driving the public discussion in many countries into an increasingly pointless and tiresome standoff. Rarely did either health authorities or the clergy win an outright victory, but the Latin American version of the culture wars blocked what could have been the opportunity provided by HIV/AIDS to tackle the ongoing transformation of sexual culture spurred by development and globalization. In the Chilean case, the Catholic-inspired resistance neutralized a nationwide move toward school-based sexuality education, which remains weak and inconsistent despite overwhelming support from parents.

With the topic of AIDS fully "condomized" and thus distanced from the arenas of human feeling, intimacy, pleasure, autonomy, and citizenship, many sexually active adults predictably tuned out the entire business. At the same time, sexual norms and attitudes were undergoing rapid change given the continent-wide demographic transition to a lower birth rate and the mass incorporation of women into the workforce (Guzman et al. 1996). Children, adolescents, and adults now are pulled in contradictory directions by an increasingly sexualized media culture on the one hand and the reiteration of stern messages to conform to traditional standards of decorum on the other. AIDS, which had emerged in the public mind as a phenomenon intimately linked with sex, stirred controversy, confusion, and conflict. The issue was primed for a re-engineered public discourse, and the advent of antiretroviral therapies would soon provide it.

ORGANIZATIONS OF PEOPLE WITH AIDS (PWAs)

Catholic influence is not solely a factor of the church hierarchy's contacts in the ministries or the frequency of the archbishop's news conferences on the cathedral steps. Latin American societies also are influenced by long-standing Catholic ways of thinking and behaving, even when individuals are quite indifferent to dogma or alienated from religious practice (Dides and Gutiérrez 2004). One example is the traditional Catholic view of charity as a highly personalized, apolitical action for both giver and receiver, and the impact of this view was felt as soon as people who had acquired HIV or AIDS emerged from the shadows to speak for themselves. This bold protagonism energized the AIDS advocacy community and challenged public opinion to reevaluate their prejudices and look to the state to answer the pointed questions raised by those affected.

At the same time, the discourse of those living with AIDS slipped neatly into a long tradition of "solving" individual tragedies with public displays of compassion while ignoring the structural factors that had produced the tragedy in the first place. Witness the oddity of a multi-million-dollar "Family Clinic" in Santiago constructed with great fanfare for dying AIDS patients by a religious charity that remained stubbornly aloof from its own patients' fight for access to HIV treatments. Furthermore, the clerical owner/operators openly fought the kinds of sexuality education that could have enabled their clinic's beneficiaries to avoid contracting the disease in the first place. The incongruence of this posture was absorbed effortlessly by public opinion over the years, and charity drives for Catholic sisterhoods ministering to AIDS babies and other freelance religious outfits purporting to help the sick rarely fail to raise impressive sums.

Meanwhile, the social movements that grew up around AIDS learned to utilize the demands of people living with HIV to force the hand of their governments. The anecdotal appeal of individuals facing a grim prognosis while life-saving medicines remained just out of reach was and is an irresistible and humane strategy. A compelling personal narrative was far more appealing than the wearying insistence on coherent prevention work and sexuality education, and those directly affected rightly assumed center stage to present it. The advocacy carried out by those with an HIV diagnosis was built on a decade of groundwork by the AIDS educators, gay rights advocates, defenders of human rights, health promoters, and feminists who insisted from the outset that people with HIV not be relegated to a passive role as "patients" or condemned as deviants, but that they speak for themselves in full possession of their dignity and rights. Eventually, some countries were pressured into providing full and universal HIV treatment, especially after Brazil did so (Berkman et al. 2005).

However, the treatment-access campaign shaped as a highly personalized narrative did not necessarily include solidarity with others facing a similar plight, and this shortcoming has had unexpected consequences. At the same time, the fight to provide life-saving medicines offered governments a familiar way out of the AIDS morass through the magic bullet of clinical medicine. The results of treatment were immediate and seemed miraculous, unlike the hard-to-measure outcomes from an inexact science such as the promotion of sexual health. Governments could shift their gaze from the knotty problem of preventing transmission of a virus to the more familiar task of battling a disease.

The results were often unfortunate. A common theme emerging in my research of AIDS in Spanish-speaking Latin America in the early 2000s is that the exclusive focus on the personal drama of living with HIV had sidetracked any deepening of the AIDS issue as a vehicle for understanding and defending the public's health or the public health system—which ironically had been an essential component of the Brazilian strategy that paved the way for treatment activism. The examples are numerous. A Guatemalan HIV-positive group found itself used as a battering ram by the government determined to discredit a local M.D. who had put the Guatemalan state's feet to the fire by demanding broader access. Facing the cut-off of their medicines, the patients were hardly in a position to resist. A Mexican activist related his frustration upon seeing medicines run short at one public hospital, while some of those who militantly demanded treatment a year before refused to sign protest petitions unless they personally were taking the unavailable drug. Chilean medical doctors told me that their attempts to incorporate the issue of health sector reform into planning for a future AIDS conference were met with stony indifference from the HIV-advocacy groups, who couldn't see what privatization of health services had to do with them. In short, while anecdote is a highly effective tool to illustrate broad principles, the principles themselves can disappear if *personalizing* the story of HIV ends up *individualizing* it.

The responsibility for these short-sighted views, however, does not lie with people trying to survive a life-threatening diagnosis but instead with the larger social movement that emerged to address AIDS and too often ceded its unique voice to those forced to deal with a personal emergency. While the personal tragedy narrative worked to increase sympathy for people with HIV and defuse the associated stigma, it also reinforced the notion that AIDS was simply a disease whose sufferers required medicines and, voilà, the End of AIDS would be at hand, just as many naively supposed had occurred in the richer countries years before (Sullivan 1995).

One area where this vision has proved to be particularly limited is the issue of how to address growing levels of heterosexual transmission and the prospect of steadily increasing proportions of women among the ranks of the HIV-infected. Women as potential victims of AIDS were a potent public concern from the start, although not out of any extraordinary sympathy for women's safety in negotiating their sexual autonomy, but rather because they could bear HIV-positive offspring. These infants, the "innocent victims" of AIDS in public discourse, were a regular counterpoint to the attempts to combat stigma against gay or drug-using HIV-positive adults, left by contrast in the category of "guilty" ones (Herek 1990).

The plight of women in societies that systematically subordinate them and restrict their options precisely in the sexual realm is a constant theme in discussions of the steady advance of heterosexual HIV (Erb-Leoncavallo et al. 2004), but the PWA narrative alone does not provide a coherent programmatic response to the problem. I have witnessed dozens of policy and media discussions of women and AIDS, which tend almost imperceptibly to morph into discussions of women *with* AIDS, their struggles and difficulties, the particular nature of the discrimination they suffer, their problems in child-rearing, the contradictions of either permitting or virtually forcing abortions on them, and so on. But this is an entirely separate category of issues. Gender inequity is relevant to these circumstances and to heterosexual transmission as well, but it does not by itself constitute a strategy for dealing with either. How heterosexual transmission is to be addressed in the future remains a conundrum that will not be solved by focusing on women with HIV alone or on women alone for that matter.

Current thinking on the topic includes a thorough discussion of the ways in which gender equity increases female vulnerability, and statements usually conclude with a summary flourish calling for changes in men's habits. But an examination of the subjectivity that might be driving male behavior and could illuminate what to do about it is usually lacking, and this disconnect is the natural outcome of viewing HIV exclusively through the lens of those facing the diagnosis.[8]

GAY MEN/NGOs

The early AIDS groups that struggled into being in the 1990s under hostile conditions fought admirably to get themselves a place at the policy table and to obtain the resources needed to do their work. They faced unusual obstacles compared with their counterparts in places like London, Los Angeles, or Barcelona. Despite the predominance of homosexual transmission, Latin American groups could build on little or no previous agitation around gay rights and therefore had no preexisting organizational base from which to branch out into AIDS prevention and care (Altman 1994). The NGOs' success in legitimizing their existence and their approach to things like peer education and the defense of human rights has been remarkable, as evidenced by the ratcheting up of AIDS-related funding and the growing insistence by donors on a strong community presence in the process of divvying up the suddenly expanded pie.[9] Innovative peer-led projects brought news of the new disease to the commercial sex scene, to gay men in heavily closeted environments, to drug injectors, and eventually to a broader public, while governments lagged behind.

But the epidemic of 1990 is not the same as that of today, and the leaders of these pioneering groups—often ten- and twenty-year veterans—have not always recognized the need to evolve along with their audiences. The groups usually moved into the vacuum left by public health authorities, who were slow to react or lackadaisical about the fate of those affected; in addition, governments simply may never have smooth access to the populations involved and thus need the storefront NGOs and advocacy groups as long-term partners.

As a result, these groups run the risk of hubris born of their own foresightedness and can succumb to recycling their habitual programming with little accountability. Since gay rights and AIDS prevention usually were born as twins in most countries of Latin America, their leaders often view sexual emancipation as equivalent to sexual health. While they were prescient in recognizing that HIV campaigns should be sex-friendly, they could also fall into the illusion that sex-friendliness was by definition enough to make a good HIV campaign.

It is a significant achievement that protective practices among homosexually active men are shown to be far more consistent than for any comparable heterosexual population (Cáceres et al. 2002). But HIV prevalence rates in the region among this population and the natural desire for relief from a lifetime of condom use make the chances of acquiring HIV for an individual gay man in Peru or Colombia very high. Maturing AIDS prevention groups now face a new set of challenges as the early adoption of condom use—never enthusiastic or majoritarian in gay Latin America—inevitably wanes, and, without a renewal of the message and independent research to keep up with shifting trends, these groups face the temptations of mechanically repeating past efforts, especially now that donor agencies are eager to address the homosexual epidemic.

But as "scaling-up" proceeds apace, one aspect rarely scaled up in tandem is rigorous examination of the effectiveness of the efforts deployed, and the long-suffering NGOs finally enjoying some financial stability are unlikely to be enthusiastic about evaluations of this sort. Programs are carried out and contracts fulfilled, but downstream outcomes remain in doubt. Transmission rates may be falling or leveling off in Latin America as a result of the boosted prevention efforts, but it is not clear that independent evaluators are fanning out to confirm whether or not this is so. (By contrast, it is quite easy to know how many people are or are not being reached by clinical treatments.)

Similarly, the mantra of "community involvement" may mean that a properly diverse panel must be appointed to oversee and advise actions in the AIDS field or that carefully inclusive NGO networks must be built to reflect all the appropriate interest groups. But UN agencies can fulfill this requirement without probing too deeply into the depth and breadth of this representation or the effectiveness of the activities of those thus elevated. Meanwhile, NGOs, being fallible human institutions, are likely to defend the successes of their opus and shift the blame for failures elsewhere.

The field of HIV testing presents an example of the resistance to change. While voluntary counseling has been a major triumph of the AIDS movement, which moved the HIV testing focus from a disease detection to a client-centered approach, the circumstances surrounding the test are now quite different from what they were in 1990. Treatments exist where there once was little to offer in the clinical setting. Where stigma dominated, courageous activism has made a dent. Where the HIV-positive individual was a rare case threatened by the public's or the news media's morbid fascination, now there are thousands of people living relatively normal lives with HIV.

Meanwhile, the need to provide universal treatment to people with HIV is a heavy burden on public health budgets even in the developed world, where new rapid-testing and home-test technologies are stirring debate and experimentation. NGOs will have to engage this discussion and defend their client-centered vision while recognizing the changed circumstances, rather than insisting on the familiar procedures simply because they are familiar. Consent, confidentiality, and partner notification issues all appear in a different light once an AIDS diagnosis includes treatment options supported by public resources. Whatever its merits, the U.S. government's drive to massively increase HIV testing is hardly surprising as health officials seek ways to streamline the process of diagnosis and treatment to reach everyone with HIV promptly and efficiently.

BRAZIL—A WELCOME ANOMALY

Brazil's achievements have been remarkable, but whether they can be replicated elsewhere on the continent remains to be seen. Despite some initial resistance Brazil eventually combined a massive, decentralized prevention model with a guarantee of free and universal clinical treatments for everyone with HIV (Galvão 2005). The country did not shrink from confronting the pharmaceutical multinationals to keep drug prices within reach and protect its universal-coverage model, a fight that only a country as big and as productive as Brazil could have won (Berkman et al. 2005). Nor was the Brazilian government cowed by Catholic or evangelical Protestant opposition.

The World Bank predicted disastrous HIV prevalence rates for Brazil in the early 1990s. But a decade later these had not materialized, and Brazilian government officials soon began to celebrate the wisdom and efficacy of their strategy as well as the savings in reduced hospitalizations. Their strategy quickly became a model even for countries with enormous social problems and poverty. All that was lacking elsewhere on the continent was the political will, which put the ball squarely back into the court of the politicians and public health authorities.

But the results in Spanish-speaking Latin America were not so impressive; in fact, those who were inspired by the Brazilian approach only haphazardly imitated it. The Brazilian activists incorporated their universal-access principle within a broader framework—that of social exclusion, poverty, the structural sins of Brazil's scandalous social and economic inequalities (Daniel and Parker 1993). This not only inspired them politically and illuminated the need to defend the public health system and the guarantee to health enshrined in the Brazilian constitution, but also kept the AIDS issue firmly grounded outside the clinical setting, even as public hospitals around the country were instituting special programs for people with HIV.

In contrast, in other countries of the region advocates for the HIV positive often saw themselves in exclusively interest-group terms: we have HIV—we need medicines; if we get them, the problem is solved. The broader AIDS movement still must speak for thousands of Latin Americans who are far from obtaining even this minimum benefit, to sustain services into coming decades and to explore effective prevention strategies. In the fight for truly universal access that can be sustained over a long period, AIDS activism requires a tighter fit with a broader struggle for health rights, which would truly constitute an imitation of the Brazilian example.

NEXT STEPS

Governments

There is no longer any excuse for Latin American governments to fail to provide universal access to HIV medicines for all those who need them. The technical knowledge and the resources to do so are available; only official probity and true commitment to public service fall short. Infrastructure is certainly inadequate in some regions, but there is considerable willingness on the part of multilateral institutions and donor agencies to help out. The only conceivable exceptions are those countries suffering from severe instability or war. The region's leaders who would be offended to hear themselves discussed in the same breath with a failed African state should prove that they do not merit the comparison.

On the trickier prevention side, however, governments must thread their way through confusing data and political minefields to assemble a coherent strategy, which will satisfy no one fully and raise the hackles of many—exactly the kind of messy social issue that politicians hate. Furthermore, public health authorities in Latin America generally arrived late to AIDS: their understanding of the epidemic and the different populations involved was blocked by their training and prejudices, while those closer to the affected populations moved ahead. Once health officials realized the difficulties of access to the most vulnerable groups, they could slip too easily into equating the presence at the table of selected representatives of gay men, sex workers, drug users, youth, women, etc., with a strategy to address the needs of these groups. Identity politics aggravated the scenario as factions naturally fought for a shot at the growing pool of AIDS-related funding.

However, the governmental role in guaranteeing that the activities they execute and support are leading to the desired outcomes requires not just consensus but evidence. It is up to governments to plot the progress of their HIV epidemics and draw the difficult conclusions from the findings about whether or not these activities are doing any good. A lack of criticism does not mean necessarily that a particular strategy is working, only that no one has managed to articulate its shortcomings.

The Catholic Church

Worldwide, institutional Catholicism has made no secret of its commitment to a fantastic vision of a desexualized Golden Age, and it is time to accept its decision and shift gears. Rather than attempting to bring religious conservatives into a broad agreement about teaching sexuality-related "values" to children and adolescents, policymakers should stop chasing the will-o'-the-wisp of consensus and produce competent, innovative, science-based sexuality education for those children and youth whose parents desire these services and are willing to defend them politically.

In Latin America any attempt to insert sensible sexuality education into private Catholic schools is now quixotic, and many public-school programs will be blocked at the national level as well. Often, however, local schools in either the public or private sector, especially those in poorer neighborhoods where parents are more realistic about sexual behavior, are eager for good programs. Governments should be spending their time and resources within these communities, not wasting energy on endless commissions aimed at bringing intransigent religious ideologues into a watery and meaningless consensus, vulnerable to immediate sabotage by even more extremist holdouts. This approach will eliminate the Catholic or evangelical veto and the resulting paralysis of governmental action and reward the majority of families who want their children to receive good preparation.

Meanwhile, the Catholic hierarchy should be challenged to get behind the fight for treatment access in countries where the clergy has been strangely silent. If Catholics view human life as sacred, archbishops and cardinals should have plenty to say about governmental incompetence and corruption in providing HIV antiretroviral therapies to those who urgently need them. This would be a far more useful and bracingly clarifying debate for AIDS organizations than more complaints about the Pope's well-known views on sex.

Organizations

Struggling NGOs shape their tactics to fit funding opportunities. Now that major Global Fund grants blanket the region, groups naturally will seek to slice off a piece of the funding pie to sustain their visions. Networks, despite their rhetoric, do not exist to articulate a comprehensive joint strategy—that's the government's job. But NGO confederations that facilitate funding access also can insist that the HIV/AIDS epidemic be understood within the broader context of what is occurring in their societies and address relevant issues such as the state of public health services, privatization and health sector reform, changing sexual culture, and the interplay of responsibilities with rights. The non-profit sector can strive for a balanced perspective that includes both individual narratives as well as the situation of the invisible and unheard populations far removed from the organizational setting. Complex and multifaceted efforts to address AIDS must be "owned" by all those affected, including those facing the diagnosis and those trying to avoid it.

In Latin America gay-oriented AIDS groups have a special role and special responsibilities. There is ample evidence from the wealthier countries that two decades of condom promotion, combined with major advances in HIV treatment, have resulted in important gains and a whole new set of problems, but the relevant lessons from the reproductive health movement are not being absorbed: just as contraceptive providers must grapple with the challenge of enabling couples and individual women to plan their children and then avoid pregnancy for decades, HIV prevention for homosexually active men faces a similar, daunting task. But AIDS projects in the region often retain their original spirit of emergency intervention combined with civil and social rights advocacy—all worthy goals, to be sure, but insufficient. Gay-oriented sexual health services need to be rethought from a lifespan, rather than a crisis-avoidance, perspective. They should build a research-driven capacity to accompany men throughout a lifetime of shifting emotional and relational circumstances in which their choices and decisions about avoiding disease continue to evolve. But now that funding levels are at historical highs, gay groups instead have the option of simply recycling their historical interventions with little fear that they will be required to show that they do much good.

CONCLUSION

AIDS arrived in Latin America accompanied by powerful symbolism and quickly spawned competing narratives with intense moral and ethical overtones. But the vigor of the struggle over how to interpret the disease and respond appropriately has colored our ability to detect interests and interest groups at work. Research results are lauded or ignored based on whether the conclusions are convenient or counterproductive to a particular audience, and, given the enormous stakes involved, it would be irrational to expect any other response. Today, AIDS in Latin America is a burgeoning industry, and this spurt of growth has set the stage for an effective challenge to the epidemic.

But twenty years since the onset of AIDS, many of the responses that emerged are less convincing than they were during the emergency phase. There are periodic alarms over the "heterosexualization" of the epidemic but a dearth of innovative proposals to address rising heterosexual transmission rates. Religious and cultural resistance blocks comprehensive sexuality education, and focalized interventions among the most vulnerable groups lack breadth. As long as the international largesse continues, hard questions about long-term prevention and sexual health do not demand an answer, and criticism remains muted. While the achievements have been extraordinary, many Latin American citizens still can only gaze at those impressive gains from afar.

NOTES

1. The Fund's website reports that it has authorized $664 million in grants to the region and disbursed $424 million (www.theglobalfund.org/en, accessed September 8, 2007).
2. The military regime in Bolivia ended in 1982, followed by those in Argentina (1983), Uruguay and Brazil (1985), Paraguay (1989), and Chile (1990). These six states were ideological cousins and shared repressive agency through the notorious Operation Condor. Peru had a left-leaning military regime until 1980. The first cases of HIV infection recorded in each country were: Brazil and Argentina 1982; Uruguay and Peru 1983; Chile and Bolivia 1984; and Paraguay 1985.
3. In 2002 the issue of access to medicines for people with HIV was brought before the Inter-American Commission on Human Rights based in Costa Rica, an indication of how deeply the human rights discourse underpinned AIDS policy and activism in the region. See Stern (1999).
4. The Mexican government's program includes the goal of eliminating "all health sector violations of human rights of persons with HIV" (Uribe et al. 1998), a typical official stance. Del Río and Sepúlveda (2002) relate how Mexico City's commercial sex workers kept HIV rates down through a cooperative approach involving city authorities without "police harrassment," thus illustrating how a rights-centered approach could achieve public health goals.
5. National statistics often did not reflect the true rate of homosexual transmission in the early years, often through a tendentious emphasis on any and all other categories. A high percentage of cases were attributed to "no known transmission route," a separate "bisexual" transmission category was used, and the frequent denial by homosexually active men of their own practices was not recognized. Health officials downplayed homosexual transmission out of a misguided desire to broaden political support for their efforts or from simple indifference.
6. Chile's AIDS program received a five-year, $38 million grant from the Global Fund in 2003. A portion of the aid enabled the government to provide universal coverage for everyone in the state-run health system, some two-thirds of the population. Now the country must shoulder the full burden of treatment for a group that is surviving much longer and steadily adding new members.
7. I had direct experience of this paradox in the early years of the epidemic. As part of a negotiation for a small subsidy from a Catholic development agency in a European country, we were required to get formal endorsement from a local bishop. Just as the church hierarchy was vigorously denouncing a government AIDS prevention campaign over the condom issue, a high-ranking official whom I visited in what I assumed would be a vain pursuit politely inquired what was the nature of the group I represented. When I told him that it was mostly homosexual men, he smiled benignly and obtained the signature in 24 hours.
8. Some "gender and AIDS" program initiatives do try to incorporate men as subjects of their own gender construction, e.g., Stepping Stones (Wellbourn et al. 1999) or those supported by the Horizons Project (Population Council 2004).
9. For example, see the Global Fund's position on the issue (http://www.theglobalfund.org/en/partners/ngo).

REFERENCES AND FURTHER READING

Altman, Dennis (1994) *Power and Community: Organizational and Cultural Responses to AIDS*. Basingstoke, UK: Taylor and Francis.

Altman, Dennis (1999) "Globalization, political economy and AIDS." *Theory and Society* 28(4): 559–84.

Atlani, Laetitia, Michel Carael, Jean-Baptiste Brunet, Timothy Frasca, and Nicholai Chaika (2000) "Social change and HIV in the former USSR: The making of a new epidemic." *Soc Sci Med* 50: 1547–56.

Atlani-Duault, Laetitia (2005) *Au bonheur des autres: anthropologie de l'aide humanitaire (For Their Own Good: The Anthropology of Humanitarian Aid)*. Paris: Société d'Ethnologie.

Berkman, Alan, Jonathan Garcia, Miguel Muñoz-Laboy, Vera Paiva, and Richard Parker (2005) "Critical analysis of the Brazilian response to HIV/AIDS: lessons learned for controlling and mitigating the epidemic in developing countries." *Am J Public Health* 95(7): 1162–72.

Cáceres, Carlos, Mario Pecheny, and Veriano Terto (eds.) (2002) *SIDA y sexo entre hombres en América Latina: Vulnerabilidades, fortalezas y propuestas para la acción*. Lima, Peru: Universidad Peruana Cayetano Heredia.

Daniel, Herbert and Richard Parker (1993) *Sexuality, Politics and AIDS in Brazil: In Another World?* London: Falmer Press.

del Río, Carlos and Jaime Sepúlveda (2002) "AIDS in Mexico: Lessons learned and implications for developing countries." *AIDS* 16: 1445–57.

Dides, Claudia and María Alicia Gutiérrez (2004) *Diálogos Sur-Sur: South-South Dialogue on Religion and Sexual and Reproductive Health and Rights. Status Reports on Argentina, Colombia, Chile and Peru*. Santiago, Chile: Universidad Academia de Humanismo Cristiano/Sociedad PROGENERO.

Dinges, John (2004) *The Condor Years*. New York: The New Press.

Erb-Leoncavallo, Ann, Gillian Holmes, Stephanie Urdang, Micol Zarb, Gloria Jacobs, Joann Vanek (UNFPA) (2004) *Women and HIV/AIDS: Confronting the Crisis*. Geneva/New York: UNAIDS/UNFPA/UNIFEM.

Family Health International/UNAIDS (2001) "FHI/UNAIDS Best Practices in Prevention Collection," ed. Makinwa and O'Grady. http://www.fhi.org/, accessed September 8, 2007.

Frasca, Tim (2003) "Men and Women–Still Far Apart on HIV/AIDS." *Reprod Health Matters* 11(22): 12–20.

Galvão, Jane (2005) "Brazil and access to HIV/AIDS drugs: a question of human rights and public health." *Am J Public Health* 95(7): 1110–16.

Gilmore, Norbert and Margaret Somerville (1994) "Stigmatization, scapegoating and discrimination in sexually transmitted diseases: overcoming 'them' and 'us.'" *Soc Sci Med* 39(9): 1339–58.

Global Fund To Combat AIDS, Tuberculosis and Malaria (2008) http://www.theglobalfund.org/en/partners/ngo, accessed January 17, 2008.

Goldman, Francisco (2007) *The Art of Political Murder: Who Killed the Bishop?* New York: Grove Press.

Gore, Charles (2000) "The rise and fall of the Washington consensus as a paradigm for developing countries." *World Dev* 28(5): 789–804.

Guzman, José Miguel, Susheela Singh, Germán Rodriguez, and Edith Pantelides (eds.) (1996) *The Fertility Transition in Latin America*. Oxford: Clarendon Press.

Herek, Gregory (1990) "Illness, stigma and AIDS," in Costa and VandenBos (eds.), *Psychological Aspects of Serious Illness*, 103–150. Washington DC: American Psychological Association.

Institute of Medicine (2004) *Scaling Up Treatment for the Global AIDS Pandemic: Challenges and Opportunities*. Washington: Institute of Medicine/National Academy of Science.

Klaiber, Jeffrey (1998) *The Church, Dictatorships and Democracy in Latin America*. Maryknoll, NY: Orbis Books.

Lernoux, Penny (1980) *Cry of the People: The Struggle for Human Rights in Latin America—The Catholic Church in Conflict with U.S. Policy*. New York: Penguin Books.

McKenna, Neil (1996) *On the Margins: Men Who Have Sex with Men and HIV in Developing Countries*. London: Panos Institute.

Orlov, Lisandro (2006) "The transforming power of a ministry to people living with HIV/AIDS," website of the Evangelical Lutheran Church of America. www.elca.org/gme, accessed September 8, 2007.

Pan American Health Organization (PAHO) (2005) "Vigilancia del SIDA en las Américas." Washington: PAHO.

Parker, Richard (2002) "The global HIV/AIDS pandemic, structural inequalities and the politics of international health." *Am J Public Health* 92(3): 343–7.

Parker, Richard, Regina Barbosa, and Peter Aggleton (eds.) (2000) *Framing the Sexual Subject: The Politics of Gender, Sexuality and Power*. Berkeley: University of California Press.

Parker, Richard, Shivananda Khan, and Peter Aggleton (1998) "Conspicuous by their absence: men who have sex with men (MSM) in developing countries: implications for HIV prevention." *Crit Public Health* 8(4): 329–46.

Population Council (2004) "Young men and HIV prevention." *Horizons Report*. December 2004.

Rico, Blanca, Maria Bronfman, and Carlos del Río-Chiriboa (1995) "Las campañas contra el SIDA en México: Los sonidos del silencio o puente sobre aguas turbulentas?" ("Campaigns against AIDS in Mexico: the sounds of silence or a bridge over troubled waters?") *Salud Pública de México* 37(6): 643–53.

Shepard, Bonnie (2006) *Running the Obstacle Course to Sexual and Reproductive Health: Lessons from Latin America*. Westport, CT: Praeger.

Steinfels, Peter (2003) *A People Adrift: The Crisis of the Roman Catholic Church in America*. New York: Simon and Schuster.

Stern, Richard (1999) "A summary of the position on HIV/AIDS work in Costa Rica, Panama, Nicaragua, Honduras and El Salvador." International Lesbian and Gay Association, www.ilgainfo.org/Information/legal_surveys/americas, accessed September 8, 2007.

Stieglitz, Joseph (1998) "More instruments and broader goals: moving toward the post-Washington Consensus." The WIDER Annual Lecture, Helsinki, Finland, http://time.dufe.edu.cn/wencong/washington consensus/instrumentsbroadergoals.pdf, accessed September 8, 2007.

Sullivan, Andrew (1995) "The End of AIDS." *New York Times Magazine*. November 10, 1995.

Terto, Veriano (1999) "Seropositivity, homosexuality and identity politics in Brazil." *Culture, Health and Sexuality* 1(4): 329–46.

Uribe, Patricia, Carlos Magis, and Enrique Bravo (1998) "AIDS in Mexico." *J Int Assoc Physicians in AIDS Care*. http://www.thebody.com/content/world/art12264.html, accessed September 9, 2007.

Welbourn, Alice, Glen Williams, and Alison Williams (1999) *Stepping Stones: A Training Package in HIV/*

AIDS, Communication and Relationship Skills. London: ActionAid.

Williamson, John (1990) "What Washington means by policy reform." In *Latin American Adjustment: How Much Has Happened*, 5–20. Washington DC: Institute of International Economics.

Wills, Garry (2001) *Papal Sin: Structures of Deceit*. New York: Doubleday.

World Bank/UNDP/Cities Alliance/UN Habitat Urban Management Programme/AMICAALL (2003) *Local Government Responses to HIV/AIDS: A Handbook*. http://www.worldbank.org/urban/hivaids/handbook/handbook.pdf, accessed September 8, 2007.

World Health Organization/UNAIDS/UNICEF (2007) "Toward universal access: scaling up priority HIV/AIDS interventions in the health sector." http://www.who.int/hiv/mediacentre, accessed September 8, 2007.

CHAPTER 20

Rollout and Rationing

Providing Antiretroviral Therapy in South Africa

Ronald Bayer and Gerald M. Oppenheimer

ABSTRACT

This chapter presents the ethical and clinical experience of public sector physicians during the post-apartheid period in South Africa, who were faced with poverty, medical scarcity, and unexpected government resistance to treating people with HIV infection. The results were garnered from oral history interviews with 79 physicians and nurses from major cities, mine clinics, and rural hospitals selected because of their long-standing commitment to treating people with AIDS. The chapter concludes that the onset of the government's "roll-out" of antiretroviral therapy (ART) in 2003, providing drugs to public sector patients, has not put an end to the rationing of care which characterized the pre-ART period.

Scarcities demand rationing. Whether implicit or explicit, whether the consequences of the market's "hidden hand" or openly embraced rules of selection, rationing is inevitable. In medicine the consequence is that some who could be relieved of suffering continue to suffer, and some whose lives might have been saved die. The central moral question posed by such selection is fairness. What social, economic, and political factors dictate the need for rationing? What patterns of inclusion and exclusion result from the rationing itself?

There is a large and important literature that examines the ethics of medical rationing both within nations and globally (Churchill 1987; Daniels 1991). There is also an empirical literature about who wins and who loses under various rationing regimes. Much less has been written about the experience of doctors who witness, and willingly participate in, or who have no alternative but to collaborate in medical rationing. The scale-up of antiretroviral therapy (ART) in very poor and relatively impoverished nations will by definition involve rationing decisions (Daniels 2005). Where HIV treatment clinics are first located will determine who will live and who will die. So too will rules about who within clinics is treated. Principles of equity will often be brought into tension with utilitarian judgments. Only when access to ART is available to all who can benefit will the need for scarcity-imposed rationing vanish. A social science of scale-up must be attentive to these issues and their impact on health care providers.

In this chapter, we turn to the experience of doctors in South Africa based on oral histories of 79 physicians and nurses from interviews we conducted in 2003–2005. These interviews were drawn from lists of names recommended by colleagues in the United States who had worked in South Africa, and from AIDS experts in that country, including members of the South African HIV Clinicians' Society. Those we interviewed worked in the major cities, in small mining towns and remote rural communities. They provided care in a number of different settings typical of South Africa: publicly operated urban medical centers and rural ex-missionary facilities, clinics run by the mining industry, and private offices and hospitals (Van Resnburg 2004). Our goal in identifying those we would interview was not to create a sample that was in any conventional sense statistically representative. Rather, we wanted to find health practitioners with varied experiences, those who could reflect on elements that were common in the encounter with AIDS in South Africa, and those who could provide insights into the utterly unique. These oral histories, to which we added 13 with nurses, also provide the basis for our book, *Shattered Dreams? An Oral History of the South African AIDS Epidemic* (Oppenheimer and Bayer 2007). This approach was one we used previously to write our study of the HIV/AIDS epidemic in the United States, *AIDS Doctors: Voices from the Epidemic* (Bayer and Oppenheimer 2000).

Our account begins before the South African government announced in 2003, after bitter resistance, that it would begin to "roll out" ART to the vast numbers with HIV. Capturing the nature of rationing in this earlier period will provide a context for understanding the experience of doctors as the scaling up of treatment began.

BEFORE THERE WAS ART

As the number of critically ill AIDS patients seeking hospital care mounted in the mid- to late 1990s, the capacity of South Africa's already strained institutions to respond eroded. Describing Johannesburg's Baragwanath Hospital, chief of neonatology Haroon Saloojee observed, "The situation has changed, mainly related to HIV. There is this enormous stress on beds. The only way you respond to that is turn people away. So you only admit the very sick."

But, although necessary, turning people away was not so easy. Triage inevitably posed moral quandaries. In Johannesburg, Pinky Ngcakani, who had, by 2004, left work in a public hospital out of sheer frustration, described the dilemmas she had previously faced in deciding whom to admit when her hospital was already full.

> So it was looking at the patients and then deciding who is sicker than the other; who can I admit and who can I not? And you knew that the ones that would not be admitted were going to be back a day or two later, because they should have been admitted, but I didn't have the space available. And how can you say really this one has chronic diarrhea and is dehydrated and I cannot admit her, that one has meningitis, and he needs more help. So they stayed in casualty overnight, or over two days, whilst waiting for an available bed.

Overcrowded tertiary care institutions, whose outpatient clinics and wards were filled to capacity, sought to shift their patients to other health care settings. Bureaucratic rigidities could serve to hold demand at bay. Themba Mabaso, a private practitioner in Durban, sardonically recounted the treatment to which he and a patient had been subject.

> I had a terrible situation where I sent a patient to King Edward VIII with a specimen bottle. He phoned to say that he had been sent away and told to go to another hospital. I told him to wait for me there, where I explained to the nurse who was doing the sorting that in Mahatma Gandhi Hospital there is no urologist, and this particular problem needs an urologist. The nurse refused. She showed me a chart which showed that if you live in this area, you go to that hospital. She said, "Now you've driven here, you can drive him to Mahatma Gandhi. Ask the doctor there to write a letter and bring him back. Then, I'll take him."

Describing the plight of those who needed inpatient care, Mabaso was even more bitter.

> There is no place for people who are dying of HIV in hospitals. If we send them to King Edward VIII in respiratory distress, they are going to die on the bench waiting to see a doctor. If they do get admitted for cryptococcal meningitis, they may be shunted to an inferior hospital after 72 hours. You don't even have clinics in those hospitals. It's just the ward where some of the most incompetent nurses or people who are tired of working go and spend

> their last days of work. You send someone there and they are going to die there, or they may send them home to die.

Some hospitals were compelled to adopt measures that represented a throwback to what had, at times, been necessary in Black institutions during the apartheid era. In rural KwaZulu-Natal at the Church of Scotland Hospital, with 350 official beds, Tony Moll told of his strategy to make room in his already filled medical wards and the institutional resistance his efforts provoked.

> We began using what we call "floor beds," which are blankets rolled out under the bed of another patient or between two beds. The patients were quite happy to accept this. What happened then was the management of the district came back to us, and said, "We see that you've got more than 100 per cent occupancy of your beds. How does this work? We can't have more than one person in a bed." We said that we were using floor beds. They said, "Well, the computer cannot accept this. There is no block to fill in the statistic for floor beds." So they actually prohibited us from making such accommodations. If we are on duty 9, 10, 11 o'clock at night, and a patient comes in and the ward is full, we have to admit that patient, put up a drip and initiate antibiotics. And what we have had to do now is to put the patient on a trolley and let them wait outside in a passage until a bed becomes available. And this is an every night's story.

Despite the existence of triage mechanisms that sought to limit admissions of those who were too sick to benefit from care, and despite the reliance on bureaucratic roadblocks to restrict the number of AIDS patients that could be admitted, those with HIV-related conditions began to displace other sick patients. "The Impact of HIV/AIDS on the Health Sector," a report prepared for the national Department of Health in 2003 (Government of South Africa 2003a), noted that, as the epidemic increased, those with HIV had begun to "crowd out" others deemed less needy. Commenting on this phenomenon at his own hospital, Tony Moll said:

> Terminally ill AIDS patients can be so sick with fulminating PCP or a cryptococcal meningitis, or have a very bad infected wound, that we try to give them priority over a diabetic or hypertensive that might not be so sick. They are ambulatory people and can be treated at home.

Given the scarcity that defined their world, even those deeply committed to the care of their patients could embrace the rationing of services as a moral imperative. For Haroon Saloojee—who would become an expert witness for the plaintiffs in a successful suit forcing the government of President Thabo Mbeki to provide antiretrovirals to pregnant women and children—deciding on who had access to limited resources was both necessary and routine:

> I believe that my role as a citizen of the community is to ensure the best utilization of resources. So it may not make sense to continue offering a baby care for five days instead of two days. Maybe the baby might have shown improvement after three or five days, but I'd rather have those three days for another baby who has a better chance. I was never uncomfortable with this, because we were often turning away babies, good, strong, big babies who only needed one day of the intensive care unit [ICU], simply because we didn't have the beds. Occasionally, those babies died in our wards. That kind of balancing act, I got into that role fairly comfortably. I hope I got the balance right; one never knows. We tried to make it as systematic and objective as possible.

Saloojee spoke frankly of his conversations with parents at Baragwanath Hospital concerning the resources that could be dedicated to their children and of their acquiescence to his judgments. "There was an issue of premature and low birth weight babies," he remembered. "I was dealing with this on a daily basis. I was very straightforward with parents." He explained that if the baby made no progress, he had no alternative but to end care. There was no need to confront parents with a series of medical options. "It was a matter of fact. We are doing this. I think most parents will accept that," he said, "because in the kind of environment we worked in, the doctor was God."

This, then, was the context within which the limits imposed on care for AIDS patients occurred. At a time when the understanding of the prognosis of children with AIDS was still evolving, when the available evidence was sparse, hospitals began to lay down restrictions. Saloojee explained how the need to limit care generated action-rules and remarkably little dispute.

> There wasn't a lot of debate on this issue, because people really didn't know how to deal with this. We had no precedent. We had a few cases of severe cancer but never on this scale. Nobody knew whether you should treat AIDS-related disorders twice, thrice, four times; where you draw the line. It was clearly perplexing to all of us not to know what we were doing. Where you draw the line wasn't a discussion going on in developed countries. So, when solutions were offered, for example, by our intensive care units, they said that the prognosis of kids admitted to the ICU was very poor and that 90 plus per cent died. We accepted that information very quickly, along with the argument that kids with HIV should not get ICU care. There wasn't intense arguments and fights. It was, okay, so that's the prognosis, alright, fine. Anecdote and experiential evidence quickly became translated into informal policy at the hospital level.

In 2003, Gary Maartens, an infectious disease physician, long dedicated to providing treatment to those with HIV, expressed his support for rule-bound rationing. He defended the explicit decision of the Groote Schuur Hospital in Cape Town to bar AIDS patients from its ICU.

> Our intensive care unit has now made an explicit policy that they will not admit HIV positive people with *Pneumocystis* pneumonia into the ICU. I think that's not unreasonable, given that they have very limited facilities. The ICU doctors had looked at the mortality rates of the other diseases they admit to ICU; they are around 20 per cent. They'd looked at their own *Pneumocystis* experience, and it's around 60 per cent. That's not a good use of resources. So they have decided to exclude that group of patients, and I don't have a problem with that as long as it's explicit. I quite like that very recent trend in rationing that we have now.

For Maartens, it was important to distinguish between the imposition of such limits and discriminatory practices that were injurious and unfair to people with HIV. While he had succeeded in crafting practices for his hospital that assured them access to surgical services that in other institutions might have been barred to them, he was compelled to acknowledge that concerns about resources were not equitably applied.

> AIDS, it's not like other diseases. This hospital does cardiac, liver, renal, bone marrow transplants. We use almost all the drugs that you would in the United States to prevent rejection. We do dialysis. So, expensive therapies are available here, but not for HIV. So there's that injustice; that is very hard.

It was precisely the extent to which the careful husbanding of resources could serve as a pretext for prejudicial acts that was so disturbing. In language that recalled the experience of doctors who had treated AIDS in gay men a decade earlier, pediatrician Dalu Ndiweni spoke with despair about the motives of his colleagues at Johannesburg Hospital, as they made decisions involving matters of life and death.

> There is an antibiotic or drug usage committee that sits, and you say, "Look, this is a child who has got AIDS, and I would like to use some of the antibiotics that we use for severe infections." Because you could not claim that next week the patient would not be back with the same infection, it felt like you were pouring money down the drain. Our budgets are not limitless. So because of that, discrimination against the patient with HIV started; you could not use this drug because you're HIV positive, because there's no hope. But you will find no one writes in black and white that you cannot give antibiotics.

Of those who could so swiftly deny access to medications that could save a child's life, he said, "You are trying to make yourself God. You have decided this one is going to die."

As the number of AIDS patients multiplied and as the deepening experience of clinicians began to permit nuanced determinations about the prospects of those infected with HIV, even those who were, in principle, committed to rationing became increasingly troubled. It became clear to them that decisions could be made in utter disregard for prognosis. In 2003, Ashraf Coovadia, a pediatrician in Johannesburg, whose interest in palliative care would make him sensitive to the need for protocols governing decisions to withdraw treatment, was highly critical of the implicit rules governing intensive care in his province.

> A child comes in very severely distressed; if it's HIV positive, that child won't go to an ICU. That is a rule right across at least Gauteng Province, and I think most provinces. That is a difficult one for us to deal with, because we argue that HIV shouldn't be looked upon as a uniform diagnosis, with everyone having the same degree of illness. For those children at death's door, it's defensible for them not to end up in the ICU unit because of the futility of the treatment. The child who has just become infected may be very healthy. But the ICU's policies throughout the country are to exempt them from care, just as it is a rule that no newborn under a kilogram will get ventilated. It is an arbitrary decision. It's an unwritten law, but it's followed by all the hospitals.

As a mother and doctor, Kogie Naidoo, who worked in Durban, felt demoralized as she confronted the intransigence of those who managed the ICU at King Edward VIII Hospital.

> You work so hard to get to a point, and then all of a sudden you are just dropping this case because there is nothing you can do. And yet, it may be a precious baby. It may be a child after eight years of infertility. It may be the third child and the other two have succumbed to HIV, and you want to keep this baby alive longer for a mother whose arms are empty. So you feel hopeless; you feel helpless. You just basically want to tell the parents and run away so you don't have to deal with it.

LIMITED ACCESS: RESEARCH AND RATIONING

Even before the South African government began its ideological campaign against antiretroviral drugs, clinicians in the public sector, who wanted to give their patients some opportunity to benefit from treatments available to AIDS patients in wealthy nations, sought to broaden the prospects of access through drug trials and other research undertakings. For pharmaceutical firms, in turn, South Africa provided an ideal setting. As Gary Maartens at Groote Schuur Hospital observed:

> We had tons and tons of patients who had never smelt antiretrovirals, so that we could get the numbers up very fast. We are a cheap place to do research. Clinicians are cheap here. Nurses are cheap here. Lab investigations are cheap here. Such trials benefited both patients and doctors. On the plus side, they enabled us to use the drugs on public sector patients; we treated several hundred. It was great for our patients to have the disease turned around instead of going downhill all the time.

Maartens also noted that money paid by pharmaceutical firms helped to fund his other research operations. Characterizing the situation, he said it was, "Win–win. Everybody was happy."

Trial participants were at the same time treated patients. As researchers, physicians could, at last, become effective clinicians. Robin Wood, working at Cape Town's Somerset Hospital, which had pioneered AIDS treatment of gay men in the 1980s, was among the first to take this route:

> It was only in 1995 and 1996 when we started performing clinical trials and the reason for that was that we recognized that this was a way of getting access to therapy in a medical system that wouldn't pay for monitoring or for drugs.

It was based on that work for which Wood and his colleagues realized that extending their efforts would necessitate going beyond hospital-based drug trials. Community based efforts—dubbed "operational research"—would permit them to gain experience in the provision of care to larger numbers without openly contravening the government antipathy to ART. By 2004 he had been able to offer treatment to 600 patients.

For Tammy Meyers at Baragwanath, it had been the experience of seeing the vitality of treated children with AIDS at New York's Harlem Hospital that had driven her to enter the world of international clinical trials.

> Why should these kids have access to this treatment that can save their lives and we see at home kids that just die? If we had clinical trials, we would be able to at least offer it to some kids. I thought that was the way to go. It was just not possible to provide antiretroviral treatment to people cared for in the public service who are mostly indigent. In 2000, the U.S.-based Pediatric AIDS Clinical Trial Group started putting out applications. We put in an application and actually got awarded the grant, and that gave us extra funding.

She then teamed up with Harlem pediatricians for a successful application to the U.S. National Institutes of Health. Hers was a small trial involving only 30 children.

For doctors working in the public sector, who had read and heard about what antiretroviral treatment could do but who had no first-hand experience of just how dramatic a clinical impact these drugs could have, the first patients brought into a trial could provide memorable moments. It was in 2003 that Tony Moll, whose rural hospital had provided a model of AIDS care with everything but antiretrovirals, started his first participants in a project jointly undertaken with veteran American AIDS clinician, Gerald Friedland, of Yale University.

> We had a small group of five patients that we started together. Three of them had very low CD4 counts, under 50. I knew that two of them would not survive another few months without antiretroviral therapy. One girl had a CD4 count of 10; she was the mother of a little child at home. She actually had Kaposi's sarcoma already in her mouth and some other places on her body. The other lady was a mother of two young boys, already school-going; her CD4 count was 38, and she was thin and wasted. We took photographs that day when they started their medication.
>
> Two weeks later they came back, and, boy, they had moans and groans. It was vomiting. It was diarrhea. It was this and that. And we sat around in a group. Everybody shared what they were feeling, what they were experiencing. We encouraged them. For us it was kind of embarking on something new for the patients. From their side it was embarking on something new. It was kind of bad, hearing all the problems and having to reassure them, not being quite sure, you see! At the end of two months, they had more or less stabilized, and it was in the third month that they all took an amazing leap forward. One guy gained six kilograms; the others gained two, three and four. That was the very first time that with our own eyes, under our own hands, with our own experience, we saw the turn-around take place. Two patients were brought back from the very brink of death.

But whatever they could mean for patients who were selected for trials that guaranteed access to antiretroviral treatment, such efforts, by definition, had to exclude many more than could be offered medication. And thus rationing potentially life-saving care characterized the world of trials as it did the world of clinical care more generally. With numbers limited, doctors and the nurses who worked at their side had to engage in a process of selection. For some it felt like "playing God."

Given the significance of these decisions, Tammy Meyers was "not proud" as she thought back on the approach she had used to choose the children for her first trial.

> We had files of the children who attended our clinic and their telephone numbers. It was probably in alphabetical order. We phoned, and whoever we got on the other end of the line was chosen. If they didn't have a phone, we couldn't get hold of them. Sometimes we did try and send messages off, but it was a rapid enrollment.

Research projects also typically entailed a series of stringent selection criteria. In the township of Guguletu outside of Cape Town, an operational research program was established to circumvent government restrictions on the provision of antiretrovirals in public clinics. A team of health workers weighed a complex set of selection guidelines before doing what Linda-Gail Bekker called "the Solomon thing." In 2003, the 41-year-old Zimbabwean-born doctor explained that, to be chosen, patients had to live within the district, had to have attended the HIV clinic for six months regularly and regularly come to its meetings. In addition, breaking the isolation imposed by the stigma attached to AIDS, candidates for treatment had to have revealed the fact that they were infected to at least one other person in the community. They also had to agree to have a counselor, who would monitor their adherence to treatment. Finally, patients had to be physically able to come to the clinic on their own. This last requirement was not simply a matter of practicality, but was also a way of excluding those who were too debilitated. Some patients, said Bekker, were just too ill to benefit. Efforts on their behalf would distract attention from individuals who might be saved. But there was a second reason for such limitations, one that was intimately connected to the precarious political context within which her clinic operated. Relentless hostility to antiretroviral treatment by the government, and the confusion such hostility sowed among ordinary men and women, imposed obligations involving institutional survival. "We had to make sure that they were not too sick. Too sick patients have a very high mortality, and that is tough on the program. It feeds the propaganda that drugs are toxic."

Like so many others involved in difficult rationing choices, Bekker believed that it was important that clear rules of selection guide the process. Such rules could prevent favoritism from intruding upon selections that were, she understood, to be matters of life and death. Nevertheless she was compelled to acknowledge that the force of an individual personality, of all-too-human emotion, could break through the constraints erected against such impulses.

> I had a young woman who had quite severe pulmonary hypertension. She was quite breathless, and the question was, Is this the reason to give her drug to somebody else who will live longer, because she has another illness which might kill her before the HIV does? So we had agreed on every other front; she was treatment ready; she was psychologically sound; she filled all the other criteria. But what about her physical state? And she must have gotten wind that she was hanging in the balance. As I walked into the clinic, she did some star jumps and jumped up and down and moved her arms, and she said, "See, I am fine; I am absolutely fine." There was just no way that I could actually say she mustn't get the drug. I mean, there are just times when somebody's needs and psychology, and the fact that they are human beings, just overwhelms every sense of better judgment. I didn't even examine her. I walked straight out and said she has to go into treatment. I can't refuse.

Ironically, clinical trials that had the potential to provide access to treatment to those who would otherwise find medication beyond reach could, at times, serve to underline the social inequalities that so defined treatment opportunity in South Africa. In Pietermaritzburg, Caroline Armstrong described a drug trial at Grey's Hospital that was only open to patients who had failed on a first-line regiment, which they had been able to pay for. Addressing the equity concerns opposed by this situation, she said, in a matter-of-fact manner, "That's right. It's all down to the money."

ROLLING OUT ART: THE PERSISTENCE OF RATIONING

In the mid-1990s ART were inaccessible to any but the most privileged in South Africa because of the price of drugs. At decade's end, as the price of drugs began to fall, the limits on access increasingly reflected government policy—a mix of concerns about capacity and almost inexplicable ideological opposition to antiretrovirals. Scarcity was thus a consequence of political choice. But rationing did not come to an end when the government announced in 2003 that it would begin a rollout of ART (Government of South Africa 2003b). When at last the list of clinics where treatment would begin was announced by the government, there were winners and losers. But, even in those settings selected to be among the first to provide antiretroviral treatment, rationing persisted. Clinical and human capacity imposed the need to limit care.

Having been accredited to provide antiretrovirals in February 2004, Tony Moll's Church of Scotland Hospital was among the very first in KwaZulu-Natal to begin the provision of medication under the rollout.

> We were very excited, and immediately things started changing. We started putting things into place to be able to give antiretrovirals on a much wider scale. We prepared a group of 9 patients very quickly, getting the CD4 counts ready and meeting entrance criteria. March 24, 2004, we announced, was going to be the day that we would actually give out antiretroviral therapy.

Once the program began, Moll and his colleagues, sensing renewed possibilities and deep urgency, surged ahead. In nine months, he, his small nursing staff, and two counselors brought 360 patients into treatment.

> After those nine, things moved very fast. The government told us, "Don't worry. Whatever you order in terms of medication we will be able to supply you." So it wasn't the medication that was a problem, and it wasn't the laboratory facilities; they were ready to receive as many CD4s as we sent them. What was particularly burdensome was that we were one of only four hospitals chosen in the province. So we had people coming from really far, hearing announcements on the radio that these are the four hospitals that are on board. The clientele built up quite a lot. Very close hospitals were starting to send buses full of patients on a weekly basis to us.
>
> What very soon became our ceiling was our own hands and our own small group of staff members. And they were incredible. On the days they were on duty, they were prepared to work through the night. But for me it was different, because I'm on duty every day. I had this conflict in myself that, if I worked a little harder, I could help a couple more people, and if I worked on a Saturday morning I could help even more people. In the end, I could see that I was just becoming chronically tired, and I wasn't doing my work properly. I was taking short cuts where I shouldn't be taking short cuts. I spoke to people and said, "You know, we could do so many more people, but we're short of staff." And even the provincial people said, "Well, Tony, then what you must do is do what you can do." That helped me to see that it was more important to have a service that was running well and run properly, where the wheel wasn't going to come off. So we just said, "OK, we'll work extra hours, but we'll stop at that time."

Serving as an additional restraint on Moll's efforts, as well as in other hospitals, was the discovery that placing large numbers of patients on ART could have unanticipated, but, in retrospect, predictable consequences for those responsible for managing the hospital's wards.

> What started happening was one or two patients came in with side effects and needed to be admitted to hospital. And these junior doctors were in charge of the wards, and they found themselves responsible for somebody who was on ART, and they themselves weren't confident in managing this. Quite correctly they came back to me and said, "Now, put the brakes on." What we did was, we brought them up to date, and they felt, "Okay, now we know when to admit; this is when to stop treatment." So we had actually run ahead of ourselves a little bit.

It was months after the adult service began to provide antiretroviral treatment that the department of pediatrics was given approval to provide drugs to children. Like his colleague Tony Moll, François Eksteen, who had, for so long, watched his patients suffer and die, approached this opportunity with zeal. Time, Eksteen knew, was not his ally, and waiting lists for very sick children were morally unacceptable to him.

> Waiting lists can go on into two months or even longer. I just feel it's a potentially fatal disease, a disease that potentially can cause severe suffering. I've got some children whose CD4s are very low, and I just feel one cannot wait with that. So I just personally feel that we must start as soon as possible.

Early on, Moll discovered how single-minded his colleague could be.

> One evening I came into his clinic, and I found the lights still on and the staff still there and François was working. And the whole waiting room was full of children with their mothers waiting. It was after 8:00 at night! It was dark outside; the public transport would have

> stopped by then. So I said, "You know, you're not going to finish. You're going to be working till 2:00 tonight if you really see everybody that's in the waiting room. Those patients who are on therapy or who are here for follow-up, finish them tonight. And those who are new patients, let them sleep over, and we will sort them out in the morning." François is right now feeling that exhilaration that I felt with the rollout, that now suddenly the children are coming in big numbers, and he is facing his own limitations in helping them.

In Pietermaritzburg, Belgium-born Paul Kocheleff had also waited—sometimes buoyed by hope, on other occasions despairing—for the moment that he could provide his patients at Grey's Hospital with antiretrovirals. Four months after Tony Moll had begun, Kocheleff believed that he done everything to make his start-up smooth, but things turned out very differently. His clinic would be dogged by the same dearth of professional staff that other locales would experience, and his ambitious plans to treat the 900 patients who qualified for ART would be thwarted by the mundane limits of a public hospital.

> Our idea was that probably we can start with ten patients a day, working five days a week. That means 50 patients per week, 200 per month. We expected that in four months, five months, everybody would be on treatment. And then we had the meeting with the pharmacy, and they had a totally different opinion about the program. They wanted to have five patients per week! That means it will take years to reach 900! And the discussion was a bit hard, but finally we agreed that maybe we can try and see what happens. So we had to slow down a little bit. But after a few weeks, we were able to increase the number of patients starting. At the moment, it's between 100 and 150 per month, so it's not far from what we wanted at the start.

By January 2005, he had enrolled 700 patients.

Even when faced with less than enthusiastic hospital administrators, those who believed that they had no alternative but to overcome obstacles were able to achieve remarkable feats. At Baragwanath Hospital, Alan Karstaedt, who oversaw the adult HIV clinic, had been able to put 1,500 patients on treatment in the six months since April 2004.

> It's been really rough, with very long hours. Sometimes, the clinics have finished at 7:30 at night. We've got more doctors now, but we've had at various times only three or four. We just committed ourselves to getting as many people on treatment as quickly as possible. We've had to cut corners.

Karstaedt had great pride in the fact that, over the years, he had been able to spend time speaking with his patients, resisting the pressure to "just turn them into faceless ciphers." But he had to acknowledge that his commitment to providing ART now compelled him to make compromises.

> Basically you're trading off, getting more people onto treatment and more people hopefully surviving longer and living independent, quality lives versus that other form of clinical interaction and satisfaction. But given the number of patients who are going to need to be put on treatment, I think this will become the model, whether it's ideal or not.

As they attempted to address the limits placed on them by the public health system's capacity, providers came to realize that the drugs which had been at the center of the bitter battle between treatment activists and the government of Thabo Mbeki no longer represented the most critical problem they faced in the massive effort to extend treatment to hundreds of thousands of patients. Rather, it was now necessary to move swiftly beyond doctor—and hospital—centered clinics in a way that did not compromise the essentials of antiretroviral treatment. Whatever role doctors would play in the future would, of necessity, be dwarfed by nurses and counselors.

Many came to believe that, once patients were stabilized, they would have to be placed in the charge of a nurse-run system, not unlike what already existed in the nation's TB program or the model developed by the huge South Africa mining conglomerate, AngloAmerican. Bernhard Gaede, working at the small ex-missionary Emaus Hospital in rural KwaZulu-Natal, was not sure that that solution would be so easy to implement. He worried that the burden, once shifted to nurses, would itself be more than the system could bear. It was not that nurses were incapable of doing the clinical work, if guided by treatment protocols. Rather, the number of available nurses would be the limiting factor. "There are not endless nurses. While it's easy to say that doctors are not coping—the nurses need to do it—who will the nurses offload to? They are at the moment our safety net, but that net is also at a breaking point."

When, in November 2003, the government had made public its antiretroviral treatment plan, it expected that almost 200,000 patients would be receiving ART by 2005. In fact, in January of that year, about 30,000 were receiving medication in the public sector. The initial plan, which embraced equity as a guiding principle, had nevertheless made clear that because of very different levels of epidemic severity and infrastructural capacity, the numbers to be brought into care would vary widely by province. In the rural Eastern Cape province, it was expected that approximately 18,000 would be in treatment by 2005, while in neighboring KwaZulu-Natal, the number would be 75,000. In Guateng, where Johannesburg is located, 45,000 would be in treatment. In the very poor provinces of Mpumalanga and Limpopo, 11,000 and 22,000, respectively, were to have been in care. But, in each instance, the numbers in treatment fell far short in practice. With 10,000 people in treatment in Guateng, the shortfall was 80 percent; in KwaZulu-Natal, only about 15 percent of the projected goal was achieved. The story was even worse in the very poorest of provinces, where between 1 and 2 percent of the target had been met. A year later, in January 2006, there had been significant improvements but the shortfall remained striking. The number of patients receiving ART in the public sector had risen to just more than 257,000 in early 2007, just more than a third of what had been promised (Hassan 2007).

In no small part the impediments were bureaucratic. Commenting on the torpid pace of the rollout, Ashraf Grimwood—who had been a public health officer in Cape Town early in his career, had gone on to private practice, and had served on the committee that prepared the rollout planned—could only express dismay over a process that had squandered the hopes of August 2003.

> The workup to the plan, getting it all done, was so amazing. We just thought it was too good to be true. You felt that we were on the brink of a major, major revolution in this country in the sense of taking the bull by the horns and saying, "Let's do it." Now you end up in bureaucratic nonsense. "We can't do that. The pharmacy's not the right size. We don't have enough fridges. We don't have enough space." This is bullshit; there are people dying out there.

Mark Heywood, a leader of the AIDS activist group Treatment Action Campaign (TAC), said in 2005:

> We still have provinces where almost nobody is on treatment. Mpumulanga Province has less than 200 people on treatment, as far as we know. Northwest Province has islands of treatment. Limpopo Province has less than 200 people on treatment—this despite the fact that in Limpopo there are health facilities with absolute capacity to run this program. One such place is Tintswalo, which is actually linked to Witwatersrand University in Johannesburg, that to this day has not been accredited to run a treatment program, so the doctors have to illicitly treat people. TAC supplies drugs now to Tintswalo, so that they can treat a limited number of people. But it's ridiculous that we have to be doing it underhandedly.

Faced with formidable institutional, material, and political constraints and a dramatically overflowing reservoir of patients requiring antiretroviral drugs, medical staff in clinics providing ART had to confront a series of morally and clinically compelling questions. These were not unlike those they had encountered earlier in the epidemic. In a resource-poor milieu, who should be treated? How should they be selected? Who should be made to wait?

Even at a quasi-private hospital like Durban's McCord (initially excluded from the government's roll out), with a large well-established treatment program, the issues had to be addressed. Said Helga Holst, its medical superintendent:

> There's some healthy tension between how best do you use the resources given to you. Do you get better results by starting patients on treatment that are well and have CD4 counts above a certain level? Then the equity issue and the justice issue come closer to the surface. Why should somebody who didn't have the opportunity to be on treatment earlier and now is very sick be refused the opportunity, granted the risk of success is less?

A few argued that a commitment to treating the greatest number demanded that the sickest, or those with the weakest immune systems, make way for patients more likely to profit from ART. In Pietermaritzburg, Paul Nijs, a Belgian ex-patriot whose initial commitment to practicing medicine in poorer countries included his willingness to accept medical limits, adopted such a stance.

> I think the first aim of an ART program is to diminish the burden of the AIDS catastrophe on the public health care system. So that means, in my opinion, that it is more fruitful and also easier to put healthy people on ART treatment than to try to put people on such treatment who already have full-blown AIDS. I'm not saying that I will refuse to put a patient who has major problems on treatment, but I sometimes say it is too late.
>
> It may sound cruel, but you must realize that if you put a very sick patient on treatment, you really have to follow him up very intensively. He will run into problems; he will develop diarrhea, vomiting, and cannot take the drugs. If you look at the time you spend with that patient, that time you could easily put, I would say, eight to ten healthy patients on treatment. So what is the choice? Here in KwaZulu-Natal, we're talking about half a million patients who we have to reach eventually. As one of my colleagues said, "You should concentrate on fruit that you can easily pick."

Others, taking a path that had been first pursued when antiretrovirals were available only in small research projects, screened out the sickest because they felt an overwhelming need to show the skeptical or dispirited in South Africa that antiretrovirals could make a difference. In her pediatric HIV clinic at King Edward VIII that treated only a fraction of those who could benefit, Raziya Bobat revealed:

> I must admit that one of our exclusion criteria for the early part of the rollout is patients who have got very severe complications like cardiomyopathy and very severe encephalopathy or any other organ failure. This is simply because we want to raise everybody's morale; you treat the child and the child starts improving, and everybody can see that they're getting better. In Malawi, they were treating the very moribund patients with ART, and they were having this very high mortality rate. And that created a problem, because people were saying, "Well, you see? The drugs are toxic and they don't work, and the patients are dying."

In contrast, at Baragwanath Hospital, pediatrician Tammy Meyers, who like Bobat treated children, was guided by a professional and moral compass that required giving priority to the sickest. The rest would follow. "We started identifying who we thought were the sicker patients who we could start immediately, as treatment became available on April 1, 2004. We identified ten children who were ready, with their low CD4s and very sick, to start treatment on that day."

Her colleague, Alan Karstaedt, also adopted a policy of moving the sickest of his adult patients to the head of the line.

> It was a fairly rough way of doing it, but if people looked reasonably well and their CD4s were in the mid to high hundreds, they were booked on a routine list. If they had a low CD4 or looked ill, then they were seen within a week or so, or at the next available clinic. You could put someone on ART within a week or two from the time they were first referred.

But for most clinicians, with patients' lives at stake, the need to ration ART and a commitment to a basic principle of equity led to a decision to treat on a first-come, first-served basis. In Kimberly, Eula Mothibi, despite external constraints imposed by inadequate provincial support, struggled to develop what was for her a just access policy.

> I get called by the assessment sites. "This person's CD4 is less than 10. This person is sick." But generally, I'm not encouraging jumping the queue, because most people come late. So I think it's unfair to those who present with a CD4 of 190; now they have to give way, lose their position in the queue. They have to give way to someone who comes in very late with a low CD4.

Like Mothibi, other clinicians often adopted a policy that appeared to obviate the need to choose. In Cape Town, Ashraf Grimwood, who directed a network of clinics jointly funded by a British charity, ARK, and the provincial government, refused to choose which patients should first receive life-sustaining drugs.

> The thing is, we're not God. We're not making those judgment calls. People who show that they'll go through the preliminary steps, the counseling, that they understand the issues—I'm going to give you a fair chance, mate, regardless of what your CD4 is, if it's 2 or 5. We've had people with CD4 counts of 2, under 2, under 1, pull back, get better and go for it. So we can't make that judgment call. Give everybody a fair chance. If they're going to die, they're going to die in six weeks, so what are you going to lose? Probably it's about a hundred dollars.

In Durban, Yunus Moosa, the head of infectious disease at King Edward VIII Hospital, had first advocated in favor of "patients that are best salvageable, so we can prove to the people out here that ART works," but the politics of such a standard made it an unacceptable strategy.

> The question had been, if a patient walked in with a CD4 count of 5, should we give him priority over the patient who walks in with a CD4 count of 150? We felt it would become a bit of a political hot potato. How do we decide who is sick enough or too well for immediate medication? So we decided on a blanket rule: whoever walks in first and is eligible for treatment gets into the program.

But fairness exacted a toll. It was difficult for clinicians, especially those in the trenches who encountered very sick and dying patients, to abide by the rule of "first come, first served." Eula Mothibi confessed, "I think it's a little bit unfair, but on occasion I do push a person in with a low CD4 count. I bring them in on a Tuesday, when I run a clinic for pregnant mothers." At McCord Hospital, Henry Sunpath, who had been drawn to HIV care because the emergency room in which he had worked in the 1990s had refused to hear the pleas of AIDS patients, recognized a similar moment now. "We have people coming here to us with their relatives, young sons and daughters, parents, and they say, 'Please do something.'" It was the same plea that had moved him years earlier—when he had seen the crowds of untreated patients at another hospital—that struck him so forcefully in 2005. He continued, "As a clinician, you're faced with the patient, and you want to do something for that patient, no matter how sick that patient is."

McCord developed a hybrid system of access, one that adhered to the principle of first come, first served, but which acknowledged the moral claims of the sickest as well. Jane Hampton described the policy that evolved in 2004.

> It's been a big change in the last year. There are always a whole lot more people that need treatment than can be treated, and so there are still people that have to wait; but now it's waiting, it's not, "Sorry, you can't afford it so you can't have it." It's not money that's the thing that's keeping people from treatment, it's waiting lists; it's the fact that you can only cope with so many people in a particular month. When the funding first came through, we thought people who are critically ill and can't wait, maybe we should try and see them first; and it turned out to be an absolute nightmare. You had to have very clear guidelines of who you should fast-track and who you shouldn't. At the moment, we've got a very limited fast-track, people that have actually been admitted to hospital and are on the wards, so they're already under care and already have been seen and worked up. One day out of the five we have a clinic for them so they don't have to wait at the end of the queue. But for everyone else there's just a queue system, first come, first served.

Whether they faced the dilemmas of

rationing directly or adopted rules that restricted their choices, the doctors we interviewed were painfully aware of the extent to which in the earliest stages of the rollout, with a large reservoir of patients waiting for ART, there would be winners and losers. Only as treatment began to meet local need—as scarcity began to vanish—did the need to ration fade.

The story was far different in those locales not yet selected to provide treatment. For clinicians in those settings geography and time had come to determine who among their patients would survive. As their patients died, practitioners would wait impotently, or press more or less aggressively to bring their clinics into the orbit of the rollout. When and if they succeeded, they, like those who came before them, would face the anguish of rationing, an anguish that in some ways was preferable to circumstances in which they could save no one.

ACKNOWLEDGMENTS

Research for this chapter was supported by the American Foundation for AIDS Research, the John M. Lloyd Foundation, the Rockefeller Foundation, and the U.S. National Library of Medicine.

REFERENCES AND FURTHER READING

Bayer, R. and Oppenheimer, G.M. (2000) *AIDS Doctors: Voices from the Epidemic*. New York, NY: Oxford University Press.

Churchill, L.R. (1987) *Rationing Health Care in America*. Notre Dame, IN: Notre Dame University Press.

Daniels, N. (1991) Is the Oregon rationing plan fair? *JAMA* 265: 2232–2235.

Daniels, N. Fair process in patient selection for antiretroviral treatment in WHO's goal of 3 by 5. *Lancet*, May 19, 2005. Published online at www.thelancet.com.

Government of South Africa, Department of Health. (2003a) "The Impact of HIV/AIDS on the Health Sector.

Government of South Africa, Department of Health. (2003b) *Operational Plan for Comprehensive HIV and AIDS Care, Management and Treatment for South Africa*. November 19.

Hassan, F. (2007) Personal communication, AIDS Law Project Monitoring Unit, May 30.

Oppenheimer, G.M. and Bayer, R. (2007) *Shattered Dreams? An Oral History of the South African AIDS Epidemic*. New York, NY: Oxford University Press.

Van Resnburg, H.C.J. (ed.) (2004) *Health and Health Care in South Africa*. Pretoria: Van Schaik Publishers.

CHAPTER 21

Understanding the Making of National HIV/AIDS Policies

The Critical Role of Health Care Institutions in the U.S. and U.K.

Tasleem J. Padamsee

ABSTRACT

This chapter discusses the critical role of national health care institutions in shaping national policy responses to the HIV/AIDS epidemic. Both the social problems HIV/AIDS creates and their potential solutions are influenced by the capacities, mechanisms, and constraints already embedded in a country's health care system. This research explores the formative influence of national health care institutions by comparing treatment-related policies in the United States and the United Kingdom, which have notably different health care systems. In both initial and ongoing phases of the response, domestic health care structures have contextualized policymaking; shaped it directly; and influenced it indirectly through interactions with other causal factors.

The story of HIV/AIDS is not merely about the spread of a deadly virus; it is about the interaction of that virus with the complexities of human life. In order to fully understand that story, we must examine the ongoing interplay between disease agents, individual behaviors, social norms, organizational action, and government choices made at local, national, and supra-national levels. Government responses to the disease are a sometimes overlooked piece of this puzzle, but they are critical to every aspect of the disease, from rates of infection to the availability of drug treatments and the quality of life of individuals living with HIV/AIDS.

As national governments have grappled with the many medical and social challenges posed by HIV/AIDS, their responses have varied dramatically in terms of both timing and content. This variation is the result of several factors which mutually determine the policies countries adopt in response to HIV/AIDS. This chapter demonstrates the critical role of one such factor: national health care institutions. The shape of national health care systems profoundly influences that country's capacity to respond to the disease. Both the social problems HIV/AIDS creates and the solutions available to be pursued are shaped by the capacities, mechanisms, and constraints already embedded in the state and the health care system.

This chapter explores the formative influence of national health care institutions on HIV/AIDS policies through a comparison of the treatment-related policy choices made by the United States and the United Kingdom since the start of the epidemic. Beginning with a brief overview of the different health care systems in these countries, the chapter then analyzes the causal dynamics that produced each nation's initial response to the treatment challenges raised by HIV/AIDS, and finally explores some of the policy choices that have been made as the epidemic continued through the 1990s and beyond. In both initial and ongoing phases of the response, domestic health care structures contextualized policymaking, shaped it directly, and influenced it indirectly through interactions with other causal factors.

OPPOSITE ENDS OF THE SPECTRUM: AMERICAN AND BRITISH HEALTH CARE SYSTEMS

The United States and the United Kingdom have the most divergent health care systems of all industrialized countries. Public health scholars position the U.S. at the market-maximized extreme of a continuum of national health systems. Here, health care is seen as a good like other goods, resources are allocated by market prices, and private and voluntary health insurance dominates. The market-minimized end of the continuum is epitomized by the U.K, where health care is understood to be distinctive in many ways, and everyone is entitled to reasonable access to care regardless of ability to pay (Anderson 1972, 1989; Field 1980; Hsiao 1992).

The market-oriented approach to health care in the U.S. results in an administratively complex system wherein both insurance and services are provided through a patchwork of mechanisms that together cover most, but by no means all, of the population. Over 60 percent of citizens have private insurance paid for primarily by their employer or the employer of a family member; a small number also purchase private insurance on their own. About a third of citizens are covered by one or more programs within the fragmented public sector. These include Medicare, which insures about 20 percent of the population and is the largest single payer in the system (Graig 1999); Medicaid, which utilizes a combination of federal and state financing to insure certain low-income people; and several smaller government programs. For the more than 40 million uninsured Americans, health care is scarce—paid for out of pocket, through public free clinics, or through charity or uncompensated care. Treatment of HIV/AIDS involves all parts of this tripartite insurance structure: over half of HIV/AIDS care is paid for by public insurance funds; many patients maintain their private insurance for at least some years of their illness; and the large proportion of PLWHAs (People Living with HIV/AIDS) with no insurance at all constitute a significant system strain that has been at the core of treatment-related policymaking.

In contrast, the U.K. treats medical care as a right, mandating not only coverage that is universal and comprehensive, but also health care provided directly through the state apparatus of the National Health Service (NHS). Vastly cheaper and administratively simpler than the U.S. approach, the British system is predicated on four basic principles: health services are universal, comprehensive, free to the patient at the point of service, and financed by general tax revenues. The budgetary process is a top-down one, with overall limits on spending set by the central government but significant control over resource allocation for local authorities and practitioners. Since the British system is universal and comprehensive, all PLWHAs have had access to care since the start of the epidemic. The smaller private health care sector, which provides services not readily available through the NHS to patients who carry supplementary insurance or pay out of pocket, is irrelevant to HIV/AIDS care. All the HIV-related expertise exists within the NHS, so British PLWHAs have had no incentive to turn to private providers and even visiting foreigners receive their treatment from NHS employees (Padamsee 2007).

EARLY BRITISH TREATMENT POLICY: RING-FENCED HIV/AIDS TREATMENT ALLOCATIONS

Treating AIDS patients has always been an expensive proposition. In the early years of the epidemic, medical care mostly revolved around fighting off opportunistic infections and acute pain in critical care episodes that recurred from the onset of AIDS until death. Because the disease first emerged among young gay men, local NHS hospitals quickly found themselves incurring huge costs to care for an ordinarily healthy population that usually drew little on health system resources. These costs were heavily concentrated within a small number of London hospitals, both because most cases were localized in these areas and because members of the gay community shared information about where to go to be treated by clinicians with the most AIDS-related experience. While most of the country was barely becoming aware of the new disease, several London hospitals were facing financial crisis: AIDS-related expenditures were draining budgets and causing deficits, jeopardizing the financial stability of local health care structures.

This financing problem was one of the first to be addressed by the policymaking circle that formed within the Department of Health and Social Services (DHSS) to deal with AIDS in the early 1980s. Awareness of the problem among the gay activists and community physicians in this circle meant that it soon became a priority. In 1985, Chief Medical Officer Donald Acheson brought the problem to Secretary of Health Norman Fowler, who wielded the power within the Thatcher government to commit extra funds for health-related issues. Fowler was persuaded that the issue must be addressed, and additional funds were allocated to the hardest-hit localities specifically to cope with AIDS (Berridge 1996; Greenaway, Smith, and Street 1992; Schramm-Evans 1990; Weeks, Taylor-Laybourn, and Aggleton 1994).

Within the next year, this quiet and low-key departmental approach to AIDS would change. During the first years of the epidemic, Conservative leaders in the Thatcher government had been profoundly uncomfortable dealing with an issue intimately related to homosexual sex and illicit drug use, and most had avoided grappling with AIDS altogether. During 1985 and 1986, however, intense media attention came to focus on infections among transfusion recipients and intravenous drug users, illustrating the spread of the disease outside the gay community. As a result, both politicians and the public began to fear that AIDS could soon affect Britons from all walks of life (Berridge 1996, 1998; Bayer and Feldman 1999; Marmor, Dillon, and Scher 1999; Schramm-Evans 1990; Weeks 1989). This discourse of generalized risk played out in the context of another prominent British discourse: that the national government has a responsibility to provide for the public health of the population. Government leaders were now compelled to act—if AIDS was a major risk for Britons in general, then they would be shirking their responsibilities unless they took a proactive role in coping with the threat.

The result of this dramatic shift in the perceptions of the disease was a late 1986 watershed in the British politics of HIV/AIDS. Still uneasy about dealing directly with sex and drugs issues, the Thatcher government decided to treat AIDS as a public health emergency—taking it upon itself to create a sense of political priority and allocate generous resources to the problem, but leaving the professional experts in the DHSS to design and implement specific interventions to deal with it (Berridge 1996; Fox, Day, and Klein 1989). Among these interventions was a dramatic expansion of the ring-fenced funding allocations.[1] In a highly publicized move, AIDS-specific allocations were made to *every* regional health authority beginning in 1987, including those that did not yet have an appreciable caseload.

The distribution of ring-fenced funds to every local health authority had an immediate and lasting impact on the treatment of PLWHAs in Britain. Clinics all over the country developed specialized services to care for HIV/AIDS patients; hard-hit regions also developed state-of-the-art treatment centers and consolidated expertise, while less affected regions raised awareness and provided prevention services.[2] By 1991, the National Audit Office reported that:

> Ring fencing is considered by health authorities to have been crucial in enabling services to respond to the HIV epidemic, especially in London (National Audit Office 1991: 17).

Ring-fenced allocations to each local health authority would remain the core of Britain's approach to guaranteeing high-quality medical services for PLWHAs well into the 1990s. As it slowly became clear that the size of the British epidemic would be smaller than initially feared, the quantity of funds and degree of political attention devoted to these allocations decreased, but the mechanism itself was retained through 2001 (Padamsee 2007).

The process of allocating ring-fenced funds to local health authorities illustrates the importance of existing health care structures to the British policymaking process, which relied heavily upon customary mechanisms and lines of communication within established health institutions. Faced with a novel set of challenges and little institutional expertise, DHSS drew physicians who knew the most about AIDS upward through the hierarchical structure of the NHS in order to help public health leaders think strategically about appropriate ways to respond. Because the NHS held centralized responsibility for national health care, conceptualizing the financing problem and initiating its solution were relatively straightforward. The problem was that NHS budgets were inadequate to cover treatment of expensive AIDS cases; a solution would therefore need to be provided by DHSS—the entity at the top of the British hierarchy of health structures. Once the Department secured additional funding, it could easily be distributed downward through the mechanisms that already existed to link local NHS units with the national Department. Later, when the national AIDS discourse shifted toward one of generalized risk, this mechanism of intervention was expanded beyond already hard-hit regions to the whole country. The hierarchical relationships between NHS levels therefore facilitated a relatively straightforward approach both to solving the hospital financing problem and to building HIV/AIDS awareness and services for the entire nation.

EARLY AMERICAN TREATMENT POLICY: LIMITED INSURANCE COVERAGE AND THE RYAN WHITE CARE ACT

The source of the financing issue surrounding AIDS treatment was the same in the United States: affected patients were mostly from groups that did not usually draw much on health care resources, and treatment was itself expensive. The very different context of U.S. health care institutions, however, made the specifics of the problem—and its possible solutions—radically different. Whereas the challenge in Britain was to provide local NHS structures with sufficient funding to provide needed services, the American challenge was to pay for the care of patients who were largely under- or uninsured.

Employment-based private insurance is the ideal and cornerstone of the U.S. system, but it has largely failed for most PLWHAs. During the 1980s, private insurance companies avoided paying for AIDS-related care by dumping patients from their rolls or refusing to cover costs associated with "catastrophic illnesses" (Padamsee 2007; Weiss and Hardy 1990). In addition, most individuals who had private coverage when they first became ill soon lost it as they became sicker and unable to work. As the years went by, HIV became increasingly concentrated in poorer communities, mostly affecting individuals who carried little or no private insurance even before they became infected.

Of the many Americans with HIV who could not rely on private insurance, only the poorest and sickest were eligible for government insurance programs. Throughout most of the 1980s, publicly insured PLWHAs were eligible either due to extreme poverty that pre-existed their illness, or because they "spent down" all their own resources after they got sick. Disability provided another pathway for PLWHAs to obtain insurance: AIDS was considered a disability and Americans who are disabled for two years become eligible for public insurance. Because most patients died within the first two years of developing AIDS, however, disability coverage was largely irrelevant to PLWHAs until activists secured a late 1980s change in federal policy that rendered any individual with a certified AIDS diagnosis *immediately* eligible for Medicaid.

Between the portion of the HIV/AIDS population with private insurance and those who qualified for public programs, there remained a pervasive gap. Traditionally, cost-shifting mechanisms (and charitable donations) were used to finance care for the uninsured. It became clear by 1990, however, that this approach would not work with AIDS in the picture: hospitals could never increase costs to paying patients enough to cover the costs of treating the medically indigent ones. Policy advocates had been pushing for a large-scale response from the federal government since the mid-1980s, and various pieces of AIDS legislation had been proposed and failed in Congress.[3] The socially conservative Bush administration preferred to avoid dealing with the growing crisis altogether, and took a resistant stance on most HIV/AIDS policy issues. Nevertheless, almost a decade into the epidemic, Congress enacted the Ryan White Comprehensive AIDS Resources Emergency (CARE) Act in 1990.

The core reason for the success of this move to take federal responsibility for HIV/AIDS care was, as in the U.K. three years earlier, the emergence of a discourse of risk to the general population. The specific understanding of this risk, however, differed notably between the two countries. American cases outside of the gay community also began to receive major publicity during 1985, occurring in a similar pattern that included intravenous drug users, transfusion recipients, and celebrities like Rock Hudson. In the U.S., however, these reports did not produce a popular perception that the whole nation was at risk. AIDS was scarier now because it seemed to be affecting a proliferating list of groups, but it was still understood as a disease of the marginal; HIV was a risk to social "others," not the national "us." This persistence of a discourse about AIDS as something largely irrelevant to the mainstream meant that legislators continued to feel little obligation to do anything about it.

By 1990, however, political leaders were motivated to take action by a different type of generalized risk: urban hospitals in hard-hit cities were in serious financial crisis. As local HIV and AIDS caseloads grew, hospital financing mechanisms were buckling under the weight of large numbers of uninsured patients accessing expensive services. With no way to recuperate the costs involved in treating them, hospitals were going from over-budget to bankrupt, and many were on the verge of closing (House of Representatives 1989).

With the growing understanding that urban hospitals were in jeopardy came a new discourse about the dangers of AIDS to the population at large. If AIDS patients deluged emergency rooms because they could not afford to get care elsewhere, occupied large numbers of beds in hospitals that cared for the poor, and caused hospitals to close down in these neighborhoods, then it was suddenly a problem for everyone. By jeopardizing the availability and standard of care for people *without* HIV, AIDS became understood as a general problem that should be addressed by the U.S. government.[4] As one of the principal authors of the CARE Act reflects:

> I can still remember the Kennedy people always referring to the *Time* magazine cover of what to do with the overcrowded hospitals and the emergency rooms. So there was a perceived . . . problem for the general community . . .; even people without AIDS are disadvantaged by having the AIDS epidemic fill up emergency rooms (I06: 211).

In addition to the emergence of an American discourse of generalized risk, two other factors contributed to making the CARE Act possible in 1990. First, the late 1980s had witnessed the first real breakthroughs in the availability of medical treatments, so the argument about providing medical care shifted from one focused on palliative and supportive care to a more compelling one about effective treatments that could "save lives."[5,6] Second, gathering the congressional support needed to pass the bill was facilitated by the strategic use of an emerging discourse about the "innocent victims" of AIDS. Policy advocates knew that gaining widespread support for federal action would require disassociating AIDS from gay men and drug users as much as possible. This was achieved in part by naming the act after Ryan White—a widely known Indiana teenager who had contracted HIV during routine treatment for his hemophilia, faced discrimination in his school and neighborhood, and died in 1990.

Once the CARE Act was authorized, it began to support a growing infrastructure of organizations and services for PLWHAs. Cities and states used these funds to pay the direct costs of treating patients, and to provide social support, home care, and case management services. Continuing these programs, however, was dependent on ongoing funding of the legislation by Congress. As a discretionary program, the CARE Act comes up for reauthorization every five years. These junctures have been openings for intense debates about issues including mandatory testing of pregnant women, formulas for distributing funds around the country, and what range of services should be supported with federal resources. Although these controversies have sometimes caused delays, the CARE Act was successfully reauthorized in 1996, 2000, and 2006, and its programs continue to thrive today. In the context of U.S. health care, the CARE Act creates a unique safety net, making PLWHAs one of the only American groups for whom income does not determine access to health care. In the words of a key congressional staffer on AIDS issues:

> Ryan White is a safety net not just under Medicaid, but also a safety net under small group insurance plans, and under people who can't get into the individual market, because it is not strictly means tested . . . [It includes] a lot of people above the poverty line, but . . . not in a large group insurance plan, and not disabled enough to qualify for Medicaid and Medicare (I06: 505).

The history of U.S. HIV/AIDS treatment policy through 1990 demonstrates the formative influence of existing health care structures on policy problems and solutions. The tripartite structure of American health care meant that, while some PLWHAs had the health care coverage they needed through private or public programs, many more found themselves uninsured. This was a problem for PLWHAs, whose quality and length of life depended heavily on health care, but it was also a major issue for the health care system itself. The default mechanism for paying for emergency care of the uninsured failed in the face of expensive HIV/AIDS cases, and the health care infrastructure for entire populations of poor urban neighborhoods was therefore jeopardized. It was this hospital financing crisis that finally galvanized the recalcitrant U.S. government to act on AIDS. The problem created by a lack of universal health care was then solved by the creation of an entirely new set of financing and delivery structures instituted by the CARE Act in 1990.

ONGOING ISSUES IN BRITISH AND AMERICAN TREATMENT POLICY: ENTRENCHED INTERESTS, HEALTH CARE REFORM, AND TENSIONS BETWEEN LOCAL AND NATIONAL CONTROL

Since 1990, new challenges have arisen stemming from the ongoing spread of disease, the changing availability of drug treatments, and the changing national contexts in which HIV/AIDS exists. As a result, each country has periodically revisited and revised its policy decisions. New choices continue to reflect the shape of domestic health care institutions and the interaction of these structures with other factors that drive the policymaking process. This section offers brief examples of three aspects of ongoing policy development that particularly reflect the causal force of health systems: HIV/AIDS policy changes that grow directly from health system changes, legacies of the institutional constraints that determined original HIV/AIDS policy choices, and the growing tension between local control and national quality standards.

Significant health system reforms began in the U.K. around 1990. One central tenet of these reforms was that local health authorities would now control the prioritization and commissioning of health care services for the population in their geographic jurisdiction. Ring-fenced allocations meant that local health authorities were obligated to spend these funds on HIV-related services,[7] a restriction which violated the core principle of local control. Ring-fencing of HIV/AIDS funds had been an unusual arrangement from the start, but now the changing shape of the NHS created a notable tension.

Suggestions that HIV/AIDS-specific allocations might be ended surfaced as early as 1992, but were politically untenable at that time.[8] The memory of prominent discussions about the risk of HIV/AIDS to the population at large was too fresh; as recently as 1989 MPs had made speeches warning that the decimating effects of AIDS on the youth of the country would result in problems finding enough workers, nurses, and soldiers.[9] Instead of an immediate end to ring-fencing, then, change began more gradually. Allocations dropped significantly in all regions except the most affected metropolitan areas starting in 1993–94, and continued as the public profile of HIV declined (Berridge 1996).[10] The sense of urgency that had motivated ring-fenced funding gradually dissipated, while ongoing health system changes increasingly devolved decision-making power to the local level.

The definitive change came in 2001 with the publication of the Blair government's *National Strategy for Sexual Health and HIV*, which addressed a range of new issues on the political scene but also fundamentally reassessed the cornerstone of British HIV/AIDS treatment policy by ending ring-fenced funding allocations. The government justified this decision in its 2002 response to protests from ring-fencing proponents:

> HIV funding has been ring-fenced for many years, and it is right that the ring-fencing should stop when services are well established. This is to avoid distortions in determining local budgets which do not reflect the reality of local need (Department of Health 2002: 7).

As a simple solution in the context of the NHS that existed at the start of the epidemic, ring-fenced treatment funds had solved an important AIDS-related financing problem when the disease was an important national priority. Once HIV/AIDS no longer occupied center stage, the program ended as a result of its inconsistency with the local-centric shape of the new, reformed NHS.

Like the U.K., the U.S. originally took the route of establishing an exceptional program to provide for HIV/AIDS treatment, and also encountered pressure to dismantle the program in subsequent years. Unlike its British counterpart, however, the American version has been reaffirmed three times since its inception and has grown exponentially in funding and political support. Among the central reasons the CARE Act has continued to thrive are the long-term consequences of the specific way U.S. legislators chose to address the AIDS treatment financing problem. While ring-fenced treatment allocations constituted an unusual funding mechanism within already-established health care institutions, the CARE Act had to establish entirely new organizations and institutions in order to achieve its goals. By building up a service infrastructure around the country, the CARE Act also created a vast network of entrenched interests heavily motivated to protect it.

HIV/AIDS policy advocacy certainly predated the CARE Act, but the organizations that are recipients of its funding have been a critical force in ensuring the passage of all three reauthorization bills, as well as many appropriations increases for CARE Act programs since 1990. The "big six" dominant AIDS service organizations in major urban areas are particularly influential in the politics of reauthorization. Alliances also exist to consolidate and represent the interests of the many other organizations around the country. These interest groups exist solely to preserve and enhance CARE Act funding, and work tirelessly to protect the legislation. In the words of a long-time policy advocate, "the stakeholder communities . . . obviously . . . want to protect their own piece of the pie" (I30: 169).

This dynamic can be seen as a long-term consequence of the same institutional features that drove the original creation of the CARE Act. Before 1990, the American health care system contained no systematic mechanisms by which to get intensive care and services to the uninsured ill. The CARE Act resolved this problem for PLWHAs by creating new service structures and thousands of jobs that depend on its funding stream. Along the way, it also created a new group of political actors, a set of entrenched interests with no British parallel. By working so far outside the confines of the pre-existing health care system, the CARE Act ensured its own future in a way ring-fenced treatment allocations to existing NHS units never did.

HIV/AIDS policy also continues to echo larger challenges endemic to both health care systems, particularly the tension between local and national control over health care funding and provision. British ring-fencing was terminated in 2001 in order to reflect the desired balance of local and national control, but the underlying problem has continued to plague policymakers. Returning decision-making power to local authorities also created the option for local NHS units to stop investing in HIV/AIDS services and the genitourinary medicine (GUM) clinics that provide them. The sexual health of the British population and the quality of relevant medical services has declined notably in recent years, and national leaders continue searching for ways to improve the situation without disempowering local decision-makers (Padamsee 2007).

The U.S. federalist system struggles with this tension between local and central control as well. In this case the strain is manifested most clearly around issues pertaining to the significant portion of CARE Act funds that are spent in state AIDS Drugs Assistance Programs (ADAPs)—individual programs through which each state purchases HIV/AIDS drugs for its patients who cannot otherwise access them. ADAPs have faced growing challenges since 2000, as the level of need in many states has outpaced the available funding. Two central problems have resulted from ADAP shortfalls: waiting lists and unequal state formularies. These problems stem partly from inadequate federal funding, but also result from variation in state-level choices. While some ADAPs run only on federal dollars, other states supplement these funds with considerable resources of their own. The result is that some state ADAPs include everyone who needs them, cover a generous range of drugs, and provide a wide range of peripheral services, while others struggle with waiting lists, have minimalist formularies, and provide few other services. Redistribution from the federal level poses a controversial question about how to reward and punish state funding choices.[11] Some policymakers and advocates argue, for instance, that a long waiting list in North Carolina is:

> North Carolina's problem because they . . . just don't put any money into AIDS programs from the state level, whereas in New York or California, they put millions of dollars into their programs (Interview with Brent Minor: 222).

From this perspective, helping North Carolina by shifting funds away from New York or California would be unfair, because "they have been doing the right thing . . . and . . . they are going to be penalized (I26: 288). On the flip side, though, others argue that it *is* appropriate for the federal government to provide for PLWHAs who cannot be helped by state policy choices.

> In New York, HIV is really a problem for them. In Kansas, the legislature doesn't prioritize it . . . and you can't blame them. Why should they? It's not a huge problem in Kansas. . . . [The federal] per case funding rate . . . needs almost to be higher there because the state legislature is never going to pony up, and they shouldn't . . . [if] I'm a Kansas legislator I just can't make that my priority, and I shouldn't if I am a decent priority setter (I12: 306–8).

CONCLUSION

In order to understand national HIV/AIDS policies, we cannot think of the policymaking process as an autonomous one influenced only by the disease, players, and politics of HIV/AIDS itself. We must also consider the critical ways in which policymaking is constrained, facilitated, and shaped by institutions and mechanisms already in place in each country. The structural features of British and American health care helped shape both the social problems the new epidemic would raise, and the options that would be available for solving these problems. Designed in response to parallel financial crises generated by the new epidemic, both Britain's ring-fenced treatment allocations and the American CARE Act treated HIV/AIDS as an exceptional health care problem that merited exceptional solutions. The contours of these national solutions, however, were quite distinct because they had to operate in the context of radically different health care structures. Even after the initial treatment policy decisions had been made, the central features and changing attributes of each health system continued to influence the shape of policymaking in response to the ongoing challenges generated by the epidemic.

The influence of health care institutions is by no means the only causal factor that determines national HIV/AIDS policy choices. As illustrated above, a range of social discourses about the epidemic and the groups most affected by it have also influenced the content and viability of policy proposals. In addition, a variety of groups have mobilized to pressure governments to recognize and grapple with the many medical and social problems HIV raises. These types of factors interact continually with the institutional conditions within which policy must be made. It is only by considering how these contexts drive policymaking that we will be able to fully understand the steps national governments have taken to address the evolving challenges of HIV/AIDS.

NOTES

1. "Ring-fencing" is a British term that is roughly equivalent to "ear-marking" in the U.S. usage. Ring-fenced funds are those within an NHS budget that can only be spent on specified types of services.
2. Interview with Brian Gazzard: 232; Interview with Saul Walker: 15; National Audit Office 1991: 17; *Hansard* 1/13/89 c. 1106–107; *Hansard* 12/20/91 c. 623. All interviews cited in this chapter were conducted by the author as part of a larger research project during 2005. Numbers after the colon indicate paragraph numbers in the interview transcript. Many informants elected to waive confidentiality and are identified by name; those who did not have been assigned informant numbers and identified as "I#" instead. *Hansard* (the printed transcripts of British Parliamentary debates) is cited by date and column number.
3. I06: 131–57.
4. I06: 161, 211; Interview with Jeffrey Levi: 250–70; I05: 374; Interview with Julie Scofield: 76.
5. In particular, aerolized pentamidine treatments helped stave off deadly pneumonias in AIDS patients, and research at this time seemed to show that AZT might delay the onset of full-blown AIDS and death.
6. I06: 209, 629–31.
7. Despite this obligation, there were many cases where local authorities diverted funds ring-fenced for HIV/AIDS work into other areas with little or no justification. Some of these choices were contested and money was sometimes recuperated or redirected toward HIV/AIDS services, but some of these instances went unchecked.
8. *Hansard* 10/22/92 c. 608; Berridge 1996.
9. *Hansard* 1/13/89 c. 1139.
10. *Hansard* 2/28/96 c. 1474.
11. I26: 370; I03: 141–9; I13: 161.

REFERENCES AND FURTHER READING

Anderson, Odin W. 1972. *Health Care: Can There Be Equity? The United States, Sweden and England.* New York, NY: Wiley and Sons.

Anderson, Odin W. 1989. *The Health Services Continuum in Democratic States.* Ann Arbor, MI: Health Administration Press.

Bayer, Ronald, and Eric A. Feldman. 1999. "Introduction: Understanding the Blood Feuds," in *Blood Feuds: AIDS, Blood, and the Politics of Medical Disaster*, edited by Eric A. Feldman and Ronald Bayer. New York, NY: Oxford University Press.

Berridge, Virginia. 1996. *AIDS in the UK: The Making of Policy, 1981–1994.* New York, NY: Oxford University Press.

Berridge, Virginia. 1998. "AIDS and British Drug Policy: A Post-War Situation?," in *Addictions and Problem Drug Use: Issues in Behaviour, Policy, and Practice*, edited by Michael Bloor and Fiona Wood. London, UK: Jessica Kingsley Publishers.

Department of Health. 2001. *The National Strategy for Sexual Health and HIV.* London, UK: Her Majesty's Stationery Office.

Department of Health. 2002. *The National Strategy for Sexual Health and HIV: Implementation Action Plan.* London, UK: Her Majesty's Stationery Office.

Field, Mark G. 1980. "The Health System and the Polity: A Contemporary American Dialectic." *Social Science and Medicine* 14: 397–413.

Fox, Daniel M., Patricia Day, and Rudolf Klein. 1989. "The Power of Professionalism: Policies for AIDS in Britain, Sweden, and the United States." *Daedalus* 118(1): 93–112.

Graig, Laurene A., editor. 1999. *Health of Nations: An International Perspective on U.S. Health Care Reform*, 3rd edition. Washington DC: Congressional Quarterly Inc.

Greenaway, John, Steve Smith, and John Street. 1992. *Deciding Factors in British Politics: a Case-Studies Approach.* London, UK: Routledge.

House of Representatives Human Resources and Intergovernmental Relations Subcommittee of the Committee on Government Operations. 1989. *The AIDS Epidemic in Newark and Detroit.* Washington DC: Government Printing Office.

Hsiao, William C. 1992. "Comparing Health Care Systems: What Nations Can Learn From One Another." *Journal of Health Politics, Policy and Law* 17(4): 613–36.

Marmor, Theodore R., Patricia A. Dillon, and Stephen

Scher. 1999. "The Comparative Politics of Contaminated Blood: From Hesitancy to Scandal" in *Blood Feuds: AIDS, Blood, and the Politics of Medical Disaster*, edited by Eric A. Feldman and Ronald Bayer. New York, NY: Oxford University Press.

National Audit Office. 1991. *HIV and AIDS Related Health Services*. London, UK: Her Majesty's Stationery Office.

Padamsee, Tasleem. 2007. "Infusing Health into the Welfare State: HIV/AIDS Policy Making in the United States and the United Kingdom." Ph.D. dissertation, University of Michigan, Ann Arbor.

Schramm-Evans, Zoe. 1990. "Responses to AIDS: 1986–1987," in *AIDS: Individual, Cultural and Policy Dimensions*, edited by Peter Aggleton, Graham Hart, and Peter Davies. London, UK: Falmer Press.

Weeks, Jeffrey. 1989. "AIDS: The Intellectual Agenda," in *AIDS: Social Representations, Social Practices*, edited by Peter Aggleton, Peter Davies, and Graham Hart. London, UK: Falmer Press.

Weeks, Jeffrey, Austin Taylor-Laybourn, and Peter Aggleton. 1994. "An Anatomy of the HIV/AIDS Voluntary Sector in Britain," in *AIDS: Foundations for the Future*, edited by Peter Aggleton, Graham Hart, and Peter Davies. London, UK: Taylor and Francis.

Weiss, Robin and Leslie M. Hardy. 1990. "HIV Infection and Health Policy." *Journal of Consulting and Clinical Psychology* 58(1): 70–76.

CHAPTER 22

Barriers to HIV/AIDS Medical Care among HIV-Infected Latinos Residing along the U.S.–Mexico Border

Antonio L. Estrada and Barbara Estrada

ABSTRACT

In response to the increasing rates of infectious diseases, including HIV/AIDS, hepatitis B, and hepatitis C, HRSA's HIV/AIDS Bureau (HAB) initiated a special funding mechanism for the U.S. Border States. The goal of the demonstration project was to develop and evaluate outreach models that increased access to specialty HIV/AIDS medical care among people living with HIV/AIDS and increase HIV testing in the region. The HIV-infected Latinos in the study were characterized as primarily male, MSM, single, born in Mexico, with low employment rates and high uninsured rates. Although the findings reported here are based on one of the largest studies conducted with Mexican-origin Latinos living with HIV disease in the U.S.–Mexico border region, much more research needs to be conducted with this vulnerable population and more health care resources need to be made available to the region.

OVERVIEW

The Latino population approximates 14 percent of the total population, making Latinos the largest ethnic minority group in the U.S. (U.S. Census Bureau 2004). Mexican-origin Latinos (Mexican, Mexican American, and Chicano), the majority of whom live in the Southwestern United States, comprise 65 percent of the Latino population, making it the largest Latino subgroup in the nation.

BORDER OVERVIEW

The U.S.–Mexico border region is legally defined as 62 miles (100 km) in either direction of the border between the United States and Mexico, and spans close to 2,000 miles (3,200 km) from the Pacific Ocean to the Gulf of Mexico (USMBHC 2003). American Border States include Arizona, California, New Mexico, and Texas. Mexican Border States include Baja California Norte, Sonora, Chihuahua, Coahuila, Nuevo León and Tamaulipas.

This region is unique in many ways. The area once belonged to Mexico; there is a shared infrastructure of economy and transport; the population is relatively young and primarily of Mexican descent/origin; high rates of poverty exist; and for the most part the U.S. counties in the border region are "Health Professional Shortage Areas" (HPSAs), a designation given by the Health Resources and Services Administration (HRSA) when a county has shortages in primary medical care, dentists, or mental health providers (HRSA 2000). In 2000, the percent of the total border population in these shortage areas was 65.9 percent in Texas, 36.1 percent in Arizona, 30.7 percent in California, and 8.1 percent in New Mexico (HRSA 2007). HRSA has noted that if the U.S.–Mexico border region were the 51st state in the nation, it would rank last in access to health care, second in mortality from hepatitis, and third in mortality from diabetes (U.S.–Mexico Border Counties Coalition 2006).

SOCIO-DEMOGRAPHIC CHARACTERISTICS

According to both the U.S. and Mexico Censuses (U.S. Census Bureau 2000; INEGI 2000), there were approximately 13 million residents in the U.S.–Mexico border region, almost evenly divided between the United States and Mexico. Close to one fourth of the U.S. border population is less than 15 years of age. The Latino border population varies from a low of 29 percent in California to a high of 84 percent in Texas. Overall, 49 percent of the U.S. border population is Latino. A paradox exists in the U.S.–Mexico border region in terms of economic status. On the one hand, the U.S. side of the border is one of the poorest in the nation. On the other, the Mexican side of the border is one of the wealthiest regions in comparison to Mexico. Similarly, educational attainment is lower on the U.S. side of the border in comparison to the nation, while on the Mexican side of the border it is higher than that in Mexico.

Overall, 19 percent of the U.S. border population lives below the federal poverty level compared to 13 percent for the nation. There are over 500 million northbound border crossings annually, with many persons having familial, employment, and educational ties in both the United States and Mexico (Bureau of Transportation Statistics 2004).

The U.S.–Mexico border is unique in another way; one that is controversial and mitigates access to health care. Homeland Security has made this region a high-priority area for potential terrorist activity. Coupled with the increasing flow of undocumented workers and drugs, this area is heavily monitored and patrolled by the U.S. Border Patrol and the National Guard. Some have called this area a region of "low intensity conflict" due to the massive mobilization of military, citizen militias, and police enforcement (Dunn 1996). As well, some Border States have passed "English Only" laws and policies, aimed at "undocumented immigrants," that have resulted in increased surveillance and detention of U.S. citizens of Mexican descent, documented Mexican nationals, and Mexican nationals in general for no other reason than fitting a profile of "illegals" or "drug traffickers."

PHYSICIAN-TO-POPULATION RATIOS

HRSA's Border Health Program provides border county health workforce profiles for each of the U.S.–Mexico border states (HRSA 2007). The physician-to-population ratio, a measure used by HRSA to designate health provider shortage areas, varies considerably among the border states. The physician-to-population ratio (per 100,000 population) was 275.6 in California (2004), 239.0 in Arizona (2004), 138.5 in New Mexico (2003), and 107.8 in Texas (2003), compared to the national average of 278 per 100,000 (2004). Clearly, access to primary care physicians is limited in the region, and those physicians who specialize are even more limited. For example, the Bureau of Primary Health Care (BPHC 2000) estimates that there were 91 primary care physicians and 115 specialty physicians per 100,000 population in counties within 62 miles (100 km) of the Mexican border. Finding a physician who specializes in HIV/AIDS medical care may be even more limited.

HRSA'S BORDER SPNS DEMONSTRATION PROJECT

In response to the increasing rates of infectious diseases, including HIV/AIDS, hepatitis B, and hepatitis C, HRSA's HIV/AIDS Bureau (HAB) initiated a special funding mechanism for the U.S. border states. The Border SPNS Project (Special Projects of National Significance) funded programs in five clinical sites along the U.S.–Mexico border: San Ysidro, California; Tucson, Arizona; Las Cruces, New Mexico; El Paso,

Texas; and Harlingen, Texas. The goal of the demonstration project was to develop and evaluate outreach models that increased access to specialty HIV/AIDS medical care among people living with HIV/AIDS and increase HIV testing in the region (Eldred, Cheever, and Parham-Hopson 2006). Almost 73 percent of the counties in the U.S.–Mexico border region are designated as Medically Underserved Areas (MUAs), and 63 percent are HPSAs for primary medical care (HRSA 2004). Hence, the need to understand the dynamics of health care, especially given the lack of specialty care for HIV disease, is important given the increasing rates of HIV/AIDS in the U.S.–Mexico border region.

HIV/AIDS STATISTICS IN THE U.S.–MEXICO BORDER REGION

The HIV/AIDS rate in the U.S. border region is almost twice the rate than that reported for the Mexican border region (USMHBC 2003). The reported AIDS rate in Mexican Border States was 5.8 per 100,000 compared to 9.3 per 100,000 in U.S. border states. The HIV infection rate in Mexican border states was 3.4 per 100,000 compared to 8.4 per 100,000 (including only Arizona, New Mexico, and Texas border counties, as California did not have confidential HIV testing at the time). Given the bi-directional flow of migrants in the region, it becomes extremely important to monitor the HIV/AIDS epidemic and intervene when and where appropriate. Increasing rates of HIV/AIDS have been found for both heterosexual transmission and male-to-male sexual transmission (MSM) in the U.S.–Mexico border region (Ruiz 2002; Ferreira-Pinto, Ramos, and Shedlin 1996).

The Centers for Disease Control and Prevention provides estimated adult/adolescent AIDS cases based on country of birth for Latinos residing in the United States (CDC 2007). Overall, among Latinos born in Mexico, 59 percent acquired AIDS through MSM, 25 percent through heterosexual sex, and 11 percent through injection drug use (IDU), (compared to Latinos born in the United States wherein 44 percent acquired AIDS through MSM, 26 percent through heterosexual sex, and 24 percent IDU). In the U.S.–Mexico border region, similar results have been obtained with the primary mode of transmission being MSM, followed by heterosexual sex (USMBHC 2003). Research conducted in the region shows that MSM and IDU are important transmission bridges to the heterosexual Latina population (Ramirez et al. 1994; Maxwell et al. 2006; Ferreira-Pinto and Ramos 1995; Strathdee et al. 2005), increasing the probability of HIV transmission among this group.

ACCESS TO CARE IN THE U.S.–MEXICO BORDER REGION

Almost 30 percent of residents in the border region have no health insurance coverage (USMBHC 2003). The fact that approximately two-thirds of the counties on the U.S. side of the border are designated as MUAs, coupled with high rates of uninsured, low income, and poverty among Latinos in the region, accessing quality health care is problematic and often beyond the financial reach of many.

Barriers to health care among Latinos in the U.S.–Mexico border region can be grouped into at least three areas: financial barriers; institutional barriers; and cultural barriers (Estrada, Treviño, and Ray 1990). Among financial barriers, factors such as cost of care, low income, poverty rates, and lack of health insurance coverage converge to make health care financially unattainable. Institutional barriers include hours of service, transportation, distance, and access based on legal residency requirements. These factors come together to make health care unavailable or inaccessible based on sociodemographic characteristics and organizational policies that limit access based on ability to pay or residency status. Cultural barriers include lack of bilingual and bicultural staff and health providers. Even with translation and interpretation services mandated by federal law (Title VI of the Civil Rights Act of 1964), many health organizations in the U.S.–Mexico border region do not have adequate translation and interpretation services.

U.S. citizens and legal U.S. residents may cross the U.S.–Mexico border legally to take advantage of the close proximity of the Mexican border to obtain medical care, dental care, and prescription medications. Undocumented immigrants have more difficulty crossing the border. Taken together, a myriad of factors converge that limit access to health care in the U.S.–Mexico border region and consequently impact the quality of life of HIV-infected Latinos residing in the region, increasing their vulnerability to opportunistic infections and not intervening in the transmission of HIV to others.

METHODS

Methodological considerations, measures, and recruitment procedures for several Border SPNS Initiative sites have been reported elsewhere (Keesee et al. 2006a, 2006b; Zuniga et al. 2006, 2007; Valverde and Felderman-Taylor 2006). Briefly, the target population was HIV-infected persons residing along the U.S.–Mexico border region. Data were collected using five standardized data collection modules (available from www.ou.edu/border). The five areas covered by the instruments included: demographics, culture and lifestyle characteristics, risk factors for HIV infection, barriers to health care, health-related quality of life, and client satisfaction with the HIV/AIDS care program at each site. The modules were completed during face-to-face interviews conducted by bilingual staff at each site between January 1, 2001 and November 30, 2004. Each site was responsible for interview training following the methodology and standards of the Border SPNS Initiative. Interviews were conducted in Spanish or English depending on the language preference of the participant. The modules were first developed in English, then translated to Spanish, then back-translated to English using professional and lay translators to ensure consistency in meaning and content. Variables with inconsistent translations were omitted from the database.

Participants in the study consisted of HIV-infected adults (18 to 64) who were receiving case management and/or HIV specialty medical care in one of the five HIV/AIDS care programs. While this sample may not provide an epidemiological profile of HIV-infected individuals residing along the U.S.–Mexico border, it may, due to the large sample size, substantially represent a majority of those HIV-infected individuals who were receiving HIV/AIDS medical treatment within 62 miles (100 km) on the U.S. side of the international border.

Individuals who tested positive for HIV had the option of being participants in one of the five HIV/AIDS care programs (either a community health center or AIDS service organization). HIV/AIDS program participants could become participants in this study by meeting all of the following criteria: living or working within 62 miles (100 km) on either side of the U.S.–Mexico international border, being HIV infected, being between the ages of 18 to 64, and voluntarily consenting to complete survey instruments. A consent form was read to each potential participant, in either Spanish or English, and was voluntarily signed by those electing to be in the study. Human subjects approval was obtained for each site. A unique identifier was provided to each study participant to protect their confidentiality.

Statistical analyses were performed using Chi-square tests and t-tests where appropriate to compare HIV-infected participants (SPSS for Windows, Version 15). Statistical significance was assessed at $p<.05$ and $p<.005$ for all analyses.

FINDINGS

As of January 2005, a total of 1,200 HIV-infected persons residing along the U.S.–Mexico border were recruited into the study. Of these, 921 self-identified as "Mexican" or "Mexican American" and 65 percent preferred to take the interview in Spanish. Among the five sites, 4.8 percent were recruited in New Mexico, 6.3 percent were recruited in Arizona, 30.4 percent were recruited in California, and 58.7 percent were recruited in Texas (32.4 percent from El

Paso and 26.3 percent from Harlingen). Selected socio-demographic and health status characteristics of the entire sample are presented in Exhibit 22.1.

The sample's average age is approximately 38 years, with 68.2 percent reporting that they were born in Mexico. The sample was predominantly male (83.8 percent), with the primary sexual orientation being gay/bisexual (58.8 percent), followed by heterosexual (40.1 percent). About half of the sample were unemployed (48 percent), 55.7

Exhibit 22.1 Selected sociodemographic and health status characteristics (N = 921)

Characteristic	*N*	*Percent*
Gender		
• Male	772	83.8
• Female	149	16.2
Sexual orientation		
• Gay/lesbian	440	47.8
• Bisexual	101	11.0
• Heterosexual	369	40.1
Employment status		
• Employed	339	36.8
• Unemployed	582	63.2
Marital Status		
• Single	513	55.7
• Married/living together	269	29.2
• Separated, divorced, widowed	136	14.8
Country of birth		
• United States	291	31.6
• Mexico	626	68.0
Age groups		
• 18–24	57	6.2
• 25–34	334	36.3
• 35–44	332	36.0
• 45–54	151	16.4
• 55–64	47	5.1
Medical insurance		
• None	671	72.9
• Private	67	7.3
• Public	183	19.9
HIV status		
• HIV positive, not AIDS	489	53.1
• HIV-positive, AIDS status unknown	190	20.6
• CDC-defined AIDS	242	26.3
Exposure category		
• MSM	533	57.9
• IDU	65	7.1
• Heterosexual	277	30.1
• Blood transfusion, blood components, tissue	33	3.6
• Other	13	1.4
Overall health status		
• Excellent	93	10.1
• Very good	197	21.4
• Good	285	30.9
• Fair	223	24.2
• Poor	95	10.3

percent were single, and 73 percent did not have health insurance coverage at the time of the interview.

The predominant HIV acquisition mode was MSM (57.9 percent), followed by heterosexual contact (30.1 percent). Slightly more than one fourth of the sample had CDC-defined AIDS and over one third (35.6 percent) reported their health status as "fair" or "poor." On average, the participants' age at diagnosis was 34 years (data not shown). HIV-infected Latinos had a mean time since HIV/AIDS diagnosis of 3.81 years compared to 2.86 years for HIV-infected Latinas ($p<.005$, data not shown).

Socio-demographic and health status characteristics were also examined by gender and country of birth of the HIV-infected Latino participants in the study (Exhibit 22.2). Statistically significant gender differences were found. A higher proportion of Latinas than Latinos were heterosexual, unemployed, and acquired HIV via heterosexual intercourse, while a higher proportion of Latinos than Latinas had no health insurance coverage, were single, and acquired HIV via male-to-male sex.

There were no gender differences found with respect to country of birth, HIV status, overall health status, or age group. In reference to country of birth, U.S.-born participants had significantly higher proportions than Mexican-born participants for acquiring HIV via injection drug use; however, Mexican-born participants had higher proportions than U.S.-born participants of being married/living together, no health insurance coverage, and being HIV positive, AIDS status unknown. There were no statistically significant differences found by country of birth for sexual orientation, gender, age groups, employment status, or overall health status.

A series of questions asked HIV-infected Latinos about health care barriers they had encountered prior to accessing care. Health care barriers were grouped into six categories: knowledge-related barriers, institutional-related barriers, personal health-related barriers, stigma-related barriers, access-related barriers, and international-related barriers (see Exhibit 22.3).

Of the 921 HIV-infected Latinos in the sample, almost two-thirds (72.6 percent) reported encountering at least one health care barrier prior to entering the study. Among the knowledge-related barriers lack of knowledge regarding cost, eligibility requirements, service availability, and HIV/AIDS specialization of medical providers were reported by relatively high percentages of the sample. Institutional-related barriers included thinking that staff did not speak Spanish, and having to wait too long for an appointment. For the personal health-related barriers, thinking that HIV medications would make them sick or believing that they were even available ranked very high. Almost one third felt that they were too ill to seek health care services. Stigma-related barriers also were also endorsed by the majority of the HIV-infected Latinos. Believing that others would think badly of them or believing that others would discover that they are gay was endorsed by upwards of 56 percent of the sample. Interestingly, access-related and international-related barriers were not encountered by the majority of the HIV-infected Latinos in the study.

In order to examine potential subgroup differences in the barriers encountered, analyses were performed comparing women to men and comparing U.S.-born to Mexican-born HIV-infected Latinos (Exhibit 22.4). Looking first at gender differences, significantly more women than men reported lack of knowledge regarding availability of health services, lack of transportation, lack of child care, and crossing the U.S.–Mexico border as barriers. Significantly more men than women reported personal health-related and stigma-related barriers such as being too sick to seek care, believing that others would think them gay, and believing their partner would become violent.

In comparing U.S.-born to Mexican-born HIV-infected Latinos, significantly more Mexican-born Latinos than U.S.-born Latinos encountered the following barriers: thought services cost too much; worried that the physician did not specialize in HIV/AIDS; thought the staff would not speak Spanish; were too sick to seek services; believed that their partner would become violent; had trouble crossing the U.S.–Mexico border;

Exhibit 22.2 Selected sociodemographic and health status characteristics by gender and country of birth of participants (N = 921)

Characteristic	*Male % (N)*	*Female % (N)*	*U.S.-born % (N)*	*Mexican-born % (N)*
Sexual orientation	**		NS	
• Gay/lesbian	57.3 (437)	2.0 (3)	46.5 (134)	49.2 (304)
• Bisexual	13.0 (99)	1.4 (2)	11.3 (70)	10.9 (31)
• Heterosexual	29.7 (226)	96.6 (143)	39.5 (244)	42.7 (123)
Employment status	**		NS	
• Employed	39.1 (302)	24.8 (37)	34.7 (102)	37.7 (236)
• Unemployed	60.9 (470)	75.2 (112)	65.3 (190)	62.3 (390)
Gender			NS	
• Male			85.2 (248)	83.2 (521)
• Female			14.8 (43)	16.8 (105)
Marital status	**		**	
• Single	62.2 (478)	23.5 (35)	60.8 (177)	53.7 (336)
• Married/living together	27.3 (210)	39.6 (59)	21.0 (61)	33.1 (207)
• Separated, divorced, widowed	10.5 (81)	36.9 (55)	18.2 (53)	13.3 (83)
Country of birth	NS			
• United States	32.2 (248)	29.1 (43)		
• Mexico	67.8 (521)	70.9 (105)		
Age groups	NS		NS	
• 18–24	5.6 (43)	9.4 (14)	6.9 (20)	5.9 (37)
• 25–34	35.5 (274)	40.3 (60)	33.3 (97)	37.7 (236)
• 35–44	38.0 (293)	26.2 (39)	37.8 (110)	35.1 (220)
• 45–54	15.9 (123)	18.8 (28)	17.2 (50)	16.1 (101)
• 55–64	5.1 (39)	5.4 (8)	4.8 (14)	5.1 (32)
Health insurance	**		**	
• None	74.7 (577)	63.1 (94)	58.4 (170)	79.7 (499)
• Private	7.4 (57)	6.7 (10)	12.4 (36)	5.0 (31)
• Public	17.9 (138)	30.2 (45)	29.2 (85)	15.3 (96)
HIV status	NS		*	
• HIV-positive, not AIDS	52.7 (407)	55.0 (82)	57.7 (168)	51.1 (320)
• HIV-positive, AIDS status unknown	20.2 (156)	22.8 (34)	15.1 (44)	23.3 (146)
• CDC-defined AIDS	27.1 (209)	22.1 (33)	27.1 (79)	25.6 (160)
Exposure category	**		**	
• MSM	69.0 (533)	0.0 (0)	53.6 (156)	59.9 (375)
• IDU	7.3 (56)	6.0 (9)	13.7 (40)	4.0 (25)
• Heterosexual	19.4 (150)	85.2 (127)	27.8 (81)	31.0 (194)
• Blood transfusion, blood components, tissue	3.0 (23)	6.7 (10)	4.1 (12)	3.4 (21)
• Other	1.3 (10)	2.0 (3)	0.7 (2)	1.8 (11)
Overall health status	NS		NS	
• Excellent	10.4 (78)	10.4 (15)	10.8 (30)	10.3 (63)
• Very good	22.6 (169)	19.4 (28)	22.3 (62)	22.0 (135)
• Good	33.1 (248)	25.7 (37)	28.8 (80)	33.3 (204)
• Fair	24.4 (183)	27.8 (40)	25.2 (70)	24.8 (152)
• Poor	9.5 (71)	16.7 (24)	12.9 (36)	9.6 (59)

* p<.05; ** p<.005

Exhibit 22.3 Health care barriers experienced by HIV-infected participants (N = 669)

Barrier categories	*N*	*Percent indicating item was a barrier*
Knowledge-related		
• Knowledge of local HIV medical care	371	55.5
• Knowledge of requirements to qualify	539	80.6
Institutional-related		
• Thought services cost too much	488	72.9
• Worried physician does not specialize in HIV/AIDS	318	47.5
• Had to wait too long for appointment	124	18.5
• Thought staff would not speak Spanish	199	29.7
• Believed HIV meds were available	282	42.2
Personal health-related		
• Too sick to seek services	208	31.1
• Medications might make sick	443	66.2
• Preferred alternative treatments	33	4.9
Stigma-related		
• Concerned others would find out HIV status	375	56.1
• Concerned others would think gay/lesbian	191	28.6
• Concerned others would think badly because HIV+	449	67.1
• Worried that family/friends would be against receiving services	141	21.1
• Believed partner would become violent	80	12.0
Access-related		
• Lack of child care	26	3.9
• Lack of transportation	185	27.7
• Lack of telephone service	48	7.2
• Caring for others prevented care	24	3.6
International-related		
• Trouble crossing the border	53	7.9
• Presence of U.S. Border Patrol	22	3.3

and presence of the U.S. Border Patrol (Exhibit 22.5). Significantly more U.S.-born than Mexican-born HIV-infected Latinos thought that HIV medications would make them sick and fewer believed that HIV/AIDS medications were available.

DISCUSSION

The HIV-infected Latinos in the study can be characterized as primarily male, MSM, single, born in Mexico, and having low employment rates and high uninsured rates. The health status of the HIV-infected participants in the study varied. Almost one fourth were diagnosed with CDC-defined AIDS, indicating late presentation of HIV disease, and about one third described their health status as fair or poor. These findings lend support to the hypothesis that HIV-infected Latinos residing along the U.S.–Mexico border region are less healthy than their non-Latino white counterparts, and present at later stages of disease due to limited financial access or availability of specialized HIV medical care.

Given the lack of health care providers in the U.S.–Mexico border region, it is perhaps not too surprising to find that the majority of HIV-infected Latinos in the study had encountered at least one barrier to obtaining health care for themselves. The specific types of barriers encountered that prevented accessing health care varied by gender and country of birth. Similar to other findings (Estrada, Treviño, and Ray 1990; HRSA 2004), women encountered more child care and transportation barriers than men. As well, financial costs and lack of health

Exhibit 22.4 Health care barriers experienced by gender of participants (N = 669)

Barrier categories	*N*		*Percent indicating item was a barrier*	
	Men	*Women*	*Men*	*Women*
Knowledge-related				
• Knowledge of local HIV medical care	295	76	52.9	68.5**
• Knowledge of requirements to qualify	446	93	79.9	83.8
Institutional-related				
• Thought services cost too much	408	80	73.1	72.1
• Worried physician does not specialize in HIV/AIDS	267	51	47.8	45.9
• Had to wait too long for appointment	105	19	18.8	17.1
• Thought staff would not speak Spanish	161	38	28.9	34.2
• Believed HIV meds were available	235	47	42.1	42.3
Personal health-related				
• Too sick to seek services	184	24	33.0*	21.6
• Medications might make sick	368	75	65.9	67.6
• Preferred alternative treatments	31	2	5.6	1.8
Stigma-related				
• Concerned others would find out HIV status	312	63	55.9	56.8
• Concerned others would think gay/lesbian	178	13	31.9**	11.7
• Concerned others would think badly because HIV+	378	71	67.7	64.0
• Worried that family/friends would be against receiving services	113	28	20.3	25.2
• Believed partner would become violent	73	7	13.1*	6.3
Access-related				
• Lack of child care	12	14	2.2	12.6**
• Lack of transportation	139	46	24.9	41.4**
• Lack of telephone service	38	10	6.8	9.0
• Caring for others prevented care	19	5	3.4	4.5
International-related				
• Trouble crossing the border	37	16	6.6	14.4*
• Presence of U.S. Border Patrol	16	6	2.9	5.4

* p<.05; ** p<.005

insurance coverage were reported in this study, again similar to other findings related to Latinos and health care utilization.

Interestingly, more HIV-infected Latinos than Latinas reported stigma-related barriers to accessing care. Perhaps this finding is related to the negative perceptions of homosexuality in Latino culture. Studies have shown that gay Mexican men, as well as other Latino males, are very aware that their culture and religion are homophobic, and usually keep their sexual orientation a secret from heterosexual relatives and friends (Magana and Carrier 1991; Diaz 1998).

The increased militarization of the U.S.–Mexico border after the terrorist attacks of September 11, 2001, coupled with stemming the undocumented migrant flow from Mexico and Central America has certainly had an impact on health care access in the region. The majority of Mexican-born participants in the study reported that the presence of the U.S. Border Patrol and the difficulty in crossing the border were barriers to accessing health care in the U.S. and Mexico.

Institutional-related barriers were also encountered by more Mexican-born than U.S.-born participants, especially believing that staff would not speak Spanish or that the physicians did not specialize in HIV/AIDS medical care, suggesting that the availability of bilingual health care services and those who specialize in HIV/AIDS medical care in the U.S.–Mexico border region continues to be limited. Lack of knowledge regarding medication side effects was also

Exhibit 22.5 Health care barriers experienced by country of birth of participants (N = 669)

Barrier categories	*N*		*Percent indicating item was a barrier*	
	Mexico	*U.S.*	*Mexico*	*U.S.*
Knowledge-related				
• Knowledge of local HIV medical care	269	102	59.3**	47.4
• Knowledge of requirements to qualify	370	169	81.5	78.6
Institutional-related				
• Thought services cost too much	349	139	76.9**	64.7
• Worried physician does not specialize in HIV/AIDS	247	71	54.4**	33.0
• Had to wait too long for appointment	89	35	19.6	16.3
• Thought staff would not speak Spanish	171	28	37.7**	13.0
• Believed HIV meds were available	163	119	35.9	55.3**
Personal health-related				
• Too sick to seek services	154	54	33.9*	25.1
• Medications might make sick	288	155	63.4	72.1*
• Preferred alternative treatments	24	9	5.3	4.2
Stigma-related				
• Concerned others would find out HIV status	265	110	58.4	51.2
• Concerned others would think gay/lesbian	136	55	30.0	25.6
• Concerned others would think badly because HIV+	311	138	68.5	64.2
• Worried that family/friends would be against receiving services	104	37	22.9	17.2
• Believed partner would become violent	63	17	13.9*	7.9
Access-related				
• Lack of child care	22	4	4.8	1.9
• Lack of transportation	134	51	29.5	23.7
• Lack of telephone service	37	11	8.1	5.1
• Caring for others prevented care	15	9	3.3	4.2
International-related				
• Trouble crossing the border	52	1	11.5**	0.5
• Presence of U.S. Border Patrol	22	0	4.8**	0.0

*p<.05; **p<.005

pronounced. These findings are similar to other research that has demonstrated that Mexican-born Latinos encounter more health care barriers than others (Levy et al. 2007; Shedlin and Shulman 2004).

More problematic is the finding that more Mexican-born than U.S.-born participants reported being too ill to seek medical care, indicating more severe symptoms of HIV disease. A medical outcomes study on a portion of the border SPNS sample was conducted that showed a similar finding (Brittingham and Williams 2005) with 39 percent of the sample having low CD4 counts and being symptomatic with 28 percent having at least one opportunistic infection, and 33 percent having no previous antiviral medications.

LIMITATIONS, IMPLICATIONS, AND CONCLUSIONS

The findings reported here are based on one of the largest studies conducted with Mexican-origin Latinos living with HIV disease in the U.S.–Mexico border region. The study used standardized measures and common data modules across the five border SPNS sites coordinated by a multi-site evaluation center that enhanced the comparability of data across all sites.

Nevertheless, sampling procedures were not probabilistic, relying primarily on outreach and word of mouth for participant recruitment. As well, the sample was drawn primarily from the California site and the two Texas sites. Thus, the sample of HIV-infected Latinos may not be representative of HIV-infected Latinos living in Arizona or New Mexico, or other more rural areas in the U.S.–Mexico border region. Further, the sample may only be representative of those HIV-infected Latinos who have attempted and succeeded in accessing medical care and not necessarily those who may have encountered too many barriers and have given up. Another limitation of the study was that the barriers elicited from the participants were a finite set, and did not include all the barriers that could be experienced. A final limitation of the study was that the research design of the border SPNS project was not longitudinal, limiting any causal inferences that can be made concerning the dynamics of health care utilization and potential barriers encountered that prevented HIV-infected Latinos from accessing or continuing with medical care.

HIV/AIDS remains a growing concern in the U.S.–Mexico border region. A lack of health care services and the lack of HIV/AIDS trained physicians contribute to the medically underserved nature of the border region. Solutions that involve bi-national cooperation between Mexico and the United States can be successful, but the current dynamics along the U.S.–Mexico border preempt cooperation and the provision of medical care in the area.

Numerous health care utilization barriers come together in the U.S.–Mexico border region, limiting access to medical care. Coupled with low income, high unemployment rates, high poverty rates, and low health insurance coverage, it is not surprising that persons living with HIV disease present at later stages of disease, experience more barriers to care, and perhaps are not receiving optimal HIV/AIDS specialty care. Clearly, much more research needs to be conducted in this unique region and with this highly vulnerable population. Focused research on health care utilization, health status, and treatment of persons living with HIV disease in the U.S.–Mexico border region are warranted. Moreover, more health care resources need to be made available to the region in order to improve upon health status and access to care, especially HIV/AIDS medical care. HIV disease does not recognize international borders.

ACKNOWLEDGMENTS

The research presented in this chapter was supported by Grant Number H97-HA00183 from the Health Resources and Services Administration (HRSA), Special Projects of National Significance (SPNS) Program. The contents of this chapter are solely the responsibility of the authors and do not necessarily represent the official view of HRSA or the SPNS Program. The authors would like to acknowledge the U.S.–Mexico Border HIV/AIDS Collaborative for providing data collection and database management: San Ysidro Health Center, San Ysdiro, California; Camino de Vida, Las Cruces, New Mexico; Centro de Salud Familiar La Fe, El Paso, Texas; Valley AIDS Council, Brownsville, Texas; Special Immunology Associates, Inc., El Rio Health Center, Tucson, Arizona; and, the University of Oklahoma, Centro de Evaluación, Norman, Oklahoma.

REFERENCES AND FURTHER READING

Brittingham, T. and Williams, L. 2005. Medical Outcomes Study. University of Oklahoma, Centro de Evaluacion. Retrieved August 20, 2007 from http://www.ou.edu/border.

Brouwer, K.C., Strathdee, S.A., Magis-Rodriguez, C., Bravo-Garcia, E., Gayet, C., Patterson, T.L., Bertozzi, S.M., and Hogg, R.S. 2006. Estimated Numbers of Men and Women Infected with HIV/AIDS in Tijuana, Mexico. *J Urban Health*, 83(2): 299–307.

Bureau of Primary Health Care (BPHC). 2000. U.S.–Mexico Border Health. Retrieved August 20, 2007 from http://bphc.hrsa.gov/bphc/borderhealth.

Bureau of Transportation Statistics. 2004. Border Crossing: U.S.–Mexico Border Crossing Data. Retrieved August 24, 2007 from http://bts.gov/programs/international/border_crossing_entry_data/us_mexico/pdf/.

Centers for Disease Control and Prevention (CDC). 2007. *HIV/AIDS Surveillance Report, 2005*, 17. Revised edition. Atlanta: U.S. Department of Health and Human Services, Centers for Disease Control and Prevention.

Diaz, R. 1998. *Latino Gay Men and HIV: Culture, Sexuality and Risk Behavior*. New York: Routledge.

Doyle, T.J., and Bryan, R.T. 2000. Infectious Disease Morbidity in the U.S. Region Bordering Mexico, 1990–1998. *Journal of Infectious Diseases*, 182: 1503–1510.

Dunn, Timothy J. 1996. *The Militarization of the U.S.–Mexico Border, 1978–1992*. The Center for Mexican American Studies, University of Texas Press.

Eldred, L., Cheever, L., and Parham-Hopson, D. 2006. Accessing Care for U.S./Mexico Border Populations Living with HIV/AIDS: The Role of HRSA's HIV/

AIDS Bureau and Special Projects of National Significance. In Herman Curiel and Helen Land (eds.), *Outreach and Care Approaches to HIV/AIDS Along the U.S.–Mexico Border*, pp. 15–35. Binghamton, New York: Haworth Press.

Estrada, A.L., Estrada, B.D., and Trujillo, S. 2006. Sexual Risks among HIV Positive Latinos: Implications for Prevention with Positives. Presented at the 134th Annual Meeting of the American Public Health Association, November 4–11, Boston, MA.

Estrada, A.L., Treviño, F., and Ray, L. 1990. Barriers to Health Care Among Mexican Americans: Evidence from the Hispanic Health and Nutrition Examination Survey. *American Journal of Public Health*, 80 (Supplement): 27–31.

Ferreira-Pinto, J.B., and Ramos, R. 1995. HIV/AIDS Prevention among Female Sexual Partners of Injection Drug Users in Ciudad Juarez, Mexico. *AIDS Care*, 7(4): 477–488.

Ferreira-Pinto, J.B., Ramos, R.L., and Shedlin, M. 1996. Migrants and Female Sex Workers: HIV/AIDS on the U.S. Mexico Border. In S.I. Mishra, R.F. Conner, and J.R. Magana (eds.), *AIDS Crossing Borders: The Spread of HIV among Migrant Latinos*, pp. 113–136. Boulder, CO: Westview.

Health Resources and Services Administration (HRSA). 2000. *Assuring a Healthy Future Along the United States–Mexico Border: A HRSA Priority*. Rockville, MD: U.S. Department of Health and Human Services.

Health Resources and Services Administration (HRSA). 2004. *U.S.–Mexico Border Health*. Bureau of Primary Health Care, U.S. Department of Health and Human Services.

Health Resources and Services Administration (HRSA). Border County Health Workforce Profiles. 2007. Rockville, MD: U.S. Department of Health and Human Services. Retrieved August 24, 2007 from http://bphc.hrsa.gov/bphc/borderhealth.

Instituto Nacional de Estadistica, Geografia e Informatica (INEGI). 2000. *XII Censo General de Poblacion y Vivienda*. (*Mexico Census*).

Keesee, M.S., Shinault, K.A., Carabin, H., et al. 2006a. Socio-Demographic Characteristics of HIV/AIDS Individuals Living and Receiving Care Along the U.S.–Mexico Border Through Five SPNS Demonstration Projects. In Herman Curiel and Helen Land (eds.) *Outreach and Care Approaches to HIV/AIDS Along the U.S.–Mexico Border*, pp. 15–35. Binghamton, New York: Haworth Press.

Keesee, M.S., Shinault, K.A., Carabin, H., et al. 2006b. Sociodemographic Characteristics of a Population of HIV/AIDS Seropositive Individuals Receiving Care through 5 Demonstration Sites along the U.S.–Mexico Border. Poster presented at the 134th Annual Meeting of the American Public Health Association, November 4–11, Boston, MA.

Levy, V., Prentiss, D., Balmas, G., Chen, S, Israelski, D, Katzenstein, D., Page-Shafer, K. 2007. Factors in the Delayed HIV Presentation of Immigrants in Northern California: Implications for Voluntary Counseling and Testing Programs. *J Immigrant Health*, 9: 49–54.

Magana, J, and Carrier, J. 1991. Mexican and Mexican American Male Sexual Behavior and Spread of AIDS in California. *J Sex Research*, 28: 425–441.

Maxwell, J.C., Cravioto, P., Galvan, F., Ramirez, M.C., Wallisch, L.S., and Spence, R.T. 2006. Drug Use and Risk of HIV/AIDS on the Mexico–U.S.A. border: A Comparison of Treatment Admissions in Both Countries. *Drug Alcohol Dependence*, 82 (Suppl. 1): S85–S93.

Ramirez, J., Suarez, E., De la Rosa, G., Castro, M., and Zimmerman, M. 1994. AIDS Knowledge and Sexual Behavior among Mexican Gay and Bisexual Males. *AIDS Educ Prev* 6: 163–174.

Ruiz, J.D. 2002. HIV Prevalence, Risk Behaviors, and Access to Care among Young Latino MSM in San Diego, California and Tijuana, Mexico. Epidemiology Branch, Office of AIDS, California Department of Health Services, Sacramento: California Office of AIDS, CA Department of Health Services.

Shedlin, M., and Shulman, L. 2004. Qualitative Needs Assessment of HIV Services among Dominican, Mexican and Central American Immigrant Populations Living in the New York City area. *AIDS Care*, 16: 434–445.

SPSS, Inc., Version 15. 2007. Chicago, IL.

Strathdee, S.A., Fraga, W.D., Case, P. Firestone, M., Brouwer, K.C., Perez, S.G., Magis, F., and Fraga, M.A. 2005. "Vivo para consumiria y la consumo para vivir" ["I live to inject and inject to live"]: High-Risk Injection Behaviors in Tijuana, Mexico. *J. Urban Health*, 82 (Suppl. 4): iv58–73.

United States Census Bureau. 2000. *State and County QuickFacts. 2000. Data derived from Population Estimates, 2000 Census of Population and Housing* (United States Census).

United States Census Bureau. 2004. *The Hispanic Population in the United States*.

U.S. Department of Health and Human Resources, Health Resources and Services Administration. 2005. *Women's Health U.S.A.*. Rockville, MD: U.S. Department of Health and Human Services.

United States–Mexico Border Health Commission (USMBHC). 2003. Healthy Border 2010: An agenda for improving health on the United States-Mexico border. October 2003. Retrieved August 24, 2007 from http://www.borderhealth.org.

U.S.–Mexico Border Counties Coalition (USMBHC). 2006. At the Cross Roads: U.S./Mexico Border Counties in Transition. Institute for Policy and Economic Development, The University of Texas, El Paso, 2006. Retrieved August 24, 2007 from http://www.bordercounties.org.

Valverde, M., and Felderman-Taylor, J. 2006. HIV/AIDS Outreach in Southern New Mexico: From Design to Implementation. In Herman Curiel and Helen Land (eds.), *Outreach and Care Approaches to HIV/AIDS Along the U.S.–Mexico Border*, pp. 55–71. Binghamton, New York: Haworth Press.

Zuniga, M.L., Brennan, J., Scolari, R., and Strathdee, S.A. 2007. Barriers to HIV Care in the Context of Cross-Border Health Care Utilization among HIV-Positive Persons Living in the California/Baja

California U.S.–Mexico Border Region. *J Immigr Minor Health*, July 26, 2007 [Epub ahead of print].

Zuniga, M.L., Organista, K.C., Scolari, R., et al. 2006. Exploring Care Access Issues for Mexican-Origin Latinos Living with HIV in the San Diego/Tijuana Border Region. In Herman Curiel and Helen Land (eds.), *Outreach and Care Approaches to HIV/AIDS Along the U.S.-Mexico Border*, pp. 37–54. Binghamton, New York: Haworth Press.

SECTION 6

Media and HIV/AIDS

FRAMING ESSAY

The Utility of "Old" and "New" Media as Tools for HIV Prevention

Seth M. Noar

OVERVIEW

The vast impact of the HIV/AIDS epidemic over the past 25 or so years, and the looming threat over the coming decades, mandates a response that is commensurate with its magnitude. As the United States (U.S.) and the world come to grips with this epidemic, public health officials and researchers have recognized that effective health communication is vital to turning its tide (Devos-Comby and Salovey 2002; Edgar, Noar, and Freimuth 2008; Freimuth, Hammond, Edgar, and Monahan 1990; Holtgrave 1997; Maibach, Kreps, and Bonaguro 1993). From basic knowledge of HIV transmission routes to behavior change messages that encourage individuals and communities to reduce sexual and drug risk behaviors, communicating key risk reduction messages in an efficient and effective manner is nothing short of a necessity. Given that no cure or vaccine is on the horizon, effective health communication across a variety of intervention contexts remains a key preventive strategy.

Since the beginning of the AIDS epidemic, traditional or "old" media have played a critical role in this effort. Although in the U.S. the news media were initially slow in reacting to the AIDS epidemic, this changed in 1985 with the high-profile cases of Rock Hudson and Ryan White (Dearing and Kim 2008). These stories put a human face on AIDS and brought news coverage of HIV/AIDS to a new level. Notwithstanding a variety of critiques of media coverage of HIV/AIDS (e.g., Biddle, Conte, and Diamond 1993), the media have since covered the epidemic in various ways and played an increasingly critical role in helping to set the HIV/AIDS public and policy agendas in the U.S. and around the world (Dearing and Kim 2008).

Old media have also been critical in the launch of scores of HIV/AIDS campaigns utilizing communication channels such as television, radio and/or print media to raise awareness about HIV/AIDS and encourage reductions in risky drug and sexual practices in countries around the globe (Bertrand and Anhang 2006; Bertrand et al. 2006; Holtgrave 1997; Myhre and Flora 2000; Palmgreen, Noar, and Zimmerman 2008; The Henry J. Kaiser Family Foundation 2006). These campaigns have been conceptualized and carried out as media-only or multi-component campaign efforts which integrate media with other communitywide components. Such campaigns aim to generate specific effects in large numbers of individuals, typically within a specified period of time, and through a coordinated set of communication activities (Rogers and Storey 1987).

Moreover, as technology has developed so rapidly and brought with it a myriad of new computer technologies, including the Internet, new ways of transmitting prevention messages have emerged (Bull 2008; Neuhauser and Kreps 2003; Noar, Clark, Cole, and Lustria 2006). While the Internet has become a double-edged sword, with some using it to meet risky sexual partners (Bull, McFarlane, Lloyd, and Reitmeijer 2004), it has also opened the door to broad access to health information (Kalichman et al. 2002; Pew Internet and American Life Project 2005) and new prevention interventions (Bull 2008). Given that aspects of the Internet such as interactivity mimic interpersonal communication still have the broad reach of mass media

(Cassell, Jackson, and Cheuvront 1998), the impact of new media on risk behaviors could ultimately be quite significant.

The purpose of the current chapter is to discuss the roles that both "old" and "new" media have played in HIV/AIDS prevention, examining the broad literature on HIV/AIDS mass communication campaigns (old media) as well as the newer emerging literature on computer-based interventions, many of which are (or potentially could be) Internet-based (new media). The primary focus is on how these media have been harnessed in HIV/AIDS prevention efforts in the U.S. and around the world.

WHAT'S CHANGED? A HISTORICAL PERSPECTIVE ON "OLD" MEDIA

How have "old" media been harnessed in the battle against HIV/AIDS? The tale of the media response to HIV/AIDS in the U.S. provides a key historical perspective for how media and media campaigns responded to the dynamics of a changing epidemic. A recent report on 25 years of HIV/AIDS campaigns in the U.S. described five eras of media response (The Henry J. Kaiser Family Foundation 2006). In the first era, "The New Threat and the Activist Response (1981–1985)," AIDS activists developed and implemented community education projects and local campaigns in San Francisco and New York, to get the word out about a new disease that was devastating the gay community. Materials utilized included informational materials and advertising, such as billboards, buttons, and leaflets. A coordinated federal response, however, did not come until the second era, "The HIV/AIDS PSA is Born (1986–1989)." During this period, the Surgeon General issued a report on AIDS and the Centers for Disease Control and Prevention (CDC) launched the first national HIV/AIDS campaign effort, known as "America Responds to AIDS." The first phase of the campaign targeted the general population, while subsequent phases (beginning in 1989) targeted a number of particular high-risk groups. In 1990, the campaign complemented its public service announcements (PSAs) with an unprecedented direct mailing of an AIDS pamphlet (titled *Understanding AIDS*) to every household in the U.S. In the third era, "Reaching Communities at Risk (1990–1995)," the media and public were shocked as Magic Johnson announced that he was HIV positive, flooding CDC's national hotline with calls and vastly increasing demand for HIV testing and condoms (Casey et al. 2003). Also at that time, the "America Responds to AIDS" campaign began to focus more specifically on risk groups such as African Americans and Latinos and the National Institute on Drug Abuse and the Ad Council collaborated on PSA campaign efforts focused on drug users.

The mid-1990s brought dramatic changes in both HIV/AIDS and the response to it. In the fourth era, "HAART Brings Hope. But is AIDS Over? (1996–2000)," new HIV treatment regimens extended life for many with HIV and began to transform AIDS into a chronic disease. "America Responds to AIDS" ended its campaign, and funding was redirected to grants that local organizations could procure to target particular high-risk groups (rather than a broader, national campaign). A storyline in the popular television show *ER* on contracting and living with HIV captured the attention of an estimated 40 million viewers. The Kaiser Family Foundation began its first of many public education partnerships aimed at collaborating with large media outlets to develop and air HIV/AIDS messages to particular target audiences. This partnership with MTV focused on combining targeted PSAs with other programming and was launched as the "BE SAFE" campaign. Subsequent partnerships included the *Staying Alive* campaign with MTV International and the *Rap It Up* campaign with Black Entertainment Television (BET). In the fifth and final campaign era, "Global AIDS (2001–2006)," the impact of AIDS around the world was widely publicized through campaigns conducted by the UN Foundation and Ad Council ("Apathy is Lethal") and Kaiser and Viacom ("KNOW HIV/AIDS"). These campaigns utilized PSAs as well as the integration of HIV/AIDS storylines into popular television programs focused on the impact of the global HIV/AIDS pandemic.

Worldwide, individual countries have had their own unique histories and responses to the HIV/AIDS epidemic, many of which have included coordinated mass communication (including entertainment education) campaign efforts (Bertrand et al. 2006; Johnson, Flora, and Rimal 1997; McKee, Bertrand, and Becker-Benton 2004; Singhal and Rogers 1999). Similar to the U.S., campaigns in a variety of countries tended to focus on HIV/AIDS knowledge and awareness early in the epidemic, with subsequent campaigns focusing more specifically on targeted groups and behavioral changes (Bertrand et al. 2006; Liskin 1990; Myhre and Flora 2000). While nowadays campaigns are in some ways ubiquitous, critical questions include how to design successful campaigns as well as whether campaigns are in fact effective at their intended purpose: improving HIV/AIDS awareness and knowledge, changing attitudes, social norms, and perceptions about HIV/AIDS, and ultimately reducing HIV/AIDS risk behaviors. In order to examine such issues, we turn next to the scientific literature on campaigns.

CONTINUITY AND CHANGE: A SCIENTIFIC PERSPECTIVE ON "OLD" MEDIA

What do we know about HIV/AIDS mass communication campaigns from a scientific perspective? The literature on this topic has grown greatly over the past two decades, and reviews have cataloged scores of campaigns that have appeared in the literature. Exhibit FE6.1 presents several key reviews of HIV/AIDS campaigns that have been conducted to date. By examining trends within and across these reviews, one can see how this literature has progressed over time. Indeed, these reviews provide evidence for what was noted above—namely, that many campaigns early in the epidemic were focused on broad, general audiences, in efforts to raise awareness about HIV/AIDS (Holtgrave 1997; Myhre and Flora 2000), while newer campaigns have been more likely to target behavioral changes in particular higher-risk groups, and thus have taken greater advantage of audience segmentation and targeting techniques (Palmgreen et al. 2008). Also, given that campaigns are increasingly focused on behavioral change rather than knowledge change, campaigns are increasingly including measures of behavior in their outcome assessments (Myhre and Flora 2000; Palmgreen et al. 2008). In addition, these reviews suggest that, while a *minority* of early campaigns were likely to be theory-based (Myhre and Flora 2000), among later campaigns (e.g., after 1998) a *majority* of such campaigns have been based upon theory (Palmgreen et al. 2008). Also promising is the fact that newer campaigns appear to be achieving better campaign exposure rates and increasingly integrating promising "new" media such as Internet websites into their design and execution (Palmgreen et al. 2008).

Although the above findings suggest progress on important elements of campaign design, including targeting, use of theory, and high audience exposure to campaign messages (Maibach et al. 1993; Noar 2006; Palmgreen et al. 2008), there are also important areas that have not moved forward. The most critical of these is the lack of robust evaluation of HIV/AIDS mass communication campaigns. In fact, despite evidence which suggests that health communication campaigns across a variety of health behaviors are capable of small behavioral effects (Bauman, Smith, Maibach, and Reger-Nash 2006; Derzon and Lipsey 2002; Snyder et al. 2004), the scientific literature on HIV/AIDS mass communication campaigns has to date yielded little strong evidence of efficacy. While some well-controlled studies have shown effects (e.g., CDC 1999; Kim, Kols, Nyakauru, Marangwanda, and Chibatamoto 2001; Vaughan, Rogers, Singhal, and Swalehe 2000; Yzer, Siero, and Buunk 2000; Zimmerman et al. 2007), as has a meta-analytic review of controlled HIV testing campaign studies (Vidanapathirana, Abramson, Forbes, and Fairley 2005), little evidence beyond such studies currently exists. This is the case *not* because such campaigns have failed, but rather because most studies have used weak outcome evaluation designs which are incapable of determining

Exhibit FE6.1 Selected reviews of HIV/AIDS mass media campaigns

Article	*Topic*	*Scope*	*Studies reviewed*	*Findings*	*Conclusions*
General HIV/AIDS campaigns					
Holtgrave (1997)	HIV/AIDS mass media campaigns	Through Fall 1996	49 studies conducted in 18 countries	• Substantial increase in literature since previous review one year before • Most campaigns targeted general populations using a variety of media • Few outcome evaluation designs included control groups • No true studies of HIV campaign cost-effectiveness	• Cost-effectiveness studies of HIV/AIDS media efforts urgently needed to help policymakers in decisions about use of campaigns • Importance of campaigns in the HIV/AIDS area will continue to increase and will require more careful evaluation
Myhre and Flora (2000)	HIV/AIDS mass media campaigns (peer-reviewed articles only)	Through 1998	41 studies conducted in 17 countries	• Majority of campaigns targeted general public (early campaigns focused on a broad, undefined audience) • Fewer than 20% used theory • Most (75%) used multiple communication channels • 62% provided a measure of campaign exposure • 17% included comparison/control groups • Knowledge and attitudes most common outcomes	• More complete reporting of campaign components needed • Greater integration of theory needed • Better measurement of outcomes and evaluation of campaigns needed • Future campaigns should incorporate community-based and communitywide efforts
Palmgreen et al. (2008)	HIV/AIDS mass media campaigns (peer-reviewed articles only)	1998–2005	25 studies conducted in 20 countries	• Campaigns are increasingly theory-based, targeted toward particular audience segments, focused on behavioral outcomes, and reporting higher campaign exposure rates • Newer campaigns are increasingly incorporating Internet websites • Campaigns used weak outcome evaluation designs. Only three studies included a control group	• Estimates of typical campaign effects are difficult to make, given weak outcome evaluation designs used • Campaign designers should increasingly follow principles of effective campaign design to increase chances of success (e.g., Noar, 2006) • New studies using multiple principles of campaign design coupled with rigorous evaluation are needed

HIV/AIDS Campaigns in Developing Countries					
Bertrand and Anhang (2006)	HIV/AIDS mass media campaigns targeting youth in developing countries	1990–2004	15 studies conducted in Africa, Latin America, and Asia	• Campaigns increased HIV knowledge, condom self-efficacy, some social norms, interpersonal communication, awareness of health providers, and condom use • Less evidence for abstinence self-efficacy, delaying first sex and decreasing sex partners • Individuals more highly exposed to campaign messages showed greater changes (dose-response)	• Work toward standardizing outcome variables • Few campaigns have been rigorously evaluated. Evaluate future large-scale campaigns using strong quasi-experimental designs that allow causality to be inferred • Conduct cost-effectiveness studies of campaigns
Bertrand et al. (2006)	HIV/AIDS mass media campaigns in developing countries (peer-reviewed articles only)	1990–2004	24 studies conducted primarily in Africa, Asia, and Latin America/the Caribbean	• Mixed results were found on outcome variables. Where effects were found, effect sizes were small to moderate • At least half of studies showed effects on HIV knowledge and reducing high-risk sexual behavior • Mixed effects on perceived risk, condom self-efficacy, interpersonal communication, abstinence, condom use	• Many studies had weak outcome evaluation designs, making strong conclusions difficult • Need alternative methods for evaluating national campaigns • Need standardized outcomes and measures to improve comparability across studies • Need better reporting of campaign components
HIV Testing Campaigns					
Vidanapathirana et al. (2005)	HIV testing campaigns using controlled designs	Through April 2004	14 studies conducted in the United States, United Kingdom, Australia, and Israel	• Short-term effects on testing behavior found in all 14 campaigns • No long-term effects were found	• Mass media can be effective in promoting HIV testing behavior in the short term • Further research is needed on the effectiveness of different types of mass media, characteristics of messages, and cost-effectiveness of campaigns

whether any observed changes in attitudes and behaviors were the result of campaign activities. Indeed, this fact is noted by every review in Exhibit FE6.1 (Bertrand and Anhang 2006; Bertrand et al. 2006; Holtgrave 1997; Palmgreen et al. 2008) except for Vidanapathirana et al. (2005), who only included studies that met stronger methodological criteria. Even in this case, more campaign studies were excluded than included in the review because of the weak outcome evaluation designs used in so many of the excluded studies (see Vidanapathirana et al. 2005). It is also noteworthy that a number of reviews have called for analyses of cost-effectiveness of HIV/AIDS campaigns (Bertrand and Anhang 2006; Bertrand et al. 2006; Holtgrave 1997; Vidanapathirana et al. 2005), and that this has not yet taken place. It may be, however, that accurate estimates of the impact of campaigns on HIV/AIDS knowledge, attitudes, and behaviors are needed in order to generate cost-effectiveness estimates.

It is certainly striking that so many reviews have called for more rigorous outcome evaluation while so few have heeded this call. For instance, the earliest review in the group, Holtgrave et al. (1997), noted that more careful evaluation of campaigns is needed, while the most recent review reports little or no progress in this area, finding, for instance, that only 3 of 25 campaign studies (12 percent) included a control/comparison community of any kind (Palmgreen et al. 2008). Discussions of HIV/AIDS campaigns that predate these reviews also had stressed the importance of rigorous evaluation (e.g., Maibach et al. 1993). The fact that so little progress has been made in this area, however, is not entirely surprising, as there are a number of barriers to rigorous evaluation of campaigns, including the costs associated with evaluation, the perception that it takes too much time or is not necessary, and the fact that some may object to evaluation on the grounds that it could interfere with campaign implementation (Valente 2001).

Moreover, the evaluation of "in the field" HIV/AIDS campaigns is a major challenge given that many campaigns are executed in entire regions or countries and as such cannot be subjected to rigorous designs such as randomized controlled trials (Do and Kincaid 2006; Hornik 2002; Noar 2006; McGrath 1991; Pettifor, MacPhail, Bertozzi, and Rees 2007). Priorities and concerns other than evaluation, such as the need to quickly roll out campaigns in countries with growing epidemics, are often front and center as well (e.g., Pettifor et al. 2007). Because of this, many campaigns use a post-only design in which a campaign survey conducted after the campaign is undertaken, and correlations among campaign exposure and HIV/AIDS attitudes and behaviors are examined (Bertrand et al. 2006; Hornik 2002; Noar 2006; Palmgreen et al. 2008). Another popular design is a pretest–posttest design, where changes from pre to post are examined as possible evidence of campaign impact. Unfortunately, these designs leave most threats to internal validity open, making the argument that *the campaign itself* led to positive changes difficult to make (Valente 2001). In these cases, alternative explanations for observed effects include: 1) reverse causality (those already engaging in the behavior are more likely to notice the campaign, resulting in an association between campaign exposure and behavior); 2) fluctuations in sample characteristics that give the appearance of campaign effects; 3) secular trends and/or historical events; or 4) a combination of these factors (Valente 2001).

More sophisticated techniques to correct for some of these problems, such as propensity scoring, have been proposed in the case of post-only designs, but to date the technique has *not* achieved widespread use in the HIV/AIDS area (Bertrand et al. 2006; Palmgreen et al. 2008). In addition, while these more sophisticated statistical methods can control for confounding factors in a way that attempts to mimic a randomized controlled design (e.g., see Do and Kincaid 2006), the extent to which methodological corrections such as propensity scoring make up for the use of weaker, evaluation designs remains unclear. For instance, while randomization disperses both known and unknown confounding factors evenly across intervention and control groups, propensity scoring can only control for confounding factors that are both known and have been adequately measured (Office of National Drug Control Policy 2002). In addition, in some areas of health research methodological corrections that were thought to correct for differences among groups have been shown to *not* make up for very basic flaws in research design (Smith and Ebrahim 2001). Indeed, a mantra in the research methods area is the fact that inferring causality is a research design issue, *not* a statistical control issue.

At a minimum, researchers and practitioners in this area should begin a dialogue about sophisticated approaches to evaluation of HIV/AIDS campaigns, given that, particularly on the international scene, the implications of HIV/AIDS are so large and many international donor agencies are investing huge sums of money into campaigns for which the effects remain largely unknown (Bertrand et al. 2006). The ongoing evaluation of the loveLife HIV prevention program in South Africa stands out as a particularly good example of beginning such a dialogue on alterative evaluation methods for large, national campaigns (Pettifor et al. 2007; also see Hornik 2002; McGrath 1991). Large-scale campaigns in other areas such as smoking cessation and exercise might also be considered in terms of evaluation methods that have been utilized in national campaign efforts (e.g., Farrelly et al. 2005; Huhman et al. 2005).

WHAT'S NEW? EMERGING PERSPECTIVES ON NEW MEDIA

While "old" media such as mass media campaigns using traditional communication channels remain vitally important, equally important are the prevention opportunities which new media technologies have introduced. A recent review of technologically based HIV prevention interventions makes the case for the growing importance of such technologies in prevention efforts (Bull 2008). In fact, a combination of factors gives these new technologies vast potential for prevention efforts. First, the Internet provides unprecedented global reach and is a technology that is increasingly used by individuals for accessing health information (Pew Internet and American Life Project 2005). Second, the Internet and other computer-based technologies (e.g., cell phones) offer opportunities not only for broad reach, but for individualized tailoring of HIV/AIDS and other prevention messages (Noar, Benac, and Harris 2007; Rimal and Adkins 2003). Third, such technologies offer interactivity, the properties of which may be persuasive with regard to health messaging (Noar et al. 2006; Street and Rimal 1997). Indeed, in the communication discipline it has long been stated that, while mass communication offers the broadest reach, interpersonal communication offers the most in terms of persuasive capabilities. The Internet and other new technologies have the potential to offer both broad reach and persuasive messaging capabilities in a way that could have a major impact on risky behaviors across a number of health domains, including HIV/AIDS (Cassell et al. 1998; Noar et al. 2006; Rimal and Adkins 2003).

Given that is the case, what kinds of technology-based applications have been tested in HIV prevention, and are such efforts showing promise in terms of impact on risky sexual outcomes? Exhibit FE6.2 lists selected applications of new technologies to HIV prevention. Although some projects are still in the early phases of evaluation (Bull 2008), these examples illustrate the diversity of approaches that have already appeared in this literature. In particular, they illustrate the use of computers to deliver a variety of intervention types, including: 1) in-person interventions delivered individually on-screen (Kiene and Barta 2006) or in group sessions (Kalichman et al. 2006); 2) interventions delivered over the Internet (Bowen, Horvath, and Williams 2007; Bull, Lloyd, Rietmeijer, and McFarlane 2004); 3) use of computers to create tailored print materials (Scholes et al. 2003); and 4) use of interactive video to simulate sexual interactions and allow "virtual" experiences in sexual decision-making (Read et al. 2006). To date, many of these interventions are showing efficacy with regard to changing critical theoretical mediators of safer sex, as well as showing impact on risky sexual behaviors (see Exhibit FE6.2). And these studies have been conducted with key infected and at-risk populations, including HIV-positive individuals, rural and urban men who have sex with men, and heterosexually active individuals.

Exhibit FE6.2 Selected applications of computer technology-based interventions in HIV/AIDS prevention

Article	*Target Population*	*Approach*	*Description*	*Outcomes*
Scholes et al. (2003)	Heterosexually active, non-monogamous young women aged 18–24	Computer-tailored self-help magazine	Intervention participants received a magazine tailored on characteristics such as condom stage of change, barriers to condom use, and partner type	At six-month follow-up, intervention participants exhibited higher condom self-efficacy, partner communication, condom carrying, and condom use compared to controls
Bull et al. (2004a)	Men who have sex with men	Internet-delivered tailored intervention	Intervention participants received three role-model stories tailored to their condom stage of change and encouraging incremental changes in condom use and STD/HIV testing	High attrition made outcome assessment problematic. At three-month follow-up, intervention participants showed more willingness to visit STD prevention websites and were more likely to get tested for HIV, compared to controls
Kalichman et al. (2006)	Men and women living with HIV/AIDS	Eight-session intervention focused on Internet skills	In group sessions, intervention participants learned about the Internet and how to evaluate websites for health information, care and support resources, and clinical trials	At nine-month follow-up, intervention participants exhibited greater Internet use for health, information coping, and social support compared to an attention-matched control
Kiene and Barta (2006)	Heterosexual undergraduate students	On-screen computer-tailored intervention	Intervention participants interacted with a computer program that provided tailored feedback on safer sex information, motivation, and behavioral skills in the form of text, quizzes, activities, and skill-building exercises	At one-month follow-up, intervention participants exhibited greater condom information, were more likely to keep condoms handy, and were more likely to use condoms compared to an attention-matched control
Read et al. (2006)	Caucasian men who have sex with men	Interactive video	Intervention participants engaged with an interactive video program that allowed them to go on a "virtual date," make decisions related to safe sex, and observe the consequences of those decisions. They also met with a counselor	At three-month follow-up, intervention participants had increased protected anal sex and reduced unprotected anal sex compared to controls (who received counseling only)
Bowen et al. (2007)	Rural men who have sex with men	Internet-delivered intervention	Intervention participants interacted with a program which included dialogue between an HIV-positive and an at-risk HIV-negative gay man, interactive activities and graphics to illustrate key points	At one-week follow-up, intervention participants exhibited increased knowledge, self-efficacy, and outcome expectancies compared to waiting-list control

While *mass* media is often concerned with broadcasting targeted messages to large audiences, many of these applications illustrate the ability of new media to narrowcast messages that are tailored at the individual level. Thus, while mass communication campaigns by necessity target messages to groups, new media is able to assess individual-level characteristics and subsequently customize messages to individuals (see Kreuter, Farrell, Olevitch, and Brennan 2000; Noar et al. 2007; Rimal and Adkins 2003). Given that this is the case, it is tempting to consider the synergy that may exist when these approaches are combined—that is, targeting messages to at-risk populations through campaigns that may serve as a "cue to action" to seek more information that would come in the form of computer-based technological interventions. Another model is to use mass media campaigns to target general sexually active populations and computer-based interventions to target higher-risk groups with interventions of greater intensity. The literature to date suggests that the synergy among mass and new media approaches is just beginning to be understood and appreciated (Bull 2008; Noar et al. 2006; Palmgreen et al. 2008), and additional studies are needed to understand how best to harness this. Given that behavioral interventions to date have clearly shown efficacy in HIV prevention (Noar 2008), while the efficacy of mass media campaigns for HIV/AIDS is much less well established, it may be wise to consider approaches that include and integrate both campaigns and behavioral interventions, including new media approaches.

A FINAL WORD: CONCLUDING REMARKS

Efforts to communicate effectively about HIV/AIDS with a variety of at-risk, HIV-positive, and general populations will continue to be critical as HIV/AIDS prevention efforts continue to be developed, tested, and brought to scale. Additional studies on the most effective uses of both "old" and "new" media for this purpose are still greatly needed. Moreover, evaluations that examine the synergy and interplay among different types and levels of interventions and media are also needed (CDC 2006; DiClemente, Salazar, Crosby, and Rosenthal 2005). As the media itself has changed and will continue to change so rapidly in the coming years, this will bring not only new challenges but incredible opportunities for both the narrowcasting and broadcasting of HIV/AIDS prevention messages to diverse audiences around the globe. Critical to these efforts will be quality research that allows us to understand effective uses of media and ultimately to maximize the use of resources that exist for HIV/AIDS prevention.

REFERENCES AND FURTHER READING

Bauman, A., Smith, B. J., Maibach, E. W., and Reger-Nash, B. (2006). Evaluation of mass media campaigns for physical activity. *Evaluation and Program Planning*, *29*, 312–322.

Bertrand, J. T., and Anhang, R. (2006). The effectiveness of mass media in changing HIV/AIDS-related behaviour among young people in developing countries. *World Health Organization Technical Report Series*, *938*, 205–241.

Bertrand, J. T., O'Reilly, K., Denison, J., Anhang, R., and Sweat, M. (2006). Systematic review of the effectiveness of mass communication programs to change HIV/AIDS-related behaviors in developing countries. *Health Education Research*, *21*, 567–597.

Biddle, N., Conte, L., and Diamond, E. (1993). AIDS in the media: Entertainment or infotainment. In S. C. Ratzan (ed.), *AIDS: Effective health communication for the 90s* (pp. 141–150). Washington DC: Taylor and Francis.

Bowen, A. M., Horvath, K., and Williams, M. L. (2007). A randomized control trial of Internet-delivered HIV prevention targeting rural MSM. *Health Education Research*, *22*, 120–127.

Bull, S. S. (2008). Internet and other computer technology-based interventions for STD/HIV prevention. In T. Edgar, S. M. Noar, and V. Freimuth (eds.), *Communication perspectives on HIV/AIDS for the 21st century* (pp. 351–376). New York: Lawrence Erlbaum.

Bull, S. S., Lloyd L., Rietmeijer C., and McFarlane, M. (2004a). Recruitment and retention of an online sample for an HIV prevention intervention targeting men who have sex with men: The Smart Sex Quest Project. *AIDS Care*, *16*, 931–943.

Bull, S. S., McFarlane, M., Lloyd, L., and Reitmeijer, C. (2004b). The process of seeking sex partners online and implications for STD/HIV prevention. *AIDS Care*, *16*(8), 1012–1020.

Casey, M. K., Allen, M., Emmers-Sommer, T., Sahlstein, E., Degooyer, D., Winters, A. M., Wagner, A. E., and Dun, T. (2003). When a celebrity contracts a disease: The example of Earvin "Magic" Johnson's announcement that he was HIV positive. *Journal of Health Communication*, *8*, 249–265.

Cassell, M. M., Jackson, C., and Cheuvront, B. (1998). Health communication on the internet: An effective channel for health behavior change? *Journal of Health Communication*, *3*, 71–79.

Centers for Disease Control and Prevention (CDC). (1999). Community-level HIV intervention in 5 cities: Final outcome data from the CDC AIDS community demonstration projects. *American Journal of Public Health*, *89*(3), 336–345.

Centers for Disease Control and Prevention (CDC). (2006). Evolution of HIV/AIDS prevention programs—United States, 1981–2006. *Morbidity and Mortality Weekly Report*, *55*(21), 597–603.

Dearing, J. W., and Kim, D. K. (2008). The agenda-setting process and HIV/AIDS. In T. Edgar, S. M. Noar, and V. Freimuth (eds.), *Communication perspectives on HIV/AIDS for the 21st century* (pp. 277–296). New York: Lawrence Erlbaum.

Derzon, J. H., and Lipsey, M. W. (2002). A meta-analysis of the effectiveness of mass-communication for changing substance-use knowledge, attitudes, and behavior. In W. D. Crano, and M. Burgoon (eds.), *Mass media and drug prevention: Classic and contemporary theories and research* (pp. 231–258). Mahwah, NJ: Erlbaum.

Devos-Comby, L., and Salovey, P. (2002). Applying persuasion strategies to alter HIV-relevant thoughts and behavior. *Review of General Psychology*, *6*(3), 287–304.

DiClemente, R. J., Salazar, L. F., Crosby, R. A., and Rosenthal, S. L. (2005). Prevention and control of sexually transmitted infections among adolescents: A socio-ecological perspective—a commentary. *Public Health*, *119*, 825–836.

Do, M. P., and Kincaid, D. L. (2006). Impact of an entertainment-education television drama on health knowledge and behavior in Bangladesh: An application of propensity scrore matching. *Journal of Health Communication*, *11*, 301–325.

Edgar, T., Noar, S. M., and Freimuth, V. S. (2008) (eds). *Communication perspectives on HIV/AIDS for the 21st century*. New York: Lawrence Erlbaum.

Farrelly, M. C., Davis, K. C., Havilan, M. L., Messeri, P., and Healton, C. G. (2005). Evidence of a dose-response relationship between "truth" antismoking ads and youth smoking prevalence. *American Journal of Public Health*, *95*(3), 425–431.

Freimuth, V. S., Hammond, S. L., Edgar, T., and Monahan, J. L. (1990). Reaching those at risk: A content-analytic study of AIDS PSAs. *Communication Research*, *17*(6), 775–791.

Henry J. Kaiser Family Foundation. (2006). *Evolution of an epidemic: 25 years of HIV/AIDS media campaigns in the U.S.* Menlo Park, CA: Kaiser.

Holtgrave, D. R. (1997). Public health communication strategies for HIV prevention: Past and emerging roles. *AIDS*, *11* (Suppl. A), S183–S190.

Hornik, R. C. (ed.) (2002). *Public health communication: Evidence for behavior change*. Hillsdale, NJ: Erlbaum.

Huhman, M., Potter, L., Wong, F. L., Banspach, S. W., Duke, J. C., and Heitzler, C. D. (2005). Effects of a mass media campaign to increase physical activity among children: Year-1 results of the VERB campaign. *Pediatrics*, *116*, e277–e284.

Johnson, D., Flora, J. A., and Rimal, R. N. (1997). HIV/AIDS public service announcements around the world: A descriptive analysis. *Journal of Health Communication*, *2*, 223–235.

Kalichman, S. C., Cherry, C., Cain, D., Pope, H., Kalichman, M., Eaton, L., et al. (2006). Internet-based health information consumer skills intervention for people living with HIV/AIDS. *Journal of Consulting and Clinical Psychology*, *74*, 545–554.

Kalichman, S. C., Weinhardt, L., Benotsch, E., DiFonzo, K., Luke, W., and Austin, J. (2002). Internet access and Internet use for health information among people living with HIV-AIDS. *Patient Education and Counseling*, *46*, 109–116.

Kiene, S. M., and Barta, W. D. (2006). A brief individualized computer-delivered sexual risk reduction intervention increases HIV/AIDS preventive behavior. *Journal of Adolescent Health*, *39*, 404–410.

Kim, Y. M., Kols, A., Nyakauru, R., Marangwanda, C., and Chibatamoto, P. (2001). Promoting sexual responsibility among young people in Zimbabwe. *International Family Planning Perspectives*, *27*, 11–19.

Kreuter, M. W., Farrell, D., Olevitch, L., and Brennan, L. (2000). *Tailoring health messages: Customizing communication with computer technology*. New Jersey: Lawrence Erlbaum.

Liskin, L. (1990). Using mass media for HIV/AIDS prevention. *AIDS Care*, *2*, 419–420.

McGrath, J. C. (1991). Evaluating national health communication campaigns: Formative and summative research issues. *American Behavioral Scientist*, *34*, 652–665.

McKee, N., Bertrand, J. T., and Becker-Benton, A. (2004). *Strategic communication in the HIV/AIDS epidemic*. Thousand Oaks, CA: Sage.

Maibach, E. W., Kreps, G. L., and Bonaguro, E. W. (1993). Developing strategic communication campaigns for

HIV/AIDS prevention. In S. C. Ratzan (ed.), *AIDS: Effective health communication for the 90s* (pp. 15–35). Washington DC: Taylor and Francis.

Myhre, S. L., and Flora, J. A. (2000). HIV/AIDS communication campaigns: Progress and prospects. *Journal of Health Communication*, *5* (Suppl.), 29–45.

Neuhauser, L., and Kreps, G. L. (2003). Rethinking communication in the e-health area. *Journal of Health Psychology*, *8*(1), 7–22.

Noar, S. M. (2006). A 10-year retrospective of research in health mass media campaigns: Where do we go from here? *Journal of Health Communication*, *11*, 21–42.

Noar, S. M. (2008). Behavioral interventions to reduce HIV-related sexual risk behavior: Review and synthesis of meta-analytic evidence. *AIDS and Behavior*, *12*, 335–353.

Noar, S. M., Benac, C., and Harris, M. (2007). Does tailoring matter? Meta-analytic review of tailored print health behavior change interventions. *Psychological Bulletin*, *133*(4), 673–693.

Noar, S. M., Clark, A., Cole, C., and Lustria, M. (2006). Review of interactive safer sex websites: Practice and potential. *Health Communication*, *20*, 233–241.

Office of National Drug Control Policy. (2002). *Evaluation of the national youth anti-drug media campaign: Fourth semi-annual report of findings*. Westat and the Annenberg School for Communication.

Palmgreen, P., Noar, S. M., and Zimmerman, R. S. (2008). Mass media campaigns as a tool for HIV prevention. In T. Edgar, S. M. Noar, and V. Freimuth (eds.), *Communication perspectives on HIV/AIDS for the 21st century* (pp. 221–252). New York: Lawrence Erlbaum.

Pettifor, A. E., MacPhail, C., Bertozzi, S., and Rees, H. V. (2007). Challenge of evaluating a national HIV prevention programme: the case of loveLife, South Africa. *Sexually Transmitted Infections*, *83* (Suppl. 1), i70–i74.

Pew Internet and American Life Project (2005). Health Information Online. Report available at http://www.pewinternet.org/pdfs/PIP_Healthtopics_May05.pdf.

Read, S. J., Miller, L. C., Appleby, P. R., Nwosu, M. E., Reynaldo, S., Lauren, A., et al. (2006). Socially optimized learning in a virtual environment: Reducing risky sexual behavior among men who have sex with men. *Human Communication Research*, *32*, 1–34.

Rimal, R. N., and Adkins, A. D. (2003). Using computers to narrowcast health messages: The role of audience segmentation, targeting, and tailoring in health promotion. In T. L. Thompson, A. M. Dorsey, K. I. Miller, and R. Parrott (eds.), *Handbook of Health Communication* (pp. 497–513). Mahwah, NJ: Lawrence Erlbaum.

Rogers, E. M., and Storey, J. D. (1987). Communication campaigns. In C. R. Berger and S. H. Chafee (eds.), *Handbook of communication science* (pp. 817–846). London: Sage.

Scholes, D., McBride, C. M., Grothaus, L., Civic, D., Ichikawa, L. E., Fish, L. J., et al. (2003). A tailored minimal self-help intervention to promote condom use in young women: Results from a randomized trial. *AIDS*, *17*, 1547–1556.

Singhal, A., and Rogers, E. M. (2003). *Combating AIDS: Communication strategies in action*. Thousand Oaks, CA: Sage.

Smith, G. D., and Ebrahim, S. (2001). Epidemiology—Is it time to call it a day? *International Journal of Epidemiology*, *30*, 1–11.

Snyder, L.B., Hamilton, M.A., Mitchell, E.W., Kiwanuka-Tondo, J., Fleming-Milici, F., and Proctor, D. (2004). A meta-analysis of the effect of mediated health communication campaigns on behavior change in the United States. *Journal of Health Communication*, *9*, 71–96.

Street, R. L., and Rimal, R. N. (1997). Health promotion and interactive technology: A conceptual foundation. In R. L. Street, W. R. Gold, and T. Manning (eds.), *Health promotion and interactive technology: Theoretical applications and future directions* (pp. 1–18). Mahwah, NJ: Erlbaum.

Valente, T. W. (2001). Evaluating communication campaigns. In R. E. Rice and C. K. Atkin (eds.), *Public communication campaigns*, 3rd edition (pp. 105–124). Thousand Oaks, CA: Sage.

Vaughan, P. W., Rogers, E. M., Singhal, A., and Swalehe, R. M. (2000). Entertainment-education and HIV/AIDS preventions: A field experiment in Tanzania. *Journal of Health Communication*, *5* (Suppl.), 81–100.

Vidanapathirana, J., Abramson, M. J., Forbes, A., and Fairley, C. (2005). Mass media interventions for promoting HIV testing (Review). *The Cochrane Database of Systematic Reviews*, *3*, 1–38.

Yzer, M. C., Siero, F. W., and Buunk, B. P. (2000). Can public campaigns effectively change psychological determinants of safer sex? An evaluation of three Dutch campaigns. *Health Education Research*, *15*, 339–352.

Zimmerman, R. S., Palmgreen, P., Noar, S. M., Lustria, M. L. A., Lu, H. Y., and Horosewski, M. L. (2007). Effects of a televised two-city safer sex mass media campaign targeting high sensation-seeking and impulsive decision-making young adults. *Health Education and Behavior*, *34*, 810–826.

CHAPTER 23

Photographic Images, HIV/AIDS, and Shifting Subjectivities in South Africa

Kylie Thomas

ABSTRACT

This chapter focuses on the photographic images of people living with HIV and AIDS by Gideon Mendel, a South African photojournalist. The chapter briefly describes how the South African state has responded to the epidemic, and how people living with HIV/AIDS have been conceptualized within state discourse; focuses on how the images in Mendel's book A Broken Landscape *(2001) intersect with these modes of representation; and concludes with an analysis of Mendel's portraits of people who have access to antiretroviral therapy. Mendel's new images both shape and reflect changing perceptions of the epidemic and of people living with HIV and AIDS in South Africa.*

In South Africa the debate about access to antiretroviral therapy has been highly politicized, and the meanings of HIV and AIDS, the efficacy of treatment, the extent, and even the existence of the epidemic, have been thoroughly contested.[1] In this context the ways in which people living with HIV and AIDS are represented has taken on an additional significance. This chapter takes as its focus the photographic images of people living with HIV and AIDS by Gideon Mendel, a London-based South African photojournalist. Mendel, who began documenting the epidemic in 1993, is one of a small group of photographers who have engaged with the issue of HIV and AIDS over time.[2] His body of work provides the most significant photographic record of the effects of the epidemic in sub-Saharan Africa, and South Africa in particular.[3]

A Broken Landscape (Mendel 2001a) chronicles the impact of HIV and AIDS on everyday life in Malawi, South Africa, Tanzania, Zambia, and Zimbabwe. A selection of photographs from the book was exhibited at the National Gallery in Cape Town from December 2001 to April 2002, and during that time Mendel began work on a new series of photographs focusing on access to antiretroviral therapy in South Africa. Through an analysis of this body of work, it is possible to trace how "AIDS," and more recently "HIV," has been imagined and represented. In particular, Mendel's work shows how the emergence of an HIV and AIDS activist movement and access to antiretroviral treatment in South Africa has led to new forms of representation of HIV-positive subjectivity.

The ways in which people living with HIV and AIDS are represented are bound up with the social, political, and economic contexts in which they live. At the same time, representation is a productive force that effectively shapes these contexts. Practices of representation can reinforce existing paradigms, but they can also reconfigure how people see themselves and how they are seen.[4] Shifts in perception affect the ways in which people live, even if the ways in which this occurs are not always easy to map. The first section of this chapter briefly describes how the South African state, both during apartheid and after, has responded to the epidemic and how people living with HIV/AIDS have been conceptualized within state discourse. I consider how the images in *A Broken Landscape* intersect with these modes of representation and then turn to an analysis of Mendel's portraits of people who have access to antiretroviral therapy. I argue that the change in Mendel's practice, evident in these new images, both shapes and reflects changing perceptions of the epidemic and of people living with HIV and AIDS in South Africa.

HIV AND AIDS IN SOUTH AFRICA

The first two cases of AIDS in South Africa were reported in 1982. For the next eight years, HIV infection rates were highest among white gay men.[5] In the early years of the epidemic state and civil society responses cast people living with HIV/AIDS as a danger to the body politic. In 1987 the South African government declared AIDS a communicable disease and proposed quarantine as a solution to the growing HIV/AIDS epidemic in South Africa.[6] The right of the state to quarantine HIV positive people was passed into legislation and, although this law was never enforced, the apartheid state's draconian approach to HIV/AIDS was made clear.[7]

In 1985 the apartheid government's Department of Health launched its first HIV/AIDS awareness and prevention campaign. Instead of conveying clear information about the means of transmission of HIV and how to avoid infection, the campaign made use of an image of coffins in graves. The campaign that followed depicted skeletons as the bed partners of sexually active couples. As Douglas Webb notes, this only served to create confusion about how HIV is transmitted (Webb 1997:74). In the context of 1980s South Africa, images of death, particularly those featured in a government campaign, were associated with political violence.[8] Even if the connections between sexual practices, HIV infection, AIDS, illness and death had been made apparent, black South Africans certainly had reason to doubt and fear the motives of the state in its attempts to control their sexual behavior.[9]

In the early 1990s the government launched the "yellow hand campaign," the logo of which depicted the outline of a yellow hand against a black background accompanied by the slogan "AIDS: Don't Let It Happen." While this approach represented a move away from the earlier campaigns in which HIV/AIDS was associated with death, it did little to prevent the rapid increase in HIV infection.

In many ways it is not surprising that the government never implemented a coherent and effective plan to prevent the spread of HIV/AIDS: the apartheid state condemned homosexuality and treated black South Africans as subhuman. In 1985, when the first deaths from AIDS occurred in South Africa, the migrant labor system was at its peak—1,833,636 South Africans were classed as migrants and half a million workers were employed in the goldmines.[10] The migrant labor system was one of the causes of the rapid spread of HIV in South Africa in the early stages of the epidemic and migrant mineworkers were among the first heterosexual men to test positive for HIV in large numbers in South Africa (Campbell 2001). Conditions of life for migrant laborers were extremely harsh; they worked for little pay, lived in single sex hostels, and were separated from their families and communities for long periods of time. The effects of the migrant labor system on sexual practices and family structures were, and continue to be, wide-reaching and have led to high HIV prevalence rates across both urban and rural parts of South Africa.[11]

The formation of the "Bantu Homelands," reserves set up by the apartheid state in the 1950s, was an integral part of the migrant labor system. The creation of the "homelands" effectively rendered all black South Africans stateless: "homeland" citizenship was imposed on all Africans in 1970 and the "homelands" were granted nominal independence from South Africa over the course of the next ten years. "By this process," South African historian Nigel Worden writes, "citizens of the 'independent' homelands lost their South African nationality, although the homelands were not recognised as independent by any other country" (Worden

1995:111). Workers ordinarily returned from their places of work in the urban centers to their families in the rural "homelands" twice a year. Conditions of life in the "homelands" were very difficult and, as rural poverty increased, more and more people sought employment in the urban centers. Able-bodied adult men were usually absent for long periods of time and the burden of providing for their families fell on women.

The crisis of HIV/AIDS in South Africa is clearly a legacy of the policies of the apartheid state but the response of the post-apartheid government has not reduced the number of new infections, nor has it addressed the needs of people living with HIV/AIDS. South Africa now has the largest country total of people living with HIV/AIDS in the world, many of whom live in conditions of extreme economic poverty without access to the treatment and care they require. State discourse on HIV/AIDS in South Africa has defined people living with HIV as responsible for their condition and at the same time has cast those who are experiencing the symptoms of AIDS as "victims" who are beyond the reach of medical care.[12]

In her essay entitled "AIDS: Keywords," Jan Zita Grover analyses the rhetorical force in naming people living with HIV/AIDS "victims." She writes that "Victims always end up revealing some tragic character flaw that has invited their tragedy" (Grover 1991:29). Grover argues that the use of the term "victim" is bound to a fatalistic approach to the epidemic that "implies that nothing, or next to nothing, can be done about the cultural, social and medical crises presented by AIDS. It denies the very possibility of all that is *in fact* being done by people living with AIDS and those working with them" (1991:29). The construction of people living with HIV/AIDS as dying subjects collapses the distinction between the sick, those who can be healed, and the dying, for whom nothing can be done. In November 2003, the South African government announced that it would begin to provide anti-retroviral drugs to patients in the public health sector. However, in spite of this change in policy the state continued to classify certain people living with HIV/AIDS as ineligible for treatment. In an article in the South African *Sunday Independent* newspaper entitled "ARV roll-out too late for majority of infected," Noelene Barbeau writes that Manto Tshabalala-Msimang, the national health minister, "criticised people who blamed the government for not handing out ARVs to people infected with HIV/AIDS." Tshabalala-Msimang is cited as saying:

> What people fail to realise is that not all of the people infected will receive ARVs, because some of them are too far gone. This is a major problem we are experiencing. People leave HIV testing for far too late. There are 5 million people infected in this country, but we are going to look at the 500 000 who are in need, if and when, we introduce the ARVs. (2004:3)

The Minister of Health's definition of people who are extremely ill with the symptoms of AIDS-related diseases as "too far gone" to receive medical care indicates that people living with HIV/AIDS continue to be positioned outside of the realms within which their right to life would be recognized.[13] Her statement also places the burden of responsibility on those who "leave HIV testing for far too late," in spite of the fact that no matter when they were tested for HIV or how ill they were, prior to November 2003 people living with HIV/AIDS would not have received antiretrovirals in the public health sector.

The discursive construction of people living with HIV/AIDS in South Africa as dying subjects for whom nothing can be done intersects with the primary mode by which AIDS in Africa is represented in the mainstream media in the west. Within such representations the everyday experiences of people living with HIV/AIDS are subsumed by sensationalised depictions of the epidemic; emaciated and diseased bodies, orphans and corpses.

PHOTOGRAPHY AND THE PRODUCTION OF "AFRICAN AIDS"

Within the popular media, photography has played a central role in how AIDS in Africa has come to be imagined and known.

Representations of HIV and AIDS in Africa have primarily focused on the bodies of people in the final stages of AIDS, often with no sign of the context in which they live. Two recent instances are James Nachtwey's photo-essay on AIDS in Africa "Crimes Against Humanity" (2001) in *Time* magazine and Geert van Kesteren and Arthur van Amerongen's collection, *Mwendanjangula! AIDS in Zambia* (2000). In both texts people living with HIV and AIDS are represented without being named and no attempt is made to record and represent the stories of those depicted. In their paper entitled "The Appeal of Experience; The Dismay of Images: Cultural Appropriations of Suffering in Our Times" (1996), Arthur Kleinman and Joan Kleinman observe that images of people in situations of crisis are often presented without reference to the social contexts in which they are situated or to the local and global economic and political forces that determine how such crises unfold. They argue that, while images play an important part in shaping international responses to humanitarian crises, omitting the social worlds of those depicted effectively reduces them to spectacle. The absence of narrative that would serve to situate images like Nachtwey's and van Kesteren's in time and place makes the causes of the epidemic appear inexplicable and positions people living with HIV/AIDS outside of Western modernity. Casting the epidemic in Africa as a natural disaster elides the possibility for the medical interventions that have transformed AIDS into a chronic manageable condition in the West.

In my analysis of the work of Gideon Mendel I show how images of dying Africans have been superseded in his oeuvre by a series of portraits that resemble passport photographs. I argue that this shift is significant in that it confounds the codes of representation through which Africans have been cast always and only as dying, and marks their claim to being recognized as living subjects by society and by the state. In the context of the epidemic in South Africa where denial and stigma has meant that so many people have died of AIDS and quite literally disappeared without a trace, documenting the experiences of people living with HIV/AIDS in ways that recognize their subjectivity is a political act. Mendel's *A Broken Landscape* powerfully evokes the devastating effects of the epidemic on the lives of people living with HIV/AIDS, their families and communities. While Mendel carefully portrays relationships, and in this sense recognizes the humanity of those he depicts, there are several images in the collection of people whose names are omitted, as too are their stories. The suffering of these individuals becomes a sign of a generalized "African" suffering.

However, *A Broken Landscape* also contains several "portraits" that are made up of a series of images of an individual living with HIV/AIDS and those who care for them. There are nineteen pages depicting the life and death of Mzokhona Malevu, a young man who lived in Enseleni Township in South Africa and who was 29 years old when he died in 2000. This series of images, the longest devoted to an individual in the collection, forms an intimate account of the days preceding his death and of the people who loved and cared for him. Of this sequence Mendel states:

> I'm proudest of a story I did this past year on one person, Mzokhona Malevu, a person with AIDS in South Africa. I think I achieved real depth. I began to photograph him in April of 2000. And I went back to visit him and his family on four different occasions over the year, leading up to attending his funeral in December. I made a strong, personal connection with him and his family, who were taking care of him with amazing love within the context of extreme poverty. Mzokhona was living in a three-room squattershack with 21 people. He was open and out about his disease. He had decided that he wanted his funeral to be an AIDS-education event and he made me promise that when he died I would come and take photographs at his funeral. He wanted to tell his story to the world and I was a sort of conduit for him to do it. The quotes which I collected from him, together with the images which tell his story from life to death, make a powerful, personalized statement. (Mendel 2001a)

Mendel's description of his relationship with Malevu and with his family, and the photographs he took of him "which tell his story from life to death," present a clear contrast to many of the other images of unnamed people dying of AIDS in the collection.

The first image in the series depicting Mzokhona Malevu is a formal head and shoulders portrait, one in which the sitter is well aware of being photographed and is posed for the camera (see Exhibit 23.1). Malevu's face and clothing are shown in sharp focus while the background of the image is blurred. His eyes are at the very center of the image and draw the viewer's attention; he appears to be looking out of the photograph, his gaze both haunting and haunted. The poignancy of the image lies in its reappearance in the book a few pages later, in an image that shows Malevu's funeral (see Exhibit 23.2), which appears after several photographs that show Malevu's daily struggles living with AIDS in conditions of extreme economic poverty, of his corpse being prepared for burial, and of his funeral procession. The photograph of the funeral shows the church choir with Malevu's coffin in the foreground. Positioned on top of the coffin is an enlarged, framed reproduction of the portrait that began the sequence of images. The appearance of this photograph within the photograph of Malevu's funeral is a haunting signifier of how, for those living with AIDS without access to treatment, ill health deteriorates rapidly into death. Time has been compressed for Malevu and his passage from life to death radically accelerated.

Malevu's lifespan has been truncated by his death from AIDS but it is also the mode of representation of his experience, one structured by the desire for narrative coherence, which abbreviates his life in this way. The reduction of Malevu's entire life story to a few frames is also that which makes possible the appearance of his story. The narrative of people living with HIV and AIDS in Africa is one that follows a sequential, predictable logic and that always ends in death. The construction of a coherent narrative of "AIDS in

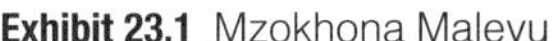
Exhibit 23.1 Mzokhona Malevu

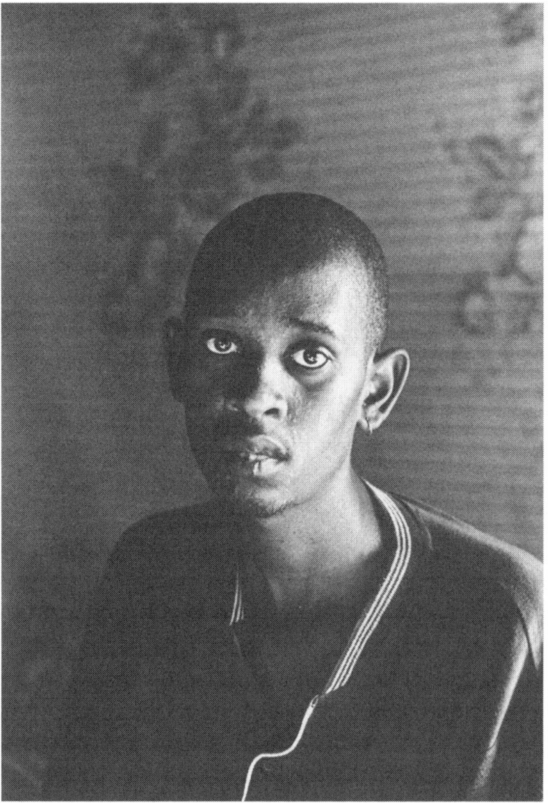

Source: Gideon Mendel

Exhibit 23.2 Malevu's funeral

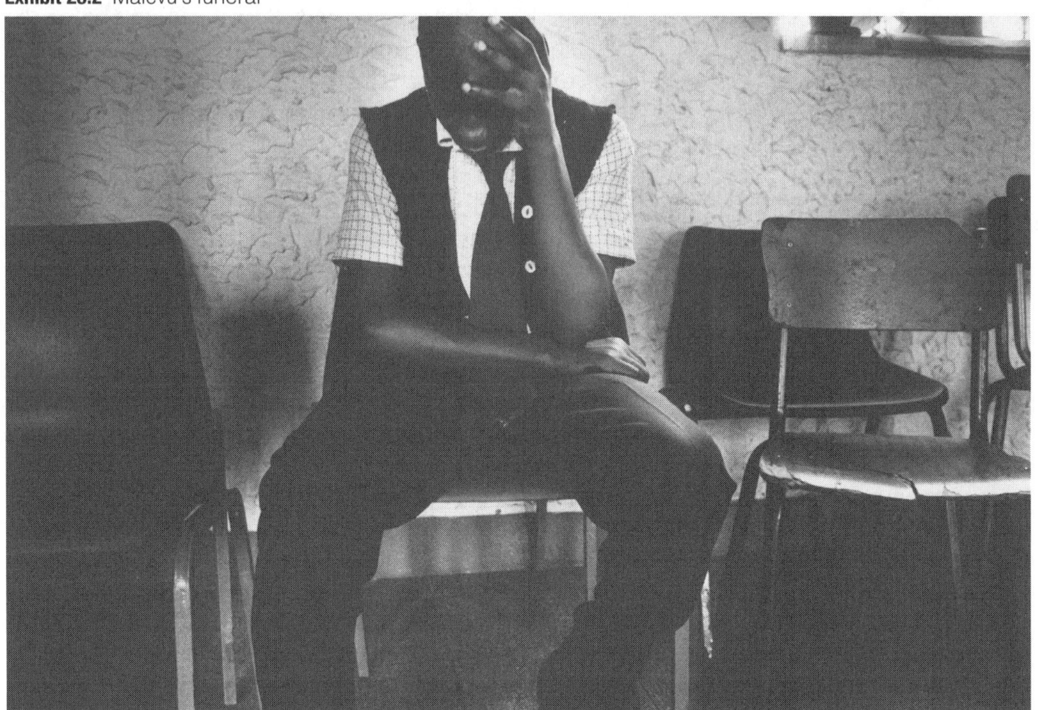

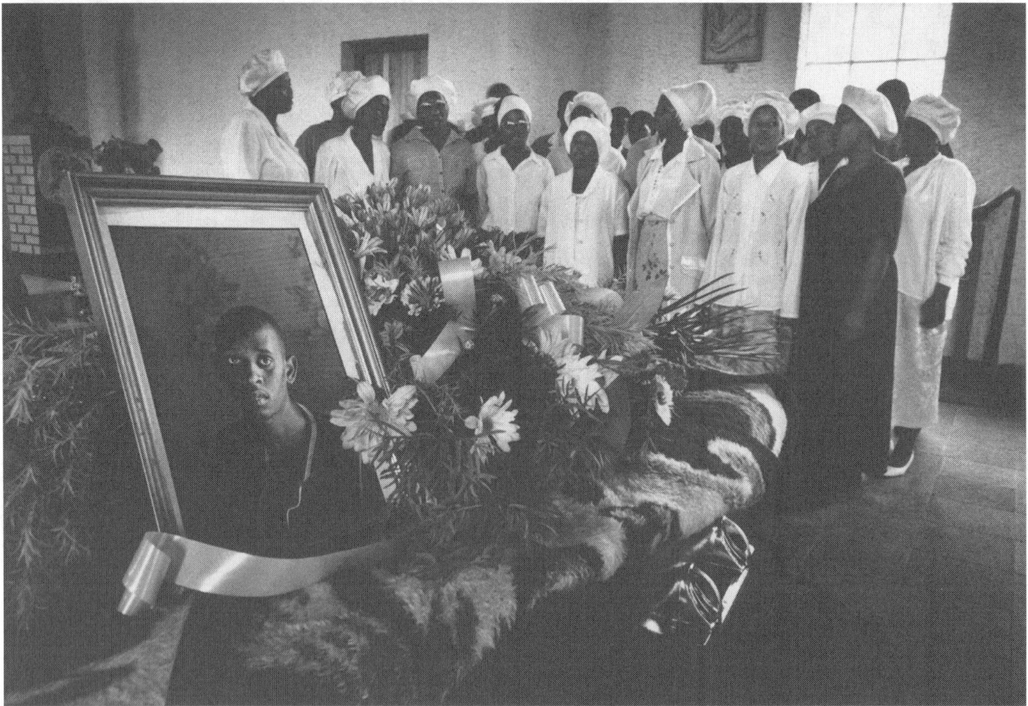

Source: Gideon Mendel

Africa," one that follows a sequential logic that is always resolved in death, restores a mode of rationality in the face of the radical unmaking of HIV and AIDS.

The extended captions that accompany the photographs in this sequence consist of two pages of Malevu's testimony and a one-page account of his death related by Nancy Khuswayo, an AIDS counselor. Mendel's photographs mirror the script of Malevu's testimony. For instance, the last section of Malevu's testimony reads as follows:

> I was given some drugs, which made me feel much better, but I cannot afford them now. I have heard that in overseas countries the government provides drugs and food free for people with AIDS, but here in South Africa there is nothing now. At the clinic they often say there is nothing they can do. You must go home. It is not fair. People overseas can get better from the good drugs they are given, while we in South Africa have to die. (Mendel 2001a:74)

The sequence of images depicting Malevu's life and illness reinforces the notion that his premature death is inevitable. The first image (Exhibit 23.1, discussed above) establishes Malevu as a man condemned, a young man but one who has glimpsed his own death, a tragic image, perhaps only made tragic by what is, inevitably, to come. Two images follow in which Malevu is shown engaged in the everyday life of the well: one an image of Malevu absorbed in a card game surrounded by smiling family members, the other a photograph in which Malevu himself is smiling, his ecstatic face appearing through the space between the arm and the body of a person in the foreground, their body large, dark, and out of focus. These images accentuate the suffering and sorrow that saturate the remaining images in the sequence. The next image is a double-page spread depicting Malevu's sleeping quarters. The photograph shows Malevu in his bed on the far right-hand side of the image; he is awake but appears in a dreamlike state, seemingly unaware of the presence of the photographer. Alongside him on the floor are the seven children with whom he shares his room, sleeping or feigning sleep, one child returning the camera's gaze. The second page of Malevu's testimony appears overleaf:

> My father is employed sometimes doing piecework on construction sites and my mother works as a maid for whites in Richard's Bay. We live in two rooms here. There is my mother, my father, their eight children and 11 grandchildren—21 of us altogether. I sleep on the bed here in this room, with seven children sleeping on the floor next to me. Sometimes we do not have enough food to go round. My father usually bathes me early in the morning before he goes to work, but since recently we have to pay for water which he collects at the communal taps. It is 60 cents for a bucket. Now even some water for washing can be a problem. (Mendel 2001a:74)

The photograph that follows Malevu's testimony is an image of Malevu's father washing his son's head. The next sequence of images portrays Malevu's deteriorating condition, his hospitalization, and the care provided him at home by his brother and sister.

These images are followed by Nancy Khuswayo's testimony, which provides an account of Malevu's death. The photograph on the facing page shows the arms and part of the legs of a man, presumably a coroner or undertaker, crouched behind Malevu's head and laying a sheet over his corpse. Only Malevu's face is visible through a hole in the heavily embroidered cloth. Malevu's lips are slightly parted and stretched over his teeth, their pearlescence and the tiny sliver of whiteness visible just beneath his closed eyelid, the only disruptions to the otherwise extreme contrast between his dark head and the white death-sheet and the white-gloved hands of the coroner, which are shown beside his face. The remaining images depict the funeral procession, Malevu's coffin being carried to the church, a grieving family member, the choir at the funeral with the coffin and portrait of Malevu in the foreground, a keening woman bent double with grief during the funeral service, and, finally, Malevu's father standing in his son's grave (Exhibit 23.3).

While the narrative of Malevu's life and death is overdetermined by the deathly logic of "African AIDS," the sequence also conveys the importance of Mendel's work in making

Exhibit 23.3 Malevu's father in his son's grave

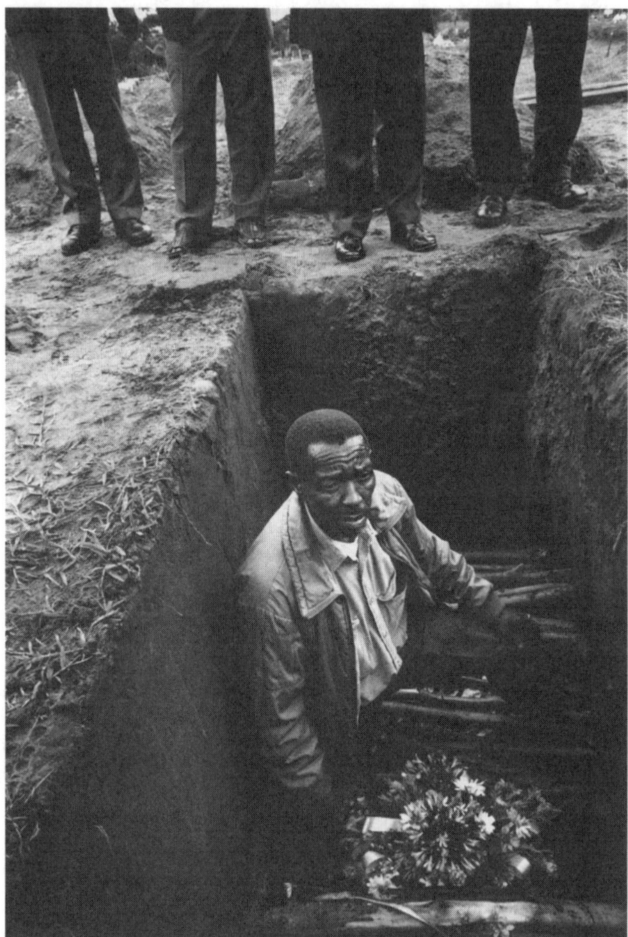

Source: Gideon Mendel

the struggles of people living with HIV/AIDS visible. Many of those living with HIV and dying of AIDS in Africa occupy a space on the social margins and their experiences are all too often invisible. Those who are left behind, frequently the elderly and very young children, often do not possess the means to make their struggles visible nor to mark the deaths of those they have lost in ways that would make them apparent to outsiders. The stigma that continues to be attached to HIV/AIDS has also meant that people's experiences of living with HIV/AIDS have been silenced and their deaths what Judith Butler has termed "publicly ungrievable" (2004). Mendel's photographs bear witness to the magnitude of loss the epidemic has caused.

The role of women as caregivers for those who are ill, as well as for the many children who are orphaned as a result of AIDS, is a central feature of several of the images in the collection. Mendel's portrait of Samkelisiwe Mkhwanazi is also a portrait of her mother and primary caregiver, Nesta, whose narrative is included alongside the testimony of her daughter. Her account, like many others in the text, relates how the burden of care for those who are ill has fallen on already impoverished families. *A Broken Landscape* also includes photographs of HIV/AIDS educators and counselors, schoolchildren who have started "Anti-AIDS clubs" in Zambia, traditional healers and religious leaders who have spoken out about the effects of the epidemic. These images, along with the photograph of AIDS activists at a protest march in South Africa, offer insight into local responses to the epidemic. Although their inclusion provides a more hopeful and complex perspective on the epidemic, these images appear at the end of the book after many images of people who are sick and dying. While *A Broken Landscape* testifies to the strength and courage of people living with HIV/AIDS and those who care for them in spite of extremely difficult circumstances, the cumulative effect of the photographs is a sense of despair.

In 2002 Mendel began work on a new series of images that moves away from his earlier work, which depicted people as helpless in the face of AIDS. The shift in Mendel's photographic practice reflects the changes that have occurred in South Africa as AIDS activists began to challenge the state and to transform how people living with HIV/AIDS are perceived.

REPRESENTING RESISTANCE

One of the last images in *A Broken Landscape* shows a group of South African AIDS activists holding hands and toyi-toying at a march at the International AIDS Conference held in Durban in 2000 (Exhibit 23.4). Alongside the image is a statement by Zackie Achmat, the chairperson of the South African HIV/AIDS activist movement, the Treatment Action Campaign (TAC):

> The importance of this march historically is that it helped to change international perceptions. The image of AIDS in Africa is usually one of powerless people, emaciated and dying. What the march showed is that there are many of us who are healthy and fighting to stay healthy. (Mendel 2001a:194)

Mendel's photograph of the march captures the energy and vitality of the activists, all of whom are wearing T-shirts issued by TAC that read "H.I.V. Positive," and who are actively campaigning for their rights as citizens to be recognized. It presents a very different perspective on HIV/AIDS in Africa from most of the other images in the book and powerfully conveys how TAC has created the space for the emergence of new and "positive" HIV-positive identities.

TAC was formed in 1998 and from its inception began to call on the state to develop and implement a comprehensive national treatment plan for people living with HIV/AIDS. Like ACTUP in the United States in the 1990s, TAC has played a crucial role in asserting the presence of people living with HIV/AIDS in a context of silence and shame. TAC has drawn on the legacy of the mass democratic movements formed during the struggle against apartheid and has successfully drawn international attention to the crisis of HIV/AIDS in South Africa. TAC has also made use of the transformed South African justice system to secure a number of important victories against the state. In 2001 TAC took the South African government to court over the issue of the provision of treatment to prevent the transmission of HIV from mother to child. TAC argued that pregnant women had a constitutional right to reproductive health care and the Pretoria High Court ordered the state to provide Nevirapine as a matter of urgency.[14] The government elected to appeal the decision in the Constitutional Court, but lost the appeal. TAC has played a crucial part in ensuring that the rights of South Africans living with HIV/AIDS are recognized and their campaign for access to treatment has also led to a marked shift in the ways in which people living with HIV/AIDS are represented.

In December 2001 *A Broken Landscape* was exhibited at the National Gallery in Cape Town as part of the "Positive Lives" exhibition. During the course of the show, which ran until April 2002, Mendel began work on a new series of images that reflected the changes that were occurring in South Africa as AIDS activists began to challenge the state and to reconfigure how people living with HIV and AIDS were perceived. These images move away from what art historian Svea Josephy, referring to *A Broken Landscape*, describes as a mode of "social documentary in its most conventionalised and traditional form" (Josephy 2005:8). In his new work, a series of portraits of people living with HIV and AIDS who have access to antiretroviral therapy through the Médecins Sans Frontières (MSF) clinic in Khayelitsha, an informal settlement outside of the city of Cape Town, and through clinical trials in

Exhibit 23.4 AIDS activists at the International AIDS Conference, Durban, 2000

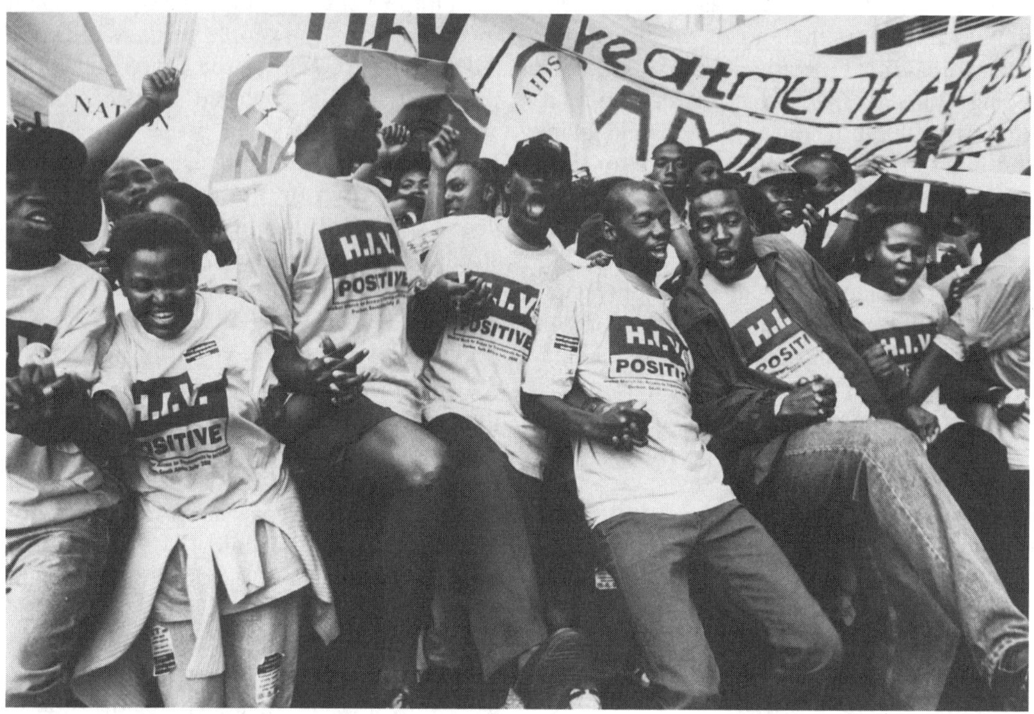

Source: Gideon Mendel

Cape Town itself, Mendel makes use of color, draws attention to the fact that the photographs are constructed, and emphasizes personal testimony.

Access to antiretroviral therapy changes the ways in which people living with HIV/AIDS are seen and also affects how people living with HIV/AIDS see themselves. Some of these shifts in individual understandings of living with HIV/AIDS are made clear in Mendel's images of people who have access to antiretroviral therapy. The people Mendel photographed were among the first in the country to access treatment outside of the private health sector. At this time high-ranking government officials were contesting both the efficacy and safety of antiretroviral drugs. Universal access to treatment for South Africans living with HIV/AIDS seemed very remote. In 2002 there were an estimated 400,000 people living in Khayelitsha, of which approximately 40,000 people were living with HIV/AIDS. MSF began their work in Khayelitsha in 1999 and set up three HIV/AIDS clinics in 2000. By the middle of 2002, MSF were treating 177 people with antiretroviral drugs.[15]

Mendel's images were intended to highlight the work of MSF and of TAC and to "both challenge the images on the walls [the photographs that constitute 'A Broken Landscape'] and explore new ways of depicting people living with HIV/AIDS" (artist's statement 2002:24). The contrast between Mendel's photographs of people who have access to treatment and his earlier work is striking. Mendel's new images are full-color portraits, each of which is accompanied by a personal narrative account that forms a central component of the image. As Josephy notes, the inclusion of testimony in Mendel's work can be connected to a more general foregrounding of narrative in cultural practice in South Africa after the Truth and Reconciliation Commission.

The change in Mendel's practice can also be understood as a response to the ways in which TAC has contested representations that cast people living with HIV/AIDS as passive victims. Of particular importance is the way in which Mendel's new works were taken. Mendel created large frames using gaffer tape and invited his subjects to position themselves within the frames in the way in which they wished to be seen. Many people chose to look directly at the camera, rejecting the conventions of traditional documentary photography and effectively returning the gaze of both the photographer and viewer. In her essay "Departures," Josephy traces how documentary photographic practice in South Africa has changed since the end of apartheid and observes that Mendel's images can be situated "somewhere between the realm of portraits and documentary (or perhaps 'self-portraits' in the sense that they reference an African tradition of studio photography where the sitter plays a crucial role in the construction of his/her identity)" (2005:8).

Mendel's use of testimony and color and the participation of those depicted in determining how they are represented contribute to the sense that people are shown to be living with HIV rather than dying of AIDS. And, indeed, as people who have access to antiretroviral therapy, the lives and stories of those who feature in Mendel's recent work are markedly different from those who do not. Their sense of being among the chosen few emerges through their testimonies, many of which valorize both TAC and MSF.

Each person's narrative recounts their experience of being extremely ill and being returned to life from the brink of death once they began to take antiretroviral drugs. What is striking about these accounts is how well versed each person is about both the medical aspects of their condition and the contested terrain of treatment access in South Africa. One of the images is of Nontsikelo Zwedala, a young woman who has access to treatment for three years through a clinical trial. She states:

> I believe the government should provide treatment for everybody. Thabo Mbeki should know that HIV causes AIDS, and it is killing people. He should know that it can be treated to allow people to live a long life with HIV. He must not stick on the resistance and side effects only. If he cannot afford to buy the treatment from the pharmaceutical companies he must talk to them to lower their prices because I know their prices are much too high now. There are options like generic producing and parallel importing. He can reduce military spending because there is no war in South Africa but people are dying of AIDS.

Zwedala, like many of those who had access to antiretroviral therapy prior to the inception of the state antiretroviral program, is a member of TAC. In the context of South Africa in 2002, where so few people living with HIV/AIDS had access to the treatment and care they required, beginning to take antiretroviral drugs and becoming an activist were often related processes. This arose because of the highly politicized debate about access to treatment in South Africa that left people living with HIV/AIDS no option but to campaign for their rights to be recognized, and as a result of the close association between MSF and TAC. The existence of TAC has led to the formation of coherent activist identities that powerfully counter stereotypical perceptions of people living with HIV/AIDS.

The pervasiveness of people's sense of the importance in raising awareness about the effectiveness of antiretroviral therapy is made clear through Mendel's portrait of a man who has not publicly disclosed his HIV positive status. The image shows his outstretched arm with his drug-adherence sheet in his hand and is accompanied by his narrative that intersects with the rhetoric of HIV/AIDS activism in South Africa. He states: "I choose to show my daily drug-adherence sheet, which I have to fill in every time I take my medication. People must know that a poor person like me living in a shack can take these drugs properly. They are my chance to live." His narrative reveals his knowledge of his condition and his familiarity with antiretroviral drug regimens:

> Tygerberg referred me to MSF here in Khayelitsha and they started looking after me with anti-retrovirals. At that point my CD4 count was 38. I had full-blown AIDS; my viral load was 1,2 million. I was given AZT and 3TC with nevirapine but I began getting a blood problem so I was changed from AZT to ddI with d4T and Efavirenz. This combination is working for me now. My weight then was very

> low. It was 38kg; but now it is 57kg. I had a lot of memory loss but my memory has come back. My viral load is now undetectable and I will get my new CD4 count results next week. These drugs have made a huge difference in my life.

Access to antiretroviral drugs significantly affects how people experience their condition—AIDS is no longer understood as a death sentence but as a chronic manageable illness, just as it is for people living with HIV/AIDS in the West. The movement for treatment access in South Africa has led to the emergence of a growing number of people living with HIV/AIDS who are resisting local and global injustice and who are determined to fight to stay alive. The courage of such people is transforming how HIV/AIDS in South Africa is both seen and lived.

NOTES

1. See Schneider and Fassin (2002) for an overview of some of the debates about HIV and AIDS in South Africa.
2. See the work of Jane Evelyn Atwood, whose photograph of "Jean Louis" appeared in *Paris Match* in 1987 and was the first publicly circulated image of a person living with AIDS in France. Maggie Steiber and J.B. Diederich photographed people living with HIV and AIDS in Haiti and in the United States. Alon Reininger, Dilip Mehta (who photographed Ryan White), Nan Goldin, and Frank Fournier were among the first photographers to document the epidemic. Reininger was also one of the first photojournalists to photograph people living with HIV and AIDS in southern Africa. Others to have worked in the region include James Nachtwey, Nick Danziger, Don McCullin, David Chancellor and Kristen Ashburn. See also Jeffrey Barbee's images of people living with HIV and AIDS in Swaziland and the work of Jide Adeniyi-Jones in Nigeria.
3. Mendel won the W. Eugene Smith Grant in Humanistic Photography in 1996. His photographs depicting people living with HIV and AIDS in Africa have been exhibited across the world. His work appeared in *National Geographic* (September 2005) and often appears in the English *Guardian* newspaper.
4. Among the foundational texts that consider the effects of representation on the course of the HIV/AIDS epidemic, see *AIDS: Cultural Analysis Cultural Activism* (1991), edited by Douglas Crimp, Ross Chambers' *Facing It* (1998), and Simon Watney's *Policing Desire* (1987). For an excellent overview of the history of the representation of the epidemic in Europe and North America, see Gabriele Griffin's *Representations of HIV/AIDS* (2000). For work that focuses specifically on representations of Africa and HIV/AIDS, see Watney's essay "Missionary Positions: AIDS, 'Africa' and race" in his collection, *Practices of Freedom* (1994), and Richard Chirimuuta and Rosalind Chirimuuta's book, *AIDS, Africa and Racism* (1989).
5. Douglas Webb, *HIV and AIDS in Africa* (1997:23).
6. Douglas Webb, *HIV and AIDS in Africa*, 1997:74.
7. In his essay, "Renegotiating Masculinity in the South African Lowveld: Male–Male Sex in Compounds, Prisons and at Home," (2001) Isak Niehaus notes that in 1987 nine people in South African prisons were found to be HIV-positive people and two people had AIDS. They were placed in isolation.
8. Webb cites Van Niftrik, who writes of the campaign depicting coffins in graves, "the general perception seemed to be that the scene portrayed victims of political violence" (1997:73).
9. Webb notes the use of Depo-Provera contraceptive injections as a form of "population control" in Namibia (1997:74) and Whiteside and Sunter state that at the Truth and Reconciliation hearings it emerged that HIV was used as a weapon by the apartheid state when HIV positive askaris were instructed to infect sex workers (2002:65).
10. Alan Whiteside and Clem Sunter, *AIDS: The Challenge for South Africa* (2002:63).
11. As Whiteside and Sunter note, HIV prevalence rates are similar in rural and urban areas in South Africa, while in African countries to the north, rural areas tend to have lower prevalence rates (2002:53). Large numbers of workers from other countries in southern Africa also formed part of the mobile labor force in South Africa. Botswana, Lesotho, Swaziland, Mozambique, and Zimbabwe all have extremely high HIV prevalence rates.
12. See, for example, the Department of Health's TB and HIV/AIDS newsletter published on their website: http://www.doh.gov.za.
13. While a category of those who are too ill to be helped by medical treatment may exist within in the medical sphere, no such category should exist in the political realm.
14. See Nawaal Deane, "AIDS: TAC vs State," *Mail and Guardian*, November 21–29, 2001, and Belinda Beresford, "Bittersweet Little Pill," *Mail and Guardian*, December 7–13, 2001.
15. "Community Anti-Retroviral Therapy: the Khayelitsha Experience," presentation at the University of Cape Town Medical School by Eric Goemare, director of MSF in South Africa, June 20, 2002.

REFERENCES AND FURTHER READING

Barbeau, Noelene. "ARV rollout too late for majority of infected." *Sunday Independent*, January 11, 2004.

Beresford, Belinda. "Bittersweet little pill." *Mail and Guardian*, December 7–13, 2001.

Butler, Judith. *Precarious Life: The Powers of Mourning and Violence*. London: Verso, 2004.

Campbell, Catherine. " 'Going underground and going after women': Masculinity and HIV transmission amongst black workers on the gold mines." In *Changing Men in Southern Africa*, Robert Morrell (ed.). Pietermaritzburg: University of Natal Press and London: Zed Books, 2001.

Chambers, Ross. *Facing It: AIDS Diaries and the Death of the Author*. Ann Arbor: University of Michigan Press, 1998.

Chirimuuta, Richard and Rosalind Chirimuuta. *AIDS, Africa and Racism*. London: Free Association Books, 1989.

Crimp, Douglas (ed.) *AIDS: Cultural Analysis Cultural Activism*. Cambridge, MA: MIT Press, 1991.

Deane, Nawaal. "AIDS: TAC vs state." *Mail and Guardian*, November 21–29, 2001.

Goemare, Eric. "Community anti-retroviral therapy: the Khayelitsha experience." Paper presented at the University of Cape Town Medical School, June 20, 2002.

Griffin, Gabriele. *Representations of HIV and AIDS: Visibility Blues*. Manchester: Manchester University Press, 2000.

Grover, Jan Zita. "AIDS: key words." In *AIDS: Cultural Analysis Cultural Activism*, Douglas Crimp (ed.). Cambridge, MA: MIT Press, 1991.

Josephy, Svea. "Departures." In *The Cape Town Month of Photography 2005*, Geoffrey Grundlingh (ed.). Cape Town: The South African Centre for Photography, 2005.

Kleinman, Arthur and Joan Kleinman. "The appeal of experience; the dismay of images: Cultural appropriations of suffering in our times." *Daedalus*. 125, 1 (1996): 1–24.

Mendel, Gideon. *A Broken Landscape*. London: Network Photographers, 2001a.

Mendel, Gideon. "Gideon Mendel." *The Digital Journalist: AIDS and Photography*. 2001b. www.digitaljournalist.org.

Mendel, Gideon. "They have given me life." *Mail and Guardian*, February 15–21, 2002, 24–25.

Nachtwey, James. "Crimes against humanity." *Time*, 157 (6), February 12, 2001.

Niehaus, Isak. "Renegotiating masculinity in the South African Lowveld: male–male sex in compounds, prisons and at home." Paper presented at the Conference for Social Research on HIV/AIDS, University of Witwatersrand, Johannesburg, 2001.

Schneider, Helen, and Didier Fassin. "Denial and defiance: a socio-political analysis of AIDS in South Africa." *AIDS*, 16 (2002): 45–51.

van Kesteren, Geert and Arthur van Amerongen. *Mwendanjangula! AIDS in Zambia*. Amsterdam: Mets and Schilts and Cape Town: David Philip, 2000.

Watney, Simon. *Policing Desire: Pornography, AIDS and the Media*. London: Methuen, 1987.

Watney, Simon. *Practices of Freedom: Selected Writings on HIV/AIDS*. London: Rivers Oram Press, 1994.

Webb, Douglas. *HIV and AIDS in Africa*. London: Pluto Press, 1997.

Whiteside, Alan and Clem Sunter. *AIDS: The Challenge for South Africa*. Cape Town: Human and Rosseau and Cape Town: Tafelberg, 2002.

Worden, Nigel. *The Making of Modern South Africa: Conquest, Segregation and Apartheid*. Oxford: Blackwell, 1995.

CHAPTER 24

Sex, Soap, and Social Change

The Sabido Methodology of Behavior Change Communication

Kriss Barker

ABSTRACT

The Sabido methodology for development of mass media entertainment-education serial dramas is designed according to elements of communication and behavioral theories for reinforcing prosocial attitudes and for motivating behavior change. These dramas communicate at the emotional level as well as the cognitive level, and further establish the conditions for social learning to take place. This chapter explores why the Sabido theory-based communication methodology has been so successful and how it differs from other entertainment-education approaches. What does the future hold for the application of the Sabido methodology to rethinking the foundation of comprehensive behavior change communication programs?

The Sabido methodology is an approach to development of mass-media serial dramas. However, unlike typical "soap operas," Sabido-style serial dramas are not used to sell sex or soap, but rather social change.

In this chapter I explore the Sabido methodology and why this theory-based approach to behavior change communication has been so successful. How do Sabido-style serial dramas differ from "soaps" and how does the Sabido methodology differ from other entertainment-education approaches? Why do audiences from the Philippines to India, from Tanzania to Ethiopia, and from Mexico to Bolivia find these dramas irresistible—and much more than merely educating in an entertaining way? And what does the future hold for the application of the Sabido methodology to rethinking the very foundation of comprehensive behavior change communication programs?

MIGUEL SABIDO: "ENTERTAINMENT WITH PROVEN SOCIAL BENEFIT"

Miguel Sabido was Vice President for Research at Televisa (Mexican television) during the 1970s, 1980s, and 1990s. While at Televisa, Sabido developed a theoretical model for eliciting prosocial attitudinal, informational, and behavioral change through commercial television programming. He called this model "entertainment with proven social benefit."

Between 1973 and 1981, Miguel Sabido produced six social content serial dramas in Mexico.[1] During the decade 1977 to 1986, when many of these Mexican soap operas were on the air, the country underwent a 34 percent decline in its population growth rate. As a result, in May 1986, the United Nations Population Prize was presented to Mexico as the foremost population success story in the world.

Thomas Donnelly, then with USAID in Mexico, wrote, "Throughout Mexico, wherever one travels, when people are asked where they heard about family planning, or what made them decide to practice family planning, the response is universally attributed to one of the soap operas that *Televisa* has done . . . The *Televisa* family planning soap operas have made the single most powerful contribution to the Mexican population success story."

> Mkwaju is a truck driver along the national routes in Tanzania. Although Mkwaju is married, he has many "girlfriends" along his route—he is quite the sexual athlete. Tunu, Mkwaju's subservient wife, stays at home to care for their children. She is becoming more and more frustrated with her husband's antics, especially the way he squanders his earnings on women and alcohol. She finally decides to take things into her own hands, and starts her own small business, selling vegetables in the market. The business does well, thus giving Tunu the self-confidence to leave Mkwaju. Mkwaju contracts HIV as a result of his high-risk lifestyle, and eventually develops symptoms of AIDS. In an act of compassion, Tunu cares for him until he dies. But, his legacy lives on through his son, Kibuyu, who is beginning to follow in his father's footsteps. He regularly smokes marijuana with his friends on the outskirts of the city, and steals money from unsuspecting passers-by. Will Kibuyu suffer the same fate as his father? Or, will he learn from his mother how to succeed in life? (Haji: 2004)

The above excerpt from *Twende na Wakati* (*Let's Go with the Times*), a radio serial drama broadcast twice weekly over Radio Tanzania, demonstrates the power of the Sabido methodology. The program was evaluated using an experimental design, pre- and post-intervention measurements of dependent variables, and measurement triangulation using an independent data source to provide more definitive evidence of the effects of the strategy on behavior change (Rogers et al. 1999). It was the first evaluation of an entertainment-education program to apply all three of these evaluation measures at a national level (Rogers et al. 1999).

RESULTS OF *TWENDE NA WAKATI*

Beginning in July 1993, Radio Tanzania broadcast *Twende na Wakati* twice weekly during prime time (at 6:30 P.M.) for thirty minutes. The radio station at Dodoma, however, did not broadcast this program, and instead broadcast locally produced programs at this time, thus serving as the comparison area in the field experiment (see Exhibit 24.1). However, the Dodoma area received all other elements of the national family planning program, including several other radio programs. Then, in September 1995, after two years of broadcasts, Radio Tanzania began broadcasting *Twende na Wakati* in the Dodoma area, starting with the first episode (Rogers et al. 1999).

By the end of 1993, *Twende na Wakati* was the most popular radio program in Tanzania, with 57 percent of the radio population listening. Independent research by the University of New Mexico and the Population Family Life Education Programme of the Government of Tanzania measured the effects caused by the program with regard to such issues as AIDS prevention behavior, ideal age of marriage for women, and use of family planning (Rogers et al. 1999; Vaughan et al. 2000). Though the population of the Dodoma comparison area was more urban than the rest of the country, a multiple regression analysis eliminated the influence such differences might have accounted for (such as increased access to information and services, higher income or educational levels, etc.). Nationwide random sample surveys of 2,750 people were conducted before, during, and after the broadcast of the program. Data were also collected from the AIDS Control Program of the government, the Ministry of Health, and the Demographic and Health Survey, all of which reinforced the findings of significant impacts on attitudes and behavior (Rogers et al. 1999; Vaughan et al. 2000; Vaughan and Rogers 2000).

Among the findings were: a significant increase in the percentage of the population who perceive that they may be at risk of HIV infection; an increase in people's belief that they can take effective action to prevent HIV/

Exhibit 24.1 Map of Tanzania showing broadcast and non-broadcast areas for *Twende na Wakati*

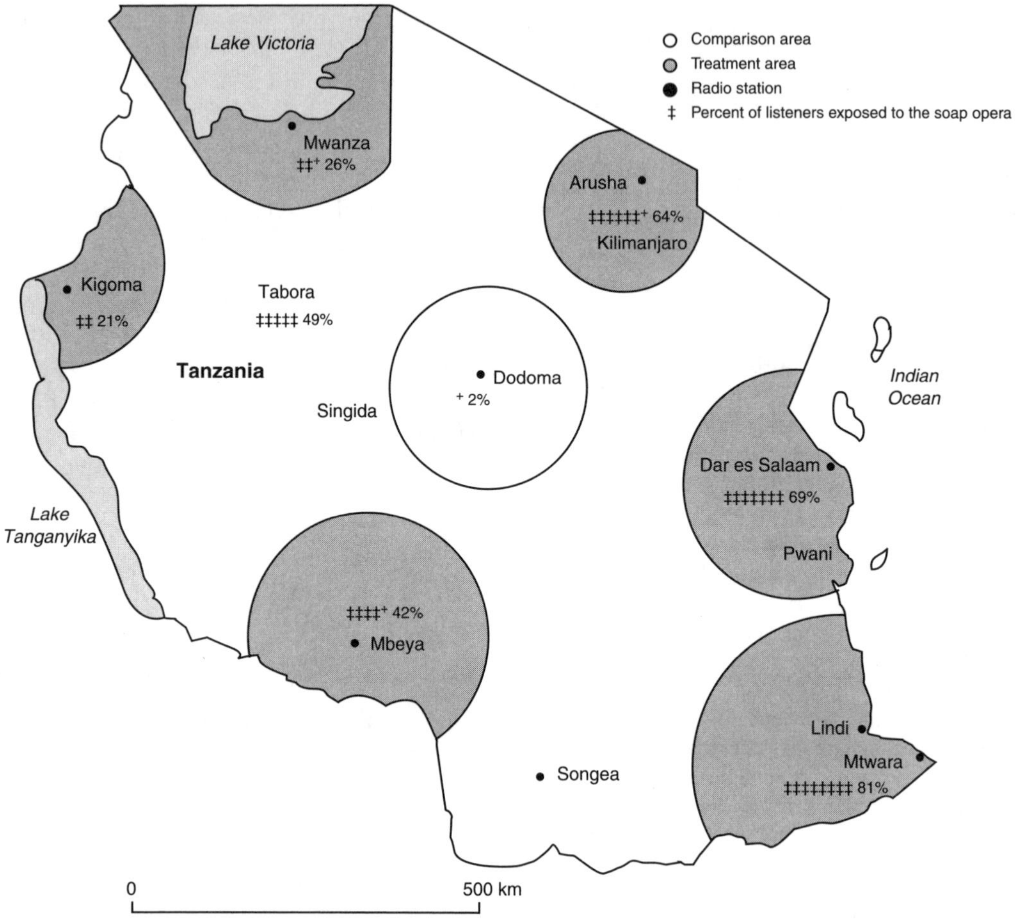

Source: Rogers et al. (1999)

AIDS; an increase in interpersonal communication about HIV/AIDS; an increase in the belief that individuals, rather than their deity or fate, can determine how many children they will have; an increase in the belief that children in small families have better lives than children in large families; and an increase in the percentage of respondents who approve of family planning (Rogers et al. 1999; Vaughan et al. 2000; Vaughan and Rogers 2000).

The study also provided evidence that the Tanzanian radio serial stimulated important behavioral changes. Of the listeners surveyed, 82 percent said the program had caused them to change their own behavior to avoid HIV infection, through limiting the number of sexual partners and through condom use. Independent data from the AIDS Control Program of the government of Tanzania showed a 153 percent increase in condom distribution in the broadcast areas during the first year of the serial drama, while condom distribution in the Dodoma non-broadcast area increased only 16 percent in the same time period (Vaughan et al. 2000).

The program was also effective in promoting family planning. There was a strong positive relationship between listenership levels by district and the change in the percentage of men and women who were currently using any family planning method. The research also showed an increase in the percentage of Tanzanians in the areas of the broadcast who discussed family planning with their spouses. The program also had a significant effect in raising the ideal age of marriage for women and the ideal age of first pregnancy (Rogers et al. 1999; Singhal and Rogers 1999).

Because of its experimental design, the evaluation results were able to disaggregate the effects of the radio serial drama from other family planning promotion and HIV/AIDS prevention programs being implemented throughout Tanzania. In regions where *Twende na Wakati* was broadcast, the percentage of married women who were currently using a family planning method increased 10 percentage points in the first two years of the program, while that percentage stayed flat in the Dodoma non-broadcast area during the time the program was not broadcast there. Then, when the program was broadcast in Dodoma, the contraceptive prevalence rate there increased 16 percentage points. In regions where the program was broadcast, the average number of new family planning adopters per clinic, in a sample of twenty-one clinics, increased by 32 percent from June 1993 (the month before the show began airing) to December 1994. Over the same period, the average number of new adopters at clinics in the Dodoma area remained essentially flat (Rogers et al. 1999).

Independent data from Ministry of Health clinics showed that 41 percent of new adopters of family planning methods were influenced by the serial drama to seek family planning. This percentage included 25 percent who cited the serial drama by name when asked why they had come to the clinic, and another 16 percent who cited "something on the radio" and then identified the serial drama when shown a list of programs currently on the air. Another family planning serial drama using a different methodology that was broadcast nationwide by Radio Tanzania at the same time was cited by just 11 percent of new family planning adopters at the same Ministry of Health clinics (Rogers et al. 1999).

Counting all the costs of the radio serial, the cost per new adopter of family planning was just under 80¢ (U.S.). The cost per person who changed behavior to avoid HIV/AIDS was 8¢ (U.S.) (Rogers et al. 1999; Vaughan and Rogers 2000).

RESULTS OF *YEKEN KIGNIT* (ETHIOPIA)

More recently, Population Media Center (PMC) produced a radio serial drama in Ethiopia using the Sabido methodology for behavior change communication. The program *Yeken Kignit* (*Looking Over One's Daily Life*) was broadcast in the Amharic language over Radio Ethiopia in 257 episodes between June 2, 2002 and November 27, 2004. *Yeken Kignit* addressed issues of reproductive health and women's status, including HIV/AIDS, family planning, marriage by abduction, education of daughters, spousal communication, and related issues.

To monitor results of the program during broadcast, PMC conducted three rounds of facility assessments (client exit interviews) in forty-eight health clinics during 2003 and 2004. The first facility assessment was completed in February 2003 and consisted of interviews with 4,084 clients. The second assessment, which included interviews with 4,858 clients, was completed in April 2004. The third round was completed in November 2004, and included interviews with 3,649 clients (Population Media Center—Ethiopia 2004a).

Each succeeding assessment report showed an increase in the percentage of both male and female clients citing radio as the primary motivating factor in seeking health services: for example, only 6.3 percent of all clients in the first assessment (February 2003) cited radio as the primary motivation for seeking services; this proportion had grown to 18.8 percent by the third assessment in November 2004 (Population Media Center—Ethiopia 2004a).

Among those who cited radio as the primary motivation to seek services, there was an increase in the percentage of clients who cited *Yeken Kignit* by name. By the time of the third assessment, 84 percent cited *Yeken Kignit*, an increase of 16 percentage points from the first assessment. There was a concurrent *decrease* of 16 percentage points among those clients who named any other radio program on the air.

One reason for the decrease between the second and third assessments in the percentage of clients naming *Yeken Kignit* as their primary motivation to seek services was the increase in the percentage citing a second PMC serial drama, *Dhimbibba*, which was in the Oromiffa language. Between the second and third assessments, the percentage naming *Dhimbibba* rose from 3.7 percent to 11.3 percent. Other than PMC's programs, by the time of the third assessment only 4.4 percent of clients named any of the other programs on Radio Ethiopia (Population Media Center—Ethiopia 2004a).

An independent research firm conducted an evaluation of the impact of *Yeken Kignit* in December 2004 (Population Media Center—Ethiopia 2004b). Preliminary findings from this study show significant results in terms of family planning and HIV/AIDS knowledge. The results also showed evidence of behavior change: most notably in terms of use of family planning methods, and in willingness to be tested for HIV. In most cases, there were significant differences in these knowledge and behavior change measures between listeners and non-listeners of *Yeken Kignit*, showing that the program had a differential effect on knowledge and behavior between listeners and non-listeners.

For example, among married women who are listeners to *Yeken Kignit*, current use of any family planning method increased from 12.3 percent to 43.5 percent (a 31.2 percentage point increase). Among non-listeners, use increased from 12.3 percent to 31.1 percent, an increase of only 18.8 percentage points. Among married men who are listeners to *Yeken Kignit*, current use of any method increased from 18.1 percent to 42.4 percent, an increase of 24.3 percentage points. Among non-listeners, use increased by only 14.6 percentage points (Population Media Center—Ethiopia 2004b).

Current use of modern family planning methods also increased significantly among listeners, compared to non-listeners. For example, use of a modern method of family planning by married women who are listeners to *Yeken Kignit* increased from 11.7 percent to 40.2 percent, a 28.5 percentage point change. Among non-listeners, use increased by only 18.2 percentage points (from 11.7 percent to 29.9 percent). Among married men who are listeners to *Yeken Kignit*, current use of modern methods increased from 15.6 percent to 41.3 percent, an increase of 25.7 percentage points. Among non-listeners, use increased by only 15.1 percentage points (Population Media Center—Ethiopia 2004b).

The evaluation also measured differences in ever use of family planning among listeners and non-listeners. Among listeners, ever use among married women increased from 26.9 percent at baseline to 79.0 percent (an increase of 52.1 percentage points). Among non-listeners, ever use increased by only 20.5 percentage points, from 26.9 percent to 47.4 percent. Among married men who are listeners to *Yeken Kignit*, ever use increased from 26.9 percent to 69.6 percent, an increase of 42.7 percentage points. Among non-listeners, ever use increased by only 17.5 percentage points (Population Media Center—Ethiopia 2004b).

The percentage of respondents who know how to determine HIV sero-status increased considerably after listening to *Yeken Kignit*. The proportion of those who said that there is "no way to determine" one's HIV status declined from 37.3 percent among women and 34.1 percent among men to 9.8 percent and 8.6 percent, respectively, after listening to *Yeken Kignit*. The proportion reporting that a blood test is a means to determine one's HIV status increased by 51.4 and 37.5 percentage points, respectively, for women and men (Population Media Center—Ethiopia 2004b).

The percentage of people who had taken a blood test for HIV after listening to *Yeken Kignit* more than tripled for women (from 7.1 percent to 28.8 percent), and more than quadrupled for men (from 6.6 percent to 28.4 percent). The percentage of respondents who had not yet been tested but were willing to be tested also increased—by 11.4 percentage points for women (from 56.8 percent to 68.2 percent), and by 22 percentage points for men (from 54.6 percent to 76.6 percent) (Population Media Center—Ethiopia 2004b).

THE SABIDO METHODOLOGY: AN EMPIRICAL AND REPRODUCIBLE APPROACH TO ENTERTAINMENT-EDUCATION

Twende na Wakati and *Yeken Kignit* produced such impressive behavior change results because they were designed using the Sabido methodology, which uses elements of communication and behavioral theories to reinforce specific values, attitudes, and behaviors (Nariman 1993; Singhal and Rogers 2002). As mentioned above, another radio serial drama, which was developed using a different methodology, was broadcast over the same period in Tanzania as *Twende na Wakati*—with significantly less impact.

Thus, the results described above demonstrate how important the design of the serial drama is to success in terms of behavior change. Sabido-style serial dramas achieve results because they are developed using an empirical and reproducible approach to behavior change communication via mass media. In fact, every detail of a Sabido-style serial drama is developed according to a theoretical and empirical research-based formula in order to reinforce a coherent set of interrelated values that is tied to specific prosocial behaviors. The Sabido methodology is also a replicable methodology that, although formularized, is still adaptable to the individual values and cultures of each country where it is used (Singhal and Rogers 2002).

The Sabido methodology is based on theoretical and social research which is used to develop mass media serial dramas that are based on the realities that people in the audience face daily. These dramas communicate at the emotional level as well as the cognitive level, and further establish the conditions for social learning to take place. Sabido-style serial dramas portray role models who realistically learn to live more fulfilling personal and interpersonal lives (Singhal and Rogers 2002).

The Sabido methodology is a comprehensive approach for reinforcing prosocial attitudes and for motivating behavior change using mass media channels. Sabido's approach comprises a theoretical dimension as well as methodologies for formative and summative evaluation research that are adaptable to varied commercial media and national infrastructures (Singhal and Rogers 2002).

The major tenet of the Sabido methodology is that education does not have to be boring—and that entertainment can be educational. Sabido originally termed his approach "entertainment with proven social benefit." Since then, many communication professionals and scholars have applied the term "entertainment-education" to the Sabido approach. However, the Sabido methodology is more than mere entertainment-education (Singhal and Rogers 1999; 2002).

Let us begin by defining entertainment-education, and then explain how the Sabido methodology differs from this approach.

> Entertainment-education is defined as the process of purposely designing and implementing a media message to both entertain and educate, in order to increase audience members' knowledge about an educational issue, create favorable attitudes, shift social norms, and change overt behavior. (Singhal and Rogers 1999: 9)

Singhal and Rogers further define entertainment-education as a performance which captures the interest or attention of an individual, giving them pleasure, amusement, or gratification while simultaneously helping the individual to develop a skill or to achieve a particular end by boosting his/her mental, moral or physical powers (Singhal and Rogers 1999). A common goal of entertainment-education programs is to entertain and educate audiences in order to catalyze social change in a socially desirable manner.

Since the 1980s, the entertainment-education strategy has been used in over two hundred health intervention programs in over fifty countries in Latin America, Africa, and Asia, dealing mainly with reproductive health issues such as HIV/AIDS prevention, family planning, environmental health, teenage pregnancy prevention, and gender equality (Singhal and Rogers 1999).

ENTERTAINMENT-EDUCATION COMES IN MANY DIFFERENT SIZES AND SHAPES

- Single films and videos have been important in Asia and Africa where they are shown from video vans as well as on national media.
- Variety shows are increasingly popular with youth in developing countries—many of these programs engage young people directly in content and production.
- Television and radio spots often include entertainment-education through short narratives or through use of familiar characters.
- Locally, street theater, community radio, indigenous storytellers, drama contests, and community rallies with local performers incorporate and/or adapt national entertainment-education productions.
- Popular songs and music videos, which are inspired by the role-modeling techniques used in Sabido-style serial dramas.

Many of these entertainment-education programs have attracted large audiences and have brought about major audience effects in knowledge, attitudes, and behavior (Singhal and Rogers 1999).

However, although they certainly produce results, these various entertainment-education programs have not demonstrated the same magnitude of effects or cost-effectiveness achieved by Sabido-style programs such as *Twende na Wakati* (Rogers et al. 1999; Vaughan et al. 2000) and *Yeken Kignit* (Population Media Center—Ethiopia 2004b).

WHAT MAKES SABIDO-STYLE PROGRAMS SO DIFFERENT THAN OTHER FORMS OF ENTERTAINMENT-EDUCATION?

Successful use of the Sabido methodology hinges on two key factors: 1) use of the serial drama format and 2) rigorous adherence to the theories underlying the methodology. Also, most entertainment-education programs are devoted to sending messages, whereas the Sabido methodology uses characters as vicarious role models, to demonstrate the desired behaviors. The use of these vicarious role models is a critical element of successful application of the Sabido approach.

Format (Long Running Serialized Drama)

First and foremost, the Sabido methodology requires the use of serial drama. Serial dramas continuing for several months or years are an extremely powerful form of entertainment-education that can influence both specific health behaviors and related social norms. Why?

- Serial dramas capture the attention and the emotions of the audience on a continual basis.
- Serial dramas provide repetition and continuity, allowing audiences to identify more and more closely over time with the fictional characters, their problems, and their social environment.
- Serial dramas allow time for characters to develop a change in behavior slowly, with hesitations and setbacks that occur in real life.
- Serial dramas have various subplots that can introduce different issues in a logical and credible way through different characters, a key characteristic of conventional soap operas.
- Serial dramas can build a realistic social context that will mirror society and create multiple opportunities to present a social issue in various forms (Coleman and Meyer 1990).

Exhibit 24.2 Theories underlying the Sabido Methodology

Theory	Function in Sabido-Style Soap Opera
Communication Model (Shannon and Weaver)	Provides a model for the communication process through which distinct sources, messages, receivers, and responses are linked.
Dramatic Theory (Bentley)	Provides a model for characters, their interrelationships, and plot construction.
Archetypes and stereotypes (Jung)	Provides a model for characters that embodies universal human physiological and psychological energies.
Social Learning Theory (Bandura)	Provides a model in which learning from soap opera characters can take place.
Concept of the Triune Brain (MacLean) and Theory of the Tone (Sabido)	Provide a model for sending complete messages that communicate with various centers of perception.

Source: Nariman (1993)

By modeling the process of change gradually, serial dramas are less likely to result in backlash, or negative reactions by the audience, than programs that try to bring about behavior change too quickly. Ideally, Sabido-style serial dramas should continue for at least 120–180 episodes (over the course of several years).

Serial dramas can present different perspectives and stimulate audience questioning that can lead to both individual health behavior change and to a change in social norms (Singhal et al. 2004). As Piotrow states, "Of all the formats for entertainment-education programs which have been adapted, developed, tested, or contributed to, serial drama—on television where possible, or on radio when access to television is limited—has proven to be a highly effective format to promote long-term changes in health behavior and to influence the social norms that can reinforce such change" (NEEF 2000: 23–24).

Second, the Sabido methodology is based on various communication theories, each of which plays an essential role in the development of a Sabido-style serial drama (see Exhibit 24.2). The application of these theories is critical to the success of the Sabido methodology in achieving behavior change.

The different theories that guide the development of Sabido-style serial dramas provide the methodology with a foundation for the structure and design of messages, settings, characters, and plots—a foundation that is based on formative research. The theories also provide a framework for articulating hypotheses for summative (evaluation) research on the impact of the program.

Communication Model: Shannon and Weaver 1949

Shannon and Weaver's Communication Model (Shannon and Weaver 1949) has five basic factors, arranged in a linear format. The components in this model are set out in Exhibit 24.3.

Sabido adapted Shannon and Weaver's linear diagram to form a communication circuit that depicted the circular nature of the communication process. He then applied this circuit to a serial drama (Televisa's Institute of Communication Research 1981a). In the case of a commercial soap opera on television, the communicator is the manufacturer of a product, the message is "buy this product," the medium is the soap opera, the receiver is the consumer, and the response is the purchase of the product and television ratings.

In the design of a social content serial drama, Sabido left the communication circuit of a commercial serial drama intact; however, he added a second communicator, a second message, a second receiver, and a second response. These additions to the communication circuit did not impede the function of the first communicator, which is still the product manufacturer, as shown in

Exhibit 24.3 Shannon and Weaver's model of communication

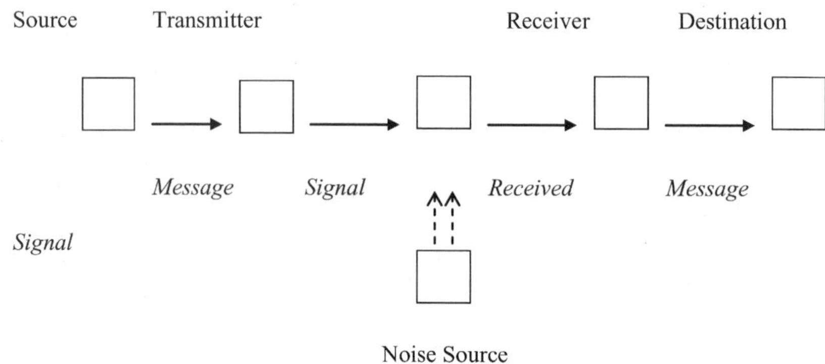

Source: Shannon and Weaver (1949)

Exhibit 24.4 Sabido's model of communication

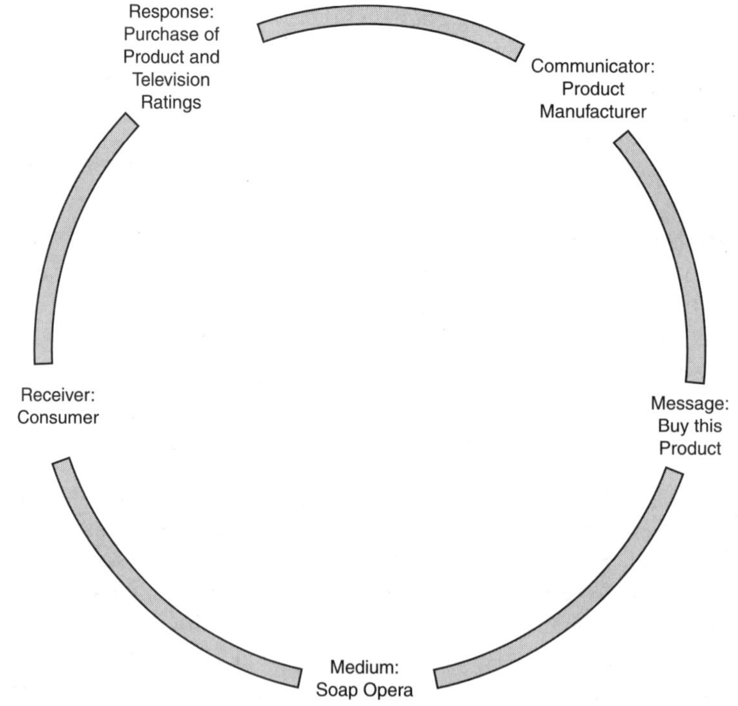

Source: Televisa's Institute of Communication Research (1981b)

Exhibit 24.5 (Televisa's Institute of Communication Research 1981a).

Dramatic Theory: Bentley 1967

Bentley's Dramatic Theory (1967) describes the structure and effects of five genres of theatre (tragedy, comedy, tragicomedy, farce, and melodrama). Among these genres, melodrama presents reality in a slightly exaggerated sense in which the moral universes of good and evil are in discord. Sabido, originally a dramatic theoretician himself, employed Bentley's structure of the melodrama genre as a basis from which to design characters and plots. "Good" characters in Sabido-style serial dramas accept the proposed social behavior, and "evil" characters

Exhibit 24.5 Additional circuit for a social content soap opera

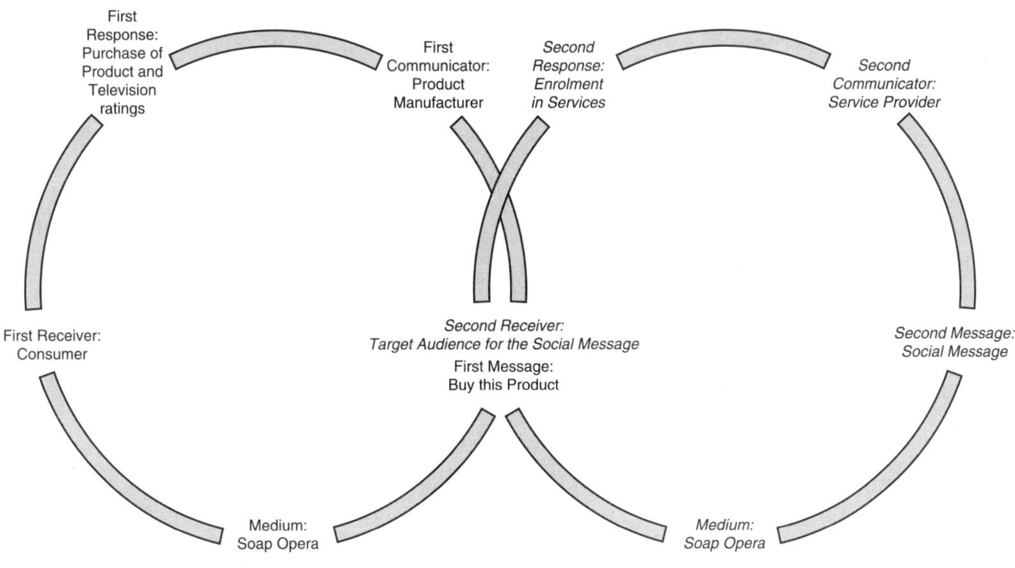

Source: Televisa's Institute of Communication Research (1981a)

reject it. Plots are then constructed around the relationships between good and evil characters as they move closer to or farther away from the proposed social behavior. Their actions encourage the audience to either champion or reject these characters accordingly.

The tension between the good and evil characters evoked by the melodrama places the audience between the forces of good and evil. But, in a twist of the typical audience role in melodrama, where audience members simply watch or listen to the battle between good and evil, Sabido inserted the audience into the heart of the action—by representing audience members through a third group, one that is uncertain about the social behavior in question. These "uncertain" characters are intended to be those with which the target audience most closely identifies. It is also these "transitional" characters who will guide the audience members through their own evolution toward adoption of desired behavior changes.

Although the three groups of characters in Sabido-style serial dramas are exaggerated, as is the case in melodrama, they are modeled on real people within the target audience and the perceptions these people might have regarding the social value and behavior being presented.

Archetypes and Stereotypes—Theory of the Collective Unconscious: Jung 1970

Jung's theory (1970) states that there are certain scripts or stories with familiar patterns and characters that people play out throughout history. These universal scripts or stories appear in myths, legends, and folktales around the world. Jung posited that these universal scripts or stories are the "archetypes of a collective unconscious" and share common characters such as "Prince Charming," "the mother," and "the warrior." Jung further suggests that these archetypes are expressions of a primordial, collective unconscious shared by diverse cultures.

Sabido used the archetypes described in Jung's theory as a basis for developing characters that embody universal psychological and physiological characteristics to address themes within the serial drama. Through these characters, the viewer finds an archetypical essence of him or herself that interacts with the social message. Sabido portrayed these archetypes as positive or negative stereotypes, representing the societal norms of the target audience.

Sabido-style serial dramas rely on extensive formative research to identify the culture- or country-specific versions of these archetypes and to identify local archetypes that represent the prosocial values (or the antithesis of these values) that will be addressed in the serial drama. If the formative research upon which the serial drama is based is done properly, the scriptwriters will be able to develop archetypical characters with which audience members will be able to identify. The formative research is used to develop a grid of positive and negative social values that these positive and negative characters will embody.

Social Learning Theory, Bandura 1977, and Social Cognitive Theory: Bandura 1986

Social Learning Theory, as articulated by the Stanford University psychologist Professor Albert Bandura (Bandura 1977), explains how people learn new behaviors from vicariously experiencing the actions of others. Bandura postulates that there are two basic modes of learning. People can either learn through the direct experience of trial and error and the rewarding and punishing effects of actions, or through the power of social modeling. Trial-and-error learning by direct experience is not only tedious but harmful when errors produce costly or injurious consequences. So, many people will short-cut this process by learning from the successes and mistakes of others. This shortcut, called vicarious learning, or modeling, is a key tenet of Bandura's Social Learning Theory.

According to Social Learning Theory, people not only learn in formal situations such as classrooms, but also by observing models. In fact, the largest portion of learning to adapt to society takes place through such observational learning. The models used in this observational learning can be people in real life or characters in mass media (such as television or radio).

A key to the use of Social Learning Theory in Sabido-style serial dramas is use of appropriate models that are visibly rewarded (or punished) in front of the audience, in order to convert the values that are being promoted by the serial drama into behavior. Social Learning Theory postulates that positive rewards have a vicarious effect upon the observer (in this case, the audience) and can motivate audience members to practice similar behavior(s). Punishing a role model for practicing a socially undesirable behavior likewise provides a vicarious experience for the observer and can inhibit his or her practice of the same behavior. This adoption is called modeling because it is based on the role model's conduct. Through modeling it is possible to acquire new forms of behavior and to strengthen or weaken certain behaviors. In Sabido-style serial dramas, characters "teach" audience members via modeling so that they are able to make a recommended response.

Sabido determined that three types of characters are fundamental to successful modeling by audience members. The first two types of characters are positive and negative role models. They embody positive and negative behaviors concerning the social issues addressed in the serial drama (and are based on Jung's theory of archetypes and stereotypes, described above). These characters will not change during the course of the serial drama, but are repeatedly rewarded or punished for their behaviors. The consequences of these positive or negative behaviors must be directly linked to the behavior in question—for example, a truck driver character that is practicing at-risk sexual behavior should suffer from a sexually transmitted infection or even contract HIV, but should not be the victim of a traffic accident.

The third type of character is the "transitional character." These characters are neither positive nor negative but somewhere in the middle. These transitional characters play the pivotal role in a Sabido-style serial drama, and are designed to represent members of the target audience. The transitional characters' evolution toward the desired behavior is that which the audience members will use to model their own behavior change.

For example, in Sabido's first social content serial drama, *Ven Conmigo* (*Come with Me*), which dealt with adult literacy, transitional characters were specifically chosen from specific sub-groups (e.g., the elderly, young adults, housewives) who represented the key target audiences for the national literacy campaign in Mexico. One of the main transitional characters was a grandfather who struggled to read the many letters he received from his favorite granddaughter. In a cathartic episode, he graduates from literacy training, and is finally able to read his granddaughter's letters, albeit with teary eyes. In the year preceding the broadcast of *Ven Conmigo*, the national literacy campaign had registered 99,000 students. Following the broadcast of this episode (and the epilogue which provided information about registration in the literacy campaign), 250,000 people registered for literacy training. By the end of the serial drama, 840,000 people had registered for the literacy program —an increase of almost 750 percent from the preceding year (Singhal and Rogers 1999).

Bandura also developed a related theory, Social Cognitive Theory (Bandura 1986), which explains that behavior change can only occur when an individual feels sufficiently empowered to change. If an individual feels that the society, culture, religion, or his or her deity (or "Fate") dictates individual behavior and its consequences, there is little that communication can do to impact behavior change. For example, if a woman perceives that Fate has determined the number of children she will ultimately bear during her childbearing years, even a well-conceived family planning communication campaign will have little effect in motivating her to plan or space her pregnancies—she feels that this decision is not hers to make. In this case, the woman's perception of self-determination must be addressed first.

Bandura termed this perception of self-determination "self-efficacy." The more self-efficacy an individual perceives, the more likely he or she will be to feel empowered to make decisions that affect his or her life and circumstances.

Research has shown that Sabido-style serial dramas can increase self-efficacy among audience members. According to Everett Rogers, the Sabido-style serial drama *Twende na Wakati* produced a marked increased in listeners' self-efficacy with regard to family size in Tanzania (Rogers et al. 1999). In fact, the series title, which means "Let's go with the times," was defined in several episodes as "taking charge of one's life." Positive and transitional role models in *Twende na Wakati* exemplified such self-efficacy and were rewarded in the storyline for taking charge of their lives by adopting a family planning method, or by otherwise taking control of, and responsibility for, their reproductive health and that of their partner(s). Negative role models like Mkwaju, who lacked such control, were punished by events.

The content of *Twende na Wakati* that dealt with self-efficacy had a marked effect on listeners' beliefs, and, indirectly, on their family planning behavior. For example, married women in the 1995 survey who believed they *could* determine the size of their family were much more likely than others (51 percent vs. 16 percent) to use a family planning method (Rogers et al. 1999).

Concept of the Triune Brain: MacLean 1973, and Theory of the Tone: Sabido 2002

The Sabido methodology is based on conveying a holistic message that is perceived by audience members on several levels of awareness. Sabido began his career as a theater director and dramatic theoretician. In his work in the theater, Sabido discovered that actors can have different effects on their audiences by channeling their energy through three different body zones. If actors focused their energy behind their eyes, the tone of the production would be conceptual. If the actor focused energy in the base of the neck, the tone of the production would be emotive. If the actor focused energy in the pubic area, the tone of the production would be primal (Sabido 2002). Sabido instinctively understood that, in order to motivate or persuade, it is necessary to provide a complete message that speaks to these three levels of perception.

Sabido's "tonal theory" describes how the various tones that are perceived by humans can be used in drama. In this theory, the producer/director serves almost the same function as an orchestra conductor, who can evoke different tones from each instrument in order to create various harmonies or tones within the body of the music and thereby inspire different moods among the audience.

Although the theory is quite complex, it can be summarized by saying that, for Sabido, the "tone" is the human communication form to which the receiver gives a tone according to his or her own genetic and acquired repertoire, thus making the "tone" the foundation of human communication (Sabido 2002). The theory has one main hypothesis: it is possible to change the tone of communication by hierarchically ordering its flow elements in a specific manner. This general hypothesis is organized into twelve sub-hypotheses, which allow us to take this abstract idea and apply it to day-to-day communication.

The producer/director uses various nonverbal elements of communication, including facial expressions, body language, lighting, music, sound effects, and tone of voice, to evoke different responses from the audience.

At first, Sabido lacked a theoretical explanation for what he was observing. He eventually discovered Paul MacLean's Concept of the Triune Brain (MacLean 1973), which presents a model of human brain structure with three levels of perception—cognitive, affective, and pre-dispositional.

Thus, MacLean's theory gave Sabido the scientific basis he needed for focusing on the emotional (second zone) and instinctive/impulse (first zone) as the basis for his serial dramas, with the third (cognitive zone) used primarily to reinforce the first and second zones' messages in the drama.

In summary, the Sabido methodology for development of mass media entertainment-education serial dramas is unique in that it is designed according to elements of communication and behavioral theories. These confirm specific values, attitudes, and behaviors that viewers can use in their own personal advancement.

NOTES

1. Between 1973 and 1981, Miguel Sabido produced six social-content serial dramas in Mexico.

    - *Ven Conmigo* (*Come with Me*) provided specific information about a study program offered by the Secretary of Public Education in 1975. Role models were used to motivate viewers to register for literacy classes.
    - *Acompáñame* (*Accompany Me*), Sabido's second entertainment-education soap opera, contained a family planning message (broadcast from August 1977 through April 1978). Role models were used in this serial drama to motivate women to use contraceptive methods, and to show wives how to negotiate contraceptive use with their spouses.
    - *Vamos Juntos* (*Let's Go Together*) promoted responsible parenthood and the active development and integration of children in the family and in society (July 1979 through March 1980). Role models were used in this program to teach parents about family integration behaviors and family life planning.
    - *El Combate* (*The Struggle*) promoted an adult education program launched in several communities outside of Mexico City (April through September 1980). Behavior models were used in this program to inform rural audiences how to dispel the myth that adults cannot go back to school.
    - *Caminemos* (*Going Forward Together*) tackled the theme of sex education for adolescents (September 1980 through April 1981). Role models in this program were used to model responsible sexual behavior for teenagers.
    - *Nosotros las Mujeres* (*We the Women*) ran from April to October 1981. Through the effective use of role modeling, this program was designed to counter traditions associated with machismo and to encourage women to become aware of their important role in the family and society.

    In 1997–98, Sabido produced one additional social-content serial drama before retiring from Televisa in 1998:

    - *Los Hijos de Nadie* (*Nobody's Children*) addressed the issue of street children. This program used role models to change opinions among audience members about the "silent conspiracy" surrounding the problem of street children in Mexico.

REFERENCES AND FURTHER READING

Albert Bandura (1977). *Social Learning Theory*. Englewood Cliffs, NJ: Prentice Hall.

Albert Bandura (1986). *Social Foundations of Thought and Action: A Social Cognitive Theory*. Englewood Cliffs, NJ: Prentice Hall.

Eric Bentley (1967). *The Life of Drama*. New York: Athenaeum.

Patrick Coleman and R.C. Meyer (1990). *Proceedings from the Enter-Educate Conference: Entertainment for Social Change*. Baltimore: Johns Hopkins University, Population Communication Services.

Rose Haji (2004). Personal communication. 2004.

Carl Jung (1970). *Archetypes and the Collective Unconscious*. Buenos Aires: Editorial Paidos.

Paul MacLean (1973). "A Triune Concept of the Brain and Behavior, including Psychology of Memory, Sleep and Dreaming." In V.A. Kral et al. (eds.) *Proceedings of the Ontario Mental Health Foundation Meeting at Queen's University*. Toronto: University of Toronto Press.

Heidi Nariman (1993). *Soap Operas for Social Change*. Westport: Praeger.

NEEF and Johns Hopkins University, Center for Communication Programs (2000). "Think Big, Start Small, Act Now." In *Proceedings of the Third International Entertainment-Education Conference for Social Change*. Arnhem/Amsterdam: September 17–22.

Population Media Center—Ethiopia (2004a). *Facility Assessment Report*. Addis Ababa: Population Media Center—Ethiopia.

Population Media Center—Ethiopia (2004b). *Final Evaluation (Preliminary Report)*. Addis Ababa: Population Media Center—Ethiopia.

Everett Rogers et al. (1999). "Effects of an Entertainment-Education Soap Opera on Family Planning in Tanzania." *Studies in Family Planning* 30(3): 193–211.

Miguel Sabido (2002). *The Tone, Theoretical Occurrences, and Potential Adventures and Entertainment with Social Benefit*. Mexico City: National Autonomous University of Mexico Press.

C.E. Shannon and E. Weaver (1949). *The Mathematical Theory of Communication*. Urbana, IL: University of Illinois Press.

Arvind Singhal and Everett Rogers (1999). *Entertainment-Education: A Communication Strategy for Social Change*. Mahwah, NJ: Lawrence Erlbaum Associates.

Arvind Singhal and Everett Rogers (2002). "A Theoretical Agenda for Entertainment-Education." *Communication Theory* 12(2): 117–135.

Arvind Singhal et al. (2004). *Entertainment-Education and Social Change: History, Research and Practice*. Mahwah, NJ: Lawrence Erlbaum Associates.

Televisa's Institute of Communication Research (1981a). "Handbook for Reinforcing Social Values through Day-time T.V. Serials" Paper presented at the International Institute of Communication, Strasbourg, France.

Televisa's Institute of Communication Research (1981b). "Toward the Social Use of Soap operas." Paper presented at the International Institute of Communication, Strasbourg, France.

Peter Vaughan et al. (2000). "Entertainment-Education and HIV/AIDS Prevention: A Field Experiment in Tanzania." *Journal of Health Communication* 5 (Supplement): 81–100.

Peter Vaughan and Everett Rogers (2000). "A Staged Model of Communication Effects: Evidence from an Entertainment-Education Radio Soap Opera in Tanzania." *Journal of Health Communication* 5(2): 203–227.

CHAPTER 25

A Cambodian Story of a Global Epidemic

Siv Cheng

ABSTRACT

The experiences of people living with HIV/AIDS (PLWHA) must be represented in media coverage of the pandemic, as they serve as both advocates and provide a "face" for the pandemic via public interest stories. In this personal narrative the author describes her life as a PLWHA and how this has had an impact on her work as a journalist in the Cambodian media since 2004. This chapter provides insight into ways to improve media coverage of the epidemic—in particular, to enhance the positive voices in the media. Journalists need to be exposed to contemporary issues affecting the lives of PLWHAs in order to become effective participants in health communications initiatives.

The events I tell below still cause a lot of pain in my heart. I dream back to the past, to the time I didn't know how to protect myself with a condom against HIV and AIDS. I experienced a nightmare for three years and I awoke with the conviction to take action because I don't want my Cambodian people to face HIV transmission without knowing, like me.

I have been living with AIDS since 2000 and working on HIV and AIDS issues with the Cambodian media since 2004. Currently based in the Capitol Phnom Penh as a Technical Advisor for the Internews Europe[1] Mekong Project, my work is to improve media coverage of the epidemic—in particular, to enhance the positive voices in the media. My previous experience was with the BBC World Service Trust[2] and the Women's Media Center[3] of Cambodia.

This chapter represents my views based on this experience. It begins with my first published print article, my personal story, "By, For and About Positive People," which ran in *Global AIDSLink*, published by the Global Health Council May/June 2007, and led to the invitation for me to write this, my second printed work. I appreciate this prestigious opportunity to tell the world about my life and my work.

PART 1

By, For and About Positive People

In 1997, I married an immigration policeman stationed at the border port of Sihanoukville, where I grew up, and expected to live happily ever after. I was 20 years old, Cambodia's seaside resort was thriving on tourism, and the Kingdom's AIDS epidemic was a mere five years old and hardly talked about.

Two years later, I gave birth to a baby girl whom the Chinese astrologers said would be clever and successful. She was thus given a name that means "Golden Cool." I breastfed her and did not know what caused her diarrhea. So I reverted to bottle-feeding with some unspoken worries about HIV infection.

Meanwhile, my husband fell sick in mid-2000, his condition worsening day to day. The drugs prescribed by both Khmer traditional healers and physicians had no effect. We sold all our belongings—two motorcycles and some jewelry—to pay for treatment, but it brought no relief.

My husband was very skinny and coughing all the time. None of the medicine I bought treated him. One day, my mother-in-law confided out loud her fear that her son was suffering from HIV-related illnesses. I was terrified. Like the majority of Khmers, all I knew about people with AIDS was that they would die soon. I didn't even know what to do with a condom. To assuage my mother-in-law's suspicions, I discreetly had my own blood tested at a nearby state-run hospital.

Although I was braced for the worst, when the day arrived, it was still shocking when the counselor, as gently as possibly, said, "You are infected with HIV—the virus that causes AIDS." I cried until all energy and hope drained from my body, and I was empty. Why had destiny punished me so? A traditional Khmer woman, I obeyed my parent's advice and, a good Buddhist, I always behaved properly and ethically.

My husband persisted in asking about my blood results. "Never mind, we aren't affected by HIV/AIDS," I smiled and lied, fearing that depression from knowing the truth would kill him. That night he ate all his dinner for the first time in weeks.

One day when my husband asked for the doctor, he simply refused to come. Having correctly concluded my husband's symptoms were from HIV-related, he gave up on treatment. My husband persisted, until one day my mother-in-law blurted out, "He does not come because you have AIDS."

My mother-in-law would soon give up on her son and banish me and her granddaughter. We were only a burden to her, despite my efforts to support my own family. By then, I had brought my husband to the capital, Phnom Penh, where I learned there were increasing services available for Cambodia's growing AIDS epidemic. I didn't have time to see the doctor about my own new joint pains. There were many obstacles to overcome, and fears to be left behind, and food to be brought to the table.

When my husband died in January 2001, I moved with my child to live with my mother in Sihanoukville. But after a few days, I couldn't move with pain throughout my joints and a fever that flared four times a day. At the hospital I was told I had syphilis. I followed the doctor's orders, but couldn't get rid of it. I thought I might die, and would never see my daughter again. My neighbors from the village came to visit me as if they were paying their last respects, with apples, oranges, and mangosteen. A month later, a hairdresser told me about a traditional herbal cure for syphilis and explained to my mother how to simmer the herbs. I drank it and the fever disappeared in a day. I drank it for a year and a half and finally recovered.

But things did not get better. My friends and my cousin avoided me. My elder sister came, tore down my room in my mother's house—the room that was mine since childhood—and claimed sole rights to the family property, even though she already had a house of her own. My mother treated me differently, let me come and go—carefree—as though I no longer had a future. My life was so isolated. I had nowhere to go. I wanted to commit suicide, but my daughter meant everything to me.

Then, one day, the sun made a rare appearance at Preah Sihanouk Hospital, where I was finally going for treatment that can prolong the lives of people with my condition—antiretroviral drugs. Little by little, it rose higher in the sky and my luck seemed to change. I finally took the plunge and tested my daughter. She was negative. I met an HIV/AIDS instructor who worked for a local group called Vithey Chivit (Road of Life) and persuaded me to work with her—to educate positive urban poor squatters about health care. As I encouraged them to stand up and demand access to medical services, fight discrimination, and get support from the community, I became braver and stronger myself.

In 2004, I met an Australian woman who had remarkably lived with AIDS for more than fifteen years. At her leadership seminar, she brought together twenty-eight women, mostly widows who had many dependents, and faced unemployment and discrimination in the workplace, family, and community. Relying only on ourselves for resources, we started the "Women for Hope Club," which became like a new or second family providing emotional support, assistance, and income generation. They elected me director with the formidable task of starting the country's first positive women's group.

A club member introduced me to the BBC World Service Trust, where I came to realize how powerful the media can be for good when it chooses to be. I wanted people to know who I was; I wanted to show through the media, that, although we are positive, we can do "anything." I also wanted to send messages to the decision-makers to fulfill their promises to positive people.

I was then accepted as a BBC World Service Trust volunteer and assigned to their AIDS radio talk show programs. A few months later, I was selected as a United Nations Volunteer in its Greater Involvement People Living with HIV/AIDS Project. My task was to inspire the local women's media center to increase its radio broadcasts on AIDS, particularly giving voice to the problems of positive people.

Later, I became a full-fledged producer, and we created a call-in show, dubbed *Hope*, targeted at discrimination and aiming to show how positive people are an invaluable resource in the response to AIDS. Yet NGOs and government HIV and AIDS projects in Cambodia were not using them. Live, on air, positive people spoke out courageously and answered questions boldly. Listeners were hearing the problems of positive people from their own lips. It was the first positive radio show—by, for, and about positive people.

When the project ended last year, I was offered a position with an international media development organization, Internews, which was launching a two-year project on HIV and the media, and seeking someone who understood the issues. Our work with journalists varies from formal training to helping them find good stories. We create opportunities for journalists, editors, and positive people to better communicate. Getting them to increase their coverage of AIDS and find new angles has been a continuing challenge. We endlessly try to address the complex issue of terminology, stigma, accuracy, and sensitivity.

I hope more positive people will become journalists, and the relationship between journalists and positive people will intertwine. Our press needs to draw more attention to AIDS issues for the sake of its people, especially those who live in the remote areas and are increasingly affected by Cambodia's epidemic, now facing the highest prevalence rate in all of Asia. Unlike the 20-year-old girl in Sihanoukville in 1997, I want them to be aware.

Sometimes my dreams do not work. But I hold onto my family and my friends—my mom, my new husband, and my "Golden Cool," who is now 9 years old. I hope that everybody can become like my family.

PART 2

Positive Work

When HIV was discovered in Cambodia in 1991,[4] people living with the virus dared not identify themselves in the media, for fear of discrimination and alienation. News media did not cover the story widely or thoroughly, and the portrayals that did emerge were almost exclusively of emaciated, hopeless, and frightening-looking people facing death.

In the years since then the situation has improved, but the media still face serious challenges in covering HIV-related issues—and positive people still struggle to find their public voice.

Cambodia has the highest HIV infection rate in Asia.[5] The epidemic is widespread, despite multi-million-dollar efforts to prevent this by donors, the United Nations agencies, Non-governmental organizations (NGOs), and the government.

Today, people living with HIV (PLHIV) face less overt contempt and discrimination. They also have greater access to information and services.

But they are still far away from achieving social equity. They still live in a society in which they are greatly stigmatized. They struggle with huge practical and psychological pressures in their daily lives. Many sell their possessions in desperation to pay for poor-quality medical treatment. People with HIV are routinely denied jobs, even in organizations working on AIDS-related issues.

They dare not complain publicly about injustices because of real fears of the consequences. They are scared to speak out against the government or to criticize NGOs and practitioners out of fear that they will jeopardize their chances of receiving good medical treatment. Most think the results of speaking out will not be good. For example, people dare not complain about bad treatment from a physician, especially one who works for the government, for fear that the physician may cut off their antiretroviral treatment, or neglect to take care of them. Vendors who work in local markets, even in the big cities, dare not speak out about their real situation because people may stop buying their goods.

Positive people need strong voices—their own voice, first—to raise both ongoing and emerging issues. They also need the support of other credible civil society groups and decision-makers who have influence, such as the donor community, Buddhist monks, parliamentarians, and health and women's organizations.

In Cambodia the donor community is especially relevant. It plays a significant role in providing social services that the government does not. There are many NGOs[6] working on HIV issues. They have varied impacts. Interestingly, PLHIV are conspicuously missing in meaningful roles in most of these organizations. Very few are paid employees, even in organizations with significant financial resources.[7] PLHIV are primarily used as "volunteers," earning about fifteen dollars per month (in most cases, not even enough for transportation to and from the workplace), though they work long hours in often difficult and stressful circumstances.

As volunteers, the ideas of PLHIV are seldom accepted by NGOs—their thoughts are met with disagreement or considered counter to NGO priorities. Many PLHIV believe this is the reason they are usually not promoted to permanent positions. They rarely have a voice in developing and implementing HIV and AIDS programs. Thus they feel "small." They think NGOs and government will not listen to "small people," and will continue to act on behalf of PLHIV, as though they know what is best for them—without having asked, consulted, or involved them. PLHIV are treated as though what they have to say is not important. Most have not been able to effectively penetrate NGOs and use them as a vehicle for getting their message across.

It is vital that PLHIV continue to develop their own leaders, advocates, organizations, and networks. It's equally important that they find ways to be the bridge between PLHIV and government and NGO resources.

One fledgling group, the Cambodian Alliance for Combating HIV/AIDS (CACHA), was formed in 2006 to be a strong network to advocate on behalf of PLHIV. This umbrella group of NGOs recognized the need for a positive organization that advocates effectively for positive people and functions as a bridge to the government and NGOs. It brings together a mix of grassroots and national and international organizations, and positive networks and groups, to coordinate and share information and to present a stronger and more united voice on issues of concern to PLHIV.

Today new messages are emerging from the grass roots as well as CACHA and other PLHIV groups—for example, that a decent continuum of care means accepting people's right to food, housing, employment, quality medical care, education, quality treatment, legal services, and the right to live in dignity in society. But these messages are seldom heard and the situation for PLHIV in regards to these rights has not improved enough, if at all. Positive people remain unskilled in getting their views across. They have justified fears that speaking out critically about government policy, NGOs, or health practitioners could compromise their services or increase discrimination against them. The process of reducing such fear is still only just beginning.

FIRST STEPS

A first step towards PLHIV voices being heard in the media has been through "positive messaging" via health and education campaigns.

One early voice to put a dent in the silence was from Ms. Penn Mony, a 27-year-old AIDS advocate living with HIV, currently a project manager responsible for strengthening women with HIV-leadership at the Cambodia for the Cambodian Community of Women Living with HIV/AIDS (CCW). "People imagine PLHIV are evil, have poor health, bad complexions, and are just skin hanging on bones," she says. To counteract such tired and negative stereotyping, she has appeared on television education spots, because she wants to show everybody, "See! PLHIV have faces just like other human beings!"

Mony helped get another important message across. Not many Cambodians realize that anyone can get infected with HIV, very often through putting misplaced trust in their partners. Mony helped challenge that dangerous assumption when she appeared on TV spots informing people—especially women—of the risks of assuming that their partners are free from HIV.

Other positive people, including myself, have been able to speak out and reach the public via sponsored radio programming. In 2006, while working as a United Nations Volunteer at the Cambodian Women's Media Center, I helped produce a series of six radio programs that were the first shows by positives, for positives, and about positive people.

We named the call-in show *Hope* because that was what we wanted to give to positive people. The aim was also to show decision-makers at all levels that, in order to effectively address the epidemic, they need to involve positive people, listen to their views, respect their rights, and make policy decisions and changes according to what PLHIV need.

The issues were broad and discussions included a wide variety of views and common needs such as food, employment, skills, and quality treatment. We invited a diverse group to contribute—including a medical expert, media representative, antiretroviral expert, and community and hospital counselors.

The program showed how PLHIV are just like others. They are part of society. They can run businesses and earn salaries. The show was an inspiration to PLHIV and NGOs. Moreover, I came to realize that "this issue is mine." Giving positive people a voice was something I had to do, I loved doing, and I had passion for.

The experience also made it clear that positive individuals and groups understand the power of media and are interested to work with media outlets. But working on information campaigns, and with journalists and media outlets directly, are in many ways very different. It feels safe to work in the relatively controlled environment of information campaigns. However it is difficult to overcome the obstacles of working with the news media. As Penn Mony put it, "I am very happy to work with journalists, but I don't trust those I don't know well."

MOVING INTO MEDIA

News journalism is undoubtedly a potentially powerful tool for disseminating information about HIV and AIDS and affecting attitudes—for good or for ill.

In Cambodia, a country with high illiteracy, most people listen to the radio. TV is gaining in popularity, particularly in public areas such as restaurants and coffee shops, where many people can view programs together. Radio and TV are popular among many housewives, farmers, and market sellers. Newspapers are enjoyed with morning noodles in urban centers, but seldom make their way to small villages. They are read by decision-makers and businesspeople, and stories in print can drive political agenda. Radio and TV often pick up and follow stories broken by the print media.

The Cambodian-language media has limitations—especially in terms of journalism skill-sets and knowledge of HIV. Of particular importance is the lack of independence and politically partisan nature of the media. Editors are customarily paid by various sources to publish or to block the publication of stories. This includes influential politicians and businesspeople, as well as many national and international NGOs that pay media outlets to run their stories or write articles. Many Cambodian people accept that journalists should pay for interviews, or that individuals and organizations should pay journalists. This corrupt system keeps the media unprofessional, and greatly reduces journalists' motivation to pursue stories on merit.

Improving the media coverage of HIV and AIDS requires taking a strategic, multi-pronged approach, with both eyes firmly focused on the local realities. For the media development organization I work for, Internews, the key methods involve building communications and networking skills among PLHIV in order that their voices be heard; building trust and contacts between PLHIV and journalists; motivating reporters; helping journalists find news angles and work through stories; combating corruption; working to overcome bias and inaccuracy; working on terminology, meeting editors, and assisting them to improve the reporting of their staff; and making information resources available.

Strengthening Positive Voices

We have worked with positive groups and individuals with limited success—for example, to build contacts with journalists, help organize media events, write press releases, and speak in public.

In 2007, we encouraged CACHA, for example, to highlight their important issues by first doing their own research by PLHIV, about PLHIV, and for PLHIV. They conducted research at the village level about food needs, an issue that affects much of the country's poor, and particularly PLHIV. The statistical and anecdotal information that resulted was relevant, interesting, clear, and illustrated various problems around food security and HIV and AIDS—including poverty, clean water, health services, and the need for jobs.

We helped CACHA identify different angles on their information, and worked with individuals who knew the various issues best. We tutored them on public speaking and in getting their messages across to the public and assisted them in practice presentations of their research findings.

A myriad of stories ideas emerged, including: "PLHIV not allowed to use village well;" "World Food Program rice donations not reaching targeted villagers;" "Community does not allow PLHIV to borrow bicycle;" "PLHIV starved to death;" "Relatives abandon orphan;" "Fertilizers and disappearing frogs cause PLHIV to go hungry." Some of the angles were used in stories published as a result of CACHA's Candlelight Memorial Day event press conference in May.

This was a good example of positive people getting their messages across, but such occasions are still pretty rare. Positive people still lack communication skills, organization, power, and influence. Most groups are too busy with their regular NGO work to devote much time to the advocacy, communication, and media liaison roles they need to play. Few PLHIV possess experience in public speaking, writing, and research. Like other Cambodians, they do not come from a literary culture or have a strong formal education. Also, unfortunately, most research documents about HIV are in English, many are very long, and are not always of relevance to the average PLHIV. There is a real need for recognized, paid, dedicated media and communications leaders to emerge in the PLHIV community and in NGOs. I want to see more PLHIV rising up like me and saying, "this issue is mine;" and people who view PLHIV as family. We have the same blood. We have to think like a positive family.

Building Trust

The main reason why such successes have been slow to grow has been the need to build trust between PLHIV and the media. Building trust is a delicate process but one that can achieve great results.

Tension often originates in a disregard on both sides for the issue of informed consent about what is and is not to be published or broadcast. On occasion, PLHIV have been clearly informed about the consequences of their speaking out, but changed their minds after publication.[8] On the other hand, journalists often do not understand informed consent, even though an HIV/AIDS law,[9] passed in Cambodia in 2002, provides some protections for the privacy of PLHIV. NGOs also do not always respect informed consent when using photographs, revealing stories, and asking people to speak in public and with the media. Indeed, even parents do not ask their children if they want to be in the public eye. Too often photographs, names, and addresses of positive people—including children—have been published in the media without the subject's informed consent.

Explaining informed consent to the media has proved extremely complex. To begin, journalists often believe they are helping vulnerable people by publishing "pity stories." They clearly identify positive people to open the possibility of the person's receiving a generous donation. They use large photos to "prove" a story is factual, perhaps an acknowledgment that media often lacks credibility with the public. Journalists may not understand that people can lose all their remaining security in life—their jobs and their relationships—as a result. Children, notably orphans, can become vulnerable to serious exploitation in school, in the community, by family, and by strangers.

An example of how children's voices can be beneficially heard was during the CACHA press campaign of May 2007. CACHA had identified two HIV-positive children with important messages about being shunned by other children and alienated from school but, like the media, had neglected to consider the issue of informed consent. We volunteered to work with the children and determine whether they wanted their stories told and, if so, how?

In the end both children decided to record anonymous messages to be broadcast at the CACHA media event. One child said she was confident that her fellow villagers would not know it was her on the radio. She said, "In my village my voice is small, but here in Phnom Penh, my voice gets big." The recordings of the two brought tears to the eyes of many in the audience filled with PLHIV, NGOs, parliamentarians, and media.

To improve media understanding of the issue of consent, we decided in February to reconvene a number of editors who had made verbal commitments to improving coverage of HIV. We invited a child rights expert to explain legal protection for children because, while Khmer theoretically know about such rights, there is little real understanding. A skilled photojournalist presented some of his creative work on the epidemic. He demonstrated various examples of images that showed PLHIV with dignity and revealed stories in themselves, without violating people's privacy. Following the meeting, we noticed that, though newspapers had not taken up all of the suggestions made by the photographer, they had significantly reduced their direct identification of children.

Our experience has been that bringing people together is the crucial ingredient in building trust and understanding each other. Joint meetings we have hosted between PLHIV and media leaders have improved understanding, created attitude and behavior change, and achieved valuable gains for both sides. PLHIV have been able to air their concerns, share their knowledge, and learn about the fair needs of media for clear, accurate, and newsworthy information. Editors and journalists have gained information, new understanding, and heightened awareness of the impacts of the stories they run, as well as new angles and useful contacts for stories.

Training that brings journalists and positive people together is also very effective. Both sides almost invariably describe such encounters as enlightening and mind-changing. Journalists are often surprised to have "scales lifted" from their eyes. Positive people are empowered by productive encounters with a powerful sector many have previously had reason to fear. Stereotypes on both sides have begun to fall away.

Journalist are now starting to initiate stories about HIV/AIDS. The frequency of reporting has risen since 2006.[10] Recent media monitoring[11] has highlighted some other improvements in media coverage. Editors and reporters have been encouraged to reduce the use of sensational and degrading headlines and controversial terminology—such as the inaccurate Cambodian expression *neak kaat AID* ("people born with AIDS") for anyone living with the virus. Today sensationalist newspaper headlines are significantly reduced. Also much reduced—but not gone altogether—are instances of journalists' employing gratuitous or inappropriate adjectives for PLHIV and their situations (i.e., "innocent" "sad," "pathetic" "angry") that flavor the tone of stories with their own personal opinions.

Getting the Stories

Helping journalists to find news angles for HIV/AIDS is challenging. Many think that AIDS is not news—it's a decade-old story. Moreover there's competition from other important "hot" issues and stories, like land ownership, politics, the Khmer Rouge Tribunal, and national elections.

On the contrary, AIDS is indeed newsworthy, both independently and as an important angle in other stories. HIV can highlight news events affecting larger communities, such as the impact of land evictions on poor communities in Phnom Penh. In separate eviction cases in 2006 and 2007, PLHIV dared to speak out about their issues, with trusted journalists. While their fight for housing was ultimately lost, public exposure of their plight helped to highlight the injustice of the evictions and need for NGO, donor and UN support for this marginalized community. HIV is an important news angle in a great range of issues and stories—for example, those about poor monitoring and treatment by medical professionals, public health policy, workers' rights, and the issues of minors affected by HIV.

Journalists have tended to restrict their interest in the HIV story to big AIDS-related events such as the annual Global AIDS Week and World AIDS Day, important government HIV awareness events, and meetings. Such events can result in very short stories, or they can be the springboard for deeper and lengthier treatment that goes beyond headline news. We are now seeing some changes with a greater variety of stories emerging in the media.

In May 2007 (a month when news coverage is typically high due to Global AIDS Week, including Candlelight Day, a commemoration of those who died with HIV), substantial newspaper stories appeared[12] on topics as varied as: the moral and practical leadership of Buddhist monks in encouraging people affected by HIV; the vulnerability of migrant workers to sexually transmitted diseases including HIV; the negative effects of discrimination against PLHIV; and the continued battle for basic survival suffered by many positive people, especially in the provinces (this issue was also exposed in the unusual story about the tragic murder of an HIV-positive infant by its penniless mother).

On rare occasions prominent features have appeared about effective PLHIV leaders whose work and personal philosophies serve as an inspiration to anyone interested in how people can successfully overcome adversity in their lives. A story about PLHIV leader Huot Totem in the daily newspaper *Rasmei Kampuchea*,[13] for example, charted one man's progression from feelings of initial desperation to a determination to live courageously, confidently, and happily and to improve the lives of positive people. The accompanying image of a smiling and serene-looking man, Huot Totem, provided the public with a very different image of positive people than many were accustomed to expect.

Such articles help encourage other positive people to feel they too can be just like Huot Totem. They also send messages to negative people in positive families. This is the kind of story I wish my mother might have read when she heard I was HIV positive, and then treated me differently, as though I had no future.

LOOKING AHEAD

There are still so many sides of the HIV and AIDS issue that have yet to see the light of day. It is true that the general reporting on the issue has changed greatly since the overwhelmingly one-sided and negative portrayals of the 1990s. Sensationalist approaches are reduced these days. Editors and reporters are becoming more aware of issues such as consent and terminology.

But there is still a great distance to go. The voices of positive people are only recently emerging. PLHIV must be empowered to make their own decisions about which issues they want and need to bring to the public —and when. PLHIV may be able to influence policies and decisions about their lives if they are able to get their messages out through the media effectively—both from without, as advocates and communicators, or from within, as journalists and editors. For its part, the news media needs to rise to its important role. Media organizations must see beyond and behind old stereotypes, dig for deeper truths, and end an old silence by bringing the issues and views of PLHIV to the public, the aid community, and leaders.

NOTES

1. Internews Europe is an international NGO working on media development globally. The DFiD (Department of Foreign International Development)-funded regional Mekong Project—including a two-year project currently underway in Cambodia—seeks to improve the quantity and quality of reporting on HIV and AIDS, and strengthening the positive voices in the media.
2. BBC World Service Trust is an independent charity promoting development through innovative use of media.
3. The Women's Media Center, a local NGO working in radio and TV, covers women and other social issues.
4. While there is controversy over the origin of HIV in Cambodia, it is commonly believed that, in 1991, "Cambodia detects HIV for the first time during screening of donated blood" and, in 1993, "Doctors diagnose the first case of HIV in Cambodia," *HIV/AIDS Media Guide* published by National AIDS Authority, Feb 2006, p. 11 (English version).
5. *HIV/AIDS Media Guide*, published by National AIDS Authority, Feb 2006, p. 36 (English version).
6. Approximately 180 NGOs currently work on HIV and AIDS projects in Cambodia, including ninety members of the HIV/AIDS Coordinating Committee (HACC); source: Dr. Kem Ley, Secretary-General, HACC.
7. Overseas Development Assistance, "Investments in HIV and AIDS grew steadily, but accelerated rapidly after 2000," with figures for 2005 at about U.S.$48 million. "Turning the Tide," National AIDS Authority, supported by UNAIDS, August 2006, pp. 21–23.
8. In May 2007, during a public press event organized by the Cambodian Alliance for Combating HIV/AIDS (CACHA), an HIV-positive community in Prey Veng Province accused WOMEN, a local NGO, of corruption in distribution of WFP rice. Before exposing the story, the community leader was clearly briefed on the possible consequences and responded, "I am not afraid because I am a soldier. This is the truth; I must speak for the sake of my sick people." After the story was published, an initial investigation was launched by World Food Program that revealed some rice was diverted from the intended PLHIV. However, later, under pressure, allegedly from the organizations involved, the informant submitted for publication a retraction of his original true story. See *Koh Santeapheap*, June 29, 2007, Radio Free Asia, June 2007.
9. The Law on the Prevention and Control of HIV/AIDS, enacted by the National Assembly on June 14, 2002; Implementing Guidelines of the Law on the Prevention and Control of HIV/AIDS, National AIDS Authority, 2005.
10. Internews Europe Mekong Project, Phnom Penh, has been monitoring print coverage of HIV/AIDS in major newspapers and magazines since July 2006. In the first six months of 2006, there were an average of ten stories per month (including twenty-four stories published in December with World Aids Day); and in the first eight months of 2007, an average of twenty-eight stories per month were published. The increase is likely to be impacted in part, by the coverage of Bun Rany Hun Sen, the wife of the prime minister, who has been speaking about HIV/AIDS in her capacity as head of the Cambodian Red Cross.
11. "HIV and the Media, Content Analysis, 2007;" Internews' Mekong Project, Bangkok, Thailand. Incorporating results from "Cambodian Radio and HIV/AIDS, 2007" and "Cambodian Press and HIV/AIDS, 2007," conducted for Internews by Media Consulting and Development (MCD), Phnom Penh, Cambodia, July 2007.
12. "HIV and the Media, Content Analysis, 2007;" Internews' Mekong Project, Bangkok, Thailand. Incorporating results from "Cambodian Radio and HIV/AIDS, 2007" and "Cambodian Press and HIV/AIDS, 2007," conducted for Internews by Media Consulting and Development (MCD), Phnom Penh, Cambodia, July 2007.
13. *Rasmei Kampuchea*, Friday, May 26, 2006, Vol. 14, Issue 3989.

REFERENCES AND FURTHER READING

Dr. Kem Ley. (2006). Personal communication. (Secretary-General, HIV/AIDS Coordinating Committee).

Mekong Project. (2007). "HIV and the Media, Content Analysis, 2007." Bangkok, Thailand. Report compiled for Internews by Media Consulting and Development (MCD), Phnom Penh, Cambodia.

National AIDS Authority. (2006). *HIV/AIDS Media Guide*. National AIDS Authority, February, pp. 11, 36 (English version).

Overseas Development Assistance. (2006). "Turning the Tide." National AIDS Authority, supported by UNAIDS, August, pp. 21–23.

National Assembly. (2005). The Law on the Prevention and Control of HIV/AIDS. June 14, 2002. National AIDS Authority, 2005.

Radio Free Asia. (2006). *Rasmei Kampuchea*. 14 (3989), May 26.

Radio Free Asia. (2007). *Koh Santeapheap*. June 29.

SECTION 7

Vulnerable Populations: Conflict, Natural Disaster, and Migration

FRAMING ESSAY

The Epidemiology of HIV among Conflict-Affected and Displaced Populations

Current Concepts

Paul B. Spiegel and Anne Rygaard Bennedsen

OVERVIEW

In 2004, 25 active armed conflicts occurred worldwide, 69 countries were affected by refugee movements and 48 countries by internal displacement of their populations. Africa was the most affected continent as well as the hardest hit by the HIV pandemic. The 2005 estimated number of refugees and internally displaced persons (IDPs) worldwide are 12 and 25 million, respectively (Alerta 2005; UNHCR 2004). At the United Nations General Assembly Special Session on HIV/AIDS (UNGASS), governments recognized that "populations destabilised by armed conflict . . . including refugees, internally displaced persons, and in particular women and children, are at increased risk of exposure to HIV infection" (United Nations General Assembly 2001). Thus, in this forum and in many others, it has been acknowledged that HIV is a critical factor to be considered in the context of conflict and forced displacement.

Many countries that are affected by conflict and host refugees are already overburdened by the scourge of AIDS. Governments affected by such situations are often unable or unwilling to provide these persons with acceptable HIV and AIDS-related services that they require, despite international obligations under Article 23 of the 1951 Convention relating to the Status of Refugees to ensure refugees lawfully staying in their territories access to the same "public relief and services" as their nationals, including medical care. For example, HIV-related needs of refugees are seldom included in National Strategic Plans and/or in national proposals submitted to major donors (Spiegel, Miller, and Schilperord 2005). By default, the international community and local non-governmental organizations often become responsible for the provision of such essential services. At UNGASS, governments called upon "all United Nations agencies, regional and international organizations, as well as non-governmental organizations involved with the provision and delivery of international assistance to countries and regions affected by conflicts . . . to incorporate as a matter of emergency HIV/AIDS prevention, care and awareness elements into their plans and programmes" (United Nations General Assembly 2001). However, a myriad of issues, such as accessibility to these populations, insufficient funds, overlapping or unclear mandates, and poor coordination often result in deficient provision of such interventions. This failure to provide HIV prevention, care, and treatment to conflict-affected and displaced populations does not only directly affect them; it also undermines effective HIV prevention, care, and treatment for surrounding host populations, and ultimately the country itself. Conflict and forced displacement can occur for years and even decades. Governments and the international community must improve coordination to provide integrated care to affected populations and host communities. Furthermore, a sub-regional approach that harmonizes HIV interventions across borders is essential for continuity of care and effective utilization of persons trained in HIV (Spiegel, Miller, and Schilperord 2005).

CYCLE OF DISPLACEMENT DUE TO CONFLICT

The cycle of displacement due to conflict is shown in Exhibit FE7.1. It has been simplified here to include three main stages of transition, though additional movement may occur during this period, and subgroups among the population may be in different phases of transition. The first is typically referred to as the *emergency phase* and is associated with the onset of a humanitarian emergency that often forces individuals to leave their homes. This phase is often marked by deprivation of food, shelter, security, and lack of access to health services and information about HIV, leaving both displaced and host population vulnerable to infection. During this phase it is essential to ensure a minimum set of HIV interventions (Inter-Agency Standing Committee 2004), even though urgent needs relating to food, shelter, and security often cause HIV-related needs to be overlooked. The second phase or *post-emergency phase* is marked by greater stability, often allowing affected persons to gain access to more comprehensive HIV and AIDS services. In the *third and final stage*, displaced persons return home or refugees may resettle in a third country or integrate in their host country (i.e., the three durable solutions). In this phase it is important to ensure that HIV and AIDS services remain available to these populations after their return, integration, or resettlement.

Exhibit FE7.1 Cycle of displacement due to conflict

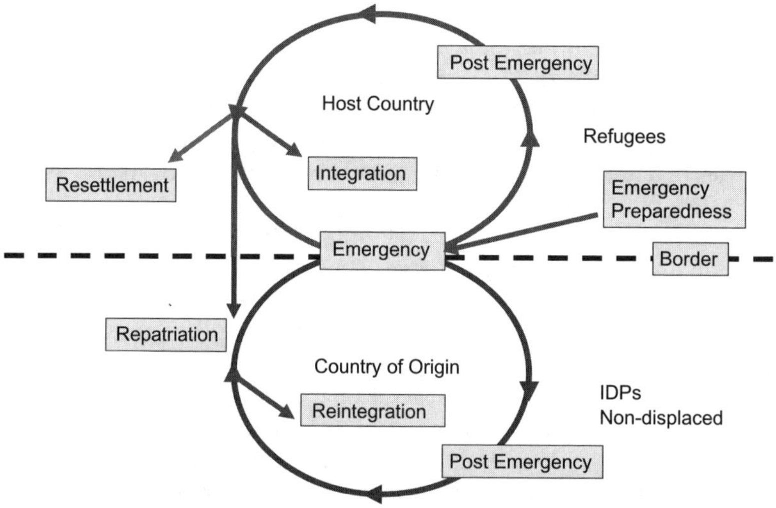

Source: Spiegel et al. (2005)

EPIDEMIOLOGY OF HIV AMONG CONFLICT-AFFECTED AND DISPLACED POPULATIONS

Conflict

Mass movement of people, as is seen during armed conflict, can cause the spread of communicable diseases, including HIV (Anderson, May, Boily et al. 1991). Until recently, it was believed that conflict increased the transmission of HIV among affected populations due to a variety of factors, including increased risky behavior, gender violence, sexual exploitation, and violence (Exhibit FE7.2). Numerous hypotheses were published on the detrimental effects of conflict causing increased transmission of HIV without much data to substantiate these claims (Anderson, Sewankambo, and Vandergift 2005; Buve, Bishikwabo-Nsarhaza, and Mutangadura 2002; Hankins, Friedman, Zafar, et al. 2002). The media reported on rape being used as a tool of war, with the consequent inevitable increase in sexually transmitted

Exhibit FE7.2 HIV risk factors for conflict and displaced persons camps

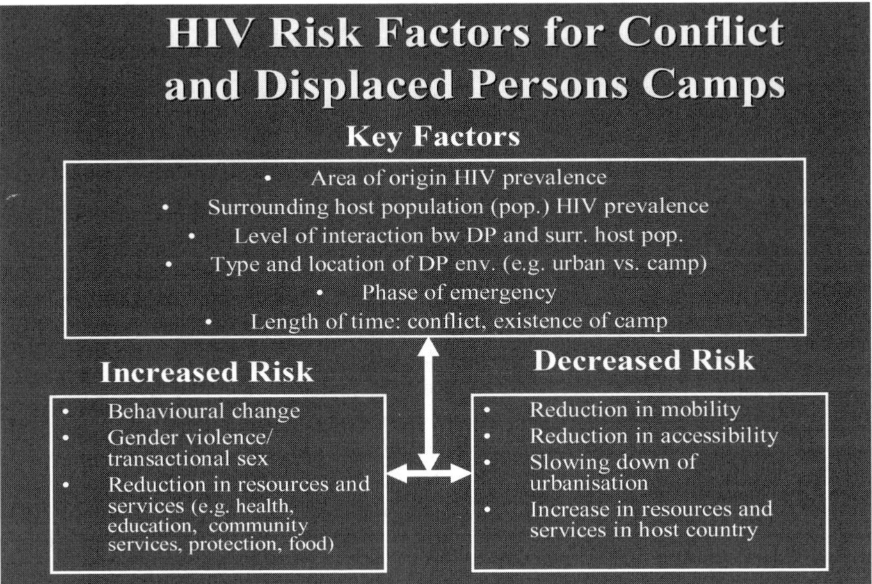

Source: Adapted from Spiegel (2004)

infections (STIs) including HIV, again without much data to support their claims (Lowicki-Zucca, Spiegel, and Ciantia 2005).

Over the past few years, a more complicated and subtle analysis of how conflict may affect HIV transmission has evolved (Mock, Duale, Brown et al. 2004; Salama and Dondero 2001; Spiegel 2004). Besides the well-known and much publicized factors that increase risk, there are other lesser recognized factors that may decrease the risk of HIV transmission in conflict, including reduction in mobility and accessibility of the population (e.g., people are caught in the bush and cannot move to larger villages and cities, visit commercial sex workers, and then return to their rural communities and infect their partners; truck drivers cannot cross borders and move around the country because there are no roads) and a decline in urbanization of a country. Essential core factors, such as the HIV prevalence of the affected population before the conflict begins, the duration of the conflict, and the interaction with outside populations, as well as the HIV prevalence of these groups, all determine the outcome of how conflict affects HIV transmission. Therefore, an interacting complex set of countervailing factors ultimately determines if conflict increases or decreases HIV transmission in a particular circumstance.

Angola and Sierra Leone are two examples where intense civil wars of a long duration began at a time when the HIV prevalence was very low among the affected populations. In both these countries, it appears as if the factors that decrease the risk of HIV transmission outweighed those that increase risk, thus allowing HIV prevalence to remain low. During the war in Sierra Leone, HIV prevalence was estimated to be much higher (7 percent nationally in 1997) (WHO, Zonal Authorities, World Bank et al. 2005) than was found to be the case when countrywide population-based surveys were undertaken post-conflict: 0.9 percent in 2002 and 1.5 percent in 2004 (Kaiser, Spiegel, Salama et al. 2002; National HIV/AIDS Secretariat 2005). Compared to the more peaceful Guinea with a national HIV prevalence of 4.2 percent in 2003 (Ministry of Health Guinea 2001), conflict-affected Sierra Leone has a lower prevalence. The HIV prevalence of Liberia, a country that has also undergone over a decade of civil war, is not known; a countrywide survey occurred in 2006/07.

In Angola, limited data on HIV prevalence during the conflict was available. However, some antenatal sentinel surveys, though not countrywide, showed lower HIV prevalence in both urban and rural areas compared to its surrounding peaceful countries of Namibia and Zambia (WHO, Zonal Authorities, World Bank et al. 2005; UNAIDS, UNICEF, WHO 2004; Asamoah-Odei, Calleja, and Boerma 2004). Preliminary post-conflict data now indicate that Angola, like Sierra Leone, has a much lower HIV prevalence than its neighboring countries. Consequently, at the end of the conflict, when countrywide surveys were undertaken in Sierra Leone and Angola, both countries had lower HIV prevalence than their respective surrounding countries that had not undergone conflict.

In contrast to Sierra Leone and Angola's conflicts, which began when the countries had a low HIV prevalence, Northern Uganda already had a high HIV prevalence when the conflict began in 1988. However, conflict does not appear, despite recent incorrect allegations (Anderson, Sewankambo, and Vandergrift 2005), to have fueled the epidemic in Northern Uganda. In fact, data show that from 1993 to 2002 the HIV prevalence in Gulu, the sentinel site in Northern Uganda, decreased from 27.1 percent to 11.9 percent (Ministry of Health Uganda 2003). Data from Kitgum and Pader, more rural areas in Northern Uganda, also show decreasing rates from 2002 to 2004 (Ciantia 2003). Some reports claim that conflict is fueling the epidemic in Northern Uganda because the 2002 HIV prevalence in Gulu is approximately double the overall HIV prevalence for Uganda. However, this high prevalence is similar to other major urban settings elsewhere in the country. A similar decrease in HIV prevalence to that of Gulu has been reported in both Kampala (24.4 percent to 10 percent) and Mbarara (18.1 percent to 10.8 percent) from 1993 to 2002. (WHO, Zonal Authorities, World Bank et al. 2005).

In another scenario, there is concern that, if the simmering instability in the Ivory Coast explodes and a large refugee crisis ensues, refugees fleeing Sierra Leone may have a higher HIV prevalence than their surrounding host countries (Lowicki-Zucca, Spiegel, and Ciantia 2005). Ivory Coast has known stability and relative prosperity in West Africa for decades. Possibly because of these factors, it also has a higher HIV prevalence than do the countries surrounding it (i.e., Ghana, Mali, Burkina Faso, and Guinea) (WHO, Zonal Authorities, World Bank et al. 2005). It is interesting to note that in sub-Saharan Africa the more affluent countries (e.g., South Africa and Côte d'Ivoire) sometimes have much higher HIV prevalence than their surrounding less affluent countries. Thus, in this hypothetical situation, factors increasing the spread may prevail in this scenario. However, this was not the case when refugees fled Burundi in the early 2000s to Tanzania. At that time, Burundi had a much higher HIV prevalence than Tanzania. However, the Burundian refugees fled from rural areas and had a lower or similar HIV prevalence to those of the surrounding Tanzanian host communities. Therefore it cannot be stated that conflict always increases or decreases transmission of HIV. The context of each individual situation must be examined carefully.

The uniformed services have often been accused of increasing HIV transmission during conflict by a variety of factors including widespread rape and other forms of sexual violence (e.g., providing services or money for sex to non-commercial sex workers as well as fueling the commercial sex business). Blanket statements that the military have two to five times the HIV prevalence of that of the general population are incorrect (McGinn, Purdin, Krause et al. 2001); each situation must be considered individually and more specific country data are needed (de Waal 2005). Although rape is prevalent in many conflict situations, such as occurred in Sierra Leone (Amowitz, Reis, Lyons et al. 2002), Liberia (Swiss, Jennings, Aryee et al. 1998), Rwanda (Donovan 2002) and Democratic Republic of Congo (Amnesty International 2006), there is no evidence that rape, even on a massive scale, has a major effect on the course of the HIV epidemic in a country. Many interacting factors must be considered, including the HIV prevalence of the rapists, the probability of transmission due to rape, and the eventual number of rape survivors who become HIV positive. This must be compared with the overall population size and HIV prevalence of the country. Although it is difficult to estimate the probability of HIV transmission during rape, it is likely higher than by consensual sex due to genital/rectal trauma, multiple assailants, and exposure to multiple receptive sites (Gostin, Lazzarini, and Alexander 1994). For consensual sex, transmission risk in discordant couples varies from 1 in 330 to 1 in 3,300 exposures (Bamberger, Waldo, Gerberding et al. 1999).

Every case of sexual violence is a horrendous event with long-term physical and psychosocial consequences. Each case must be provided with respect and appropriate treatment in a dignified manner (Inter-Agency Standing Committee 2004; UNHCR 2003; WHO, UNHCR 2004). In a low prevalence epidemic, uniformed service personnel with a higher HIV prevalence than the population with whom they are interacting may "seed" the virus throughout the country; this may cause the spread of the virus among the population over a wide geographic area which could lead to a generalized HIV epidemic in the future. This may have occurred in Uganda and Guinea-Bissau (Smallman-Raynor and Cliff 1991; Poulsen, Aaby, Jensen et al. 2000; Lemey, Pybus, Wang et al. 2003). However, once again, there is no evidence, despite repeated assertions, that uniformed services have increased the overall HIV prevalence of a country at the population level; this is true even for Cambodia, despite claims otherwise (Beyrer 1998a, 1998b). For example, what would be the effect on the HIV epidemic in a country of 20 million people with an HIV prevalence of 10 percent in the horrific event that 50,000 women were raped? Numerous complex and competing factors listed above would need to be examined, including the HIV prevalence of the perpetrators and the sexual networks of the women who were raped. The fact that one adult in ten in that country is already HIV positive is a major factor that may mitigate the overall effects on a population level. Therefore, the common assumption that uniformed services and widespread rape fuel the HIV epidemic at a population-based level (as opposed to an individual level) during conflict is not substantiated by data; the context of each individual situation must be examined carefully.

Forced Displacement

A common misperception is that refugees bring HIV with them and infect the host population. This has negative consequences for the affected populations, including the aggravation of xenophobic fears, the possible imposition of mandatory HIV testing by authorities to regulate immigration or refugee inflows, refoulement (forced return of refugees to their country of origin), the hampering of reconciliation processes and creating obstacles to their integration in host communities (Lowicki-Zucca, Spiegel, and Ciantia 2005).

Refugees are often displaced from countries with a low HIV prevalence when the conflict began (e.g., Sierra Leone and Angola) and, thus, they often have a lower HIV prevalence than the surrounding host communities. In these circumstances, refugees are a vulnerable group, at risk of contracting HIV from their surrounding host populations (Spiegel 2004). In other circumstances, when the HIV prevalence was high when the conflict began in a country, refugees may have higher HIV prevalence than their surrounding host communities. This could be the case if the situation in Côte d'Ivoire explodes and refugees flee to neighboring countries that have lower HIV prevalence. It is interesting to note that Côte d'Ivoire is the most affluent country in West Africa; it is this affluence and its consequences that may have aided this country to have the highest HIV prevalence in West Africa. However, despite the magnitude of HIV in a country at conflict, refugees often come from low prevalence rural settings rather than the higher prevalence urban settings. Thus, for example, although Burundi had a higher HIV prevalence than Tanzania in the early 1990s, the Burundian refugees have a similar or lower level than the surrounding Tanzanian host populations (UNHCR data). Once again, every context is unique and must be considered individually.

Since 2003, the United Nations High Commissioner for Refugees and its partners have conducted HIV sentinel surveillance among pregnant women in more than 20 camps/settlements consisting of approximately 800,000 refugees in Kenya, Rwanda, Tanzania, Sudan, Uganda, and Zambia. In all circumstances, refugees had a similar or lower HIV prevalence than their surrounding host populations. However, from the limited time trend data available, the prevalence of the refugees appears to be increasing to that of the surrounding host population. In all situations, tracking HIV prevalence trends over time among refugees and surrounding host populations is essential in examining the long-term effectiveness of HIV/AIDS programs.

In general, there is a lack of sufficient data on HIV prevalence among IDPs. In Sudan, HIV prevalence amongst IDPs was collected during a national survey conducted by the Sudan National Aids Control Program in 2002; the HIV prevalence among IDPs did not differ from that among non-displaced people. Another HIV survey was conducted in 2002 in Lubumbashi, Democratic Republic of Congo (Mulanga, Bazepeo, Mwamba et al. 2004). HIV prevalence amongst IDP pregnant women were higher than non-displaced pregnant women but there was no statistically significant difference. Future studies with sufficient statistical power among IDPs, surrounding populations, and among the populations in the IDP's area of origin, are needed in differing contexts.

Return

Concerns have arisen that refugees residing in host countries with higher HIV prevalence rates than those of their country of origin may increase the spread of HIV when they repatriate. This may be a legitimate concern. However, it is difficult to substantiate, because many factors may affect the HIV prevalence in a post-conflict/reconstruction country; these include refugee and IDP return as well as demobilization of soldiers, and increased mobility and accessibility of the population as roads are rebuilt and shipping and trucking resume and intensify throughout the country. It has been postulated that the return of Contra troops, their families, and refugees to Nicaragua may have helped to increase the HIV prevalence of that country post-conflict. (Arauz, Low, Gorter et al. 1991; Low, Smith, Gorter et al. 1990; Summerfield 1991).

Although there is the possibility that refugees may have higher HIV prevalence than the populations of origin, many refugees receive training and develop important HIV skills during their displacement that can be used in their country of origin, thus contributing to halting the epidemic there. Some behavioral surveillance surveys by UNHCR show that refugees have better HIV knowledge and practices than surrounding host populations and area of origin populations. This highlights the importance of refugees accessing HIV services and training during their displacement. Once again, every situation is unique and must be examined according to the context.

CONCLUSION

Recent epidemiological evidence is now challenging old assumptions about the link between conflict and the increase of HIV transmission. Many previous assumptions were based on insufficient, biased or badly reported data; and some conclusions were not even based on data at all. It is essential to critically examine data reported during conflict situations, which may often be biased due to the difficult situation in which it is gathered, and triangulate it with post-conflict data to assess the former's validity.

The well-documented factors that increase the vulnerability to HIV among conflict-affected and displaced populations must be considered alongside other essential factors, such as reduced mobility and accessibility of the population that may work to decrease HIV transmission. HIV prevalence among displaced persons and surrounding host communities also influence HIV transmission, as do the level of interaction between these two communities. In many countries, when the conflict began when the HIV prevalence was low, the HIV prevalence remained relatively low as compared with neighboring countries at peace (e.g., Sierra Leone and Southern Sudan). Refugees who fled from these countries often had a lower HIV prevalence than their surrounding host populations. Over time, the HIV prevalence among these refugees appears to have increased towards that of the host population.

Assessing the impact of rape by uniformed services in conflict situations on the HIV epidemic at a population level in a conflict-affected country can be difficult for various reasons, listed above. It appears that in countries with a very low HIV prevalence, uniformed services may "seed" the virus, allowing it to spread to populations that would not otherwise have been affected at the current stage of the epidemic. However, there is no evidence that wide-scale rape has increased the overall HIV prevalence of a country. Mathematic modeling should be undertaken in order to assess the potential effects according to numerous different factors.

As a more complex view of the connection among conflict, displacement, and HIV prevails and more data become available, HIV programming for these affected populations may change and be more contextual. It is essential that the context-specific circumstances in which refugees, displaced persons, and surrounding host populations live is examined and used to guide HIV/AIDS policies and programs.

REFERENCES AND FURTHER READING

Alerta 2005: Informe sobre conflictos, derechos humanos y construccion de paz. Barcelona: Escola de Cultura de Pau—UAB, 2005.

Amnesty International. "Mass rape: time for remedies." http://web.amnesty.org/report2005/cod-summary-eng. Last accessed April 2006.

Amowitz, L.L., Reis, C., Lyons, K.H. et al. "Prevalence of war-related sexual violence and other human rights abuses among internally displaced persons in Sierra Leone." *JAMA* 2002;287(4):513–521.

Anderson, R., May, R., Boily, M., Garnett, G., and Rowley, J. "The spread of HIV-1 in Africa: sexual contact patterns and the predicted demographic impact of AIDS." *Nature* 1991;352:581–589.

Anderson, R., Sewankambo, F., and Vandergrift, K. *Pawns of politics—children, conflict and peace in Northern Uganda.* Kampala: World Vision, 2005.

Arauz, R., Low, N., Gorter, A., and Davy Smith, G. "AIDS in Nicaragua." *Lancet* 1991;337:1290–1290.

Asamoah-Odei, E., Calleja, J., and Boerma, J. "HIV prevalence and trends in Sub-Saharan Africa: no decline and large subregional differences." *Lancet* 2004;364:35–40.

Bamberger, J., Waldo, C., Gerberding, J., and Kats, M. "Postexposure prophylaxis in immunodefienciency virus (HIV) infection following sexual assault." *American Journal of Medicine* 1999;106(323–326).

Beyrer, C. Burma and Cambodia. "Human rights, social disruption, and the spread of HIV/AIDS." *Health and Human Rights.* 1998a;2(4):84–97.

Beyrer, C. *War in the blood: sex, politics and AIDS in Southeast Asia.* London: Zed Books, 1998b.

Buve, A., Bishikwabo-Nsarhaza, K., Mutangadura, G. "The spread and effect of HIV-1 infection in sub-Saharan Africa." *Lancet* 2002;359(9322):2011–2017.

Ciantia, F. "HIV seroprelavence in Northern Uganda: the complex relationship between AIDS and conflict." *Journal of Medicine and The Person* 2003;2(4):172–175.

de Waal, A. *Issue paper 1: HIV/AIDS and the military.* The Hague, 2005.

Donovan, P. "Rape and HIV/AIDS in Rwanda." *Lancet* 2002;360 Suppl:s17–s18.

Gostin, L., Lazzarini, Z., and Alexander, D. "HIV testing, counseling and prophylaxis after sexual assault." *JAMA* 1994;271(1436–44).

Hankins, C.A., Friedman, S.R., Zafar, T., and Strathdee, S.A. "Transmission and prevention of HIV and sexually transmitted infections in war settings: implications for current and future armed conflicts." *AIDS* 2002;16(17):2245–2252.

Inter-Agency Standing Committee (IASC). *Guidelines for HIV/AIDS interventions in emergency settings.* Geneva: IASC Reference Group, 2004.

Kaiser, R., Spiegel, P., Salama, P. et al. *HIV seroprevalence and behavioral risk factor survey in Sierra Leone.* Atlanta: Centers for Disease Control and Prevention, 2002.

Lemey, P., Pybus, O., Wang, B., Salemi, M., and Vandamme, A. "Tracing the origin and history of the HIV-2 epidemic." *PANAS* 2003;100(11):6588–6592.

Low, N., Smith, G.D., Gorter, A., and Arauz, R. "AIDS and Migrant Populations in Nicaragua." *Lancet* 1990;336:1593–1594.

Lowicki-Zucca, M., Spiegel, P., and Ciantia, F. "AIDS, conflict and the media in Africa: risks in reporting bad data badly." *Emerging Themes in Epidemiology* 2005;2:12.

McGinn, T., Purdin, S., Krause, S., and Jones, R. *Forced migration and transmission of HIV and other sexually transmitted diseases: policy and programmatic responses.* UCSF Center for HIV Information, 2001.

Ministry of Health Guinea, USAID. *National HIV seroprevalence study.* GOG, USAID, FHI, Stat-view International, 2001. www.usaid.gov/gn/health/news/021011_hivsurvey/index.htm. Last accessed April 2006.

Ministry of Health Uganda. *STD/HIV/AIDS surveillance report.* Kampala, 2003.

Mock, N.B., Duale, S., Brown, L.F. et al. "Conflict and HIV: a framework for risk assessment to prevent HIV in conflict-affected settings in Africa." *Emerg.Themes.Epidemiol.* 2004;1(1):6.

Mulanga, C., Bazepeo, S., Mwamba, J. et al. "Political and socioeconomic instability: how does it affect HIV? A case study in the Democratic Republic of Congo." *AIDS* 2004;18(5):832–834.

National HIV/AIDS Secretariat, Ministry of Health and Sanitation. *National population based HIV seroprevalence survey of Sierra Leone in 2004.* Freetown, 2005.

Poulsen, A.G., Aaby, P., Jensen, H., and Dias, F. "Risk factors for HIV-2 seropositivity among older people in Guinea-Bissau. A search for the early history of HIV-2 infection." *Scandinavian Journal of Infectious Disease* 2000;32(2):169–175.

Salama, P., and Dondero, T.J. "HIV surveillance in complex emergencies." *AIDS* 2001;15 Suppl 3:S4–S12.

Smallman-Raynor, M.R., and Cliff, A.D. "Civil war and the spread of AIDS in Central Africa." *Epidemiology of Infectious Disease* 1991;107(1):69–80.

Spiegel, P.B. "HIV/AIDS among conflict-affected and displaced populations: dispelling myths and taking action." *Disasters.* 2004;28(3):322–339.

Spiegel, P., Miller, A., and Schilperord, M. *Strategies to support the HIV-related needs of refugees and host populations: UNAIDS Best Practice Collection.* Geneva: UNHCR, UNAIDS, 2005.

Spiegel, P., and Nankoe, A. "UNHCR, HIV/AIDS and refugees: lessons learned." *Forced Migration Review* 2004;19:21–23.

Sudan National AIDS Control Program. *Situation analysis: behavioral and epidemiological surveys and response analysis.* Khartoum, 2002.

Summerfield, D. "Nicaragua: the ending of war and AIDS." *Lancet* 1991;337(8747):967–968.

Swiss, S., Jennings, P.J., Aryee, G.V. et al. "Violence against women during the Liberian civil conflict." *JAMA* 1998;279(8):625–9.

UNAIDS, UNICEF, WHO. *Angola Epidemiological Fact Sheet on HIV/AIDS and Sexually Transmitted Infections.* 2004 Update. Geneva: UNAIDS, 2004.

United Nations General Assembly. *Declaration of commitment on HIV/AIDS.* Geneva: United Nations and UNAIDS, 2001.

UNHCR. *Sexual and gender-based violence against refugees, returnees, and internally displaced persons.* Geneva, 2003.

UNHCR. *Refugee Trends: 1 January–30 September 2004.* Geneva, 2004.

WHO, UNHCR. *Clinical management of rape survivors: developing protocols for use with refugees and internally displaced persons.* Geneva, 2004.

WHO, Zonal Authorities, World Bank, UNAIDS, UNICEF, UNDP. *Somalia 2004 first national second generation HIV/AIDS/STI sentinel surveillance survey.* Mogadishu, 2005.

CHAPTER 26

The Potential for PTSD, Substance Use, and HIV Risk Behavior among Adolescents Exposed to Natural Disasters

Implications for Hurricane Katrina Survivors

Karla D. Wagner, Deborah J. Brief, Melanie J. Vielhauer, Steve Sussman, Terence M. Keane, and Robert Malow

ABSTRACT

Adverse psychosocial outcomes can be anticipated among youth exposed to natural disasters, such as Hurricane Katrina. Adolescents are particularly vulnerable to the impact of catastrophic events and may suffer lasting psychological consequences. We review existing literature on the effects of exposure to natural disasters and similar traumas on youth and, where data on youth are unavailable, on adults. The effect of natural disasters is discussed in terms of risk for three negative health outcomes: Post-Traumatic Stress Disorder, substance use disorder, and HIV-risk-taking behavior.

Fall 2005 proved to be one of the most devastating hurricane seasons in recent years for the Gulf Coast of the United States. Hurricane Katrina made landfall on August 29, 2005, ravaging communities in Louisiana, Mississippi, and Alabama and acutely impacting an estimated 700,000 people (Gabe et al. 2005). While the full consequences of Katrina and its aftermath (e.g., evacuation and relocation of residents and repopulation of the area), as well as possible exposure to subsequent hurricanes, are still being assessed, adverse psychosocial outcomes can be anticipated among the area's youth. Not only are affected youth at risk for Post-Traumatic Stress Disorder (PTSD) and other psychological consequences of exposure to a natural disaster, but they may also engage in a variety of problem behaviors in response to this trauma, such as substance use and sexual risk taking. Thus, assessment and care of adolescent Gulf Coast hurricane survivors will have significant implications for their long-term physical and psychological wellbeing. In the years following Hurricane Katrina, it will also be important to understand the factors that may put exposed adolescents at increased risk for chronic psychological morbidity due to their trauma exposure.

The aim of this chapter is to describe the current state of knowledge about the effects of hurricanes and similar natural disasters on adolescent psychological wellbeing, with a particular focus on psychological morbidity and negative health behaviors in the form of PTSD, substance use, and HIV-risk behavior. In reviewing these topics, we draw upon literature from both the United States and international experience that investigates the associations between trauma, PTSD, substance use disorders (SUD), and HIV-risk behaviors in adolescents and, when similar research on adolescents is unavailable, in adults.

TRAUMA EXPOSURE

There is a large body of literature on exposure of adolescents to traumatic events, most of which focuses on interpersonal victimization (e.g., Giaconia et al. 1995; Ward et al. 2001). Epidemiological data indicate that adolescents are at high risk for experiencing traumas such as assault, rape, and robbery (Centers for Disease Control and Prevention 2000; Boney-McCoy and Finkelhor 1995). However, a few studies have provided information on prevalence of lifetime exposure to another form of trauma among youth: natural disasters. For example, Giaconia et al. (1995) found a lifetime prevalence rate of approximately 2 percent for exposure to a natural disaster among a sample of 18-year-olds from a predominantly white, working-class community in the northeastern United States, while Breslau et al. (2004) reported a prevalence of 8.6 percent among a cohort of urban youth from a mid-Atlantic U.S. state who were enrolled in the 1985–86 school year and followed up in 2000–02. Costello et al. (2002) conducted a longitudinal general population survey of youth in western North Carolina and found that rates of lifetime exposure to a natural disaster were 1.9 percent for girls and 2.3 percent for boys. In Japan, a survey of female college students aged 18 to 29 found that 65.6 percent of women had experienced a natural-disaster-related trauma in their lifetime, with 34 percent reporting exposure to a natural disaster during adolescence (Mizuta et al. 2005). For most of these women, the natural disaster was likely the Kobe earthquake of 1995.

POST TRAUMATIC STRESS DISORDER

One potential outcome of exposure to traumatic events is the development of PTSD, a debilitating disorder that may have long-term consequences for adolescent survivors. PTSD is an anxiety disorder of at least one-month duration that is characterized by symptoms of re-experiencing (e.g., intrusive memories or thoughts), avoidance and/or emotional numbing, and hyperarousal. It is often accompanied by feelings of anxiety and depression, social alienation, and mistrust of family, friends, and systems (Keane and Barlow 2002). PTSD is generally considered to be acute if symptoms last for less than three months, while individuals with symptoms lasting more than three months are characterized as having chronic PTSD. Delayed onset PTSD may occur with onset of symptoms up to six months after the stressor (American Psychiatric Association 2000).

As in adults, the types of traumas that are most frequently linked to PTSD in adolescents are those involving interpersonal violence (Giaconia et al. 1995; Cuffe et al. 1998; Kessler et al. 1995). However, there is also evidence of psychological morbidity in the form of PTSD among adolescents exposed to natural disasters including bushfires (McFarlane, Plicansky, and Irwin 1987), hurricanes (Garrison et al. 1995; La Greca et al. 1996; La Greca and Prinstein 2002), and earthquakes (Asarnow et al. 1999).

Prevalence

Rates of PTSD among adolescents and young adults have been provided across several large-scale community samples. For example, in the U.S. National Comorbidity Survey, 8 percent of 15- to 24-year-old participants met lifetime criteria for PTSD (Kessler et al. 1995). In a nationally representative sample of U.S. youth aged 12–17 years, Kilpatrick et al. (2000) found that 5 percent of youth met criteria for a current diagnosis of PTSD. Of note, these rates do not reflect subthreshold yet clinically significant symptomatology experienced by some trauma-exposed youth. There is some evidence that the concept of post-traumatic stress can be applied to adolescents cross-culturally (Charney and Keane 2007). Ruchkin et al. (2005) surveyed 14- to 17-year-olds in New Haven, Connecticut and Arkhanglesk, Russia. Associations between symptom and trauma severity were similar in the two groups, as were levels of comorbid psychopathology. While the majority of youth in this study reported traumatic events related to community violence, rather than natural disasters, its results support the cross-cultural application of PTSD assessment.

In studies focusing specifically on natural disasters, PTSD has been identified as a common reaction in youth (Vernberg et al. 1996). In a review of studies investigating rates of PTSD among youth exposed to devastating hurricanes (e.g., Hurricane Andrew in 1992 or Hurricane Hugo in 1989), La Greca and Prinstein (2002) reported that, across studies, approximately one third to a half of youth reported moderate to severe PTSD symptoms. Estimates of PTSD symptoms among youth exposed to the 1999 Athens earthquake ranged from 4.5 percent of youth in the affected area three months after the earthquake (Roussos et al. 2005) to 78 percent six months following the event (Kolaitis et al. 2003). Among Armenian youth exposed to the 1988 earthquake, rates of PTSD 1 to 1/2 years after the event ranged from 26 percent in a minimally affected area to 95 percent in the most severely affected area (Goenjian et al. 1995). Estimates of PTSD symptoms among youth two months after the Indonesian tsunami of 2004 range from 11 percent in minimally affected villages in Thailand (Thienkrua et al. 2006) to 70.7 percent in southern India (John, Russell, and Russell 2007).

Research indicates that once PTSD develops in youth it may persist over time. La Greca and Prinstein's (2002) review indicated that some children exposed to hurricanes and earthquakes may exhibit symptoms up to one year after the event. Other investigators such as Shaw et al. (1995) found that Hurricane Andrew-exposed youth continued to report PTSD symptoms up to 32 weeks post-disaster. Similarly, among 7- to 14-year-old Thai children exposed to the Indonesian tsunami in 2004, rates of PTSD ranged from 11 percent to 13 percent in affected areas two months after the tsunami and did not decrease significantly at the nine-month follow-up (Thienkrua et al. 2006). Given the long-term morbidity that can be associated with PTSD among youth, in the aftermath of Hurricane Katrina we should expect that the psychological morbidity among adolescents will present over an extended period of time, and at varied prevalence rates in a variety of sub-populations. Certain subgroups of adolescents may be at particularly elevated risk of developing morbidity and problem behaviors in response to this disaster. Youth exposed to several risk factors will have a greater chance of developing PTSD in the wake of Hurricane Katrina and may be at increased risk as they enter future hurricane seasons. These predictors of PTSD are discussed next.

Predictors

La Greca and colleagues (1998, 1996) have outlined an integrated conceptual model of predictors of children's post-disaster reactions that includes: 1) characteristics of the stressor (e.g., life threat and loss, or disruption), 2) characteristics of the child (demographics and pre-disaster functioning), 3) features of the post-disaster environment (level of support and occurrence of major life stressors), and 4) the child's efforts to cope with disaster-related distress. Over several studies described below, each of the proposed factors in this model was shown to account for a unique portion of the variance in predicting post-traumatic stress symptoms in children (La Greca et al. 1996; Vernberg et al. 1996).

Important characteristics of the stressor have been evaluated in studies of youths' reactions to natural disasters. These include perceived life threat, number of life-threatening experiences, and loss experienced in the disaster (Vernberg et al. 1996). Others have also found that level of exposure accounts for a significant portion of the variance relative to the other predictors (La Greca, Silverman, and Wasserstein 1998; La Greca et al. 1996; Vernberg et al. 1996). Several other investigations around the globe have also supported the importance of the level of threat in explaining PTSD reactions among youth in response to a variety of natural disasters (Groome and Soureti 2004; Roussos et al. 2005; Bokszczanin 2007; John, Russell, and Russell 2007; Thienkrua et al. 2006; Kar and Bastia 2006). For example, Goenjian et al. (2001) found that level of impact, objective and subjective features of the event, and thoughts of revenge accounted for 68 percent of the variance in the severity of post-traumatic stress reaction in a sample of

Nicaraguan adolescents exposed to Hurricane Mitch in 1998.

Characteristics of the child such as age, gender, and ethnicity have also been investigated as possible predictors of PTSD in youth, but results have been equivocal. Age-related differences in PTSD symptoms following disasters have been observed in comparisons between youngsters of varying age cohorts (Green et al. 1991; Bokszczanin 2007; Nader et al. 1990). La Greca and colleagues failed to find age differences in PTSD symptoms following Hurricane Andrew, but this may have been due to the fact that they were studying this question among children within a narrower age range (third- to fifth-graders; La Greca et al. 1996).

Several studies suggest that gender may be related to a child's risk for post-traumatic stress symptoms (Famularo et al. 1996; Bokszczanin 2007; John, Russell, and Russell 2007; Groome and Soureti 2004; Ruchkin et al. 2005; Giaconia et al. 1995; Zink and McCain 2003), although the data are mixed. For example, Shannon et al. (1994) found higher levels of symptoms in girls than boys following Hurricane Hugo. In contrast, after controlling for level of exposure, La Greca, Silverman, and Wasserstein (1998) failed to find gender differences in post-traumatic stress responses among young children following Hurricane Andrew. Russoniello et al. (2002), on the other hand, found that the effect of female gender on PTSD symptoms persisted even after controlling for level of flooding associated with Hurricane Floyd in a sample of fourth-graders.

The role of ethnicity in children's PTSD symptoms following a disaster has also been examined. Some studies in the United States suggest that minorities are at elevated risk for PTSD compared to other racial or ethnic groups (Garrison et al. 1995; Kilpatrick et al. 2003; La Greca et al. 1996; La Greca, Silverman, and Wasserstein 1998; Lonigan et al. 1991). It has been suggested that ethnic differences may relate to socioeconomic status; minority families who are already financially compromised may be more adversely affected by the economic consequences of a hurricane (La Greca et al. 1996). Thus, the possible role that minority status and socioeconomic factors play in the emergence of PTSD following a trauma clearly warrants further investigation.

There is also some evidence that suggests that a prior trauma history may affect the development of PTSD following subsequent trauma exposure. This relationship has been examined among adults (King et al. 1999) and, more recently, among children. Neuner et al. (2006) surveyed Sri Lankan 8- to 14-year olds three to four weeks after the 2004 Indonesian tsunami and found that a history of traumatic events (mostly exposure to civil unrest and violence) was associated with preliminary PTSD symptoms. Thus, it may be important to investigate whether psychological responses to an earlier trauma influence the development of PTSD following Hurricane Katrina and whether exposure to Katrina will affect the development of PTSD following subsequent traumas.

Pre-trauma environmental factors (e.g., socioeconomic status and family instability) have also been shown to exert indirect effects on the development of PTSD in adults through post-trauma recovery variables (e.g., availability of social support; King et al. 1999); that is, individuals from a pre-trauma disadvantaged environment may have insufficient resources to deal with the aftermath of the trauma and additional stressors. Not only will these findings regarding pre-existing psychosocial problems assist in the ongoing assessment and care of adolescents exposed to Hurricane Katrina, but they will also inform community response as the Gulf Coast enters future hurricane seasons and residents prepare for additional storms.

Evidence also suggests that certain elements of the post-disaster environment, including the functioning of significant others and access to supportive relationships, exposure to additional life stressors, and use of coping strategies, may influence the emergence of PTSD in youth (La Greca and Prinstein 2002; La Greca et al. 1996). For example, Vernberg et al. (1996) found that children with higher levels of social support from various sources, including parents, teachers, and classmates, reported fewer PTSD symptoms after Hurricane Andrew than did those with less social support from these sources. Following an event of the magnitude of Hurricane Katrina, the availability of social support from these important sources may be diminished. This is particularly relevant among those affected youth from lower socioeconomic status neighborhoods, some of which were the hardest hit, most badly damaged, and slowest to repopulate. These neighborhoods suffered loss of infrastructure, including homes, and other community resources, which has severely impacted the support available to adolescents after the storm. Further, school closures and relocations may limit access to other sources of support. It is also important to note, however, that disasters of this magnitude may also mobilize other sources of community support. In a survey of mostly New Orleans residents housed at the Houston convention center after the hurricane, 26 percent said that they were rescued from their homes by friends or neighbors (Brodie et al. 2006). Displaced families were also housed by families in non-affected areas, which likely enhanced the availability of social and psychological resources among affected individuals.

Parental reactions to a trauma such as a natural disaster may influence the likelihood that children will develop PTSD (Hamblen 2006). Wickrama and Kaspar (2007) found that positive mother–child relationships served a protective function in mitigating both PTSD and depressive symptoms among tsunami-exposed adolescents in Sri Lanka, while high levels of depressive symptoms amongst mothers negatively influenced adolescent outcomes. Similarly, the severity of PTSD in children exposed to an earthquake in Bolu, Turkey was associated with the presence of PTSD and severity of depression in their fathers (Kilic and Ulusoy 2003). Parents who are experiencing a high level of distress may not be able to serve important functions for their children in the post-disaster environment, such as modeling coping and providing nurturance and a sense of physical safety (Vernberg et al. 1996).

Additional environmental stressors and adversities often follow trauma and loss experiences (National Child Traumatic Stress Network 2006). For survivors of natural disasters this might include a lack of supplies, food, medications and shelter, a destabilization of routines, and a loss of community infrastructure. Estimates of the number of individuals displaced by Hurricane Katrina range from 600,000 to 1.5 million. Over 265,000 applications for temporary housing payments and just under 12,000 temporary housing trailers had been provided by the federal government as of October 19, 2005, partially indicating the scope of the displacement (Gabe et al. 2005). This displacement may be particularly disruptive for children, who represented approximately one fourth of affected individuals (Gabe et al. 2005). Since the hurricane struck at the beginning of the school year, children's routines, social networks, and support systems were also disrupted.

Exposure to new, major life events in the months following a disaster is also thought to be a significant contributor to post-disaster stress reactions among youth. La Greca et al. (1996) found that exposure to additional stressful life events predicted increases in PTSD symptoms in children over the year following Hurricane Andrew. While the mechanism remains unclear, the authors hypothesize that exposure to further life events may limit social support available to the child, or serve to magnify symptoms in an additive manner. Further, they suggest that additional work is needed to disentangle these subsequent life events from hurricane-related sequelae (e.g., death of a relative).

The data on coping responses following a natural disaster and their relationship to PTSD symptoms in youth is fairly limited. There is some evidence to suggest that self-reported coping styles and PTSD symptoms are strongly associated. Data indicate that this association is stronger for some types of coping than others. For example, La Greca et al. (1996) found that the use of certain negative strategies (i.e., blaming, angry responses) best predicted post-traumatic stress symptoms over time. In a survey six months after Hurricane Floyd, Russoniello et al. (2002) found that 95 percent of fourth-grade children reported some PTSD symptoms. The most common coping strategies used by youth were wishful thinking (hope), cognitive restructuring, social support, distraction, emotional regulation, and problem solving. Social withdrawal, resignation, blaming others, and self-criticism were less frequently used but, similar to the findings of La Greca et al. (1996), were more strongly associated with PTSD symptoms. Evidence among adults exposed to the Indonesian tsunami suggests that support seeking may serve a protective function, predicting better adjustment six months after the disaster (Tang 2006).

Another type of coping that is common following a trauma, but that is maladaptive, is substance use (Giaconia et al. 2003). The development of negative health behaviors such as substance use as a result of trauma exposure is of particular concern among adolescents because the formation of maladaptive behavioral patterns in adolescence may contribute to further psychosocial morbidity and to long-term chronic health problems in adulthood. Findings relevant to the relationship between trauma, PTSD, and substance use are discussed below.

COMORBIDITY OF TRAUMA EXPOSURE, PTSD, AND SUD

Several studies with adults have shown that trauma exposure increases the risk for alcohol and drug use (Rheingold, Acierno, and Resnick 2004; Stewart 1996; Kilpatrick et al. 1997). Limited data suggest that traumatized adolescents are also likely to have high rates of substance use disorders (SUDs; Giaconia et al. 2003). In a study with Dutch adolescents, those exposed to a café fire were significantly more likely than those not exposed to engage in excessive use of alcohol 12 months after the fire (Reijneveld et al. 2005). In a sample of German adolescents and young adults aged 14 to 24 years, a history of trauma exposure was linked to a lifetime SUD in 35 percent of participants (Perkonigg et al. 2000). This rate exceeds lifetime rates of SUD found among adolescents in general community samples. Thus, while middle to late adolescence may be the peak risk period for first onset of serious substance use problems (Burke et al. 1991; Kessler et al. 1994), trauma exposure appears to increase this risk. These data suggest that exposure to a natural disaster such as Hurricane Katrina might put adolescents at risk for developing a SUD.

Among trauma survivors, PTSD has also been shown to increase the risk for problematic drinking and drug use in adults (Kessler et al. 1995; Kulka et al. 1990) and adolescents (Schroeder and Polusny 2004). Moreover, research indicates that PTSD may mediate the relationship between trauma exposure and severity of substance use problems (Epstein et al. 1998). Among individuals with PTSD, the chronicity of PTSD symptoms has also been found to predict an increased risk for comorbid substance use problems beyond PTSD alone (Breslau and Davis 1992).

Rates of trauma exposure and PTSD have also been examined in adolescents with an SUD. In Giaconia et al.'s (2000) study of 18-year-olds, approximately 56 percent of participants with an SUD reported at least one lifetime trauma and 11 percent met criteria for lifetime PTSD. Further, across studies researchers have found that adolescents with an SUD are at heightened risk for experiencing any lifetime trauma (two- to fivefold) and for developing PTSD (four- to ninefold) (Clark et al. 1997; Giaconia et al. 2000; Kilpatrick et al. 2000) compared to adolescents in the community without an SUD. Giaconia et al.'s (2000) community study reported that, even after controlling for cumulative lifetime exposure to trauma, adolescents with an SUD continued to be at greater risk (twofold) for developing PTSD than their peers without an SUD. Risk for PTSD may also vary across drugs of abuse (fourfold for alcohol, sixfold for marijuana, and ninefold for other drug abuse or dependence; Kilpatrick et al. 2000). These data suggest that the association between trauma, SUD, and PTSD is likely to become evident among exposed youth, and that the potential for the further development of maladaptive coping strategies such as SUD is cause for concern among this population.

INTERSECTION OF TRAUMA, PTSD, SUBSTANCE USE, AND HIV RISK

Another negative health behavior that has been associated with both trauma exposure and PTSD is HIV risk-taking behavior, either in the form of risky sex or drug use. The destabilizing effects of natural disasters may lead to increased use of injection drugs and subsequent HIV transmission, though effects have varied depending on local context (Strathdee et al. 2006). This relationship has been studied in adults, but fewer studies have examined it among adolescents. Retrospective studies of individuals living with HIV have documented high rates of victimization and other types of trauma in this population. There is also growing evidence that PTSD is prevalent among individuals living with HIV (Brief et al. 2004). Further, data indicate that trauma exposure and/or PTSD may increase an individual's risk for becoming infected with HIV. For example, Zierler and colleagues (1991) found that college-aged men with a history of sexual abuse had a twofold increase in the prevalence of HIV infection relative to men who had not been abused, regardless of their sexual preference.

There are several mechanisms through which trauma exposure might increase risk for HIV in adolescent trauma victims, particularly in the context of PTSD or PTSD-SUD. First, there is evidence of an association between trauma exposure (Johnsen and Harlow 1996; Lodico and DiClemente 1994), early onset PTSD (Stiffman et al. 1992) and involvement in high-risk drug use behaviors for some types of trauma survivors (e.g., sexual abuse). Survivors of early childhood abuse show higher rates of using drugs that are likely to be injected (Johnsen and Harlow 1996), an earlier initiation of needle use (Holmes 1997), and a higher incidence of needle sharing (Lodico and DiClemente 1994). Any increase in needle use following a natural disaster, particularly among adolescents, is reason for concern. Sharing contaminated needles is a primary or secondary risk factor in a large proportion of HIV infections; 17 percent of new HIV diagnoses in the United States between 2001 and 2004 were among injection drug users (IDU) and 4 percent were among men who are IDU and have sex with men (Centers for Disease Control and Prevention 2005b). However, it is important to note that increases in substance use, in general, and injection drug use, in particular, have not been noted in all regions exposed to natural disasters. For example, preliminary evidence from the Aceh province of Indonesia following the 2004 tsunami indicate that there has been little change in drug use as a consequence of the natural disaster (Strathdee et al. 2006).

Studies with trauma survivors also find higher rates of participation in high-risk sexual activities that can lead to HIV infection (e.g., unprotected intercourse, high numbers of sexual partners, and sex with riskier partners) (Rheingold, Acierno, and Resnick 2004). Trauma survivors who develop an alcohol or drug problem even in the absence of IDU may also increase their risk for HIV through participating in high-risk sexual activities while intoxicated (Centers for Disease Control and Prevention 2005b). Whether adolescent survivors of Hurricane Katrina will show increased participation in either high-risk drug or sexual behaviors, similar to survivors of sexual abuse, is unclear. Further research is needed to examine these relationships in Hurricane Katrina survivors and in particular to determine whether those who experienced some type of interpersonal violence in the aftermath of the hurricane are at greater risk for engaging in HIV-related drug and sexual behaviors.

IMPLICATIONS FOR HURRICANE KATRINA-EXPOSED ADOLESCENTS

Several risk factors for PTSD are present among the population exposed to Hurricane Katrina. One early study with 124 adult Hurricane Katrina evacuees in the two weeks after the hurricane found that 39 percent of study participants reported moderate, and 24 percent reported severe, PTSD symptoms (Coker et al. 2006). Rates of PTSD symptoms among adolescent survivors are also expected to be high. Many of the individuals who were affected by the hurricane experienced direct exposure to the hurricane and floodwaters, witnessed the injury or deaths of family members, or in the aftermath of the hurricane were directly exposed to violence or were stranded in their homes (Coker et al. 2006). Furthermore, many families were separated, had their homes destroyed, and were prohibited from returning to their homes due to safety issues. Lack of instrumental (e.g., insurance, medical care, employment, and housing) and social resources (e.g., social support and adequate coping) may further impede the post-disaster recovery of adolescents and their families. Moreover, the duration of the upheaval created by the hurricane and high-profile media coverage may be significant factors in predicting the level of vulnerability to negative mental health outcomes. Thus, rates of PTSD should be expected to be high among exposed youth, and symptoms may be sustained for many months, and perhaps years, beyond the hurricane.

Rates of substance use among youth in New Orleans, Mississippi, and Alabama were generally comparable to national rates before the hurricane (Centers for Disease Control and Prevention 2005b). Intensification of use and/or transitions from lower- to higher-risk drug use behaviors (e.g., initiation of injection) may be expected among youth as a result of their exposure to the trauma, especially among those who develop PTSD. In addition, exposure to Hurricane Katrina and the subsequent development of PTSD either alone or in combination with an SUD may lead to high-risk behavior patterns, including sexual risk taking that may put youth at risk for HIV.

Thus, adolescents exposed to Hurricane Katrina may be at elevated risk for numerous negative health outcomes, both in the immediate aftermath of the hurricane and in the long term. Comprehensive care for adolescents exposed to Hurricane Katrina will require attention to additional trauma exposure in the aftermath of the hurricane, PTSD, and SUD, as well as HIV risk behaviors. Without intervention, there is concern that an early pattern of poor self-care, established in many young trauma survivors, may persist into adulthood (Allers and Benjack 1992). With attention to the provision of sensitive and widespread assessment and care of traumatized adolescents, however, communities and care providers will have the opportunity to make a lasting impact on the health and wellbeing of affected adolescents.

ACKNOWLEDGMENTS

This work was supported, in part, by a grant from the National Institute on Drug Abuse (Grant R03-DA 21982) and by the National Center for PTSD.

REFERENCES AND FURTHER READING

Allers, C. T., and K. J. Benjack. 1992. "Barriers to HIV Education and Prevention: The Role of Unresolved Childhood Sexual Abuse." *Journal of Child Sexual Abuse* 1 (4):69–81.

American Psychiatric Association. 2000. *Diagnostic and Statistical Manual of Mental Disorders*, 4th edition, text revision.

Asarnow, J., S. Glynn, R. S. Pynoos, J. Nahum, D. Guthrie, D. P. Cantwell, and B. Franklin. 1999. "When The Earth Stops Shaking: Earthquake Sequelae Among Children Diagnosed for Pre-Earthquake Psychopathology." *Journal of the American Academy of Child and Adolescent Psychiatry* 38 (8):1016–18.

Bokszczanin, A. 2007. "PTSD Symptoms in Children and Adolescents 28 Months after a Flood: Age and Gender Differences." *Journal of Traumatic Stress* 20 (3):347–51.

Boney-McCoy, S., and D. Finkelhor. 1995. "Psychosocial Sequelae of Violent Victimization in a National Youth Sample." *Journal of Consulting and Clinical Psychology* 63:726–36.

Breslau, N., and G. C. Davis. 1992. "Posttraumatic Stress Disorder in an Urban Population of Young Adults: Risk Factors for Chronicity." *American Journal of Psychiatry* 149 (5):671–5.

Breslau, N., H. C. Wilcox, C. L. Storr, V. C. Lucia, and J. C. Anthony. 2004. "Trauma Exposure and Posttraumatic Stress Disorder: A Study of Youths in Urban America." *Journal of Urban Health* 81 (4):530–44.

Brief, D. J., A. R. Bollinger, M. J. Vielhauer, J. A. Berger-Greenstein, E. E. Morgan, S. M. Brady, L. M. Buondonno, and T. M. Keane. 2004. "Understanding the Interface of HIV, Trauma, Post-Traumatic Stress Disorder, and Substance Use and its Implications for Health Outcomes." *AIDS Care* 16 (Suppl. 1):S97–S120.

Brodie, M., E. Weltzien, D. Altman, R. J. Blendon, and J. M. Benson. 2006. "Experiences of Hurricane Katrina Evacuees in Houston Shelters: Implications for Future Planning." *American Journal of Public Health* 96 (5):1402–408.

Burke, K. C., J. D. Burke, D. S. Rae, and D. A. Regier.

1991. "Comparing Age at Onset of Major Depression and Other Psychiatric Disorders by Birth Cohorts in Five U.S. Community Populations." *Archives of General Psychiatry* 48 (9):789–95.

Centers for Disease Control and Prevention. 2000. "CDC Surveillance Summaries." *Morbidity and Mortality Weekly Report 2000* 49 (No. SS-5).

Centers for Disease Control and Prevention. 2005a. "Trends in HIV/AIDS Diagnoses-33 States, 2001–2004." *Morbidity and Mortality Weekly Report 2005* 54 (45):1149–53.

Centers for Disease Control and Prevention. 2005b. "Youth Risk Behavioral Surveillance Survey, Youth Online: Comprehensive Results." http://apps.nccd.cdc.gov/yrbss/ (accessed September 27, 2005).

Charney, M. E., and T. M. Keane. 2007. "Psychometric Analyses of the Clinician-Administered PTSD Scale (CAPS)–Bosnian Translation." *Cultural Diversity and Ethnic Minority Psychology* 13 (2):161–8.

Clark, D. B., N. Pollock, O. G. Bukstein, A. C. Mezzich, J. T. Bromberger, and J. E. Donovan. 1997. "Gender and Comorbid Psychopathology in Adolescents with Alcohol Dependence." *Journal of the American Academy of Child and Adolescent Psychiatry* 36 (9):1195–9.

Coker, A. L., J. S. Hanks, K. S. Eggleston, J. Risser, P. G. Tee, K. J. Chronister, C. L. Troisi, R. Arafat, and L. Franzini. 2006. "Social and Mental Health Needs Assessment of Katrina Evacuees." *Disaster Management and Response* 4 (3):88–94.

Costello, E. J., A. Erkanli, J. A. Fairbank, and A. Angold. 2002. "The Prevalence of Potentially Traumatic Events in Childhood and Adolescence." *Journal of Traumatic Stress* 15 (2):99–112.

Cuffe, S. P., C. L. Addy, C. Z. Garrison, J. L. Waller, K. L. Jackson, R. E. McKeown, and S. Chilappagari. 1998. "Prevalence of PTSD in a Community Sample of Older Adolescents." *Journal of the American Academy of Child and Adolescent Psychiatry* 37:147–54.

Epstein, J. N., B. E. Saunders, D. G. Kilpatrick, and H. S. Resnick. 1998. "PTSD as a Mediator Between Childhood Rape and Alcohol Use in Adult Women." *Child Abuse and Neglect* 22 (3):223–34.

Famularo, R., T. Fenton, R. Kinscherff, and M. Augustyn. 1996. "Psychiatric Comorbidity in Childhood Post Traumatic Stress Disorder." *Child Abuse and Neglect* 20 (10):953–61.

Gabe, T., G. Falk, M. McCarty, and V. W. Mason. 2005. *Hurricane Katrina: Social-Demographic Characteristics of Impacted Areas*. Washington DC: Congressional Research Service, Library of Congress.

Garrison, C. Z., E. S. Bryant, C. L. Addy, P. G. Spurrier et al. 1995. "Posttraumatic Stress Disorder in Adolescents After Hurricane Andrew." *Journal of the American Academy of Child and Adolescent Psychiatry* 34 (9):1193–201.

Giaconia, R. M., H. Z. Reinherz, A. C. Hauf, A. D. Paradis, M. S. Wasserman, and D. M. Langhammer. 2000. "Comorbidity of Substance Use and Post-Traumatic Stress Disorders in a Community Sample of Adolescents." *American Journal of Orthopsychiatry* 70 (2):253–62.

Giaconia, R. M., H. Z. Reinherz, A. D. Paradis, and C. K. Stashwick. 2003. "Comorbidity of Substance Use Disorders and Posttraumatic Stress Disorder in Adolescents (Chapter 12)." In *Trauma and Substance Abuse: Causes, Consequences, and Treatment of Comorbid Disorders*, edited by P. Ouimette and P. J. Brown. Washington DC: American Psychological Association.

Giaconia, R. M., H. Z. Reinherz, A. B. Silverman, B. Pakiz, A. K. Frost, and E. Cohen. 1995. "Traumas and Posttraumatic Stress Disorder in a Community Population of Older Adolescents." *Journal of the American Academy of Child and Adolescent Psychiatry* 31 (10):1369–180.

Goenjian, A. K., L. Molina, A. M. Steinberg, L. A. Fairbanks, M. L. Alvarez, H. A. Goenjian, and R. S. Pynoos. 2001. "Posttraumatic Stress and Depressive Reactions Among Nicaraguan Adolescents After Hurricane Mitch." *American Journal of Psychiatry* 158 (5):788–94.

Goenjian, A. K., R. S. Pynoos, A. M. Steinberg, L. M. Najarian, J. R. Asarnow, I. Karayan, M. Ghurabi, and L. A. Fairbanks. 1995. "Psychiatric Comorbidity in Children After the 1988 Earthquake in Armenia." *Journal of the American Academy of Child and Adolescent Psychiatry* 34 (9):1174–84.

Green, B. L., M. Korol, M. C. Grace, and M. G. Vary. 1991. "Children and Disaster: Age, Gender, and Parental Effects on PTSD Symptoms." *Journal of the American Academy of Child and Adolescent Psychiatry* 30 (6):945–51.

Groome, D., and A. Soureti. 2004. "Post-Traumatic Stress Disorder and Anxiety Symptoms in Children Exposed to the 1999 Greek Earthquake." *British Journal of Psychology* 95 (Pt. 3):387–97.

Hamblen, J. 2006. "Terrorist Attacks and Children: A National Center for PTSD Fact Sheet." http://www.ncptsd.va.gov/ncmain/ncdocs/fact_shts/fs_children_disaster.html?opm=1&rr=rr54&srt=d&echorr=true (accessed January 4, 2006).

Holmes, W. C. 1997. "Association Between a History of Childhood Sexual Abuse and Subsequent, Adolescent Psychoactive Substance Use Disorder in a Sample of HIV Seropostive Men." *Journal of Adolescent Health* 20 (6):414–19.

John, P. B., S. Russell, and P. S. Russell. 2007. "The Prevalence of Posttraumatic Stress Disorder Among Children and Adolescents Affected by Tsunami Disaster in Tamil Nadu." *Disaster Management and Response* 5 (1):3–7.

Johnsen, L. W., and L. L. Harlow. 1996. "Childhood Sexual Abuse Linked with Adult Substance Use, Victimization, and AIDS Risk." *AIDS Education and Prevention* 8 (1):44–57.

Kar, N., and B. K. Bastia. 2006. "Post-Traumatic Stress Disorder, Depression and Generalised Anxiety Disorder in Adolescents After a Natural Disaster: A Study of Comorbidity." *Clinical Practice and Epidemology in Mental Health* 2:17.

Keane, T. M., and D. H. Barlow. 2002. "Posttraumatic Stress Disorder." In *Anxiety and Its Disorders*, edited by D. H. Barlow. New York: Guilford Press.

Kessler, R. C., K. A. McGonagle, S. Zhao, C. B. Nelson et al. 1994. "Lifetime and 12-month Prevalence of DSM-III–R Psychiatric Disorders in the United States: Results from the National Comorbidity Study." *Archives of General Psychiatry* 51 (1):8–19.

Kessler, R. C., A. Sonnega, E. Bromet, M. Hughes, and C. B. Nelson. 1995. "Posttraumatic Stress Disorder in the National Comorbidity Survey." *Archives of General Psychiatry* 52:1048–60.

Kilic, C., and M. Ulusoy. 2003. "Psychological Effects of the November 1999 Earthquake in Turkey: An Epidemiological Study." *Acta Psychiatrica Scandinavica* 108 (3):232–8.

Kilpatrick, D. G., R. Acierno, H. S. Resnick, B. E. Saunders, and C. L. Best. 1997. "A 2-year Longitudinal Analysis of the Relationships Between Violent Assault and Substance Use in Women." *Journal of Consulting and Clinical Psychology* 65 (5):834–47.

Kilpatrick, D. G., R. Acierno, B. E. Saunders, H. S. Resnick, C. L. Best, and P. P. Schnurr. 2000. "Risk Factors for Adolescent Substance Abuse and Dependence: Data from a National Sample." *Journal of Consulting and Clinical Psychology* 68 (1):19–30.

Kilpatrick, D. G., K. J. Ruggiero, R. Acierno, B. E. Saunders, H. S. Resnick, and C. L. Best. 2003. "Violence and Risk of PTSD, Major Depression, Substance Abuse/Dependence, and Comorbidity: Results from the National Survey of Adolescents." *Journal of Consulting and Clinical Psychology* 71 (4):692–700.

King, D. W., L. A. King, D. W. Foy, T. M. Keane, and J. A. Fairbank. 1999. "Posttraumatic Stress Disorder in a National Sample of Female and Male Vietnam Veterans: Risk Factors, War-Zone Stressors, and Resilience-Recovery Variables." *Journal of Abnormal Psychology* 108 (1):164–70.

Kolaitis, G., J. Kotsopoulos, J. Tsiantis, S. Haritaki, F. Rigizou, L. Zacharaki, E. Riga, A. Augoustatou, A. Bimbou, N. Kanari, M. Liakopoulou, and P. Katerelos. 2003. "Posttraumatic Stress Reactions Among Children Following the Athens Earthquake of September 1999." *European Child and Adolescent Psychiatry* 12 (6):273–80.

Kulka, R. A., W. E. Schlenger, J. A. Fairbank, R. L. Hough, B. K. Jordan, C. R. Marmar, and D. S. Weiss. 1990. *Trauma and the Vietnam War Generation: Report on Findings from the National Vietnam Veterans Readjustment Study*. New York: Brunner/Mazel.

La Greca, A. M., and M. J. Prinstein. 2002. "Hurricanes and Earthquakes." In *Helping Children Cope with Disasters and Terrorism*, edited by A. M. La Greca, W. K. Silverman et al. Washington DC: American Psychological Association.

La Greca, A. M., W. K. Silverman, E. M. Vernberg, and M. J. Prinstein. 1996. "Symptoms of Posttraumatic Stress in Children after Hurricane Andrew: A Prospective Study." *Journal of Consulting and Clinical Psychology* 64 (4):712–23.

La Greca, A. M., W. K. Silverman, and S. B. Wasserstein. 1998. "Children's Predisaster Functioning as a Predictor of Posttraumatic Stress Following Hurricane Andrew." *Journal of Consulting and Clinical Psychology* 66 (6):883–92.

Lodico, M. A., and R. J. DiClemente. 1994. "The Association Between Childhood Sexual Abuse and Prevalence of HIV-Related Risk Behaviors." *Clinical Pediatrics* 33 (8):498–502.

Lonigan, C. J., M. P. Shannon, A. J. Finch, T. K. Daugherty et al. 1991. "Children's Reactions to a Natural Disaster: Symptom Severity and Degree of Exposure." *Advances in Behaviour Research and Therapy* 13 (3):135–54.

McFarlane, A. C., S. K. Plicansky, and C. Irwin. 1987. "A Longitudinal Study of the Psychological Morbidity in Children Due to a Natural Disaster." *Psychological Medicine* 17 (3):727–38.

Mizuta, I., T. Ikuno, S. Shimai, H. Hirotsune, M. Ogasawara, A. Ogawa, E. Honaga, and Y. Inoue. 2005. "The Prevalence of Traumatic Events in Young Japanese Women." *Journal of Traumatic Stress* 18 (1):33–7.

Nader, K. O., R. Pynoos, L. Fairbanks, and C. Frederick. 1990. "Children's PTSD Reactions One Year After a Sniper Attack at their School." *American Journal of Psychiatry* 147 (11):1526–30.

National Child Traumatic Stress Network. 2006. "Hurricanes." http://www.nctsnet.org/nccts/nav.do?pid=hom_main (accessed January 4, 2006).

Neuner, F., E. Schauer, C. Catani, M. Ruf, and T. Elbert. 2006. "Post-tsunami Stress: A Study of Posttraumatic Stress Disorder in Children Living in Three Severely Affected Regions in Sri Lanka." *Journal of Traumatic Stress* 19 (3):339–47.

Perkonigg, A., R. C. Kessler, S. Storz, and H.-U. Wittchen. 2000. "Traumatic Events and Post-Traumatic Stress Disorder in the Community: Prevalence, Risk Factors and Comorbidity." *Acta Psychiatrica Scandinavica* 101 (1):46–59.

Reijneveld, S. A., M. R. Crone, A. A. Schuller, F. C. Verhulst, and S. P. Verloove-Vanhorick. 2005. "The Changing Impact of a Severe Disaster on the Mental Health and Substance Misuse of Adolescents: Follow-Up of a Controlled Study." *Psychological Medicine* 35 (3):367–76.

Rheingold, A. A., R. Acierno, and H. S. Resnick. 2004. "Trauma, Posttraumatic Stress Disorder, and Health Risk Behaviors." In *Trauma and Health: Physical Health Consequences of Exposure to Extreme Stress*, edited by P. P. Schnurr and B. L. Green. Washington DC: American Psychological Association.

Roussos, A., A. K. Goenjian, A. M. Steinberg, C. Sotiropoulou, M. Kakaki, C. Kabakos, S. Karagianni, and V. Manouras. 2005. "Posttraumatic Stress and Depressive Reactions Among Children and Adolescents After the 1999 Earthquake in Ano Liosia, Greece." *American Journal of Psychiatry* 162 (3):530–37.

Ruchkin, V., M. Schwab-Stone, S. Jones, D. V. Cicchetti, R. Koposov, and R. Vermeiren. 2005. "Is Posttraumatic Stress in Youth a Culture-Bound Phenomenon? A Comparison of Symptom Trends in Selected U.S. and Russian Communities." *American Journal of Psychiatry* 162 (3):538–44.

Russoniello, C., T. Skalko, K. O'Brien, S. McGhee, D. Bingham-Alexander, and J. Beatley. 2002. "Childhood Posttraumatic Stress Disorder and Efforts to Cope after Hurricane Floyd." *Behavioral Medicine* 28 (2):61–71.

Schroeder, J. M., and M. A. Polusny. 2004. "Risk Factors for Adolescent Alcohol Use Following a Natural Disaster." *Prehospital and Disaster Medicine* 19 (1):122–7.

Shannon, M. P., C. J. Lonigan, A. J. Finch, and C. M. Taylor. 1994. "Children Exposed to Disaster: I. Epidemiology of Post-Traumatic Symptoms and Symptom Profiles." *Journal of the American Academy of Child and Adolescent Psychiatry* 33 (1):80–93.

Shaw, J. A., B. Applegate, S. Tanner, D. Perez, E. Rothe, A. E. Campo-Bowen, and B. L. Lahey. 1995. "Psychological Effects of Hurricane Andrew on an Elementary School Population." *American Academy of Child and Adolescent Psychiatry* 34 (9):1185–92.

Stewart, S. H. 1996. "Alcohol Abuse in Individuals Exposed to Trauma: A Critical Review." *Psychological Bulletin* 120 (1):83–112.

Stiffman, A. R., P. Doré, F. Earls, and R. Cunningham. 1992. "The Influence of Mental Health Problems on AIDS-Related Risk Behaviors in Young Adults." *Journal of Nervous and Mental Disease* 180 (5):314–20.

Strathdee, S. A., J. A. Stachowiak, C. S. Todd, W. K. Al-Delaimy, W. Weibel, C. Hankins, and T. L. Patterson. 2006. "Complex Emergencies, HIV, and Substance Use: No 'Big Easy' Solution." *Substance Use and Misuse* 14:1637–51.

Tang, S. C. 2006. "Positive and Negative Postdisaster Psychological Adjustment among Adult Survivors of the Southeast Asian Earthquake-Tsunami." *Journal of Psychosomatic Research* 61 (5):699–705.

Thienkrua, W., B. L. Cardozo, M. L. Chakkraband, T. E. Guadamuz, W. Pengjuntr, P. Tantipiwatanaskul, S. Sakornsatian, S. Ekassawin, B. Panyayong, A. Varangrat, J. W. Tappero, M. Schreiber, F. van Griensven, and Thailand Post-Tsunami Mental Health Study Group. 2006. "Symptoms of Posttraumatic Stress Disorder and Depression Among Children in Tsunami-Affected Areas in Southern Thailand." *JAMA* 296 (5):549–59.

Vernberg, E. M., A. M. La Greca, W. K. Silverman, and M. J. Prinstein. 1996. "Prediction of Posttraumatic Stress Symptoms in Children After Hurricane Andrew." *Journal of Abnormal Psychology* 105 (2):237–48.

Ward, C. L., A. J. Flisher, C. Zissis, M. Muller, and C. Lombard. 2001. "Exposure to Violence and its Relationship to Psychopathology in Adolescents." *Injury Prevention* 74 (4):297–301.

Wickrama, K. A., and V. Kaspar. 2007. "Family Context of Mental Health Risk in Tsunami-Exposed Adolescents: Findings From a Pilot Study in Sri Lanka." *Social Science and Medicine* 64 (3):713–23.

Zierler, S., L. Feingold, D. Laufer, P. Velentgas et al. 1991. "Adult Survivors of Childhood Sexual Abuse and Subsequent Risk of HIV Infection." *American Journal of Public Health* 81 (5):572–5.

Zink, K. A., and G. C. McCain. 2003. "Post-Traumatic Stress Disorder in Children and Adolescents with Motor Vehicle-Related Injuries." *Journal for Specialists in Pediatric Nursing* 8 (3):99–106.

CHAPTER 27

Africa's Globalization

Colonial Labor Economy, Migration, and HIV/AIDS

Ezekiel Kalipeni, Joseph R. Oppong, and Jayati Ghosh

ABSTRACT

This chapter identifies some pathways of the impact of globalization on HIV/AIDS, including internal and international migrant labor flows and the consequences for HIV proliferation, the role of globalization in fostering inequality and poverty in weaker economies, and its impact on gender and vulnerability to HIV. Specific examples of how globalization promotes vulnerability to HIV and ways in which such vulnerability can be mitigated are offered. The chapter's central argument is that unequal economic and social conditions that globalization has promulgated across the world was the engine behind the proliferation of HIV/AIDS in Eastern and Southern Africa.

OVERVIEW

By any measure, Africa is the region that has experienced the worst of the scourge of HIV/AIDS. Statistics from UNAIDS are astounding, beyond comprehension. With only about 10 percent of the world's population, Africa has about 70 percent of the world's AIDS cases, 80 percent of AIDS deaths, and 90 percent of AIDS orphans (UNAIDS 2007). In 2005, an estimated 24.5 million people, 64 percent of the global total, were living with HIV in sub-Saharan Africa. Three-quarters of the world's women and 90 percent of the world's children living with HIV in 2005 were living in sub-Saharan Africa. Women outnumbered men, comprising 59 percent of all adults living with HIV in sub-Saharan Africa. The world's highest number of AIDS orphans, an estimated 12 million children under the age of 17 (just under 10 percent of children) living in sub-Saharan Africa had lost one or both parents to AIDS. Despite these disturbing statistics, Africans have the least access to life-saving HIV/AIDS medications. Around 72 percent (or 4.7 million) of all people in need of antiretroviral therapy live in sub-Saharan Africa, but in 2005 around one in six people in need of treatment in the region were receiving it (i.e.,17 percent or 810,000 people).

Such statistics have led to the characterization of Africa as a diseased continent, often based on shoddy scholarship that creates the erroneous impression that Africa and Africans are universally afflicted with the disease due to universal promiscuity and polysexual behaviors (see, for example, Rushing 1995). Yet, there is a very clear geography to the HIV/AIDS pandemic in Africa. Generally, beginning at the northern extremity of the continent, the severity of HIV/AIDS increases with increasing distance south across the region (see Exhibit 27.1).

South Africa with about 5 million HIV-positive people has the second largest number of people living with HIV/AIDS in the entire world. Botswana, Lesotho, and Swaziland, with an urban adult prevalence exceeding 25 percent, are the regions with the most severe crisis. In contrast, at the other end of the spectrum are such countries as Senegal

Exhibit 27.1 Distribution of HIV/AIDS in Africa in 2003

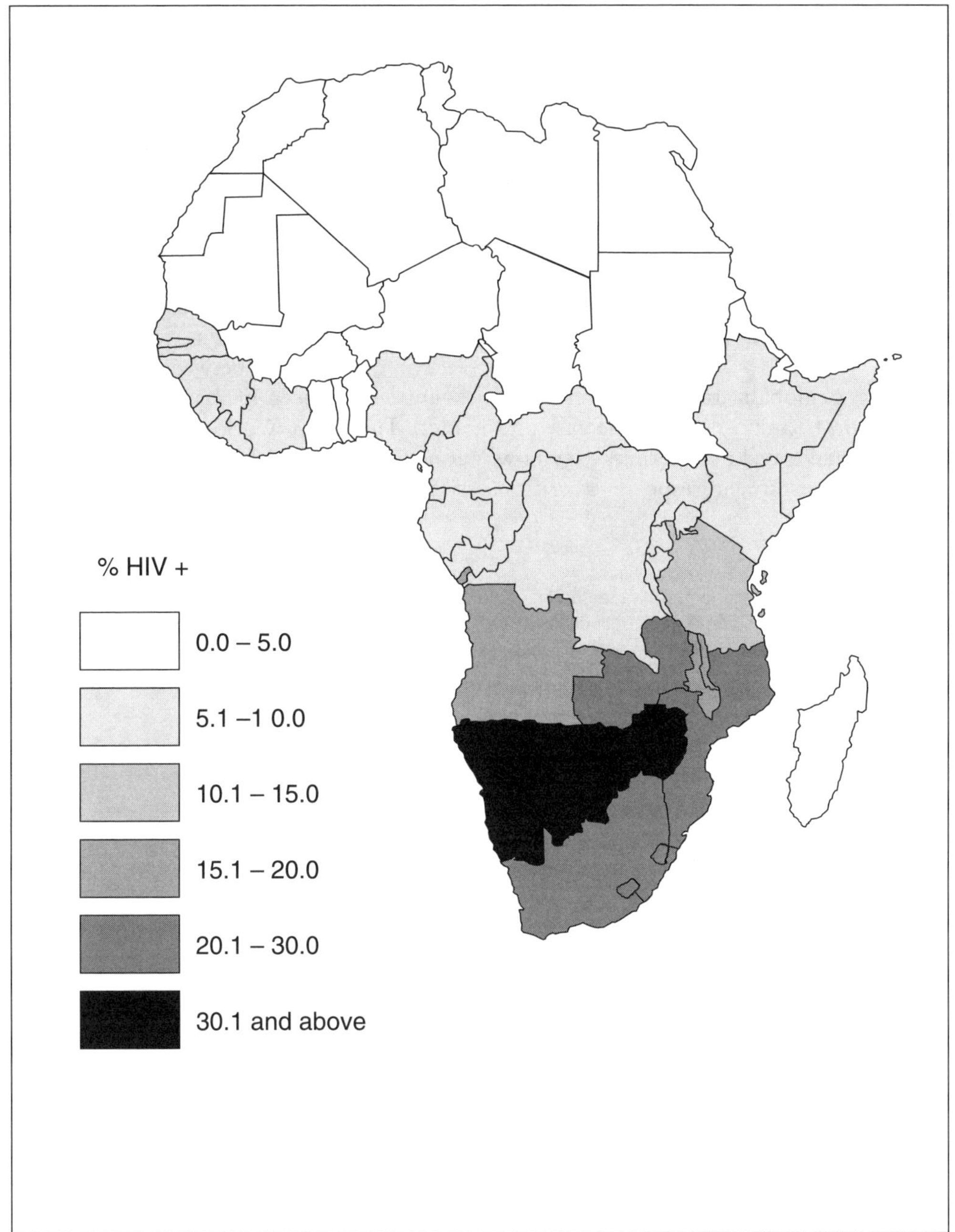

Source: Authors (2007)

and Mali, with an adult prevalence of less than 1 percent. Ghana has 3 percent, Nigeria has 5 percent, but Côte d'Ivoire has about 9 percent. However, this general pattern of prevalence conceals important regional variations. For example, pockets of high HIV rates persist in countries with low national prevalence rates. Similarly, countries with high national prevalence rates such as South Africa have regions where HIV prevalence is so extremely low, it is almost undetectable.

Many researchers agree that Africa's HIV/AIDS crisis is a complex and regionally specific phenomenon rooted in global and local economies, deepening poverty, migration, gender and cultural politics (Kalipeni et al. 2004). Consequently, it cannot be stemmed until issues of sexuality, empowerment and vulnerability as well as social, gender, and economic inequities are addressed in meaningful ways at both local and global levels.

GLOBALIZATION, INEQUALITY, AND POVERTY

Proponents of globalization, such as the IMF and the World Bank, often cite the ease and speed of global travel that permits easy flow of capital and investment resources as critical developments that will promote global trade, create jobs, and spread wealth. However, both the IMF and the World Bank clearly admit that there is a problem with this way of conducting business; that globalization and its attendant development trajectory does not benefit rich and poor countries equally (International Monetary Fund 2000). Poor countries are usually left worse off. As clearly illustrated in Exhibit 27.2, while global average per capita income rose significantly during the twentieth century, considerable variation existed between countries.

The income gap between rich and poor countries has been increasing for many decades. The 2003 World Economic Outlook concludes that, while output per capita has risen appreciably, the distribution of income

Exhibit 27.2 Output performance and trade shares: developing countries and newly industrialized economies of East and Southeast Asia income gaps between rich and poor countries

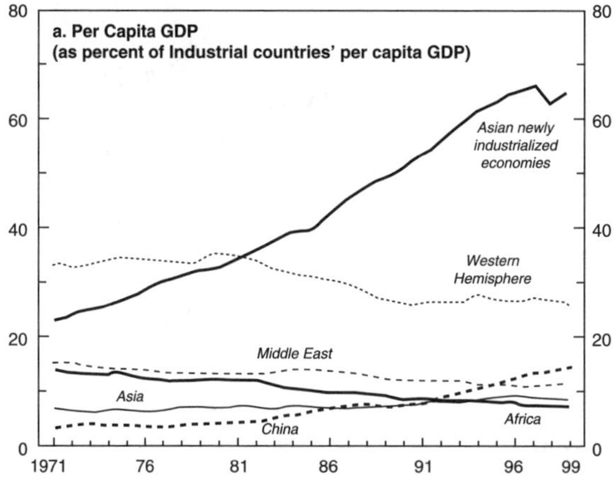

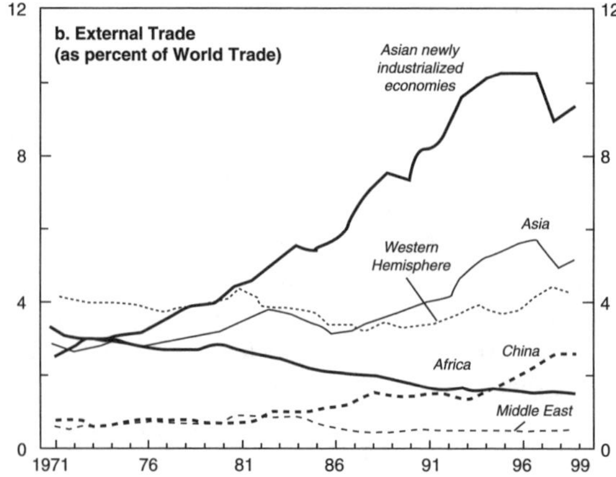

Source: International Monetary Fund (2000)

among countries has become more unequal than at the beginning of the century (International Monetary Fund 2003). Some countries are integrated into the global economy more quickly than others. Countries that have been able to integrate are seeing faster growth and reduced poverty. With reference to the developing world, these are few in number and mostly concentrated in East and Southeast Asia (see Exhibit 27.2).

Globalization produces economic benefits by promoting painful change, the elimination of opportunity for some and creation of opportunity for others, as well as the rise and fall of different industries and economic activities. Individuals and families who are able to adapt quickly to the change benefit, but those who feel threatened and unable to cope with the process of change, or resist it, lose the expected economic benefits. Thus poor countries who lack resources that are demanded heavily worldwide will receive little benefit from globalization, as they proceed to remove barriers to global trade. Without adequate investment in the human capital of the poor—increasing their access to health, education and economic opportunity, and strengthening safety nets—the poor suffer adversely from globalization.

The crises in the emerging markets in the 1990s have made it quite evident that the opportunities of globalization do not come without risks—risks arising from volatile capital movements and the risks of social, economic, and environmental degradation created by poverty (International Monetary Fund 2000). Indeed, many of these poor countries also happen to be in Africa. Not because they are naturally poor but because of the manner within which African countries have been drawn and integrated into the international community over the past 500 years beginning from the era of slavery, to colonial exploitation and to the post-independence one-sided and subordinate integration of Africa into the global economy. This is one-sided integration in the sense that Africa continues to provide raw materials for the industries of the highly developed parts of the world, raw materials which fetch very little at international markets but greatly enhance the wealth of the highly developed economies. According to the IMF, while global per capita incomes have increased over the past century, the gaps between rich and poor countries, and rich and poor people within countries, have grown. The richest quarter of the world's population saw its per capita GDP increase nearly sixfold during the century, while the poorest quarter experienced less than a three-fold increase (Exhibit 27.3). In the era of globalization, income inequality has clearly increased. Indeed the verdict on the consequences of globalization with reference to Africa is clearly negative and its performance in enhancing African livelihoods has been dismal.

AFRICA'S GLOBALIZATION: THE COLONIAL LABOR ECONOMY, MIGRATION AND HIV/AIDS

The historical and geographical context of Africa is critical to understanding the spread of the HIV/AIDS epidemic. Since the arrival of the Portuguese in West Africa in the fifteenth century, the continent has seen one crisis after another. Thus globalization for Africa is nothing new to this rich continent; it dates back to the first encounter with Europeans hell bent on extending their empires globally. First, it was slavery at unprecedented rates and then outright colonization by European settlers and traders ushering in a new economic system based on exploitative labor migration. Independence from colonial rule in the 1960s was exciting, as it meant a new dawn for the African peoples. Soon these hopes were dashed as the links to the international market forces that had been put in place during the colonial era were intransigent and meant Africa would continue to be in a subservient position within this arrangement. Indeed, it is possible to prove the significance of colonization via the use of surrogate variables such as labor migration, geographic interaction, and flows of people from one country to another.

As Yeboah (2007) points out, the physical geography of the region has had more pervasive effects on HIV/AIDS than the mere opportunities that the tropical environment

Exhibit 27.3 Twentieth-century world income trends

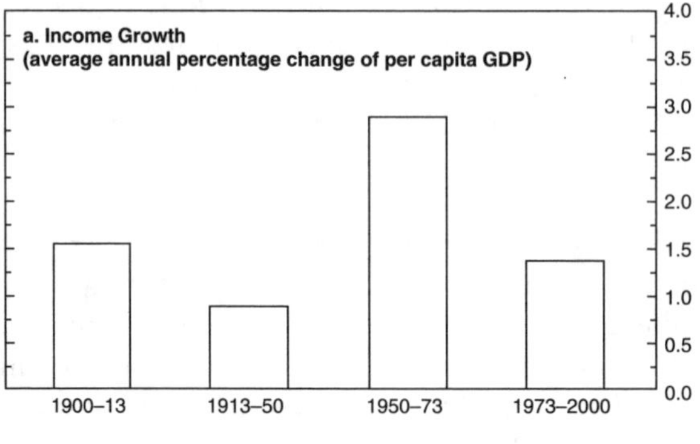

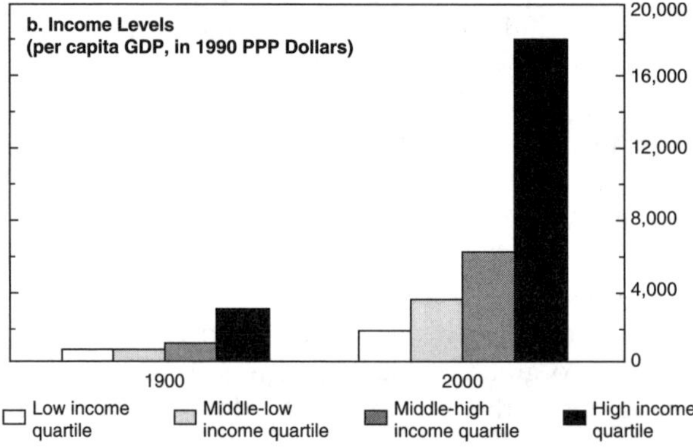

Source: International Monetary Fund (2000)

may provide for the breeding of bacteria, viruses, fungi, and other parasites. He argues that Africa's physical environment has been both a blessing and a curse. He points out that when a map of HIV/AIDS rates is juxtaposed to a topographic map of sub-Saharan Africa, we clearly see that southern and eastern Africa (high Africa) have the highest HIV/AIDS prevalence rates and higher land. West and central Africa (low Africa) have the lowest of both phenomena in the region. He points out that this relationship between HIV and higher land may look spurious, but a further analysis shows that this relationship can be used to explain what is happening in the region. The high prevalence of HIV/AIDS in the AIDS belt (southern and eastern Africa) is strongly related to the interconnectedness of physical environment, history, international migration, and Eurocentric views of the region (Yeboah 2007). Because of the excellent climate in eastern and southern Africa conducive to European settlement, rich soils, presence of numerous minerals (gold and diamonds among them) and other resources, Europeans came to settle in this part of Africa in contrast to tropical West Africa. In doing so, they established islands of economic development setting in motion massive movements of labor from rural areas to these areas in high Africa. The intermixing of peoples on a grand scale meant also the spread of various diseases from one part to another, particularly sexually transmitted diseases.

An excellent example here is South Africa. The high prevalence and incidence rates of HIV/AIDS in South Africa are illustrative of the lingering impact of colonial rule and its economy. South Africa has a long history of political unrest as well as racial and social tensions. The legacy of colonization and apartheid includes a large population of economically disenfranchised people. During apartheid, about 80 percent of the people lived on 13 percent of the land, which was devoid of resources and, thus, economic opportunities (Desmond 2001; van Niekerk

2001). This lack of economic prospect has forced many black people to commute daily to towns and cities from the peri-urban settlements. In many instances, they were forced to migrate further distances in search of employment (Desmond 2001). With the end of apartheid over a decade ago, South Africa has emerged as a leading economic power, but continues to struggle with the economic marginalization of selected population groups. This struggle has indirectly contributed not only to South Africa's rapid increase in HIV/AIDS cases but also to the challenges facing the country in combating the epidemic.

The major economic factor contributing to the rapid spread of HIV/AIDS in South Africa are migrant workers. In South Africa, migrant workers include rural to urban migrants, foreign workers, truck drivers, young women, and mine workers. Due to the dearth of job opportunities and very low incomes in rural areas, many heads of households, mainly young men, may be forced to migrate to urban areas in order to find employment. It is generally assumed that when young men leave rural homes in search of work in urban areas, they may engage in sex with women who are at high risk, thus putting themselves at higher risk of infection. When they return to their rural homes, those infected with HIV infect their rural partners as well. This circular migration is typical of the patterns of movement of young men throughout South Africa (Horowitz 2001).

Migrant laborers working in the South African gold and diamond mines, especially, have been identified as a major facilitator for HIV transmission. The mining industry accounts for 50 percent of export earnings, as well as 20 percent of the country's total Gross Domestic Product (GDP) (Williams et al. 1999). Mining as a vitally important economic activity began with the British in the 1880s. After South Africa gained independence, the significance of the industry continued as the profits greatly benefited the country. Moreover, the mining industry is a major source of employment for South Africans and neighboring countries such as Malawi, Mozambique, Lesotho, and Swaziland (Kalipeni 2000). During the 1990s the mining industry employed over 350,000 workers, the vast majority of whom were migrant workers. Over 90 percent of the industry's black employees are migrants; the vast majority live in single-sex hostels and can only visit their rural families occasionally. Few facilities exist for wives and families to visit the mines (Campbell 1997; Desmond 2001). Prolonged separation from their wives encourages miners to have sexual relationships with other women, and for that matter other men, and, since miners are relatively well paid, they are targets for commercial sex workers. Not surprisingly, an estimated 10 to 20 percent of South African miners are HIV positive, and another 7 percent are living with AIDS (Calitz 2000). As Gilgen et al. (2001) indicate, sex with commercial sex workers provides comfort and intimacy that helps mine workers cope with their fears and stresses. Because of the severe sex imbalance in the mining areas, most miners are unable to find a stable partner in the mining communities and so sexual relations with several commercial sex worker partners may be common (Campbell 1997).

HIV/AIDS knows no international boundaries. Out of the total population of gold-mining workers in South Africa, 40 percent are foreign workers originating from Zimbabwe, Malawi, Botswana, Lesotho, and Swaziland (Campbell 1997). Foreigners generally return home even less frequently than their South African mining counterparts, and their partners are even less likely to visit them on the mines. This illustrates how migrant workers in South Africa may facilitate the rapid spread of HIV/AIDS, and also supports the view that the HIV/AIDS pandemic knows no international boundaries and is truly a global problem (Campbell 1997; Kalipeni 2000).

In spite of the attention that is paid to the mining industry, the majority of migrant workers are employed in other sectors in South Africa or they are in the process of seeking work. Large gaps exist in the knowledge of the other forms of migration in South Africa, particularly for those engaged in the informal sector. While single-sex hostels are quite common in the mining areas, they are also prevalent outside the mining industry, as well. For example, within a twenty-mile radius of Durban, there were at least seven men's hostels with an excess of 43,000 officially registered beds, one women's hostel with over 1,000 beds and one mixed hostel with 11,000 beds (Webb 1997).

A substantial amount of research has also focused on the role of truck drivers in southern and eastern Africa as a major player in the rapid spread of HIV/AIDS in the globalized context (Gilgen et al. 2001). It is often argued that truck drivers may spend long periods of time on the road and away from their families. Much like the mine workers, a sense of loneliness and depression may result, which could increase the likelihood of patronizing commercial sex workers who frequently target them. Indeed several detailed studies on the relationship between truck drivers, commercial sex workers, and the spread of HIV/AIDS highlight this dimension as one of the multiple dimensions in the spread of the epidemic throughout high Africa from Ethiopia down to South Africa (Gould 1993; Bwayo 1994; Mbugua et al. 1995; Lankoande et al. 1998; Laukamm-Josten et al. 2000; Marcus 2001). To summarize, the colonial economy that was introduced in southern and eastern Africa during colonial rule bringing Africa into the global world economy has fostered a fertile environment in which men and women find themselves vulnerable to the rapid spread of HIV.

MIGRATION, GENDER, AND VULNERABILITY TO HIV/AIDS

Study after study has found out that women's vulnerability to HIV is closely related to globalization, gender relations, economic dependency, and cultural factors. Women and girls are particularly vulnerable due to their lower social status, which in turn influences their economic status. Social factors including unequal access to education, training, and assigned roles in society contribute towards vulnerability (Travers and Bennett 1996; Akeroyd 1997; Lamptey et al. 2002; Delay 2004; Kalipeni et al. 2004; Campbell and Mzaidume 2001). Based on social and cultural norms, women and young girls from different socioeconomic backgrounds occupy a subordinate position in society and are required to play a submissive role (Wojcicki 2005). In Islam, for example, females involved in extramarital sex face harsh penalties but their male partners are seldom penalized. In fact, in many societies, extramarital sex by men is condoned if not outright approved (Venkataramana and Sarada 2001). Lack of education and training, as evident from the high level of illiteracy among females, begins at a much younger age, forcing women to follow the norms of society. Due to their economic and social subordination, women and girls are more vulnerable to HIV because of their limited ability to negotiate protective sex. Also, without access to antiretrovirals, infected women are likely to pass the virus on to their children (Merchant and Lala 2005).

An increasingly mobile local and global population exacerbates the risk of HIV transmission. The increasing volume of international travel within Africa contributes to the spread of sexually transmitted infections, including HIV (Rogstad 2004). If we take the case of southern Africa as an example, although males dominate employment-related international migration to resource rich areas such as Botswana and South Africa, young women also migrate, seeking work as domestic servants and in other types of informal sector work. Some may even be forced to make a living as commercial sex workers. Female migrants who do not work in the commercial sex industry are still at risk of contracting HIV/AIDS, due to the degree of rape that might occur in the hostels where the women stay. Furthermore, HIV/AIDS in southern Africa needs to be understood in the context of poverty and social structure. The social factors leading to the widespread increase of HIV/AIDS in southern Africa have been mainly due to gender issues (van Niekerk 2001). Women carry a heavier burden than men in terms of rate of HIV infection because of the stigmatization that results from their being blamed for HIV/AIDS. Yet, disclosure of women's HIV status usually results in abuse or abandonment by their families and loss of rights to children and property (Division for the Advancement of Women 2000).

Women also find themselves at higher risk of contracting the disease due to biological reasons. Their relative lack of power over their bodies and sexual lives supported and reinforced by social and economic inequality increases their vulnerability to HIV/AIDS. Other factors that increase young women's vulnerability to HIV infection include some cultural and religious entrapments (Akeroyd 2004), including the strong desire to have children, yielding to men's desire for "flesh-on-flesh" intercourse and "dry sex," and other fears about condoms. Finally, sex trafficking and poverty are critical factors of HIV vulnerability (Ackerman and de Klerk 2002; Craddock 2000a, 2000b; Susser and Stein 2004; van Niekerk 2001).

It is important to note that the greatest burden of care also rests on the shoulders of women. Families often remove girls from school to care for sick relatives or assume more family responsibilities, jeopardizing the girls' education and future prospects. Thus, the effect on girls' development is especially detrimental, leaving girls even more vulnerable to HIV infections. Ghosh and Kalipeni (2005) note that girls who are forced to abandon their schooling are less likely to achieve the earning power required to increase their economic independence. Furthermore, reduced education for women also impedes national development (Division for the Advancement of Women 2000). Thus, a careful examination of the status of women in these days of a globalized context in sub-Saharan Africa is crucial to our understanding of the impact of globalization on gender in the rapid spread of the epidemic.

INDIVIDUAL LEVEL IMPACTS OF GLOBALIZATION: SPECIFIC EXAMPLES OF VULNERABILITY

The Migrant Labor Industry and Vulnerability to HIV

Mark Lurie, a prominent scientist at the Medical Research Council of South Africa, notes the following:

> If you wanted to spread an STD, you'd take thousands of young men away from their families, isolate them in single-sex hostels, and give them easy access to alcohol and commercial sex. Then, to spread the disease around the country, you'd send them home every once in a while to their wives and girlfriends. And that's basically the system we have with the mines. (Schoofs 1999)

As noted above, the mining industry, fueled by the insatiable appetite for gold, diamonds, and other minerals globally, has resulted in the wide proliferation of HIV/AIDS in eastern and southern Africa. During the heyday of apartheid, this industry employed more than three-quarters of a million men from as far north as Tanzania. As Schoofs (1999) points out, this system laid the foundation for the spread of STDs and HIV. Indeed it has been well documented that over the past 100 years migrant labor on the gold mines, with its signature single-sex hostels, bred epidemics of syphilis, gonorrhea, and other sexually transmitted diseases. One study after another is finding out that migrant workers and their partners are about twice as likely to be infected with HIV as nonmigrant couples. Thus the international labor migration system—coupled with other factors such as poverty, poor health care, illiteracy, and female powerlessness—have resulted in such a huge HIV/AIDS epidemic in southern Africa. These factors result in situations of powerlessness of individuals and communities at large. Below we offer specific scenarios or cases in which people become vulnerable.

In a micro-level study in Malawi, Kalipeni and Ghosh (2007) conducted interviews with men in poor income areas of Lilongwe, the capital city of Malawi. One of the gentlemen, who was in his late thirties, noted the following:

> I completed standard 8 long time ago in the early 1980s at Ntakataka in Dedza District. Immediately I completed my standard 8 studies, I left for South Africa on WENELA in those days, they call it THEBA now. I was working in gold mine in Joburg. You know, with WENELA, we used to stay there for three years nonstop without coming home. But I had to go to earn money because I wanted to marry

> this girl. I came back after three years, married my wife and went back again. You know WENELA wouldn't allow us to bring our wives with us. In South Africa I had this *kazintombi* [girl] that I used to visit from time to time. I think I made her pregnant but I can't be sure because she had other men but she pointed me out. I came back for good to Malawi in 1995. Since then I have been very sick, my wife just died last year and I am now taking care of my kids all by myself. One is in secondary school and the other two are here with me. I think it is this *kachilombo* disease.

More discussion with this gentleman revealed that it was not just in south Africa that he was moving with other women, but also in his poor income residential areas of Chinsapo. It is likely he might have gotten the disease from South Africa, brought it back to Malawi, and infected his wife and others in Chinsapo. Indeed the major driver of the HIV/AIDS epidemic in southern Africa is thought to be the colonial labor migration system as amply discussed in this chapter.

Gender and Poverty

In the same study of Lilongwe's low socioeconomic residential areas, Ghosh and Kalipeni (2005) interviewed women about their perception of risk to HIV among men and women in Lilongwe. In this study, a young woman, age 17, who had migrated from a rural area of Mchinji District, 54 miles west of Lilongwe City, told us the following story (see Ghosh and Kalipeni 2005):

> I was in grade 6 at Guillimme Catholic Primary School when my father died in 2002. He used to grow tobacco to pay my school fees. Without him around, and coming from a family of 6 children, four boys and two girls, I was forced to drop out of school. My mother could now only afford to send the two boys to school. My mother asked me to see if I come here in Lilongwe to look for a job. I came to stay with my aunt who lives in Area 10. But after 6 months I couldn't find a job and I was forced to move out of my aunt's house as they have their own children to look after. A friend of mine took me in here at Chinsapo. She also doesn't have any employment. During the day we go to Lilongwe Market to sell second hand goods, but there is a lot of competition there. At night we try to do all we can do to get a little income. Sometimes we stand by the roadside to see if we can be picked, at other times we go to Lilongwe Hotel, Lingadzi Inn and other such places when there is a conference. If we are lucky in a night we might come back home with about K200 (U.S.$1.50). Some men they just use us without paying us and we are afraid of being beaten to ask for the pay. Life is tough here in the city, but it is even tougher in the village where I came from. From time to time I am able to send a little money to my mother but I don't reveal how and where I get it.

It is easy to see that poverty and the low status of women have resulted in this girl's precarious situation. In further interviews with her she revealed that she was scared that she might get infected with the HIV virus. She indicated that some men like to use condoms and others do not like condoms and she has to oblige in both instances since she needs the money badly. The HIV infection rate among commercial sex workers in Malawi is very high, as many of the clients are HIV infected and pass the virus on to the girls who in turn pass it on to other clients. But as noted by this girl, they are forced into these acts by their untenable circumstances.

Political Instability, Refugees, and Vulnerability to HIV

Throughout Africa, civil wars, many of them instigated by foreign powers, powers that are clamoring for Africa's precious resources, have resulted in forced movements of millions of people, particularly women and children, as refugees and displaced persons. Thus globalization which has prompted the international need for Africa's raw materials has also spawned internal conflicts, popularly known as "blood diamonds" conflicts. Fights for diamond control in Sierra Leone and Angola, fights for rich oilfields in the region of Darfur in Sudan, fights for control of mineral resources in the Democratic Republic of Congo, are just but a few examples. The consequences and potential for the spread of disease has been tragic. AIDS is particularly worrisome among refugee populations, particularly powerless children, young girls and women. Even more disturbing is the fact that war and civil strife have restored diseases such as malaria that were once thought to be conquered (Kalipeni and Oppong 1998).

More importantly, however, sexual violence and exploitation are a shockingly frequent experience for refugee women before or during flight and even in refugee camps. A recent scandal in the Democratic Republic of the Congo has revealed that girls, as young as 10 years old, are not immune to rape by even United Nations soldiers supposedly posted at the camps to protect them from marauding rebels (Holt 2004). Where political instability is rife, sexual violence is routinely an element of the persecution of women. During flight, sexual exploitation or violence may be part of their experience with border officials, other refugees or people in the host region. Unfortunately, a high risk of infection with sexually transmitted diseases including HIV/AIDS accompanies all sexual violence against women and girls. Yet, as Kalipeni and Oppong (1998) observe, refugee women commonly lack even the most basic elements of reproductive health care while facing unwanted pregnancies, unsafe abortions, and other risks such as sexually transmitted diseases. The breakdown of health services worsens the impact of such diseases and the chances for treatment and escalates the risk involved in pregnancy. At many refugee camps most of those who become pregnant are considered to be in high-risk groups: adolescents, women over 40, women with many existing children, and women who are physically and emotionally exhausted and undernourished.

Thus, civil strife amplifies the effects of poverty and vulnerability, accelerating the spread of the virus. Exchanging sex for money to buy food is common in or around refugee camps, putting both sex workers and their clients at high risk. Mixing of populations in refugee camps compounds the problem. Sexual contact between people who have migrated from areas with high HIV rates with others from a low HIV rate area spreads the virus among all groups.

As reported by Holt (2004) on the recent rape by UN soldiers of helpless girls:

> Faela is 13 and her son Joseph is just under six months old. The refugee camp is just meters from the peacekeepers' base. Sitting on the dusty ground in Bunia's largest camp for Internally Displaced People (IDP), with Joseph in her arms, she talks about how she ensures that she and her son are fed: If I go and see the soldiers at night and sleep with them then they sometimes give me food, maybe a banana or a cake, she explains. I have to do it with them because there is nobody to care, nobody else to protect Joseph except me. He is all I have and I must look after him.

Holt (2004) writes:

> It is a story that might not sound out of place in any part of the war-ravaged Democratic Republic of Congo but for one thing, the soldiers Faela is talking about are not the rebel groups who devastated Ituri Province, in north -eastern DR Congo, during the last four-and-a-half years of conflict. "Every night the soldiers would come to our hut and make my sisters and I do it with them," Faela, Bunia camp resident. The soldiers are part of the UN peacekeeping force, Monuc, and are stationed next to the IDP camp in Bunia on UN orders.

TRAGIC CONSEQUENCES OF GLOBALIZATION AND HIV/AIDS

Globalization which has fueled labor migration and civil strife in Africa has resulted in increasing socioeconomic inequality and the rapid spread of HIV/AIDS. Differences in health levels and vulnerability to HIV across gender and socioeconomic standing are mainly a result of exacerbated inequality resulting from unequal global socioeconomic health determinants (Leon 2001; Craddock 2000b; Rives and Yousefi 1997; Turshen 1991). Global economic changes can contribute towards a drop in the purchasing power of households at the local level, leading to migration, a decline in public sector resources, and a restructuring of both private and public sectors in response to growing competitiveness. These in turn affect an individual's job security, access to health care, education, and thus increase the vulnerability to HIV (Turshen 1997; Turshen and Twagiramariya 1998). A decline in public sector resources can further place restraints on promotion of HIV/AIDS awareness programs. As we have amply illustrated in this chapter, the determinants of vulnerability are rooted in poverty, social disruption associated with migration, underemployment, gender, and access to resources. For women, vulnerabilities to HIV are exacerbated by widespread gender based social inequities in a globalized and volatile world (Oppong 2003; Kalipeni 2000; Craddock 2000a).

We conclude this chapter by highlighting the tragic consequences of deepening poverty and marginalization of African peoples in the era of HIV. One of the channels through which HIV/AIDS affects overall poverty levels is its effect on economic growth. Because the disease claims lives primarily from the working age segments of the population, severely affected countries experience major reductions in their workforces and, thus, gross domestic product (GDP) growth rates. Higher domestic production costs make the country less attractive to foreign direct investment (see Haacker 2004). Also, HIV/AIDS adversely affects the availability and the accumulation of human capital (Bell et al. 2004).

Whiteside (2002) concludes that, at the household level, the final effect of HIV/AIDS depends on the resources available to households and in the general community. With poorer access to resources, the poor are less able to cope with the sudden and substantial increase in expenditures and reduction in income caused by HIV/AIDS. Steinberg and others (2002) conclude that, despite considerable efforts in South Africa, home-based assistance from the government rarely reaches the poorest segments of society. Booysen (2003) in turn shows that in South Africa the incidence, depth, and severity of poverty are higher among households affected by HIV/AIDS, and their members are more likely to experience chronic poverty and income variation.

To compound the matter, the food crisis in southern Africa during the past few years has caused increased vulnerability to HIV infection. The food shortage took place in the context of a severe epidemic which increased the vulnerability of children, of young people, and women to infection. Some of the strategies taken by people affected by a food crisis often included finding additional sources of food or income, migrating, dropping out of school, engaging in hazardous work, and exchanging sex for food or money. In southern Africa a number of such coping mechanisms facilitate the spread of HIV, putting young people, especially girls, at high risk of infection. The only way for some HIV-positive people to support themselves and their families may be to sell sex, thereby furthering transmission.

In this same vein or line of thinking, UNICEF offers the following examples of vulnerability to HIV/AIDS:

> HIV/AIDS continues to strain communities in southern Africa by killing some of the most productive members of society, including civil servants, teachers, farmers and parents. The HIV epidemic has resulted in more households headed by women, children, or the elderly. These households are particularly vulnerable as they have fewer opportunities to earn an income or grow crops. Families fostering orphans have greater demands on their scant resources. The impact of the drought on these families is particularly severe. If the only caring adult is an elderly grandparent, assisting them with food aid may be the only mechanism for survival of the children. (UNICEF n.d.)

> Diminished agricultural productivity and ability to work for cash, may lead families to sell their assets, reduce levels of child care and spiral into a cycle of increased poverty and deprivation. As a result, children are withdrawn from or drop out of school to care for ailing family members and help with earning an income and getting food. Children may have to care for themselves and their siblings, and are often hidden, voiceless and excluded from society. Many turn to the streets or to hazardous work to make ends meet, placing them at risk of violence and HIV infection. (UNICEF n.d.)

The World Health Organization (WHO) notes that HIV/AIDS is undermining the benefits of globalization for many countries (World Health Organization n.d.). The WHO further notes that, between 1960 and 1990, life expectancy in Africa increased by a total of nine years. The impact was to add between 1.7 percent and 2.7 percent a year to the growth rate of per capita GDP. The HIV/AIDS epidemic, however, is reversing these gains. According to a World Bank report, HIV/AIDS may subtract an additional 1 percent a year from GDP economic growth in some sub-Saharan African countries, owing to the continuing loss of skilled and unskilled workers in the prime of life. In South Africa HIV/AIDS may depress GDP by as much as 17 percent over the next decade (World Bank 1997; Centers for Disease Control and Prevention 2002).

THE WAY FORWARD: LESSENING VULNERABILITY TO HIV/AIDS

As Stock (2004) points out, Africa is one of the most important producers of minerals that symbolize opulence and solid, inflation-proof wealth. About 25 percent of gold and over 50 percent of diamonds in the world come from Africa. Yet, as Stock (2004) laments, the continent is known for its poverty rather than its prosperity. For Africa the dimensions of vulnerability in a globalized economy are deep-rooted and they are here to stay. The historical context of colonialism and its long-lasting effects cannot be done away with overnight. However, for some of the factors, there are certain actions which could be implemented at the local level with genuine government commitment and well-meaning international support. Below we offer several important general recommendations to remove some of the obstacles that put men, women, and children in vulnerable positions in Sub-Saharan Africa.

The historical context of labor migration is here to stay with us and will continue into the unforeseeable future. However, the consequences of migration on family and the proliferation of HIV and other diseases can be mitigated through corporate social responsibility. For example, in the case of the mining industry in South Africa companies could inform truck drivers and migrant laborers about the risk factors and thereby increase awareness. This will help to reduce the cases of HIV/AIDS, medical cost, and improve productivity. In addition, living quarters for migrant laborers could be dramatically improved. Improvements might include, for example, building of apartment blocks to allow families to come with the men to places of work from their home countries.

As noted above, Africa is a rich continent but sadly it continues to be a basket case. Years of exploitation and neglect during the colonial era and the post-independence era have seen untold suffering on the continent. We recommend continued support from the international community in one form or another. Examples might include appropriate forms of aid and technology, provision of affordable medications to treat all forms of maladies, not just HIV, provision of assistance to educate the population on how to avoid being infected with HIV, and so on. As we have argued elsewhere, the only way African countries are going to move through the various stages of the epidemiologic transition is through the eradication of communicable diseases on a sustainable basis. Indeed advances in the development of vaccines and chemotherapeutic agents have brought many communicable diseases under control (see Kalipeni 2000). But these need to be made available widely to those that need them, particularly those afflicted with HIV/AIDS. With reference to poverty, lender and donor nations should continue their programs leading to debt forgiveness so that African countries can begin to focus on investing in education, health, and real development to end poverty and hunger. In the areas of international trade there is great need for fair and equitable treatment of African products and incomes derived from those products to benefit African societies who toil to produce them for international consumption.

An aspect that lends itself well in the fight against the proliferation of diseases including HIV is female autonomy and empowerment. This is also the easiest to tackle, and yet many African countries lag behind. It has been shown throughout the world that educating women has great benefits for the rest of society. We recommend that researchers, policymakers, international donors, and African governments should take on greater responsibility for the total cost of girls' education, particularly for those who have lost their parents and are therefore unable to afford an education on their own. Education should also be structured in such a way that it caters to the needs of young women who have to stay at home to take care of their sick parents and relatives. Distance education, for example, could be one option. But (more importantly) governments in partnership with the international community should endeavor to develop and implement a responsive and appropriate curriculum that caters to the adolescent girls who often drop out of the formal educational system in rural areas of Africa (see, for example, Hogle et al. 2002). Such a curriculum could teach these rural girls basic education in terms of reading and writing and also include hygiene and health, particularly how to avoid getting infected with HIV.

The thinking here is that the limited education of girls increases their vulnerability because it limits their options for acquiring knowledge to protect themselves from sexually transmitted diseases and limits their options of employment, thus resulting in their having to resort to informal employment, which at best may be domestic work and at worst may be selling sex. Any form of employment, whether it overtly involves selling sex or not, places women at risk of sexual abuse because of the limited physical and social power that women have in the employment arena and the lack of monitoring or regulations in such employment. Ensuring that women have access to education and have the opportunity to complete their education is, therefore, one way of reducing their vulnerability. Education for women often means economic independence and the ability to freely choose from the various employment opportunities available, many of which do not expose them to HIV infection. In short, specific emphasis should be placed on protecting and educating vulnerable groups, particularly infants, children, women, and the very poor. All efforts should be made to ensure the care of orphans, particularly females, who are vulnerable to sexual abuse in order to reduce their risk to HIV.

Another recommendation in this line is increasing the availability of microcredit loans to women. Many women remain in relationships in which they are at high risk for HIV because they are economically dependent on their promiscuous partners. Having an alternative source of income that allows women to be economically independent gives them the freedom to disengage themselves from an unhealthy relationship if they are concerned that the relationship places them at risk for HIV infection.

Political instability is an intractable problem in many African countries that are experiencing or have experienced civil strife. Nevertheless, stronger political and economic commitment and action by local, regional, and international actors can certainly help to achieve long-lasting solutions. In this regard, we recommend continued political reform and peace accords, engagement and empowerment of Pan-African organizations, foreign policy changes by Western governments and greater vigilance of nongovernmental organizations (NGOs) in the surveillance of disease outbreaks and allocation and distribution of relief aid in refugee camps. As Kalipeni and Oppong (1998) suggest, Pan-African organizations such as the African Union at the continental level, and ECOWAS, Southern African Development Coordination Conference (SADCC), the Arab League, etc. at the regional level should be empowered not only to keep peace at the continental level and in their respective regions but also to prevent escalation of political violence and conflict. We also strongly recommend that there be accountability of peacekeepers guarding refuge camps to make sure that abuse of vulnerable groups such women and children (as recently happened in the Democratic Republic of Congo) does not occur.

CONCLUSION

We could highlight many examples where HIV/AIDS spread has been enhanced in Africa because of the unequal integration of the continent into the modern global economy. Migration (be it international migration for labor within southern African countries, internal migration from rural to urban areas in search of jobs in eastern and southern Africa, or forced migration as a result of civil strife) has combined with other local factors resulting in the rapid proliferation of HIV/AIDS. We are cognizant of the fact that no single factor can cause an epidemic as huge as AIDS in southeastern Africa. The migrant labor system in southern Africa is simply one of the many dimensions that have resulted in HIV's fertile ground in this region. Poverty, poor health care, illiteracy, and female powerlessness mark the region and work in sync with the migrant labor system in amplifying HIV. Indeed, the case in point here is the explosive growth of the epidemic in South Africa over a very short period of time. This explosive growth was not just simply due to poverty and commercial sex work, which are rampant throughout the continent, but also to migration. There is no question that migration tears families apart and corrodes social cohesion, leading to increased numbers of sexual partners, thereby sustaining the very epidemic it helped inflame (Schoofs 1999).

Globalization, which can be traced back to the initial encounters between Africa and Europeans about 500 years ago, has tragically resulted in both macro- and micro-conditions of vulnerability to various diseases, including HIV/AIDS. The dimensions of this vulnerability are deeply rooted in the history of the continent, especially its colonial interlude. The historical context of colonialism and its economy based on labor migration, contemporary gender issues that are exacerbated by the global forces and its unfairly skewed economy, poverty and disease burden, lukewarm government commitment, and the cultural context have all intertwined in complex ways to put peoples of sub-Saharan Africa at risk of contracting HIV. Indeed, a closer look at globalization might offer an informative framework for understanding vulnerability, as argued in this chapter. While individual behaviors and actions are inherently important in vulnerability to HIV, the context is even more critical. Such individual behaviors and actions occur in a social and spatial context, and usually in response to larger global, social and cultural phenomena, and other dictates or pressures. Thus, any assessment of HIV vulnerability has to include global, national, regional, and community factors that influence or exacerbate personal vulnerability.

REFERENCES AND FURTHER READING

Ackerman, L. and de Klerk, G. W. 2002. "Social Factors that Make South African Women Vulnerable to HIV Infection." *Health Care for Women International* 23: 163–172.

Akeroyd, Anne. 1997. "Sociocultural Aspects of AIDS in Africa: Occupational and Gender Issues." In G. C. Bond, J. Kreniske; I. Susser; and J. Vincent (eds.), *AIDS in Africa and the Caribbean*. Boulder, CO: Westview Press, pp. 11–30.

Akeroyd, Anne. 2004. "Coercion, Constraints, and 'Cultural Entrapments:' A Further Look at Gendered and Occupational Factors Pertinent to the Transmission of HIV in Africa." In E. Kalipeni, S. Craddock, J. Oppong and J. Ghosh (eds.), *HIV/AIDS in Africa: Beyond Epidemiology*. Malden, MA: Blackwell Publishers, pp. 89–103.

Bell, C., S. Devarajan, and Gersbach, H. 2004. "Thinking about the Long-Run Economic Costs of AIDS." In M. Haacker (ed.), *The Macroeconomics of HIV/AIDS*. Washington DC: International Monetary Fund, pp. 96–133.

Booysen, Frederick le Roux. 2003. "Poverty Dynamics and HIV/AIDS Related Morbidity and Mortality in South Africa." Paper presented at an international conference on "Empirical Evidence for the Demographic and Socio-Economic Impact of AIDS," Health Economics and HIV/AIDS Research Division, University of KwaZulu-Natal, South Africa, March 26–28.

Bwayo, J. 1994. "Human Immunodeficiency Virus Infection in Long-Distance Truck Drivers in East Africa." *Archives of Internal Medicine* 154: 1391–1396.

Calitz, J. M. 2000: *Provincial Population Projections, 1996–2021: High HIV/AIDS Impact*. Halfway House: Development Bank of Southern Africa.

Campbell, Catherine. 1997. "Migrancy, Masculine Identities and AIDS: The Psychosocial Context of HIV Transmission on the South African Gold Mines." *Social Science and Medicine* 45(2): 273–281.

Campbell, M. C. and Mzaidume, Z. 2001. "Grassroots Participation, Peer Education, and HIV Prevention by Sex Workers in South Africa." *American Journal of Public Health* 91(12): 1978–1986.

Centers for Disease Control and Prevention. 2002. *Protecting the Nation's Health in an Era of Globalization: CDC's Global Infectious Disease Strategy*. Atlanta, GA: Centers for Disease Control and Prevention, Department of Health and Human Services.

Craddock, Susan. 2000a. "Disease, Identity, and Risk: Rethinking the Geography of AIDS." *Transactions of the Institute of British Geographers* 25: 153–168.

Craddock, Susan. 2000b. "Scales of Justice: Women, Inequity, and AIDS in East Africa." In I. Dyck, S. MacLafferty and N. D. Lewis (eds.), *Geographies of Women's Health*. London: Routledge Press.

Delay, P. 2004. "Gender and Monitoring the Response to HIV/AIDS Pandemic." *Emerging Infectious Diseases* 10(11): 1979–1983.

Desmond, J. 2001. "Health and Development in South Africa: From Principles to Practices." *Development* 44(1): 122–128.

Division for the Advancement of Women. 2000. "The HIV/AIDS Pandemic and its Implications." Online version at www.un.org/womenwatch/daw, retrieved June 25, 2007.

Ghosh, Jayati and Kalipeni, Ezekiel. 2005. "Women in Chinsapo, Malawi: Vulnerability and Risk to HIV/AIDS." *Journal of Social Aspects of HIV/AIDS* 2(2): 320–332.

Gilgen, D., Williams, B. G., MacPhail, C., van Dam, C. J., Campbell, C., Ballard, R. C. and Taljaard, D. 2001. "The Natural History of HIV/AIDS in a Major Goldmining Centre in South Africa: Results of a Biomedical and Social Survey." *South African Journal of Science* 97: 387–392.

Gould, P. 1993. *The Slow Plague: A Geography of the AIDS Pandemic*. Boston: Blackwell Publishers.

Haacker, Markus. 2002. "The Economic Consequences of HIV/AIDS in Southern Africa." IMF Working Paper WP/02/38. Washington DC: International Monetary Fund.

Haacker, Markus (ed). 2004. *The Macroeconomics of HIV/AIDS*. Washington DC: International Monetary Fund.

Hogle, J. A., Green, E., Nantulya, V., Stoneburner, R. and Stover, J. 2002. *What Happened in Uganda? Declining HIV Prevalence, Behavior Change, and the National Response*. Washington DC: Office of HIV/AIDS, Bureau for Global Health, U.S. Agency for International Development.

Holt, K. 2004. "DR Congo's Shameful Sex Secret." *BBC News*, Thursday, June 3. Online http://news.bbc.co.uk/2/hi/africa/3769469.stm, retrieved June 10, 2007.

Horowitz, S. 2001. "Migrance and HIV/AIDS: A Historical Perspective." *South African Historical Journal* 45: 103–124.

International Monetary Fund. 2000. *Globalization: Threat or Opportunity?* Washington DC: International Monetary Fund. Online http://www.imf.org/external/np/exr/ib/2000/041200.htm), retrieved July 23, 2007.

International Monetary Fund. 2003. *World Economic Outlook*. Washington DC: International Monetary Fund.

Kalipeni, Ezekiel. 2000. "Health and Disease in Southern Africa: A Comparative and Vulnerability Perspective." *Social Science and Medicine* 50(7): 965–985.

Kalipeni, Ezekiel and Ghosh, Jayati. 2007. "Concern and Practice Among Men about HIV/AIDS in Low Socioeconomic Income Areas of Lilongwe, Malawi." *Social Science and Medicine* 64(5): 1116–1127.

Kalipeni, Ezekiel and Oppong, Joseph. 1998. "The Refugee Crisis in Africa and Implications for Health and Disease: A Political Ecology Approach." *Social Science and Medicine* 46(12): 1637–1653.

Kalipeni, Ezekiel, Craddock, Susan, Oppong, Joseph R. and Ghosh, Jayati (eds.). 2004. *HIV/AIDS in Africa: Beyond Epidemiology*. Malden, MA: Blackwell Publishers.

Lamptey, P., Wigley, M., Carr, D. and Collymore, Y. 2002. "Facing the HIV/AIDS Pandemic." *Population Bulletin* 57(3): 1–39.

Lankoande, S., Meda, N., Sangare, L., Compaore, I. P., Catraye, J., Zan, S., Dyck, E. Van, Cartoux, M. and Soudre, R. 1998. "HIV Infection in Truck Drivers in Burkina Faso: A Serologic Study." *Médecine Tropicale: Revue du Corps de Santé Colonial* 58(1): 41–47.

Laukamm-Josten, U., Mwizarubi, B. K., Mwaijonga, C. L., Outwater, A., Valadez, J. J., Nyamwaya, D., Swai, R., Saidel, T. and Nyamuryekung'e, K. 2000. "Preventing HIV Infection Through Peer Education and Condom Promotion Among Truck Drivers and Their Sexual Partners in Tanzania, 1990–1993." *AIDS Care* 12(1): 27–40.

Leon, D.A. 2001. "Common Threads: Underlying Components of Inequalities in Mortality between and within Countries." In D. A. Leon and G. Walt (eds.), *Poverty, Inequality and Health*. Oxford: Oxford University Press, pp. 58–87.

Marcus, T. 2001. "Is There an HIV/AIDS Demonstration Effort? Findings from a Longitudinal Study of Long Distance Truck Drivers." *Society in Transition* 32(1): 110–120.

Mbugua, G. G., Muthami, L. N., Mutura, C. W., Oogo, S. A., Waiyaki, P. G., Lindan, C. P. and Hearst, N. 1995. "Epidemiology of HIV Infection among Long Distance Truck Drivers in Kenya." *East African Medical Journal* 72(8): 515–518.

Merchant, R. H. and Lala, M. M. 2005. "Prevention of Mother-to-Child Transmission of HIV: An Overview." *Indian Journal of Medical Research* 121(4): 489–501.

Oppong, Joseph R. 2003. "Medical Geography of Sub-Saharan Africa." In S. Aryeetey-Attoh (ed.), *Geography of Sub-Saharan Africa*, 2nd edition. Upper Saddle River, NJ: Pearson Education, pp. 324–362.

Rives, J. M. and Yousefi, M. 1997. *Economic Dimensions of Gender Inequality: A Global Perspective*. Westport, CN: Praeger.

Rogstad, K. E. 2004. "Sex, Sun, Sea, and STIs: Sexually Transmitted Infections Acquired on Holiday." *British Medical Journal* 329: 214–217.

Rushing, William A. 1995. *The AIDS Epidemic: Social Dimensions of an Infectious Disease*. Boulder, CO: Westview Press.

Schoofs, Mark. 1999. "All That Glitters: How HIV Caught Fire in South Africa—Part One: Sex and the Migrant Miner." *Village Voice*, April 28–May 4, pp. 46–49. Internet resource at http://www.villagevoice.com/news/9917,schoofs,5176,1.html, retrieved on July 20, 2007.

Steinberg, M., Johnson, S., Schierhout, G. and Ndegwa,

D. 2002. *Hitting Home: How Households Cope with the Impact of the HIV/AIDS Epidemic.* The Henry Kaiser Family Foundation.

Stock, Robert. 2004. *Africa South of the Sahara: A Geographical Interpretation.* New York: Guilford Press.

Susser, I. and Stein, Z. 2004. "Culture, Sexulaity, and Women's Agency in the Prevention of HIV/AIDS in Southern Africa." In E. Kalipeni, S. Craddock, J. Oppong and J. Ghosh (eds.), *HIV/AIDS in Africa: Beyond Epidemiology.* Malden, MA: Blackwell Publishers, pp. 133–143.

Travers, M. and Bennett, L. 1996. "AIDS, Women, and Power." In L. Sherr, C. Hankin and L. Bennett (eds.), *AIDS as a Gender Issue: Psychosocial Perspectives.* Bristol, PA: Taylor and Francis, pp. 64–98.

Turshen, Meredeth. 1991. *Women and Health in Africa.* Trenton, NJ: Africa World Press.

Turshen, Meredeth. 1997. "The Political Ecology of AIDS in Africa." In M. Singer (ed.), *The Political Economy of AIDS.* Amityville, NY: Baywood, pp. 167–182.

Turshen, Meredeth and Twagiramariya, Clotilde. 1998. *What Women Do in Wartime: Gender and Conflict in Africa.* London: Zed Books.

UNAIDS. 2007. *Report on the Global AIDS Epidemic 2006.* Geneva: UNAIDS.

UNICEF. n.d. "HIV/AIDS: Crisis Causes Increased Vulnerability to HIV Infection. Online http://www.unicef.org/emerg/southernafrica/index_hiv_aids.html, retrieved July 20, 2007.

van Niekerk, A.A. 2001. "Moral and Social Complexities of AIDS in Africa." *Journal of Medicine and Philosophy* 27(2): 143–162.

Venkataramana, C. B. S. and Sarada, P.V. 2001. "Extent and Speed of Spread of HIV Infection in India through the Commercial Sex Networks: A Perspective." *Tropical Medicine and International Health* 6(12): 1040–1061.

Webb, D. 1997. *HIV/AIDS in Africa.* Pietermaritzburg: University of Natal Press.

Whiteside, Alan. 2002. "Poverty and HIV/AIDS in Africa." *Third World Quarterly* 23(2): 313–332.

Williams, B.; Campbell, C. and MacPhail, C. 1999. *Managing HIV/AIDS in South Africa.* Aukland Park: Council for Scientific Industrial Research.

Wojcicki, J. M. 2005. "Socioeconomic Status as a Risk Factor for HIV Infection in Women in East, Central and Southern Africa: A Systematic Review." *Journal of Biosocial Science* 37(1): 1–36.

World Bank. 1997. *Confronting AIDS: Public Priorities in a Global Epidemic.* New York: Oxford University Press.

World Health Organization. n.d. "Globalization, Trade and Health." Online resource at http://www.who.int/trade/glossary/story051/en/index.html, retrieved on June 30, 2007.

Yeboah, Ian E. A. 2007. "HIV/AIDS and the Construction of Sub-Saharan Africa: Heuristic Lessons from the Social Sciences for Policy." *Social Science and Medicine* 64(5): 1128–1151.

CHAPTER 28

Mobile Populations, Vulnerability, and HIV/AIDS in a Globalized World

The Case of the English-Speaking Caribbean

Roger McLean

ABSTRACT

This chapter addresses the topic of HIV/AIDS and migration in the region, with specific reference to those mobile groups that are classified as high risk based on their vulnerability to contracting and possibly spreading the virus. Research in the context of the English-speaking Caribbean has highlighted the need to expand this range from the traditional groups such as commercial sex workers (CSW) to include men who have sex with men (MSM). This expended range should also include a growing young mobile group, which includes students and street children. In the final analysis, the key to truly arresting the growing vulnerability of these groups to the virus is a continued assessment at both the supply and demand sides of the topic, addressing the socioeconomic and cultural driving factors that determine and ultimately impact on the environment.

OVERVIEW

Globalization is now widely regarded as virtually inevitable by most international economists. It involves the intensification of linkages across a wide sphere involving such areas as transnational corporate business structures, international finance, global cultural exchanges and environmental issues, technology and communications as well as the key area of population mobility (Barnett 2002, 10). Globalization, while not a new phenomenon,[1] has, in this present era, certain key features and processes that impact significantly on the character and nature of mobile populations and international migration both positively and negatively. These negative effects have been proven to pose serious challenges to the wellbeing of mobile populations thereby increasing their vulnerability to a number of social ills, chief of which is the risk of contracting HIV/AIDS. The HIV/AIDS epidemic is seen as one of the few global epidemics for which there has been a global political and public consciousness (Barnett 2002) and there has been increasing evidence on the relationship between mobile populations and HIV/AIDS.

The chapter addresses this topic with specific reference to the situation as it relates to the English-speaking Caribbean in general and Trinidad and Tobago specifically. In addressing this topic, the chapter examines the literature on those mobile groups that are classified as high risk based on their vulnerability to contracting and possibly spreading the virus. This entails a review of the criteria used in identifying these groups as high risk, and an assessment of the applicability of this classification to the Trinidad and Tobago context in particular and the Caribbean context in general. The chapter also reviews the key enabling factors that are responsible for, and continue to drive, the perceptions and practices of these groups.

APPROACH TO THE CHAPTER

In approaching the topic, the methodology employed drew upon both primary and secondary data collection techniques. The former involved the conduct of key informant interviews and small group discussions with a number of experts and other practitioners in the area, as well as those who comprise the mobile population. The latter approach involved a comprehensive review of the literature on migration and related areas locally, regionally and internationally, including studies conducted by key agencies. This information was also supplemented with data compiled from a number of the key statistical agencies. A major challenge in the conduct of this study was the paucity of data on the subject area both regionally and in particularly at the national level. As such the methodology had to draw not solely on quantitative data, but also heavily on qualitative approaches, including anecdotal reports, in addressing the key areas of the chapter.

PROFILE OF THE EPIDEMIC

By the end of 2006, the HIV/AIDS pandemic had infected roughly 40 million adults and children, with an estimate of just over four million infected (4.3 million) and 2.9 million deaths from AIDS in the year 2006 alone (UNAIDS 2006a). The Caribbean continues to hold the unenviable position as the region with the second highest prevalence rate after sub-Saharan Africa. In this region, the epidemic, which began to rear its head in the early 1980s, continues to grow, with roughly 250,000 persons estimated to be infected with the virus at the end of 2006. From this figure an estimated 27,000 new infections and 19,000 deaths were reported in 2006 alone.

In spite of the fact that nearly three-quarters of the number of reported cases are to be found in the island of Hispaniola, which comprises the countries of Haiti and the Dominican Republic, adult prevalence rates remain high throughout the region (1 percent to 2 percent). Haiti is the worst affected of the Caribbean nations, with an adult HIV prevalence estimated at 2 percent (UNAIDS 2006, 44). In the Bahamas HIV prevalence among pregnant women was estimated at 3 percent in 2002, while in the Dominican Republic and Guyana the adult prevalence rate stood at 1 percent and 2.4 percent respectively in 2005. AIDS continues to be the leading cause of death among those aged 15 to 44 years (UNAIDS 2006b).

Among the key characteristic of the epidemic that has evolved over the years is its feminization, as reflected in the increased rate of infection among women and young girls. This is reflected in a shift in the male to female ratio, which in the case of Trinidad and Tobago moved from 3:1 in 1986 to roughly 1:1 seventeen years later. This trend is also clearly captured in Exhibit 28.1 through the merging of the male and female trend lines.

A similar pattern emerges when we assess the reported AIDS cases (see Exhibit 28.2). Beginning with eight initial cases in 1983, here again the trend is an upward one, with over 5,000 cases of AIDS being diagnosed by June 2004. A decrease in the number of new AIDS cases has been reported since 2002 after peaking in 2001 at 446 cases. While the fall in both AIDS cases and AIDS-related deaths points to the inroads that have been made in the treatment, care and support program, it also highlights the increasing number of persons living with the virus.

Another dimension of the gender dynamics associated with the epidemic is high risk of contraction among young people and in particular the high degree of vulnerability among young women in the age group 15–24 years. It is estimated that this cohort accounts for more than two-thirds (69 percent) of all young people estimated to be living with HIV/AIDS in the Caribbean (Kaiser Family Foundation 2007). This trend is captured in Exhibit 28.3. In terms of age group, while the epidemic continues to be firmly positioned on the productive segments of the population, it is observed that women are being exposed to the virus at a younger age than their male counterparts.

Exhibit 28.1 New reported HIV cases by year and sex, Trinidad and Tobago 1983–2005

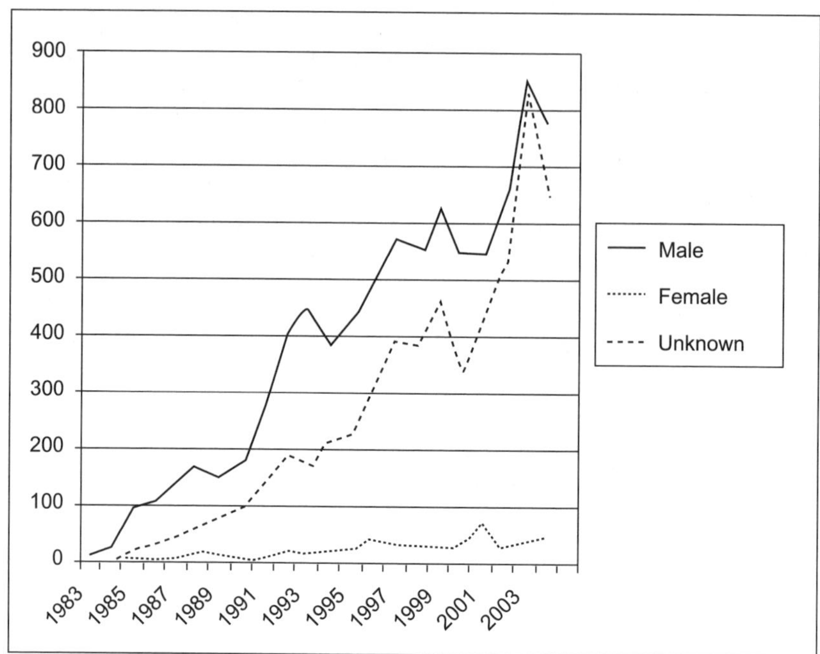

Source: Trinidad and Tobago National Surveillance Unit, Annual Reports (2004 and 2007).

Exhibit 28.2 Reported AIDS cases by year: Trinidad and Tobago

Year	*Male*	*Female*	*Unknown*	*Total*	*Total number of persons with AIDS (cumulative)*
1983	8	0	0	8	8
1984	13	0	0	13	21
1985	32	7	0	39	60
1986	60	13	0	73	133
1987	58	20	0	78	211
1988	97	36	0	133	344
1989	84	36	0	120	464
1990	119	57	0	176	640
1991	159	79	0	238	878
1992	200	78	0	278	1156
1993	207	74	0	281	1437
1994	154	90	0	244	1681
1995	215	111	0	326	2007
1996	225	99	2	326	2333
1997	195	102	0	297	2630
1998	230	131	2	363	2993
1999	278	174	0	452	3445
2000	266	145	0	411	3856
2001	281	177	9	467	4323
2002	248	167	3	418	4741
2003	198	120	3	321	5062
2004	152	92	1	245	5307
2005[a]	123	66	0	189	5696

Note: [a] Data presented as at September 30, 2005.
Source: Trinidad and Tobago National Surveillance Unit date file (2007).

Exhibit 28.3 New HIV cases by sex by age group 2002

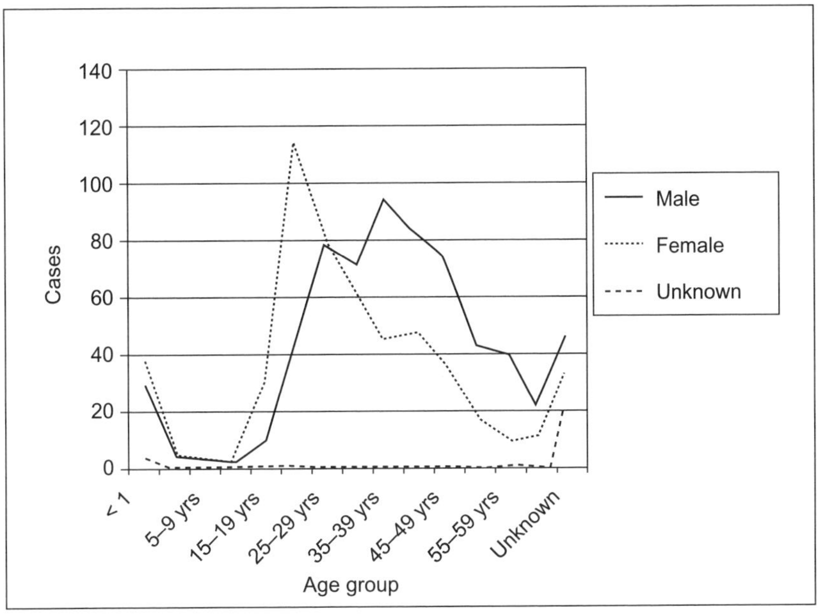

Source: Trinidad and Tobago National Surveillance Unit date file (2004).

Notable advancement has, however, been made in the antiretroviral therapy programs in a number of Caribbean territories, which has manifested itself in an increased number of persons accessing treatment. This has resulted in significant inroads being achieved in reducing AIDS-related mortality in such countries as the Bahamas, Jamaica, and Trinidad and Tobago, as illustrated earlier.

In the face of this trend, the key challenge to the region and specifically the national community is to address the needs of those who are living with the virus by continuing to provide a comprehensive package of care, treatment, and support, while simultaneously implementing an effective and broad-based prevention program.

A number of key factors continue to drive the HIV/AIDS epidemic across the region. These include:

1 poverty and unemployment
2 sociocultural influences
3 inconsistent knowledge of HIV/AIDS (particularly among the high-risk groups)
4 wealth and equity
5 stigma and discrimination
6 gender inequalities
7 absence of sustained political will and leadership in both public and private sectors

These factors have manifested themselves in such forms of risky activities as multiple partnering, particularly among the youth; the inconsistent use of condoms among the sexually active; the inability of females to negotiate the use of condoms in their relationships; and the stigmatization of persons living with HIV/AIDS (PLWHA) and men who have sex with men (MSM). The latter has ultimately resulted in members of these vulnerable groups isolating themselves from the "mainstream."

An examination of the above factors highlights areas of influences that are known to also act as key push factors for mobile populations and migrants in the Caribbean. Major among them are stigma and discrimination, poverty and unemployment, and gender inequality.

CARIBBEAN MIGRATION—AN OVERVIEW

The terms "migrants" and "mobile populations" are sometimes used interchangeably.

However, for this chapter I will draw on the definition used by UNAIDS (2001, 3): "Mobile people can be described broadly as people who move from one place to another temporarily, seasonally or permanently for a host of voluntary and/or involuntary reasons . . . Migrants are mobile people who take up residence or who remain for an extended stay in a foreign country."

The concept of migration is by no means new to the region, as the Caribbean population, by its very nature, can be classified as migratory, beginning with the initial encounter between Europe and the Caribbean in 1492 and followed by a series of immigrant waves during the period of indentureship that saw the movement of labor mainly from Asia. Migration has been responsible for, and continues to contribute to, the diversity that characterizes the islands of the Caribbean.

Migration in general is a very complex issue, as exemplified by the fact that it can, in large part, be driven by a combination, or any one, of a number of personal, national, regional, and international factors and circumstances. These circumstances can be classified as economic, social, demographic, and political and have been classified as those factors that drive persons from the source (push factors) as well as those that provide an incentive to the destination point (pull factors). These push and pull factors are critical to what is seen as the main types of migratory patterns displayed in the Caribbean:

- *External migration*: which encapsulates movement at the intra-regional level concentrated within the islands of the Caribbean and extra-regional movement towards international destinations with emphasis on key metropolitan centers in North America and Europe.
- *Internal migration*: with the main trend being the movement from rural areas to urban centers within country.

External Migration—A Historical Overview

Prior to the 1970s, the Caribbean was considered a region of significant immigration. The eighteenth century, for example, witnessed selective emigration streams and inter-regional immigration that manifested itself in the movement of labor to North America, as well as destinations in Central and South America in response to the economic hardships that were being experienced across the colonies due to depressed export prices and markets. Emigration from the British West Indies during the period 1955–61 saw as much as 6 percent of the islands' population leaving for the imperial homeland to take advantage of educational and employment opportunities in Great Britain.

Many of the same factors that resulted in the movement of Caribbean people prior to the 1970s continued in the decades to follow as captured by Conway (2003, 242):

> The globalization of the world's economic order in accordance with market principles, which began in the 1970s, continued through the 1980s and 1990s and is still imposing neo-liberal policies today, brought about these changes in population trends. Wholesale indebtedness, recession, increasing polarization of classes, and declines in standards of living, among other things, were the structural realities that the region suffered during this time. This has prompted more diasporas, more transnational circulation, and the formation of more multi-local networks.

In particular, a greater number of Trinidadians, Guyanese, and Antiguans moved to the United States in the 1970s compared to the United Kingdom during the peak period (1955–61), many of them choosing New York City as their preferred destination. What developed as a result of this process were a series of well-established Caribbean communities in such urban centers as Miami, New York, Washington DC in the United States, London in Great Britain, and Montreal and Toronto in Canada. By the 1990s a significant percentage of the region's population resided in the United States and Canada, as illustrated in Exhibit 28.4.

More recent developments have witnessed a wave of anti-immigrant policies being imposed by the United States. This was evident in the 1996 passing of the Illegal Immigration Reform and Immigrant

Exhibit 28.4 Population who immigrated annually to North America 1990–91 (by Caribbean country of origin)

	Population from the Caribbean (Thousands as part of the Census)			
	1990/91 Census count	*Canada 1991*	*United States 1990*	*Percentage that live in North America*
Antigua	64	2.0	–	3.01
Bahamas	255	1.1	21.6	8.19
Barbados	257	14.8	43.0	18.43
Belize	187	1.0	30.0	14.19
Bermuda	61	1.7	–	2.78
Cuba	10,628	1.8	737.0	6.58
Dominican Republic	7,110	2.8	347.9	4.92
Grenada	91	2.8	17.7	20.09
Guyana	795	66.1	120.7	19.38
Haiti	6,486	39.9	225.4	3.95
Jamaica	2,366	0.2	1,200.0	24.10
St. Lucia	133	1.8	–	1.37
St. Vincent and the Grenadines	114	–	2.1	5.64
Trinidad and Tobago	1,236	49.4	115.7	12.00

Source: Pan American Health Organisation (PAHO), *Health in the Americas*, vol. 1, Washington DC, PAHO, 1998.

Responsibility Act, which made possible the rapid deportation of "criminal" resident aliens and stiffer penalties for overstayers.

Intra-regionally, migration continued as well from the 1970s onward, with those countries that were experiencing economic prosperity in such areas as tourism and oil being the preferred destinations. These countries provided opportunities not only for professionals and semi-professionals, but also to such downstream sectors as the construction and service sectors for the less skilled. To this end, well-established paths emerged in the intra-regional migration routes. These included the movement of Nevisians and Kittitians to Antigua, St. Thomas and the U.S. Virgin Islands, St. Lucians to Barbados, and the well-established movement between Guyana and Grenada and Trinidad. The latter pattern has continued to the present day in the Trinidad and Tobago context, with Barbados also featuring prominently in the migration route.

Based on data from the Commonwealth Caribbean Population and Housing Census (1994), Trinidad and Tobago heads the list of countries with the largest concentration of immigrants, while others included the U.S. Virgin Islands and Barbados, as illustrated in Exhibit 28.5.

Internal Migration

Caribbean economies in the post independence period were characterized by a small highly capital-intensive non-agricultural sector existing side by side with the more labor-intensive agriculture sector. In Trinidad, for example, the former is represented by the petrochemical sector. The changing global environment, which manifested itself in lower export prices in the traditional agriculture sector, was in large part responsible for the urban–rural shift over the last two decades. This was accompanied by developments in the services sector, driven in large part by advances made in the tourism sector.

Internal migration as reflected in the rural to urban shift is, however, driven not only by wage differentials between the agricultural and non-agricultural sectors, but expectations about access to employment, social and cultural amenities, housing, social services, and the overall quality of life in the urban areas. Migration from rural to urban areas will be rational, even in situations of high and rising urban unemployment, whenever the expected net long-term economic prospects in urban areas exceed those in rural regions. This is in large part responsible for what has been the constant urban–rural

Exhibit 28.5 Regional migration rates for selected Caribbean countries 1990 and 1991

		Migrants		*Migrant rates*	
Selected countries	*Natives ('000)*	*In migrants*	*Out migrants*	*In migrants*	*Out migrants*
Antigua/Barbuda	55,056	8,287	5,620	15.1	10.7
Bahamas	210,590	4,047	109	1.9	0.1
Barbados	236,322	12,847	4,240	5.4	1.9
Dominica	67,624	871	7,507	1.3	10.1
Grenada	82,155	2,806	18,687	3.4	19.1
Guyana	698,950	1,003	13,453	0.1	1.9
Montserrat	9,928	1,362	1,958	13.7	18.6
St. Kitts and Nevis	38,886	1,553	8,309	4.0	18.2
St. Lucia	130,723	2,996	8,483	2.3	6.2
St. Vincent	104,980	2,734	18,169	2.6	15.1
Trinidad/Tobago	1,105,325	37,071	8,735	3.4	0.8
U.S. Virgin Islands	92,232	23,280	1,524	25.5	2.2

Source: Caribbean Community Regional Census Office (1994).

Exhibit 28.6 Urban and rural populations for selected Caribbean countries (1980 and 1995)

	1980			*1995*		
Country	*Urban ('000)*	*Rural ('000)*	*% Urban*	*Urban ('000)*	*Rural ('000)*	*% Urban*
Bahamas	123	87	59	185	91	67
Barbados	100	149	40	121	140	46
Guyana	232	527	31	299	535	36
Haiti	1,272	4,081	24	2,243	4,935	31
Jamaica	1,017	1,116	48	1,534	1,013	60
Trinidad and Tobago	616	466	57	866	440	66

Source: IDB Economic and Social Progress in Latin America (1996).

shift that has been observed over the last two decades across the region, as illustrated in Exhibit 28.6.

PROFILE OF THE CARIBBEAN MIGRANT

In her assessment of the subject area, Elizabeth Thomas-Hope (2000, 1.2.2) identified Caribbean migration as a reflection of variations based upon the purpose for the movement (work, education, accompanying persons), combined with length of stay at the destination.

The Caribbean migrant is likely to display some degree of variation on the basis of sex and occupational status as we moved from the intra-regional migrant to those targeting international destination. The latter is more likely to be male and associated more with labor-intensive occupations, while the former is more likely to be female. The intra-regional migrant is also inclined to be classified more into the professional, technical, and related categories in terms of occupational status (Villa and Pizarro (2001, 2).

The discussion thus far has focused on the migration patterns and profiles that have been captured through official sources. There is, however, a significant number of people who migrate both internationally and intra-regionally, but are not recorded either in the censuses or in any systematic way through any of the official statistical agencies. This important form of migration includes informal commercial activities of various types, including drug trafficking and commercial sex work. The movement of groups involved in the latter is of particular importance due in large part to what has been described in the literature as their vulnerability to HIV/AIDS. This relationship will be addressed in more detail in subsequent sections.

HIV/AIDS AND MIGRATION

The discussion on migration, mobility, and HIV/AIDS focused initially on the movement of mobile populations between and within countries spreading the virus. This focus has since shifted with the recognition that migrants may be at least at equal risk or more vulnerable to HIV/AIDS through their interactions while away than the non-mobile population, and are therefore more likely to return to their home with the infection (UNAIDS 2001, 2). In the Caribbean clear evidence of this pattern is seen in Guyana, where miners who work for prolonged periods away from families have been known to get infected away from home and infect the home in the process. In a Study by Palmer et al. (2002), involving gold miners in the Amazon region in Guyana, 6.5 percent of the men were found to be HIV positive. The continued movement by miners between the city and the Amazon jungle, as well as their interaction with the indigenous communities, has serious implications for the spread of the virus.

The vulnerability of migrant populations to HIV/AIDS is linked to their socioeconomic and cultural circumstances, as well as changes in the accessibility and availability of health and other support services in the host country. Even in cases where health and social services would be prepared to assist migrant populations, they often encounter great difficulties in reaching them. For the migrant who is HIV positive and likely to be the subject of stigmatization and discrimination, the situation is further aggravated, as he or she is likely to hide their status for as long as possible, thereby exposing themselves and others in the process.

According to the International Organisation on Migration (IOM), the magnitude of this vulnerability as it relates to mobile populations can be linked to whether the movement of the migrant group is voluntary or involuntary.[5] Examples of the former classification includes displacement for professional or personal reasons, while the latter refers to movement driven by such factors as poverty, wars, human rights abuses, ethnic tensions or through forced labour.[6] The movement of mobile and migrant populations in the English-speaking Caribbean can be classified as largely voluntary and includes agricultural and other casual workers, the business traveler, members of the military, students and teachers, tourist, commercial sex workers (CSW), and petty traders. A great deal of emphasis has been placed over time on the latter three, and in particular on CSW, due to the obvious high-risk nature of this profession in general and as it relates to HIV/AIDS. The extension of the list is a recognition that the dialogue must be expanded to go beyond the "traditional high-risk groups" and include those groups that a engaged in "high-risk activity" but whom may not fall readily into a clearly defined "high-risk group." To this end the inclusion of students and business travellers represents an important move. To this I would like to add the group of MSMs. A more detailed look at the highlighted groups will be conducted in the sections to follow.

Tourism

The tourism sector continues to be among the largest growing sectors worldwide and is the economic mainstay of many of the islands of the Caribbean, bringing over 15 million visitors to the region annually of which the English-speaking islands account for just over 6 million, according to The World Bank (2000, 10).

According to Kempadoo (1999, 14), the Caribbean has positioned itself as a "pleasure destination" in the tourism market, and this is clearly portrayed in the promotional material and other advertisements that portray Caribbean men and women as providers of services and (sexual) pleasure. It is therefore no surprise that accompanying the growth in tourism in the region has been growth in the sex tourism industry.

Transactional sex catering to the needs of sex-seeking tourists continues to grow in Tobago. Similar to the "rent-a-dread" concept in Jamaica, this growing industry involves both men and women travelling to the island seeking the services of a "beach-boy" for a few days (CAFRA 2004). Wesley Gibbings, in an article that addressed the topic of sex tourism in Tobago made the following observation:

> Sex tourism in Tobago mainly involves European and North American women and local men. The trade is run with business-like efficiency by "tourist agents" and unlisted guest houses, with advertisements in European magazines announcing "package deals" including the services of a local male or female. (Gibbings 1997)

In an environment that is largely rural, with high levels of unemployment particularly among the youth, commercial sex work of this nature presents the opportunity to earn foreign currency quite easily. The risks involved are however quite significant as Tobago is presently grappling with an HIV/AIDS epidemic that continues to grow, as evidenced by the increase in the number of reported AIDS cases from a mere 10 in 1990 to 66 just six years later. During this period a total of 276 persons had tested positive for HIV in this, the sister isle of Trinidad (CAREC 2004, 120).

Commercial Sex Workers

In general, commercial sex workers (CSW) tend to be extremely mobile, coming from a variety of source countries. Most appear to come from within the region, though Colombia and Venezuela and Guyana are repeatedly mentioned. In some cases, the migration of CSWs appears to reflect general migration and mobility patterns, and in many cases the CSWs enter into countries as tourists (IOM 2004). The link between tourism and commercial sex work is clearly highlighted above and represents an important feature of most of the heavily visited destinations. The area of commercial sex work, however, goes beyond the topic of tourism and is very central to the discussion on mobile populations.

Prostitution is illegal in most countries in the English-speaking Caribbean, with persons found guilty of such an offence liable on conviction to imprisonment for as much as five years in the case of the Trinidad and Tobago Sexual Offences Act. Despite the presence of such laws, commercial sex work continues to thrive across the region.

Commercial sex work in Caribbean is usually facilitated through a number of avenues, ranging from the street "hustler" to well-organized networks that include hotels, nightclubs, fashion houses, and escort services. There is reported to be a significant foreign clientele among the organized networks, which include Taiwanese, Europeans, and North Americans who are hotel guests and "yachties." Commercial sex workers are, in general, a very mobile group, moving not only regionally, but also within country as well. The local CSWs are likely to be the ones whose movements are typically confined to within country, while the CSWs who are external migrants are usually engaged in intra-regional and extra-regional travel.

The more mobile CSWs are known to come from the South American continent, as explained in an interview with a former sex worker and manager of an escort service:

> Most of my foreign girls came from Venezuela, Columbia and Cuba. Some of them commute between their homes and Trinidad regularly . . . Some of them were students or just tourists and got involved in the business to augment their income or in order to purchase a particular item.

In terms of the intra-regional movement of the CSWs, there is known to be a significant degree of movement between Suriname, Guyana, Belize, and Trinidad in the industry by those located in Trinidad and Tobago and Guyana (CAREC 2000, 17). CSW located in Barbados and the Eastern Caribbean were likely to travel to and from destinations like Antigua and Barbuda, St. Vincent, St. Lucia, St. Maarten, and Martinique for work. There were also reports of CSWs coming as far as Haiti and Dominican Republic to ply their trade.

A study conducted by the Caribbean Epidemiology Centre (CAREC) on female sex workers in Guyana in the year 2000 found that roughly one in every three CSWs worked outside of Georgetown. From this group, among the key countries visited were Suriname, French Guyana, Trinidad, and to a lesser extent Barbados (CAREC 2000, 17). The significance of this can be appreciated when one considers that the study also reported that 31 percent of the street and brothel-based women sampled were found to be HIV positive.

Condom use in general, however, appears to be high among the CSW sub-population in the study. A significantly high 84 percent of the sample of female sex workers in the Guyana study claimed to always use condoms with their clients. This pattern appears to have also taken root in the local landscape, as condom use was found to be widespread among the locally based CSWs. They have in most cases been advised to use or insist on the use of protection by their clients. As indicated by the former escort service manager,

> My girls always used protection, that is never an issue . . . I allow my girls the option of denying their clients once they refuse to comply with the their request that a condom be used.

For persons who are infected, the high degree of mobility by this group increases the likelihood of the virus being spread, particularly in cases where they may not be aware of their status. In an environment that still outlaws the soliciting of sex, some CSWs, particularly those who work on the streets, remain marginalized, and are unlikely to willingly access health and related social services that are available for fear of discrimination, both as a person living with HIV/AIDS and as a commercial sex worker if their status is revealed. In other cases sex workers have been known to function as part of a well-organized network that sees to the needs of their employees. The externally based CSWs fall readily into the latter category are known to operate, in some cases, in a heavily protected environment.

Students

Students represent another mobile group that is particularly important in the Caribbean context. This is evident, as students in the Caribbean are known to display in-country internal movements, as well as inter-regional and international migratory patterns. In the Trinidad and Tobago context, the institutions around which a significant portion of this migration patterns takes place are the University of the West Indies and the Schools of Languages.

The St. Augustine Campus of the University of the West Indies accommodates over 8,500 students, of which approximately 13 percent come from other Caribbean countries, as shown in Exhibit 28.7.

Students attending these institutions, in general, have reported a high degree of sexual activity. This is driven in part by the absence of the rigid controls that are normally associated with the standard school system and supported by the ease of access to alcohol in particular and other drugs, in and around the institution. The following quote came of a focus group discussion involving students at the St. Augustine Campus on the topic of the behaviour of the more mobile students on the campus during the conduct

Exhibit 28.7 The University of the West Indies, St. Augustine campus: On-campus enrollment by nationality

	ACADEMIC YEAR					
NATIONALITY	*1997–98*	*1998–99*	*1999–2000*	*2000–01*	*2001–02*	*2002–03*
Trinidad and Tobago	5,388	5,609	5,815	5,982	6,743	7,723
Other UWI Caribbean Contributing Countries	678	710	735	714	683	710
Non Contributing Countries	237	299	310	271	215	196
Total	6,303	6,618	6,860	6,967	7,641	8,629

Source: University of the West Indies, OPD Annual Report (2004).

of the Trinidad and Tobago Situation and Response Analysis on HIV/AIDS (The University of the West Indies 2001):

> There are party tendencies . . . freedom and experiences that go with being on your own for the first time. Some students live in San Fernando, for instance and daily travelling is not an option, so they move onto one of the (student) halls or surrounding apartments. Without parent supervision, there is a certain amount of freedom that is gained and explored.

During group discussions with representatives of the student body, mention was made of the "matrix"—the environment where one keeps their love interests concealed so as to facilitate more than one partner. The foreign student was also seen as having the upper hand among the students, as indicated below:

> Foreigners appear to score more with the girls . . . there is a lot of foreign–local interaction. Foreigners are amazed at the amount of attention that they get when they come to this campus. Guys talk among themselves about how they share girls.

Despite the heightened sexual activity on the campus, contraceptive use was, however, reported to be inconsistent at the very best:

> Guys still take a chance as long as the girl looks "safe" and "quiet." Unless a girl is strong enough to demand that the guy use a condom, it will not be used. Guys hesitate to use a condom because they say it reduces their sensitivity.

Men Who Have Sex With Men (MSM)

The act of sex between men is illegal and is a criminal offense in Trinidad and Tobago, as it is in all countries in the English-speaking Caribbean. These relationships are highly stigmatized and are frowned on by many across the Caribbean landscape, particularly those among the religious community, and are at times treated with a great deal of aggression among others. Faced with such an environment, men who engage in same sex relationships typically resort to assuming heterosexual lifestyles, even getting married in some cases in order to conform to the social norm, or simply remain "in the closet." According to the CAREC/PAHO study on Gay Research (CAREC 1998), what results among a segment of this group is therefore a "double role"—a public one which involves heterosexual relations, and a private life in which they engage in intimate relationships with men. It has been stated that the rapid increase in the prevalence of AIDS among women in the last ten years is due in large part to infection by male partners who also belong to MSM communities (De Groulard, et al. 1998).

The MSM groups are known to be quite mobile in the Caribbean. The importance of this is seen, as it presents the ideal opportunity to be "open" with their partners in an environment where they are not known. As a result there is regular movement of MSM around the region, with travel often scheduled around key sporting events like cricket and key festivals like carnival. It was revealed, during the interviews with members of the MSM community, that the more mobile MSMs come from across the region but mainly from St. Vincent, Barbados, Grenada, Venezuela, and Guyana. Given the mobility associated with the group, migration typically assumes both internal and external dimensions.

The internal migration pattern is found to be bi-directional between rural areas and urban centers, with the main objective being the avoidance of discrimination and to be in an environment where they are not known, more accepted or better able to congregate with their partners and peers. For the MSMs who are HIV positive the move to urban centers is also made to better gain assess to facilities and medications. The move to rural areas interestingly may also involve a return to one's home village, as explained by a member of the MSM support group:

> The only time they (MSM) would return home in the rural areas will be when it is at the last stages of AIDS and they go home to be taken care of.

Like internal migration, external migration trends are driven by the need to be away from a familiar environment.

> MSMs from Trinidad go to other countries to hide their relationships, or the fact that they just found out their HIV status and don't want their families to know. Just as some leave Tobago and Toco to come to Port of Spain, those who can afford it, leave Trinidad and go to Barbados, for example.

In the face of growing stigmatization the MSM community face a particularly daunting situation. For the HIV-infected MSM, the situation is further exaggerated as the combined social stigma of same sex relationships and HIV infections present what can be termed a double stigma that is confronted by this group. This limits open communication with MSMs and has given rise to what has been termed a growing culture of silence and secrecy (CAREC/PAHO/WHO 1998).

Street Children

Another of the growing vulnerable groups that are engaged in and exposed to a high degree of risky activity including sexual activity is street children. These children, comprised largely of boys, are in most cases either homeless or running away from home and come from impoverished surroundings. Based on the findings of a report by Lee and Felix (1997, 19), the pattern of movement displayed by this group easily classifies them among the migrant population due to their tendency to gravitate towards the urban centers (Port of Spain, Kingston). The capital stands out, however, as the preferred venue. The boys, whose ages range from 11 to 14 years, are sometimes picked up in cars and taken to various venues where they are known to exchange sexual favors for food, brand-name clothing, but in most cases money. Runaway adolescent girls who are recruited from the streets, children and adolescents involved in formal prostitution, and the sexual exploitation of primarily male street children are evidence of a vibrant sex trade that is firmly rooted in this group.

Petty Traders

While identified among the list of at-risk groups in the dialogue on mobile and migrant populations, in the Caribbean context, however, the petty trader is found to be less inclined to fall into the above category. A study done by the International Organization on Migration (IOM) on mobile populations in the Caribbean in 2004 assessed the extent to which these traders were involved in commercial sex, thereby increasing their risk of contracting HIV/AIDS (IOM 2004). Based on the study, petty traders in the English-speaking Caribbean were found in general to be extremely mobile, traveling often with stays of short duration in-country. Some traders are known to average roughly four visits per year to destinations, staying on longer than two weeks per visit. In the other cases they entered more frequently, sometimes more than once weekly, but stayed for only a few days each time. The source countries for most of these traders mirror the general migration patterns for the countries in the region.

While in the literature petty traders are identified among the high-risk mobile groups, largely due to their links with commercial sex work, in the case of the English-speaking Caribbean, the petty trader did not feature among this classification. The petty trader in the Caribbean context was typically a mature person (40 years or more), likely to be either married or in a common law relationship. In addition these traders were found in general to have had one sexual partner and be less likely to be engaged in risky sexual encounters of any nature while working (IOM 2004).

SUMMARY AND CONCLUSION

The vulnerability of migrants and mobile populations to the virus is linked to the high-risk behavior that is characteristic of some mobile groups, such as miners, truckers, and professionals who work away from home for both short and long periods; and high-risk groups that are by their very nature mobile, which include Commercial Sex Workers and petty traders.

With this in mind a clear distinction was made between what was identified as high-risk groups and mobile groups engaging in high-risk behavior. Without devaluing the importance of the former groups, this distinction allowed for the revisiting of the list, with greater emphasis being placed on the latter (high-risk behavior). This repositioning will therefore see the inclusion of the MSM group among the migrant population and greater emphasis placed on students as a mobile group engaging in high-risk sexual activity, with less emphasis played on petty traders.

The IOM has identified the environment faced by the migrant as characterized by high levels of poverty, discrimination, and exploitation, alienation and sense of anonymity, limited access to social, education, and health services, separation from families and partners, and separation from the sociocultural norms that inform behavior in stable communities. In the presence of this environment mobile populations are likely to engage in wealth-seeking behavior that is typically high risk by nature, thereby exposing themselves to abuse, exploitation, and exposure to HIV/AIDS. In a more positive environment characterized by increased access to information and services, better opportunities and livelihood, these groups are likely to yield benefits at the individual, family, and community level, and at the wider economy. Increased earning capacity on the path of these groups in a nonthreatening environment is likely to result in increased income, the benefits of which will be felt at both the source and destination points in the form of transfers and remittances. The latter has, over the last decade, emerged as a key source of capital inflow and foreign exchange for a number of Caribbean territories (Nurse 2004).

In a less supportive environment for migrant workers and mobile groups the resulting negative impact is likely to see an upsurge in the spread of HIV among this group. In the absence of coordinated and sustained policy interventions to address needs of these high-risk groups, what will follow is continued attempts at coping in a hostile and less enabling environment for the mobile PLWHA. These circumstances are likely to result in an increase spread of the epidemic at both the source and destination points as survival strategies are attempted. This is in turn likely to see a reinforcement of the push factors, which further perpetuates the negative environment faced by mobile groups and migrant workers. This path is captured below in the form of a decision tree (Exhibit 28.8). Investing in a positive and enabling environment early is therefore seen as the most cost-effective and efficient intervention option and one that is likely to yield larger benefits, in terms of fewer persons infected, and fewer costs in terms of resources required to address the health and related needs of a growing number of new infections that would have otherwise resulted.

CLOSING REMARKS

From this review of HIV/AIDS and mobile populations it is clear that the two are inextricably linked. This relationship should not be seen as cause and effect or linear, but more lateral in type. HIV is a manifestation of a number of socioeconomic ills, which are represented in inequalities and deprivation, in lack of access to key services, information, and social support systems. This environment in turn breeds behaviors that increase vulnerability and susceptibility to HIV/AIDS among those most at risk, which includes the migrant and mobile populations. Migration in itself is not a driver of vulnerability for HIV/AIDS; it is the unsafe practices that result from the conditions faced by migrants and mobile populations that create conditions of vulnerability and susceptibility. In a world that is facing increased globalization, the key to addressing this complex link between migration and HIV lies, therefore, in addressing the socioeconomic environment that drives this phenomenon.

This includes, for example, the adoption of a broad-based approach that goes beyond the lop-sided and largely punitive supply side measures that are usually implemented to curb the activities of such high-risk groups as MSM and CSW. Such measures have over the years brought little or no value added and have in most cases reinforced the negative environment, thereby driving these critical target groups underground and making them more inaccessible to critical program interventions.

Exhibit 28.8 The pathway of HIV-AIDS and mobile populations and vulnerability

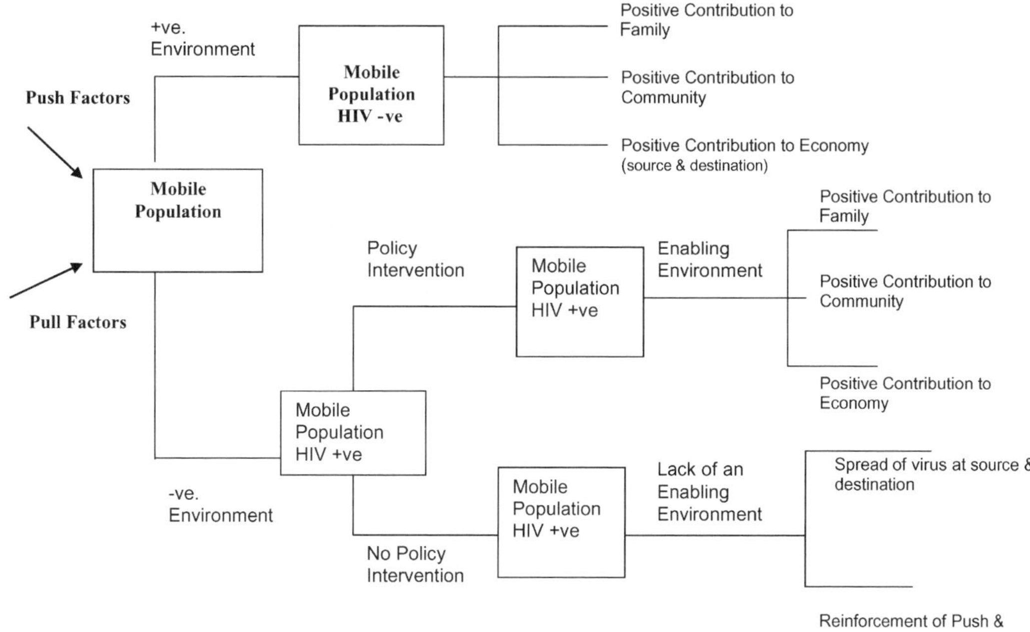

A more broad-based approach also involves demand side initiatives that address the causal factors behind the high-risk behavior and practices of the vulnerable mobile groups.

NOTES

1. The sixteenth and late nineteenth centuries are both characterized by advancements in communication, transportation and production systems that have been associated with increased globalization.
2. The IOM defines migrants as people who move from one place to another temporarily, seasonally or permanently for a host of voluntary and/or involuntary reasons.

REFERENCES AND FURTHER READING

Anderson, H., Marcovici, K., and Taylor, K. (2002). *The UNGASS, Gender and Women's Vulnerability to HIV/AIDS in the Latin America and the Caribbean.* Washington: PAHO.

Barnett, Tony. (2002) "HIV/AIDS and Globalization, What is the Epidemic Telling Us About Economics, Morality and Pragmatism?" in Forsythe, Steven (ed.), *State of the Art: AIDS and Economics*, Washington DC: The Policy Project.

Brown, Dennis A. V. (2002). *Socio-Demographic Vulnerability in the Caribbean: An Examination of the Social and Demographic Impediments to Equitable Development with Participatory Citizenship in the Caribbean at the Dawn of the Twenty-First Century.* Santiago, Chile: ECLAC—Latin American and Caribbean Demographic Centre (CELADE).

Camara, Bilali. (2001). *Eighteen Years of the HIV/AIDS Epidemic in the Caribbean: A Summary.* Port of Spain, Trinidad: CAREC.

Caribbean Association for Feminist Research and Action (CAFRA). (2004). *Situation Analysis of Commercial Sex Work in Trinidad and Tobago – Support to the National Response to HIV/AIDS: Addressing a vulnerable group in Trinidad and Tobago.* Port of Spain: CAFRA/UNAIDS.

Caribbean Community Regional Census Office (CCPHC) (1994). *Commonwealth Caribbean Population and Housing Census, 1991*, Port of Spain. Trinidad.

Caribbean Epidemiology Centre (CAREC). (2000). *HIV Infection and HIV Risk Practices among Female Sex Workers in Georgetown, Guyana—A Follow-Up Survey.* Port of Spain, Trinidad: CAREC/GTZ.

Caribbean Epidemiology Centre (CAREC). (2004). *Status and Trends: Analysis of the Caribbean HIV-AIDS Epidemic 1982-2002.* Port of Spain: CAREC/PAHO/WHO.

Caribbean Epidemiology Centre/German Technical Cooperation. (2000). *HIV Infection and HIV Risk practices among Female Sex Workers in Georgetown, Guyana.* Port of Spain, Trinidad: CAREC.

Caribbean Epidemiology Centre (CAREC)/PAHO/WHO. (1998). *An Analysis of Discussions with Men who Have Sex with Men (MSM), A Technical Report.* Port of Spain, Trinidad: CAREC.

CARICOM Secretariat. (2002). *A Plan of Action for the CARICOM Secretariat in Response to the HIV/AIFD Pandemic in the Caribbean*. Georgetown: CARICOM Secretariat.

Carlier, Jean-Yves, and Schiffino, Graciela. (1999). *The Free Movement of Persons Living with HIV/AIDS*. Luxembourg: European Commission.

Conway, Dennis. (2003). "The Caribbean Diaspora," in Hillman, Richard and D'Agostino, Thomas (eds.), *Understanding the Contemporary Caribbean*. Kingston: Ian Randle Publishers.

De Groulard, M., et al. (1998). *Analysis of the Situation of HIV/AIDS in CAREC Member Countries*. Port of Spain, Trinidad: Caribbean Epidemiology Centre.

Gibbings, Wesley. (1997). "Trinidad and Tobago—Health: The High Cost of Sex Tourism." *Inter Press News (IPS)*. March 4.

Harawa, N., Bingham, A. et al. (2002). "HIV Prevalence Among Foreign- and U.S.-Born Clients of Public STD Clinics." *American Journal of Public Health*, 92(12).

Inter American Development Bank. (1996). *Economic and Social Progress in Latin America*. Washington DC: IDB.

International Organisation for Migration (IOM). (2002). *IOM Position Paper on Migration*. Santo Domingo, Dominican Republic: IOM.

International Organisation for Migration (IOM). (2004). *Baseline Assessment: HIV/AIDS and Mobile Populations in the Caribbean*. Santo Domingo, Dominican Republic: IOM.

Kaiser Family Foundation. (2007). *The Global Impact of HIV/AIDS on Youth*, Fact sheet, January.

Kempadoo, Kamala. (1998). "The Migration Tightrope in Kempadoo," in Kempadoo, Kamala, and Doezomia, Jo (eds.), *Global Sex Workers—Rights, Resistance and Redefinition*. New York and London: Routledge.

Kempadoo, Kamala. (1999). "Continuities and Change—Five Centuries of Prostitution in the Caribbean," in Kempadoo, Kamala (ed.), *Sun, Sex and Gold Tourism and Sex Work in the Caribbean*. London: Rowman and Littlefield Publishers, Inc.

Lee, A., and Felix, J., (1997). *Child Prostitution Child Pornography and the Sale of Children*. June.

Martindale, Carol. (2003). "Risky Business." *Weekend Nation, Barbados*. July 25.

Ministry of Health, the Republic of Trinidad and Tobago. National Surveillance Unit. (2004). "*HIV/AIDS Morbidity and Mortality Report.*" *Quarterly Report, 2004*, Ministry of Health, Port of Spain.

Ministry of Health, the Republic of Trinidad and Tobago. National Surveillance Unit. (2007) "*HIV/AIDS Morbidity and Mortality Report.*" *Quarterly Report, 2007*, Ministry of Health, Port of Spain.

Nurse, Keith. (2004) *Diaspora, Migration and Development in the Caribbean*. Canadian Foundation for the Americas, Policy Paper, Ontario, Canada. June.

Palmer, C., Validum, L., Loeffke, B., Laubach, H., Mitchell, C., Cummings, R., and Cuadrado, R. (2002). "HIV Prevalence in a Gold Mining Camp in the Amazon Region, Guyana." *Emerging Infectious Diseases*, 8(3), March.

Pan American Health Organisation. (1998). *Health in the Americas*, Vol. 1. Washington DC: PAHO.

Thomas-Hope, Elizabeth. (2000). "Trends and Patterns of Migration to and from Caribbean Countries." Presented at Simposia Sobre Migración International en Las Americas, San José, Costa Rica, September 4–6, 2002.

Trinidad and Tobago Central Statistical Office. (1999). *Annual Statistical Digest*. Port of Spain: CSO.

Trinidad and Tobago Ministry of Community Empowerment, Sport and Consumer Affairs. (2001). *Country Report to the Regional Governmental Congress on Sexual Exploitation of Children.*

Trinidad and Tobago. (1986). *The Sexual Offences Act*, No. 27 Sections 22–24.

Trinidad and Tobago. (2006). *The Immigration (Caribbean Community Skilled Nationals) Act, 1996.*

UNAIDS. (2000a). *HIV and AIDS in the Americas: An Epidemic with Many Faces*. Geneva: Joint United Nations Programme on HIV/AIDS.

UNAIDS. (2000b). *Report on the Global HIV/AIDS Epidemic 2002*. Geneva: Joint United Nations Programme on HIV/AIDS.

UNAIDS. (2001) *Population Mobility and AIDS, UNAIDS Technical Update*. Geneva: Joint United Nations Programme on HIV/AIDS.

UNAIDS. (2006a). *Report on the Global HIV/AIDS epidemic*, Geneva, December.

UNAIDS. (2006b). "Caribbean," Fact sheet, May.

UNAIDS/UNESCO. (2000). *Migrant Populations and HIV/AIDS—The Development*. Geneva: UNAIDS/UNICEF.

United Nations General Assembly. (2001). "Declaration of Commitment on HIV/AIDS: Global Crisis—Global Action." United Nations Special Session on HIV/AIDS, New York, June 25–27.

University of the West Indies, Health Economics Unit (HEU). (2001). *Situational and Response Analysis of HIV/AIDS in Trinidad—Final Report*. St. Augustine: HEU/UWI, April.

University of the West Indies, Health Economics Unit (HEU). (2002). *The Republic of Trinidad and Tobago. Five-Year National HIV/AIDS Strategic Plan 2003–2007, Final Report*. St. Augustine: UWI/HEU.

University of the West Indies. (2004). *Office of Planning and Developments Annual Report*. St. Augustine: UWI.

Villa, Miguel, and Jose Martínez Pizarro (2001). "Trends and Patterns of International Migration in Latin America and the Caribbean." Paper presented at APEC-HRD-LSP International Workshop on International Migration and Structural Change in APEC Member Countries.

Wolfe, Scott A. (2002). *The Shared Burden: Toward an Assessment of the Impact of Caribbean Migration on Comprehensive HIV/AIDS Care*, Background Document for the PAHO/HRSA Consultation, Draft 18–19, 2002, Washington DC.

World Bank. (2000). *Tourism and the Environment in the Caribbean: An Economic Framework*. Washington DC: CGCED, The World Bank.

CHAPTER 29

Framing HIV Prevention Discourse to Encompass the Complexities of War in Northern Uganda

Michael J. Westerhaus, Amy C. Finnegan, Yoti Zabulon, and Joia S. Mukherjee

Reprint from American Journal of Public Health (2007) 97:1184–1186.

ABSTRACT

In northern Uganda, physical and structural violence (political repression, economic inequality, and gender-based discrimination) increase vulnerability to HIV infection. In settings of war, traditional HIV prevention that solely promotes risk avoidance and risk reduction and assumes the existence of personal choice inadequately addresses the realities of HIV transmission. The design of HIV prevention strategies in northern Uganda must recognize how HIV transmission occurs and the factors that put people at risk for infection. A human rights approach provides a viable model for achieving this aim.

Uganda, a country that has demonstrated dramatic success in reducing national HIV prevalence, remains at the center of the current debate between the proponents of risk avoidance and harm-reduction strategies for the prevention of HIV transmission (Green 2003; Okward et al. 2005). In this debate, enormous energy and expenditures are invested in efforts that pit abstinence and behavior change against condom promotion. However, both strategies rest on the assumption that individual behavior and personal choice are to blame for HIV transmission. Neither strategy acknowledges that poverty, political instability, and gender inequality are driving forces in the epidemic (Farmer et al. 1996; Smallman-Raynor and Cliff 1991; Tarantola and Mann 1995; Zwi and Cabral 1991). The experience of those living in northern Uganda, where HIV prevalence stands at nearly double that of the rest of the country, challenges the supposition that individual choice determines HIV transmission risk (Uganda Ministry of Health 2005).

NORTHERN UGANDA AND VULNERABILITY TO HIV INFECTION

For 21 years, northern Uganda has experienced a particularly brutal conflict between an insurgent group called the Lord's Resistance Army (LRA) and the army of the Ugandan government (Médecins Sans Frontières 2004). The war has been characterized by child abductions, frequent rapes, attacks on civilian camps, deliberate maiming, and ruthless killings. Three unique exigencies of the war in northern Uganda make traditional HIV prevention programs ineffective: the mass abduction of children into the LRA, the phenomenon of night commuting, and the existence of internally displaced people's camps.

First, child abductions create increased vulnerability to HIV infection among the young. During the war, more than 66,000 children have been abducted to fight as soldiers or serve as sex slaves (Survey of War Affected Youth 2006). Males abducted into the LRA are coerced through physical violence to use rape as a weapon of war, and many of the girls are forced into sexual slavery as "wives" to LRA commanders, with some eventually contracting HIV.

Second, tens of thousands of "night commuters," most of whom are children, flee the insecurity of their communities each evening and traverse northern Uganda unsupervised to seek safety in hospitals and city shelters (Women's Commission for Refugee Women and Children 2004). These children are often sexually victimized, and even when the sexual activity is consensual it often occurs at an early age and without the benefit of information abut safe sexual practices. This reality creates an environment ripe for HIV transmission (Anderson et al. 2004). (Currently, because of a cessation of hostilities while the government and the LRA are negotiating peace, the number of night commuters has dramatically fallen. However, night commuting has been a factor that has contributed to HIV vulnerability.)

Third, the 1.8 million people currently living in internally displaced people's camps are vulnerable to HIV infection because of both insecurity and severely limited economic opportunity. Women who tend crops and collect firewood on the perimeters of the camps are frequently attacked and raped by both Ugandan soldiers and members of the LRA (Akumu et al. 2005). Additionally, women are frequently driven to transactional sex (i.e., providing sexual services for money) in order to provide for their children and attain the means to provide educational opportunities for their children.

EXPANDING THE FRAME FOR HIV PREVENTION

The sole promotion of traditional forms of HIV prevention (abstinence, behavior change, and condom prevention) will not reduce the prevalence of HIV in northern Uganda. The unique and interconnected realities of child soldiers, night commuters, and the internally displaced people's camps that entangle the population in a dangerous web of physical and structural violence (i.e., political repression, economic inequality, and gender-based discrimination—structures that disadvantage certain populations) must be accounted for to design successful HIV prevention programs.

Condom promotion does not adequately minimize HIV transmission for women and children who are raped by members of the LRA and government soldiers, because women in this situation lack power to negotiate condom use. Furthermore, condom promotion programs fail to protect women who have limited negotiation power and are driven into transactional sex to meet basic living necessities. Abstinence and behavior change strategies ignore how poverty and war strip individuals of personal choice essential to avoid HIV transmission. Although some may argue that individuals never lose personal agency—the ability to affect one's surroundings and personal relationships in a manner consistent with personal desires—the situation in northern Uganda demonstrates that settings permeated by war and poverty obstruct the expression of such agency.

Given the context of conflict in northern Uganda, it is imperative that efforts to prevent HIV transmission expand beyond traditional risk avoidance and reduction strategies to include the need for personal, political, and economic security in such communities. Child soldiers, night commuters, and life in the internally displaced people's camps create widespread vulnerability to HIV infection in northern Uganda. To reduce HIV transmission in this region, the social and political forces that underpin risk must be understood, a task that rests on attentiveness to the local and global contexts. A human rights approach to HIV prevention promotes recognition of the ways in which a lack of basic social and economic rights—including the right to food, shelter, heath, education, and economic opportunity—augment HIV risk significantly in northern Uganda.

With a human rights approach in mind, it is clear that poverty eradication and income generation activities are essential for effective HIV prevention among women at internally displaced people's camps, where livelihoods are severely limited or nonexistent.

If options for income generation existed, women could avoid transactional sex as a means for meeting basic human needs, thereby diminishing their risk of HIV infection. Furthermore, HIV prevention programs must also target men. In northern Uganda, displacement has compromised male gender roles, creating frustration that manifests itself in violence against women (Liu Institute for Global Issues 2005). HIV prevention programs must acknowledge these realities and attempt to counter this violence by working with men to reshape their gender roles in ways that are acceptable to both men and women (see Exhibit 29.1).

TOWARD A HUMAN RIGHTS APPROACH

Further, Uganda and countries with significant influence in East Africa, such as the United States and Great Britain, must focus on interventions that provide real security for vulnerable populations, such as the deployment of peacekeepers and the establishment of well-protected centers of education, heath care, and shelter, which will decrease not only HIV risk but also the overall morbidity and mortality in the region. Conflict resolution and peace advocacy efforts must also form a critical component of strategies to reduce HIV transmission in northern Uganda, because resolution of the war will diminish the social pressures that contribute to HIV transmission. Such interventions will require significant funding, a collective responsibility of the United Nations, wealthy countries, the Ugandan government, and both local and global nongovernmental organizations.

These lessons from northern Uganda's experience have applicability on a global scale, particularly in conflict settings where risk of HIV infection clearly extends beyond individual choice (Hankins et al. 2002; Mock et al. 2004). Without understanding of local contexts and the impact of global forces upon those contexts, HIV prevention efforts risk failure on a grand scale. A rigorous incorporation of social, political, and eco-

Exhibit 29.1 Internally displaced people's camp in Northern Uganda 2004.

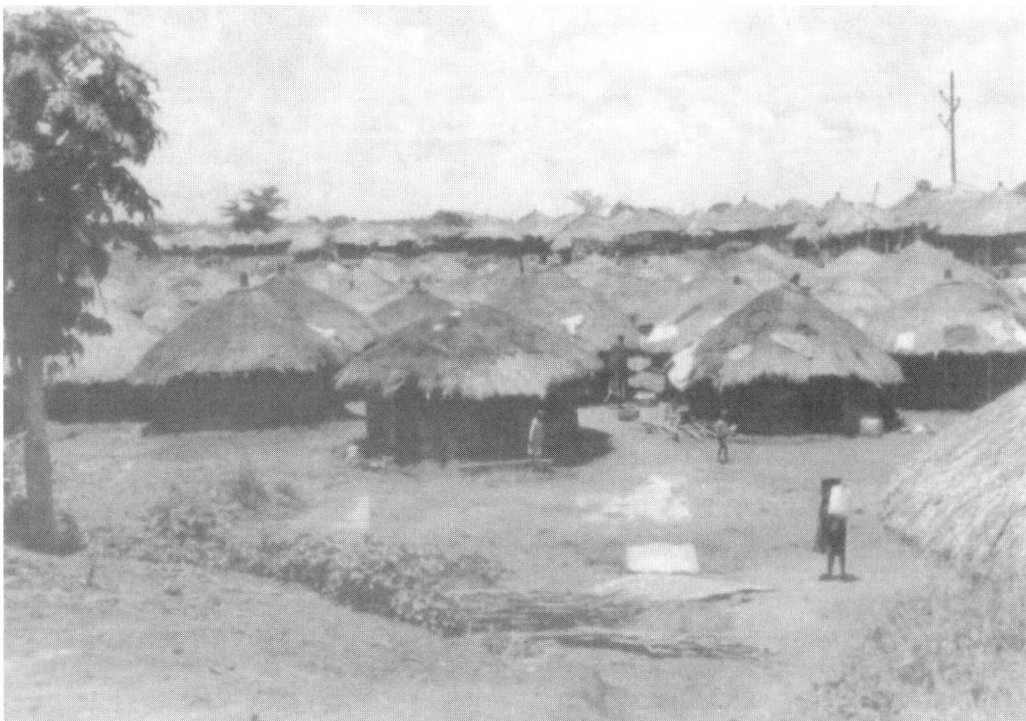

Source: Photo courtesy of A. C. Finnegan

nomic context into HIV prevention strategies promises a new dawn in curbing HIV transmission.

ACKNOWLEDGMENTS

We would like to thank the staff of both Lacer Hospital and Human Rights Focus in Gulu, Uganda, who facilitated the research and provided critical insights. We are also grateful to the staff of Partners in Heath, who provided useful commentary on the ideas presented here.

REFERENCES AND FURTHER READING

Akumu, C.O., I. Amony, and G. Otim. *Suffering in Science: A Study of Sexual and Gender Based Violence in Pabbo Camp, Gulu Disrict, Northern Uganda*. Geneva, Switzerland: UNICEF, 2005.

Anderson, R.E., F. Sewankambo, and K. Vandergrift. *Pawns of Politics: Children, Conflict, and Peace in Northern Uganda*, 2nd ed. Kampala, Uganda: World Vision International, 2004.

Farmer, P.E., M. Connors, and J. Simmons. *Women, Poverty, and AIDS: Sex, Drugs, and Structural Violence*. Monroe, MN: Common Courage Press, 1996.

Green, E.C. *Rethinking AIDS Prevention: Learning from Successes in Developing Countries*. Westport, CT: Praeger Press, 2003.

Hankins, C.A., S.R. Friedman, T. Zafar, and S.A. Strathdee. "Transmission and prevention of HIV and sexually transmitted infections in war settings: implications for current and future armed conflicts." *AIDS* (2002) 16:2245–2252.

Liu Institute for Global Issues, Gulu District NGO Forum, Ker Kwaro Acholi. *"Roco Wat Acholi:" Restoring Relationships in Acholi-land: Traditional Approaches to Justice and Reintegration*. Vancouver, British Columbia: Liu Institute for Global Issues, 2005.

Médecins Sans Frontières. *Life in Northern Uganda: All Shades of Grief and Fear*. Geneva, Switzerland: Médecins Sans Frontières, 2004.

Mock, N., S. Duale, L. Brown et al. "Conflict and HIV: a framework for risk assessment to prevent HIV in conflict-affected settings in Africa." *Emerging Themes in Epidemiology* 1(2004) 6:11–14.

Okward, S., J. Kinsman, S. Onyango, A. Opio, and P. Kaggwa. "Revisiting the ABC strategy: HIV prevention in Uganda in the era of antiretroviral therapy." *Postgraduate Medical Journal* (2005) 81:625–628.

Smallman-Raynor, M.R. and A.D. Cliff. "Civil war and the spread of AIDS in Central Africa." *Epidemiology of Infectious Diseases* (1991) 107:69–80.

Survey of War Affected Youth. *Research Brief 1*. Gulu, Uganda: Survey of War Affected Youth, 2006.

Tarantola, D. and J. Mann. "AIDS and human rights." *AIDS and Society* (1995) 6(4):1, 5.

Uganda Ministry of Health. *Uganda HIV/AIDS Sero-Behavioural Survey 2004–05*. Kampala, Uganda: Ministry of Health, 2005.

Women's Commission for Refugee Women and Children. *No Safe Place to Call Home: Child and Adolescent Night Commuters in Northern Uganda*. New York, NY: Women's Commission for Refugee Women and Children, 2004.

Zwi, A.B. and A.J. Cabral. "Identifying 'high risk situations' for preventing AIDS." *British Medical Journal* (1991) 303:1527–1529.

SECTION 8

Living and Caring for Individuals with HIV/AIDS

FRAMING ESSAY

Multiplicity of Meaning

Living with HIV/AIDS

Todd Faubion

As this chapter and section will show, diagnosis with HIV/AIDS continues to catalyze a seismic shift in the lives of those it strikes. Living with HIV/AIDS carries markedly different implications for individuals of varying socioeconomic strata, geographical locations, cultures, genders, and sexual orientations, among other anthropogenic forces forming the fabric of everyday life. Prevention, transmission, and survival can hinge upon cultural sensitivity of taboo topics or candid discussion of the disease and transmission mechanisms. For some, living with HIV/AIDS revolves around adherence to three dozen pills a day, while for others symptom management and palliative care in an environment of sustained crisis related to poverty and marginality is the best possible option. Still yet, for others, living with HIV/AIDS means constructing an illusion of good health and wellbeing lest stigma come to dominate their lives. This chapter reviews current literature relating to the broad topic of living with HIV/AIDS or, more specifically, the experiences of people living with HIV/AIDS (PLWHA). I draw from the experiences of all PLWHA and engage the many lenses through which perceptions of and experiences with the disease can be captured.

This chapter's goal is to capture current writing pertaining to this topic. It attends to *all* PLWHA while acknowledging the flattening effect of trying to synthesize such a varied group of experiences into a few pages. Nonetheless, it crosses space, socioeconomics, race/ethnicity, gender, and sexual orientation in an effort to illustrate the myriad implications of living with HIV/AIDS and thematic similarities among disparate groups in disparate places around the world.

Researchers studying HIV/AIDS are keenly aware that the risk of contracting and suffering from HIV/AIDS more intimately relates to social stressors, such as poverty, gender power imbalances, migration status, low educational attainment, and stigma than to inherent biological risk or susceptibility associated with biology or race/ethnicity. Literature has progressively transformed to a more nuanced and informed understanding of how and why such stressors impact the lives of people living with HIV/AIDS. Such studies are now being integrated, where possible, with biomedical research such that synergy can occur amongst often vertically established academic disciplines and research foci.

I am reviewing this literature as an activist in the arena of HIV/AIDS advocacy in the city of Seattle, taking great pride in contributing to a continuum of care of exemplary quality and compassion. I am in a unique position in that I know for certain that this chapter cannot adequately capture the breadth of issues faced by PLWHA in Seattle, though the articles do an exemplary job of advocating for improved care for and treatment of PLWHA, especially for those finding themselves on the margins of their respective social contexts. In Seattle we observe that a frightening rebound appears to be occurring whereby men who have sex with men (MSM) are beginning to perceive HIV as a chronic or curable disease versus the lethal threat it remains. A substantial amount of literature herein analyzes the multiple dimensions of highly active antiretroviral therapy (HAART) adherence, yet none addresses this simple and intuitive element of adherence: people cannot adhere to a medication regimen without stable housing and a supportive environment, especially those with addiction or mental health issues. Such observations are part of my appeal to continue to listen carefully to the voices of PLWHA and their care providers, advocates, families, and social networks.

Encouragingly, a substantial body of current literature relates specifically to the experiences of vulnerable and marginalized groups. A few examples include: pregnant women in rural southern India (Rogers et al. 2006), the geriatric community (Emlet 2006), Asians and Pacific Islanders living in the United States (Kang 2006), the unique needs of youth (de Carvalho Mesquita Ayres 2006), and gender differences in survival between men and women on antiretrovirals (ARVs) in Brazil (Braga et al. 2007). Marginality remains a primary risk factor in contracting HIV and often translates to enduring the ravages of HIV/AIDS with little support or ability to access available care options. Capturing such voices and experiences highlights spaces of intervention and possibility for a population highly vulnerable to infection, debilitation, and transmission. The considerable attention to micro-level analysis of vulnerable and marginalized groups highlights the scholarly community's clear recognition that environments of risk are nuanced and related to social, economic, political, and cultural structures that uniquely manifest across space. More heartening still, this literature not only identifies concurrent crises challenging the livelihoods of marginalized groups, but much of it tracks in the direction of understanding *how* and *why* the HIV-positive status of particular individuals reflects far more than contact with a fatal pathogen—it reflects social and structural constraints to wellbeing and good health.

Literature reviewed for this chapter falls into three broad categories. First, I discuss the unmistakable theme of stigma that continues to compound diagnosis with HIV/AIDS globally. There is a clear need for researchers to be insistent on returning to this theme and contributing to projects aimed at undercutting stigma or providing HIV-positive individuals with resources and faculties to mediate the adverse impacts of hostile responses to the disease. Within this section, I also emphasize the theme of vulnerability that emerges from the literature—not in relation to vulnerability to contracting the virus but rather vulnerability manifesting after HIV diagnosis. Such vulnerabilities include job loss, social marginalization, chronic illness, and other livelihood shocks challenging the very possibility of leading a "normal," safe, and healthy life post-diagnosis. I follow with a review of the current biomedical and clinical literature relating to the topic of PLWHA, giving due attention to developments in research relating to the disease's clinical manifestations and biomedical interventions that can be enormously effective in improving the lives of PLWHA. The savior of countless millions of lives after its introduction, HAART earns the major focus of biomedical research. A fuzzy line exists in this subsection in relation to HAART; adherence is integral to the effectiveness of the regimen but hinges upon myriad factors, most of which are social in nature. I nonetheless include most references to HAART here because it is, above all, a pharmacological regimen that remains the only known way to significantly extend the lives of PLWHA. The last section of this framing chapter examines the provider–patient relationship. These relationships remain the conduit to good health and must be founded upon principles of trust, candor, and non-judgment if HIV-positive individuals are to achieve optimal health outcomes and prevent disease transmission. Yet, as the literature demonstrates, much work remains in ensuring that such relationships and interactions serve the patient well. Those providing care to PLWHA must embody the idea of care as a social compact and exercise the principles of sympathy, compassion, commitment, and non-judgment.

STIGMA AND VULNERABILITY

The first unequivocal theme to emerge from current literature relates to the ever-present purveyor of fear and self-loathing: stigma. Stigma and social exclusion are perpetual fixtures in places where the epidemic has only recently emerged as a crisis. More discouragingly, abundant literature reviews stigma experiences in places where the epidemic has entered its third decade. Some of the most frequent contemporary literature relates to China's exploding epidemic (Zhou 2007; Li et al. 2006; Chen et al. 2007) as well as India's (Rogers et al. 2006; Chakrapani et al. 2007; Sri Krishnan et al. 2007). Current writing makes plain that even in places with established epidemics, stigma continues to factor heavily in the lives of PLWHA. For example, in South Africa, infamous for its cataclysmic HIV/AIDS epidemic, Simbayi et al. found that 60 percent of their sample in Cape Town "said that they had not told people about their HIV infection because of fear of their reactions" (2007: 1829). Similarly, in a powerful analysis of interviews conducted with HIV-positive active drug users, Ware et al. found that, among a group of mostly male American study participants, "interviewees invested considerable effort in concealing their HIV status. Some made long commutes to clinics and pharmacies so as not to risk being seen getting care for HIV in their own neighbourhoods" (2006: 907). Ichikawa and Natpratan found that community acceptance was the determinant of the quality of life for many Thai PLWHA (2006). In essence, stigma and HIV/AIDS continue to be intimately connected regardless of the location, population, or maturity of the epidemic.

Literature about the impact of stigma often relates to what, at a cursory glance, appears to be antiquated social norms or knowledge gaps. South Africa has an older epidemic, yet researchers have found that in Cape Town, a place lauded for its open and candid discussion of HIV/AIDS' presence in the community, "more than 40% [of study participants] had experienced discrimination resulting from having HIV infection and one in five persons with HIV/AIDS had lost a place to stay or a job because of their HIV status" (Simbayi et al. 2007: 1829). China's latent epidemic is now surging in a context where disclosure of HIV/AIDS status carries potentially grave consequences for PLWHA. Zhou argues that "the dominant discourses of HIV/AIDS in China are still morality-centered, and PLWHA are constructed as morally problematic *others*" (2007: 293). The duality of moral judgment and othering compounds the devastation of HIV diagnosis and is itself a reflection of the type of anthropogenic power structure making certain people more vulnerable to contracting the virus in the first place. Rogers et al. (2006), in a study of pregnant women in southern India, provide a robust analysis of the reasons women are disinclined to be tested, disclose a positive status, or pursue prevention of mother-to-child transmission options. A woman may choose to keep her HIV-positive status secret due to harsh societal reprisals, but the choice to abstain from breastfeeding infant children would subject her to a widespread belief of infidelity and an assumption of HIV-positive status without her ever having made that disclosure herself.

Attempts to critically interrogate stigma examine how stigma relates to poverty, institutional policies, racism, social status, gender, and age, all of which are social constructs perceived and experienced through particular sociological lenses. In a study of children on HAART medication in Brazil, Abaídia-Barrero and Castro (2006) found that there is a need to broaden the scale of analysis beyond individual perceptions and attitudes to structural factors shaping belief and value systems. Chakrapani et al. found that Indian MSMs expressed remarkable vulnerability and victimization related to stigma at the hands of draconian laws criminalizing sex between men in India. The Indian government must take elementary steps, including decriminalization of same sex behavior and "enforcing anti-hate crime legislation that would hold individuals accountable for violence and abuse targeting" (2007: 360) MSM before the prospect of undermining transmission will become a genuine possibility. Sri Krishnan et al. (2007) encourage basic information gathering in an effort to better understand the epidemic and target interventions and resources in a manner informed by the realities of Indians with HIV/AIDS.

Beyond the psychological trauma of stigma, exciting research by Remor et al. (2007) indicates that "perceived stress significantly predicts CD4+ cell count decline" among PLWHA. Low CD4+ cell counts are the benchmark through which the biomedical community diagnoses AIDS; stigmatization that drives the disease underground no doubt induces a remarkable amount of stress. When compounding factors are taken into account, stigma is a morbidity in itself. This type of research by Remor et al. reflects a synergy that can happen between biomedical and sociological research.

A corollary to stigma is the notion of vulnerability. The theme of vulnerability emerges robustly from the current literature as an element in the constellation of impediments to good health amongst PLWHA. The concept of vulnerability, or the potential to succumb to tangible or social stressors as a result of HIV/AIDS status, speaks to the fragile situation of those living with HIV/AIDS and is, in some ways, a perpetuation of the stigma issue. Vulnerability is an extension of the idea that marginalized individuals lose control of their life course. Diagnosis with HIV/AIDS is no exception. Elsewhere in this anthology, authors have addressed vulnerability to infection with the HIV virus. However, here I highlight the vulnerabilities that arise as a consequence of diagnosis with HIV. I do so because the clinical course of the disease reflects just part of the experience of living with the disease, perhaps only a modest part for some individuals for whom their everyday context is one of risk and vulnerability post-diagnosis. PLWHA face the need to disclose their status to families and the challenge of existing in a community potentially hostile to this status. Women face significantly greater vulnerability as HIV-positive status can be seen as a sign of infidelity, promiscuity, and risk taking—sentiments upon which especially male counterparts may act. Women are often vulnerable to domestic violence if their partners learn of their HIV status, as the Rogers et al. study (2006) of women living in southern India demonstrates. Women choosing to disclose their HIV status faced not just judgment, but potentially harsh and life-threatening reactions from their husbands, parents, and community.

For many, attending an HIV/AIDS clinic increases vulnerability to job loss, judgment, or simply "outing" the individual as a carrier of the virus (Ware et al. 2006). For the impoverished majority living with HIV/AIDS globally, a crucial vulnerability lies in the cost associated with ARV procurement. Further, the necessity of having strong family support and ability to take time away from employment responsibilities should he or she fall ill from adverse treatment outcomes belies another type of vulnerability that has arisen in the neoliberal global order where states vigorously retreat from the provision of human and social services. Harawa et al. (2006) capture an additional vulnerability faced by minority populations amongst their study of African-American men who have sex with both men and women. This already sexually stigmatized group has the added burden of minority and oppressed racial status in the United States, facing yet another layer of marginality if they choose to disclose their HIV-positive status. An obviously appealing option is to keep HIV-positive status secret. The corollary to this self-imposed secrecy is danger and vulnerability of transmission for their sexual partners. The association of HIV/AIDS with promiscuity, uncouth behavior, homosexuality, and lower socioeconomic status, among others, bears disproportionately upon the lives of these already vulnerable individuals and stands as a foremost impediment to good health.

SOME CLINICAL AND BIOMEDICAL APPROACHES

Surprisingly, or perhaps as a reflection of a shift in the epistemology of HIV/AIDS research, proportionate to the whole of search hits on this topic, relatively few articles published of late analyze clinical issues facing PLWHA. Surely an immense body of literature currently exists examining clinical manifestations of the disease, symptom management, medication development and adherence, the long-term impact of HIV/AIDS on mental and neurological health, and co-morbidities. That said, the issue may be indicative of research not necessarily engaging the idea of "people living with HIV/AIDS" but rather treating the human body as a scientific capsule, not a being circulating in the world for whom the social and embodied consequences of living with a disease carry infinitely more importance than the disease's biological and pathological processes. Whilst the minority of hits responding to this search were clinical in nature, there are nonetheless several current studies that are important to review in order to gain a robust understanding of the meaning of living with HIV/AIDS.

Of the literature currently available, the discernible trend is for an examination of the symptoms associated with HAART, particularly after long-term usage; the other distinct theme relates to adherence to the medication, particularly reasons for non-compliance with prescribed regimens. Currently researchers are unsure of the boundaries of HAART's benefits, the result being that HIV/AIDS need not be treated as a swift death threat any longer. Since its unveiling in Vancouver in 1996, HAART has extended the lives of millions of PLWHA. The regimen can be equated with enduring chemotherapy for life, and profoundly impacts the health of the body by both extending life through regaining health and as an impediment to good health related to adverse outcomes. HAART often leads to metabolic effects limiting the utility of the medications currently available (Gallagher 2006). While HAART has mercifully reduced HIV-related morbidity and mortality drastically among those with access to the therapy, adverse outcomes can make adherence a challenge and can limit the efficacy of this medication (Gallagher 2006).

The great majority of PLWHA reside in settings of material deprivation where the health care infrastructure is inadequate or nonexistent; access to therapies and treatments highlighted in this section remains illusive for the majority population. Those PLWHA finding themselves, through the accident of birth and geography, on the periphery of scientific progress simply *live* with HIV/AIDS and the symptoms associated with the virus's march towards debilitation. More work is needed to understand how people engage alternative medicine, seek family support for palliative care, attempt to maintain a semblance of normalcy as they suffer in silence and exclusion, and how entire social and cultural networks respond to the disease when the only option may be to watch it progress untreated. Traditional medicine will continue to be used in these contexts and more studies of this variety are important when addressing the health needs of PLWHA without adequate financial resources to access ARV therapy or even routine medical care.

Research describing how HIV-positive status and adverse impacts of HAART impede the health of the individual is becoming increasingly important. The most prominent clinical manifestation of HAART is lipodystrophy, or fat redistribution within the body, a development that often leads to atrophy of fatty tissue in the face, limbs, and buttocks. Another type of lipodystrophy is lipohypertrophy, a condition where fat accumulates in excess quantities around the abdomen, breast, and dorsocervical regions of the body. Lipodystrophy is a risk factor for heart disease. Evidence also suggests that the risk of heart disease is compounded by HIV-positive individuals' increased risk for Type II diabetes and insulin resistance (Gallagher 2006).

We now know that HIV and tuberculosis (TB) are one another's primary risk factor. Those on ARV therapy are granted a reprieve in terms of slower disease progression and are also at a reduced risk of acquiring TB because their immune systems are fortified by HAART. Bonnet et al. (2006) examine a particularly dangerous time period for those with HIV: after the initiation of HAART, there is a period known as immune reconstitution where the risk for TB may increase. The authors conclude that a global health priority must be the integration of HIV and TB care such that care of one does not increase the risk of, nor compromise the care of, the other. With increasing HIV and TB burdens globally, this type of focus carries significantly greater importance outside the so-called "developed countries" of the West and illuminates a vital point of intervention if those advocating for improving global health as a priority are to aim for integrated health systems (as opposed to the "siloed" or individual disease focus commonly found in donor-funded initiatives) well beyond HIV/AIDS and TB care.

Porche and Willis (2006) investigate the co-morbidity of mental illness associated with HIV/AIDS; such psychosocial factors complicate the care of HIV-positive people and can arise for myriad reasons, including harsh societal judgment, AIDS-related dementia, or pre-existing conditions that are only exacerbated by the life-altering shock of HIV-positive diagnosis. Recognition of affective disorders is yet another way to improve adherence to ARV therapy. Arendt (2006) reviews evidence that HAART-associated affective disorders like depression catalyzed by efavirenz, a component of HAART, have an adverse impact on HAART adherence. Toro et al. assessed HIV/AIDS services in the western region of Puerto Rico and found that "depression symptoms were present in 98.1 percent of the people living with HIV/AIDS and were significantly associated with the number of needs reported" (2006: 998). This number highlights the fact that HIV can be the first in a coalescence of morbidities threatening health and wellbeing.

PLWHA AND RELATIONS WITH HEALTH CARE PROVIDERS

An emerging and promising theme evident from the literature relates to the patient–provider dynamic; namely, the relationship between the HIV-positive individual and his or her physician. Especially in a context where the trend (or aspiration at least) is towards ARV access for all, an analysis of patient–physician interactions is essential. Physicians can embody any number of roles from compassionate advocate and informer to gatekeeper and hindrance to good health. At a basic level, physicians are responsible for the sharing of information and serving as the initial link between PLWHA and community resources. The relationship between physician and patient must be one founded upon the principles of trust, candor, and non-judgment. Such a statement is especially true for drug addicts, prostitutes, sexual minorities, those who have been incarcerated or are homeless, and those whom the broader society might judge harshly for past and current choices. Physicians have the capacity to sever trends in transmission by virtue of their roles as disseminators of knowledge. Beyond physicians, this subsection also speaks more broadly to "social and psychological services, individual guidance, community intervention, health education, and appointment coordination as services that [need] to be improved" (Toro et al. 2006: 998) if individuals and entities committed to HIV/AIDS care are to fully embody that goal.

Of the myriad problems individuals have adhering to an ARV regimen, Fehringer et al. (2006) found that the physician–patient interaction rarely addresses the scope of the patient's concerns. While physicians are concerned with matters of adherence, their questions are closed-ended and mostly follow a biomedical line of inquiry, attempting to flesh out diagnosable problems and clinical developments. Rarely can such questioning address the psychosocial dimensions of living with AIDS. This doubly challenges the patient to troubleshoot or endure non-clinical issues and forces internalization of important psychosocial concerns that can have the effect of leading to poor medication adherence and a lower CD4 count (Remor et al. 2007), among others. Fehringer et al. (2006) concur that an atmosphere of honesty and non-judgment as well as an environment open to all patient concerns will address many so-called "non-compliance" issues and ensure better health of PLWHA. This theme, as well as any, is expressed across space with recent articles being written about people in Puerto Rico (Toro et al. 2006), Rio de Janeiro (Fehringer et al. 2006), the United States (Williams et al. 2006), and Mexico (Campero et al. 2007). Non-compliance discussions have an ugly history of racism, paternalism, and the type of insidious judgment that often blames the victim of social injustice for his or her inability to achieve more in life; fortunately, the current literature challenges this trend, examining factors external to the patient contributing to non-compliance.

Williams et al. conducted a study of the effects of home-based care with visits by nurses and peer support workers, concluding that such visits lead to "medication adherence greater than 90 percent among a vulnerable population of people living with HIV/AIDS in the northeastern United States" (2006: 319). The Campero et al. study provides a series of conclusions that should be loudly broadcast to HIV/AIDS providers. Claiming that, "in general, the PLWHAs in [their] study understood neither the physicians' motivations for prescribing, changing, or suspending their antiretroviral medication nor the underlying logic or mechanisms of action of ARV therapy" (2007: 608), the researchers encourage making great strides to enhance the patient–physician relationship by virtue of this relationship's demonstrated association with better ARV adherence. These researchers excel in their insistence that provider–patient relationships must be focused on health and wellbeing—in all spheres and as fully as can possibly be obtained. Scolding a patient for not taking medications or leveling threats of ill-health does not inspire patients to take their medications appropriately, but rather focuses on individual failures and further deflates self-image and desire to be healthy. They challenge care providers to develop "a comprehensive long-term treatment education model that focuses on wellbeing and healthy living" (2007: 609). As this book endeavors to do, we must treat wellbeing as significantly more than a clinical phenomenon, lest we run the risk of objectifying human beings and inaccurately addressing the origins of disease and ill-health.

CONCLUSION

As is bound to happen when attempting to capture in a short chapter the current literature available speaking to the experiences of people living with HIV/AIDS, the sections may seem somewhat artificial. They are, alternatively, tightly related in the sense that all are part of the constellation of forces impacting the life course of PLWHA. To reduce research on the disease to any one discipline refutes a mountain of evidence that the disciplines must more effectively coordinate and work collaboratively to find creative solutions, even when those solutions require new modes of inquiry and action. PLWHA have seen remarkable changes in the trajectories of their lives but certain threats have a stalwart presence thirty years into the pandemic. The advent of ARV therapy heralded a new era of optimism for PLWHA, but new challenges have arisen related to adherence and adverse outcomes. Synthesizing articles reviewed for this chapter, HAART and the challenges of adherence (from medication-induced metabolic changes to socioeconomic challenges to adherence) is perhaps the strongest theme of all. I also wish to stress again before closing that most PLWHA are not experiencing these symptoms, given access limitations; in this sense, the literature ignores the most challenged and vulnerable PLWHA. Unfortunately, PLWHA remain amongst the most vulnerable on earth (as their initial infection makes plain), and living with HIV/AIDS stigma is a persistent and grinding casualty of the human tendency to do violence to those already marginalized.

REFERENCES AND FURTHER READING

Abadía-Barrero, Cesar Ernesto and Arachu Castro. (2006). "Experiences of Stigma and Access to HAART in Children and Adolescents Living with HIV/AIDS in Brazil." *Social Science and Medicine* 62(5): 1219–1228.

Arendt, Gabriele. (2006). "Affective Disorders in Patients with HIV Infection: Impact of Antiretroviral Therapy." *CNS Drugs* (20)6: 507–518.

Bonnet. Maryline et al. (2006). "Tuberculosis after HAART Initiation in HIV-Positive Patients from Five countries with a High Tuberculosis Infection." *AIDS* (20(9): 1275–1279.

Braga, Patricia et al. (2007). "Gender Differences in Survival in an HIV/AIDS Cohort from Sao Paulo, Brazil." *AIDS Patient Care* (21)5: 321–328.

Campero, Lourdes et al. (2007). "Bridging the Gap Between Antiretroviral Access and Adherence in Mexico." *Qualitative Health Research* (17)5: 599–612.

Chakrapani, V. et al. (2007). "Structural Violence Against Kothi-Identified Men Who Have Sex With Men in Chennai, India: A Qualitative Investigation." *AIDS Care and Prevention* (19)4: 346–364.

Chen, J. et al. (2007). "The Effects of Individual- and Community-Level Knowledge, Beliefs, and Fear on Stigmatization of People Living with HIV/AIDS in China." *AIDS Care* (19)5: 666–673.

de Carvalho Mesquita Ayers, José Ricardo. (2006). "Vulnerability, Human Rights, and Comprehensive Health Care Needs of Young People Living With HIV/AIDS." *American Journal of Public Health* (96)6: 1001–1006.

Emlet, Charles. (2006). " 'You're Awfully Old to Have *This* Disease': Experiences of Stigma and Ageism in Adults 50 Years and Older Living With HIV/AIDS." *The Gerontologist* (46)6: 781–790.

Fehringer, Jessica et al. (2006). "Supporting Adherence to Highly Active Antiretroviral Therapy and Protected Sex among People Living with HIV/AIDS: The Role of Patient–Provider Communication in Rio de Janeiro, Brazil." *AIDS Patient Care STDs* (20)9: 637–648.

Gallagher, Donna. (2006). "Current Clinical Issues Impacting the Lives of Patients Living with HIV/AIDS." *Journal of the Association of Nurses in AIDS Care* (18)1S: S11–S16.

Harawa, Nina et al. (2006). "Perceptions Towards Condom Use, Sexual Activity, and HIV Disclosure among HIV-Positive African American Men Who Have Sex with Men: Implications for Heterosexual Transmission." *Journal of Urban Health: Bulletin of the New York Academy of Medicine* (83)4: 682–694.

Ichikawa, M. and C. Natpratan (2006). "Perceived Social Environment and Quality of Life Among People Living with HIV/AIDS in Northern Thailand." *AIDS Care* (18)2: 128–132.

Kang, Ezer. (2006). "Are Psychological Consequences of Stigma Enduring or Transitory? A Longitudinal Study of HIV Stigma and Distress Among Asians and Pacific Islanders Living with HIV Illness." *AIDS Patient Care and STDs* (20)10: 712–723.

Li et al. (2006). "Understanding Family Support for People Living with HIV/AIDS in Yunnan, China." *AIDS and Behavior* (10)5: 509–517.

Porche, Demetrius and Danny Willis (2006). "Depression in HIV-infected men." *Issues in Mental Health Nursing* 27(4): 391–401.

Remor, Eduardo et al. (2007). "Perceived Stress is Associated with CD4+ Cell Decline in Men and Women living with HIV/AIDS in Spain." *AIDS Care* 19(2): 215–219.

Rogers, Alexandra et al. (2006). "HIV-Related Knowledge, Attitudes, Perceived Benefits, and Risks of HIV Testing Among Pregnant Women in Rural Southern India." *AIDS Patient Care STDS* (20)11: 803–811.

Simbayi, Leickness et al. (2007). "Internalized Stigma, Discrimination, and Depression Among Men and Women Living with HIV/AIDS in Cape Town, South Africa." *Social Science and Medicine* (64): 1823–1831.

Sri Krishnan, A. K. et al. (2007). "Sexual Behaviors of Individuals Living with HIV in South India: A Qualitative Study." *AIDS Education and Prevention* (19)4: 334–345.

Toro, Gloria Asencio et al. (2006). "Using a Multisectoral Approach to Assess HIV/AIDS Services in the Western Region of Puerto Rico." *American Journal of Public Health* (96)6: 995–1000.

Ware, N.C. et al. (2006). "Social Relationships, Stigma and Adherence to Antiretroviral Therapy for HIV/AIDS." *AIDS Care* (18)8: 904–910.

Williams, Ann et al. (2006). "Home Visits to Improve Adherence to Highly Active Antiretroviral Therapy: A Randomized Controlled Trial." *Clinical Science* (42)3: 314–321.

Zhou, Yanqiu Rachel (2007). " 'If You Get AIDS . . . You Have to Endure it Alone': Understanding the Social Constructions of HIV/AIDS in China." *Social Science and Medicine* (65): 2007.

CHAPTER 30

A Word to Policymakers and Pilgrims

Mary Fisher

ABSTRACT

This chapter advocates for people living with HIV/AIDS and calls for a more collectivist and empathetic approach to building alliances across political, economic, racial-ethnic, and national boundaries. This can be accomplished by developing an AIDS infrastructure, challenging myths and stigma, coordinating public responses to the pandemic and drawing on private enterprise. This personal narrative highlights the author's experience in a variety of spheres—cultural, social, political—and draws on her experiences as an HIV-positive heterosexual woman since she first publicly acknowledged her serostatus during a keynote address at the 1992 Republican National Convention.

We have learned something in over twenty-five years—not enough, but something. We've learned that the media cannot continue a story when people have heard enough of it. So, for example, 15 million children orphaned by AIDS isn't seen as 15 million stories; it is one story told 15 million times. Old news. Doesn't sell papers or attract advertisers.

We've learned that people who are sick and dying cannot continue to lead. Nearly the entire early generation of AIDS advocates is dead; Larry Kramer, the founder of ACT-UP, has outlived the vast majority of his followers and bemoans an AIDS community that is willing to die "with a whimper, not a bang."

But we've also learned the massive importance of two audiences: policymakers, especially in Washington DC, who can do massive good and corresponding degrees of evil, and people who are HIV positive, my fellow pilgrims on the road to AIDS. Looking back at a quarter-century of this epidemic, hoping that this work will find readers in both camps, I want to say a word to those who are at work in each.

Policymakers need to know that AIDS has not gone away in America; it has gone underground among communities of poverty and color, communities of youth and women. It's gone exactly the same place globally: to those with the least social standing and fewest economic resources—typically, the young and always the women. When American young people who are most at risk—African Americans, women, drug users—are asked about AIDS, they respond in overwhelming numbers with the conviction that "Magic Johnson is cured and there is no risk." That ignorance is going to kill them.

I recently visited several African nations where life expectancy has dropped fifteen years since 1990 because of AIDS. I stood with a grandmother raising orphaned grandchildren. Where once she had a garden next to her home, now she has a graveyard—grave after grave, she lined them up as she buried her children one by one as they fell to AIDS.

In Rwanda, the genocide of 1994 left a legacy of AIDS. A full 60 percent of those who survived torture and rape were left HIV positive. When the killing was over, 100 doctors were left to care for the nation's 17 million people.

What dominates the African landscape is orphans. Acres of orphans—orphans raising orphans, because there is no one else left to do it. Tough children take to the streets. Weak children die of starvation. Many just sit, docile and sick, a vast, human ocean of orphans, mostly infected and doomed.

I've labored for over a decade with the label "The lady who told the 1992 Republican convention she had AIDS." They remember it because they were surprised; most of them didn't believe women could get AIDS—and some of them didn't believe Republicans could. It's no sillier, really, than the commonplace belief today that AIDS in Africa or Asia can be kept out of the United States. Every new strain of virus can and apparently does find its way across our borders within days, if not hours. With regard to AIDS, we live in a Flat Earth society denying that the world is round, and the virus is prolific.

Perhaps our racism traps us into indifference. I want not to believe it, but the evidence is hard to deny. Walking Rwanda, stepping in the trail of torture and blood that crisscrossed that country, I couldn't help but wonder why, knowing what we knew, we did so little. How do we escape the fear that because they were dominantly Black, and we are dominantly White, we simply did not care?

And what do we say to 15 million or more orphans that we did not say to 5 million a few years ago, or that we will not say to 20 million in a year or two? Is it because my children are White and American that I receive so many letters of concern for them, and because Rwanda's children are Black and African that we can say, "They are not ours?"

I am most grateful for the leadership shown by Secretary of State Colin Powell and his colleagues during early days of this century. They have, in many ways, reversed the image and reality that America did not care how many people died, so long as they died of AIDS. But we have hardly begun. We spend less fighting AIDS in America than we spend, annually, on potato chips and popcorn. We are investing less in the international battle against AIDS each year than we spend on weapons research in a month. So long as our national priorities put expertise in killing ahead of research into lifesaving, we are—as a nation—in trouble.

If I could move national and legislative priorities, I would do these few things.

First, I would develop a coordinated response at home and abroad. The fragile international coalition woven together by Secretary Powell and others is strained to breaking—and America's immoral "morality tests" for effective AIDS policy is part of what's straining it. Even here, within the U.S., we have never approved a single, comprehensive strategy that includes effective education, prevention, research, and care. Twenty-five years into this epidemic we have a piecemeal national program with more loose seams than the now-retired NAMES Project AIDS Memorial Quilt.

Second, I'd create an infrastructure for fighting AIDS. The infrastructure must be broad. In America it ranges from school curricula to public health care, from advertising policies to immigration reform. In Africa it embraces everything from roads to clinical care facilities, from clean water to medical supplies. If we don't understand the need for infrastructure, our ignorance will be measured in a staggering cost of human life.

Third, I'd engage private enterprise. In the U.S. we are prohibited by law from the frank classroom instruction needed to teach children how to save their own lives. Here and internationally, the most effective support and prevention structures have risen from peer-based programs. Those with AIDS must talk to those who do not, yet, have AIDS. But they will not be trusted if they represent the government.

Fourth, we need to eradicate the myths. There is no cure for AIDS, including ARVs. They promote extended life but they do not prevent death. And Americans hate death. Our culture does all it can to deny its reality. If we can't defeat death, we often retreat to "There's nothing we can do." We can't afford to have our policymakers do this, because some of our best options will be helping people die with greater comfort.

Given science, it's the best we can do; given morality, it's the least. For example, people with AIDS have begged me for skin creams to treat the sores on their body; we could provide massive doses of comfort for the dying at a cost of about $4 per dose. Simple antibiotics, clean water, nutrition—here is where we must begin, not with an expensive and nonexistent cure.

Policymakers who are humane, compassionate, and smart will make and keep AIDS a national and international priority. They'll recognize that the most critical issue impacting the economy, and therefore security, of the African continent is AIDS. We cannot win a war against a strategy (terrorism) so long as we allow hundreds of millions of people to grow increasingly hopeless. Without compassion, there will be no security.

And, while policy is the role for those elected to leadership in this nation, there is also a key role to be played by those of us who are infected with the AIDS virus.

Many in this community have experienced deep and terrifying rejection. Homes in which we were raised have been closed against us, sometimes for reasons of our sexual orientation, sometimes for reasons of our infection, sometimes for reasons we cannot ferret out. For gay men and marginalized women, for at-risk youth and the most vulnerable in communities of color, AIDS has often been the *final* indignity, not the first—the *next* reason for suffering, not the only.

To be effective in calling for change, we need to avoid self-pity and begin engaging in activism. As a person with AIDS, I need the unity of our community. As a woman with AIDS, enduring every side effect and drug-stimulated symptom known to the medical community, I need hope. And, as a Republican with AIDS, God knows I need humor.

Being a Republican has its advantages. Like you, I may wake every morning to that arsenal of pills and persistent nausea. But unlike many of you, I can wrap my arms around the cold base of a nearby stool knowing that, at that very moment, the Reverend Pat Robertson needs to admit that I am a still member of his Party.

National policy is driven by politics, but politics are driven by crises. Without crises, we can move neither public policy nor public will. The American government—because of election cycles and the power of marketing—does not, cannot, respond to chronic issues. It tackles only crises that matter to a sizable voting block. This is why, for example, we have more uninsured Americans today than when the Clintons launched their famous reform effort the same year I talked to some Republicans in Houston.

It was the AIDS-induced economic and political crises in Africa overlaid by "September 11" that produced the Administration's response to Africa. It wasn't the milk of human kindness that moved policy; it was the image of airplanes flying into landmark buildings full of my fellow Republicans. It was the belief that, now, we have a crisis.

The day the *Washington Post*, the *New York Times*, and CNN all claim that AIDS in America threatens us economically, politically, and socially—that's the day American AIDS policy will be transformed. And it's up to those of us with AIDS, now, in this nation, to tell a story of crisis for America, because it is the truth. The fact that Hollywood starlets have moved on to the next fad, and that headline writers have stopped dressing page one with our disease, does not change the truth that more people died of AIDS in September 2001 than died at the World Trade Center and the Pentagon combined. We have a crisis and its name is "AIDS." We just don't have editorial writers, corporate executives, and lawmakers who believe the truth.

The truth is this. In clinics across America, people are showing up to be tested too late in the course of infection. By the time they present, they've reinfected others and they can't benefit from most life-prolonging drugs. Some people do not know they have been at risk. Even more know the risk, but dread the stigma that follows diagnosis. They can imagine what life will be like if they are dirty people with a dirty disease contracted through dirty needles or dirty sex. A quarter of a century into the American epidemic, ignorance, stigma, and shame are driving people away from testing, thus swelling the ranks of the infected. No wonder infection rates in the county where I have lived—the lovely West Palm area of Florida—are up a staggering 44 percent. No one wants to be tested and found positive because they know they will be judged and stigmatized.

We who have AIDS are ethically responsible for protecting life in our relationships. But when the social environment says people with AIDS are guilty, not sick, and calls for policy built on "personal responsibility", this echoes policies for German Jews in 1933. I'll gladly accept personal responsibility for my behavior. But I'll go to my grave denying that I—or any of my brothers and sisters in this family—are made morally inferior by a virus. And efforts to build public policies on the platform of such whispered suspicions are evil.

We have a crisis. But we'll never persuade others unless we can capture headlines that demonstrate the crisis to those who legislate. Until then, both the virus within us and the environment of shame around us will continue to grow.

I shudder at the thought of an AIDS superorganization. But at the least, we need a Congress or coalition with enough permanence and stability to meet with policymakers and speak on our behalf. We need partnerships based on shared values between the infected and the uninfected, and we need leadership from both sides of that partnership: scientists standing with activists, journalists bound to physicians, hospice-bound patients sitting in field offices of Washington-bound politicians. We need more than a few heroic individuals; we need a collection of leaders speaking as a common voice.

We may not need to institutionalize, but we do need to organize. Because, if we cannot achieve at least this level of unity and organization, we will never convince those who drive public policy that we are a community, that there is a crisis, and that it matters.

To play on Norman Vincent Peale's famous maxim, "The Power of Positive Thinking," we who are positive need to think more about power. When we do, we'll discover that power comes in looking to the needs of the entire community. Power is found in defending others, in protecting those not yet infected, in reminding naive editorial writers that "prevention efforts" will not extend the life of those already infected. Power comes in surprising Health and Human Services with an invitation to dialogue, offering the improbable opportunity to start building trust and communication. Until we get to this point as a community, those of us who are positive are wishing—we are not really thinking.

Nothing so confounds judgmental bigots as a joyful community of people. It wasn't a fat bankroll or great lobbyists that drove the civil rights movement to its great gains of the 1960s—these gains came by way of two factors: community organization and an increasingly sympathetic media. What moved both the media and the bigots was the power of people who sang while being jailed, prayed while being beaten, and laughed in the face of evil. A joyful community can matter when nothing else will do.

Dark hours will come. In those hours, we will be saved by unity, hope, and humor. Unity assures us that, when we can no longer lift our hand to write a check or touch a lover, then others will gently raise them for us. Hope promises that, when I can no longer lift my voice, then others must raise theirs. And humor maintains our sanity, reminding us that we are a community that was conceived in funerals, birthed in cemeteries, warmed by a Quilt too large to manage.

If there is any divine purpose for us, it is this. That we have been welcomed into a community, not a company of victims; that we are a congregation disciplined by AIDS to call for justice and compassion.

If we can be faithful to such a calling, then in the still, soft moment of our most difficult hour we will hold each other, whisper a word of comfort and joy, and listen together to a distant voice saying quietly, "Grace to you, and peace."

CHAPTER 31

Mending the Safety Net

Women Community Activists in AIDS-Affected Regions of East Africa

Helen Ruth Aspaas

ABSTRACT

The family safety net has been stretched to the point of breaking as extended families desperately try to care for children orphaned by HIV/AIDS in sub-Saharan Africa. Women in rural communities, small towns, and cities have responded to this crisis in caregiving by taking on roles as community activists. Using longitudinal research in Uganda and Kenya, this chapter demonstrates that, as community activists, women move above and beyond the reproductive and productive responsibilities set by society for household maintenance and provisioning. These women seek to serve the common good of their neighborhoods and communities.

OVERVIEW

The twenty-first century finds Africans facing the continuing reality of caring for orphans. Large population growth in the latter half of the twentieth century coupled with natural disasters and civil unrest created large numbers of orphans. Over time, the traditional safety net of the extended family along with assistance supplied by international donors provided care for children who lost families and homes. The AIDS pandemic that is sweeping across sub-Saharan Africa is not a short-term devastating natural crisis nor the immediate outcome of civil strife. Slowly, steadily, the pandemic has killed immense numbers of adults, leaving in its wake children and elders as survivors. The traditional safety net provided by kin networks has not been able to support these ever-increasing numbers of orphans. It has become frayed as it stretches to the breaking point. Innumerable orphans can no longer expect to receive care from their own extended family networks. In response, non-family members of their communities are stepping forward to provide care.

This chapter examines efforts by Kenyan and Ugandan women who, with limited connection to formal organizational structures, have developed strategies for helping to alleviate the precarious circumstances of AIDS orphans and other destitute people in their communities. By examining these grassroots efforts by women in four case studies, we see a collective picture emerge of women who have used a range of resources and skills to create a balance between their reproductive and productive roles and their dedication to the needs of their communities, particularly in service to families and children in poverty exacerbated by the AIDS pandemic.

WOMEN'S ROLES IN DEVELOPING SOCIETIES

When the study of women in developing societies took root in the 1960s, the focus was on reproductive and productive roles. Reproductive roles center around bearing and rearing children and, by extension, include women's responsibilities for feeding and clothing their children in a safe, protective home environment. The last half of the twentieth century witnessed a broadening of the reproductive role to insure children's education and access to formal health care (Brydon and Chant 1989). This literature enlightened the world about women's activities within the confines of their households, often hidden from view and study as they reproduced the next generation of their respective cultures and societies.

As the world's rural societies took on the trappings of urbanization and moved from subsistence to cash economies, women, too, became intimately intertwined in the productive dimensions of their local communities. Cash became a necessary reality for survival as women struggled to maintain their responsibilities toward their homes and children, but could do so only through access to cash incomes.

In sub-Saharan Africa, women's access to cash has been circumscribed by cultural and social practices. Cultural norms in rural African communities stipulate that women are granted usufruct rights to farmland belonging to male family members or to land allocated by the local male leader. Ever-increasing rural populations have diminished access to tracts of land for growing food, while cash crops owned by men receive priority over the food crops that are grown by women. Rural women turn to other options that yield cash incomes in order to fulfill roles as family food providers (Blumberg 1988, 1991).

Throughout much of sub-Saharan Africa, household earnings are controlled through the practice of separate purses. Tradition dictates that husband and wife are under no obligation to pool cash resources and other earnings. Household budgeting decisions are not made as a result of open dialogue between husband and wife. Hence, African women have no expectations of guaranteed access to their husband's resources for help in raising and providing for their children (Fapohunda 1988). From an optimistic perspective, we note that women's incomes become their own, for which they can make independent decisions regarding allocation.

The emergence of women-headed households is a more recent phenomenon, which grew out of labor needs during the colonial regimes. The demand for male workers for colonial projects siphoned men away from rural areas. The trend continues today, resulting in many rural households that are headed by women if only on an ephemeral basis. Accurate data are not available, but at any given time as many as 50 percent of sub-Saharan households may be headed by women (Aspaas 1998). De jure women-headed households are easier to identify, since these include women who are widowed, legally divorced, or never married. De facto women-headed households are more problematic to label since some women in rural communities only see their husbands once a year on their return home for annual leave from their urban employment. In some cases, the length of time between visits stretches further and further apart as some men take on urban wives and set up homes in the cities.

The interplay between their reproductive and productive roles is highly complex for African women. Yet, despite the challenges of meeting day-to-day survival needs for their own families, women make commitments to come to the assistance of community people in need. They express this commitment through the contribution of their resources and their time toward garnering scarce resources to provide material goods or services that meet community needs. These same activists supervise distribution or access to the resources according to fair and equitable rules. These resources, not otherwise available, may include provision of day-care facilities, soup kitchens, health clinics, or access to clean water supplies. In a sense, then, these activists are extending their societal roles of reproduction out into their own communities (Reed 2000; Moser 1987, 1991). In most cases, these women, by necessity, are also themselves consumers of the goods or services that they help to provide. This role as activists at the community level was recognized by Caroline Moser in the late 1980s as the third vital role of women in developing societies and equal in importance to their reproductive and productive responsibilities (Moser 1991, 1993).

Case studies from developing countries have earned international respect. Among these are the food kitchens organized by women in the barrios of Central and South American cities (McFarren 1992; Kusterer 1993; Blondet 1995) and the Chipko Movement in India where women guard forest and timber reserves upon which they rely for fuel, building materials, artisans' supplies, food, and medicinal plants (Sharma et al. 1985, Kumar 1995). In Africa, Nigerian women have mobilized to confront large multinational oil companies whose operations destroy environments (Turner 1997). Ugandan women have formalized services to AIDS victims through the indigenous organization TASO (The Aids Support Organization), which respects all AIDS sufferers and seeks to give them dignity even in the face of certain death (www.tasouganda.org). In African markets, women organize into rotating savings and credit associations so that small savings by individuals become relatively large purses distributed at scheduled times to participating members (Aspaas 1992).

While one could focus on the immediate outcomes of these efforts that provide scarce resources to community members, long-term evaluation is equally important. Moser suggests that by participating as community organizers, women become acutely aware of their roles in the development process of their communities. The visibility and skills gained through grassroots action yield a keener sense of problem solving and long-term planning for the future of their communities (Moser 1987, 1991, 1993; Martin 2002). Women begin to demand action from developmental plans that respect the needs of households, children, and women. They make a transition, then, from organizing to secure and distribute scarce resources in the short term to becoming activists who focus on long-term solutions to community problems.

COMMUNITY ACTIVISTS AND THE AIDS PANDEMIC

When the impacts of AIDS were first felt in sub-Saharan African communities, the age-old safety net of the extended family and practice of child fostering came to the assistance of the growing number of orphans whose parents were stricken by the disease. Child fostering is a culturally sanctioned practice in Africa, where natal families send their children to live with relatives. Such a practice is rooted in numerous rationales, but the benefits are perceived as accruing to both the sending family and the accepting one (Isaac and Conrad 1982; Isiugo-Abanihe 1985; Bledsoe 1990; Castle 1995, 1996; Page 1989).

Various situations stimulate child fostering. The natal family may experience close births of infants and perceive the need to foster out a young child to insure that every child receives good care (Aspaas 1999). Some child fostering occurs when urban parents want their children to develop ties with the home village and its traditions. Conversely, rural families may send their children to urban relatives to insure access to better education.

In the early stages of the AIDS pandemic, many families relied on child fostering. However, as increasing numbers of reproductive-age adults succumbed to the disease, leaving numerous orphaned children, crisis fostering became the norm. Unlike traditional child fostering practices, crisis fostering has little or no reciprocity function. Rather, those who are willing, but not always able, take on the care of orphaned kin. They do so because of a keen sense of moral obligation to their kinship networks (Goody 1982; Bayles 2002). While AIDS profoundly affects incredibly large numbers of families throughout sub-Saharan Africa, poverty remains a broader issue. One cannot easily separate an AIDS-stricken family from one in deep poverty. Other issues associated with low productivity, high joblessness, low levels of literacy, and other issues linked with human resources all play into the struggles faced by individuals, families, and communities where AIDS is rampant (Ndege 2001).

As the extended family safety net stretches tighter and tighter, strands begin to unravel. Aged grandparents have limited resources for their grandchildren. Aunts and uncles may themselves succumb to AIDS. These kin networks then become unreliable for providing care, and in the face of a large number of orphans may become discriminatory in the distribution of limited resources (Aspaas 1999). When providing basic care for these children becomes impossible for caregivers, capable, caring women in the communities may step in to fill the void. These women have no kinship to the children but still draw on their maternal roles to take in orphans or to see that they receive nurturing care.

EAST AFRICAN CASE STUDIES OF WOMEN ACTIVISTS

Four case studies of women who contribute to their communities by caring for AIDS orphans and other destitute individuals now validate an emerging source of community, grassroots activism. I have met the women in these case studies as a consequence of living in small towns and villages while conducting field studies in Uganda or working at a rural university in Kenya. None of these women were ever subjects in my research projects. Rather, I came to know them through the informal settings and personal contacts that blossom out of everyday life in rural Africa, especially in small towns and villages where all contacts are highly personal.

These women's activism became a part of my own life as I learned more about their efforts and then began to serve as a catalyst for linking them with resources and donors in the developed world in which I live and work. I maintain regular correspondence with them and visit them whenever I return to East Africa. The level of intimacy which brings me into their homes for visits and long conversations allows me to evaluate the efficacy of their projects and the impacts, both short term and long term, on their communities.

In the following case studies, I will describe the socioeconomic, geographic, and cultural settings of each woman. I include a description of their home settings and a listing of the personal skills that the women bring to their activism. Then I describe their community efforts along with my participation in them. Pseudonyms are given to the women and their settings.

Alicia in Uganda

Alicia is a widow, approximately 40 years old, and has four children ranging in age from 10 to 20 years old. All children are in school. Alicia has completed O levels in school and works as a secretary for a local manufacturing firm in the nearby town, a principal manufacturing region of Uganda. Her home is currently a rented house in a bedroom community. Besides her education, Alicia has an excellent command of written and spoken English, is a skilled typist, and has learned to use email, faxes, cell phones and can scan documents. She can access Western Union and controls her bank account.

As a pastor's wife in Africa, Alicia had many extra responsibilities and expectations placed upon her outside of her productive work as a secretary and her reproductive work as a mother to four children. This is common for pastors' wives throughout the continent. They are expected to entertain, provide housing as needed for travelers, and keep their homes available for church meetings. Alicia continues to do this even after the death of her husband.

Her activism is a continuation of her husband's dream of building a school for children in a low-income neighborhood of their community. In addition, the school would serve as a church on Sunday and provide access for community gatherings. Following her husband's untimely and tragic death, Alicia moved ahead with his plans, supported by members of her church. She worked closely with the government of Uganda's Ministry of Education, the local town council, and with her own church members. The combined effort resulted in the donation of land for the building by the town council, provisions of teacher salaries by the National Ministry of Education and labor provided by the church members supplemented by visiting work teams from a sister church in Northern Ireland.

The school is now fully occupied with six classrooms, and additional classrooms are being built because of ever-increasing school enrollments in the neighborhood. The children who attend the school represent the under-served of Ugandan families. The children are from impoverished households and would not have opportunities for education otherwise. The impact of AIDS in this particular district was strongest in the early 1990s, and, while the AIDS rate for Uganda has diminished to an adult prevalence rate of 4.1 percent (www.cia.gov/library/publications/the-world-factbook/), the loss of wage earners leaves children dependent on non-family networks for guarantees of education and basic survival.

The school is evidence of Alicia's commitment to realizing her husband's dream and to serving the educational needs of the marginalized children in her community. My connection with the school derives from having worshiped there while doing research in the district. I have helped to build connections between church women's groups in the U.S.A. and the women's group at Alicia's church. Primarily the connections serve to provide resources to develop income-generating projects for the women.

Annetta in Kenya

Annetta is in her early thirties and has two children, one of whom she adopted. In addition to these two daughters, she has taken in six orphaned children from two separate families ravished by AIDS. All of the orphans are girls ranging in age from 20 years to six years.

Annetta's home is a one-bedroom apartment with electricity and access to a water tap a few blocks away. The apartment is not considered safe, especially for the teenaged girls, because of the proximity to heavy traffic on a main trunk road connection between Kenya and Uganda and an active market place close by. Annetta has never married, has a primary school education and supports herself with her successful hair salon. Much of her salon's success is a function of proximity to a rural university from which Annetta draws students and faculty members for her clients.

Annetta is skilled with spoken English but usually has a translator help her with written English. Annetta can use email, has established a checking and savings account at a respected bank, can access Western Union, and knows how to send facsimile messages and scanned items. She owns and uses a cell phone on a regular basis.

Annetta's community efforts are an extension of her own unmet desire to complete her secondary education. Through numerous contacts she identifies teenage girls who have no resources to attend secondary school. These are usually young women whose families are directly affected by AIDS and, in most cases, have lost both parents to the disease. Without extended family members who are able to provide school fees, bright, capable young women are doomed to lives of drudgery, early marriages, or prostitution. Annetta, working with my contacts in the U.S., has been successful in putting six young women through secondary school. Annetta is adamant about helping these young women to lead moral lives as well and is fearless in lecturing them about proper behavior and studying hard in order to pass their secondary school exams. She maintains this self-identified community watch program throughout the market where she lives.

Annetta has taken on the guardianship role for a family of four children who lost their parents to AIDS. Their grandmother is HIV positive and unable to provide care. Annetta checks on the older children, now in their teens, on a regular basis and takes food and farming materials so that they can grow some of their own food crops. She has worked tirelessly to help the children keep their rightfully inherited land from the clutches of greedy and ruthless relatives. She assesses the children's school performance, making sure they attend regularly. With resources acquired from a U.S. patron, she has enrolled the first-born son in carpentry school and pays school fees for the others along with providing substantial supplements of food and clothing.

Janet in Uganda

Janet lives in the large Ugandan manufacturing town mentioned above. She is in her late forties, is a widow and has three children. The two older sons are independent, and her daughter has just completed secondary school exams. Janet has completed O levels and has an excellent spoken and written command of the English language. She lives in a spacious, though old and deteriorating, apartment near to her work and rents some of the exterior rooms to workers in the town.

Janet supports herself and her family by knitting sweaters and accessories that are part of local high-school uniforms. Her hand-loomed knitting machine occupies a sunny location in a shop that she shares with a woman tailor. The shop, located on one of the town's main streets, is enlivened by frequent visits by clients and other shopkeepers in the general vicinity. Janet's knitting skills are supplemented by her technology skills. She owns a cell phone, can use email, manages a bank account, accesses Western Union and knows how to send items by international airfreight. She can use scanners and facsimile machines.

Janet's community activism arose out of her concern for incarcerated women in one of the national prisons located on the perimeter of her town. Her efforts to visit the women have flowered into a successful endeavor to provide them with resources that help them to build skills for self-support upon release. Through resources acquired from international donors, she has placed two treadle sewing machines and sewing supplies in the women's section of the prison. The women now spend their time productively by learning tailoring skills. In addition, Janet visits the women's families in rural communities and ascertains the status of their children who are in the care of relatives. For those women who deliver babies while in prison, Janet provides infant clothing and accessories. Women who are released often come to Janet's shop seeking basic assistance which she does her best to provide. Her connection with her church and with missionaries allows her to seek out additional resources to assist not only the incarcerated women but destitute women who come to her for help. Funds from the U.S. have helped in the purchase of the sewing machines and for ongoing purchases of fabric and sewing supplies.

A RURAL WOMEN'S GROUP IN UGANDA

The final case study, unlike the three previous examples, is a collective endeavor by a rural women's group in southern Uganda. The group has approximately forty members ranging in age from early twenties to late seventies. Household circumstances, education, and livelihoods of the women all vary. However, they are all mothers with children and grandchildren who depend upon them for various resources. Like women throughout Africa, they realize the impact of the phenomenon of separate purses and so reach out for opportunities to earn income over which they have their own control. To do so, they create crafts unique to their cultural region including basketry, reed mats, and bark cloth accessories. Bark cloth is a material closely resembling a stiff fabric or a lightweight leather, dark brown in color and useful for items that would otherwise be made from heavy fabric or leather. The cloth is prepared by pounding the bark of a local tree.

The women's group operates under a charter that is filed with the state granting them official status. They hold elections for officers and through the skill of their officers have developed a successful endeavor to export high-quality crafts to the U.S., where they are sold at holiday bazaars and fairs. The women in turn use the income to pay school fees for their own children and to support a small local school that caters to AIDS orphans. The women have hired a teacher for the school and provide school supplies as well as a noon meal for the orphans. They oversee the school's activities and monitor the children's education progress and living conditions.

The group's leaders are skilled with email communication, banking, international shipping processes through airfreight and access to Western Union. Their president can readily speak and write English and owns a cell phone.

ANALYSIS OF THE CASE STUDIES

Common characteristics of these women activists are evident. Some are innate and others have been acquired through formal and informal education. Regardless of the source of these characteristics or skills, the women put them to work to further their activist efforts.

The women in these case studies are neither wealthy nor destitute. While they do, at times, face periods of shortfall in resources, all have a productive base that gives them nearly adequate income to meet daily household needs. I assert that, by having a minimal guaranteed monthly income, the women are then freed up in time to address their community activities.

The one personal innate characteristic of all four case studies is that these women are very hard-working. Despite challenges of work, family, social obligations, and economic uncertainties, they never seem to grow weary and show incredible ability to find one more bit of energy to meet the demands of their reproductive, productive, and community roles. They work long days in order to meet these triple demands on their time, energy, and resources.

Other skills have been honed through formal education or through work in informal settings. First of all, the women are adept at multitasking and certainly can manage their time well. This is validated by Mehra (1993) who acknowledges women's skills at structuring their work and labor responsibilities to fill a finite body of time. For example, the women crafters can produce their traditional wares within the home. This gives them opportunity to attend to reproductive obligations at the same time that they are producing products for sale. Janet's and Annetta's shops are settings not only for economic gain but where idea exchange occurs. Some of Annetta's clients are university professors, and she has become skilled at seeking their advice on numerous issues. Janet's shop location allows for the casual contact on a daily basis that provides seed for new ideas. Women in distressed circumstances can easily seek Janet out to acquire assistance.

Quality parenting is another skill that the women rely on for their extension out into the communities in which they live. Annetta, whose own education was interrupted by lack of resources to pay school fees, is known as an advocate for many teenage girls in her small village. She investigates their home circumstances and does follow-up research pertaining to availability of school fees. If she finds that young women are orphans or have no support for education, she seeks out resources for assistance. In addition, she readily advises young women about the value of education, and helps them to develop visions for their future.

Janet opens her home to young women who are destitute. They may be orphaned or have such poverty in their homes that they leave in search of better opportunities and then find themselves alone and struggling in an unfamiliar town. Janet often houses as many as three young women at a time, training them to be skilled knitters and seamstresses like herself.

The women's group's efforts to provide schooling, a noon meal and a teacher for AIDS orphans along with carefully monitoring of home situations exemplifies this same extension of parenting and maternal roles into the communities.

Technological skills are well developed among these women. All are skilled with using email, have purchased cell phones if at all possible, and use these modern communication devices on a regular basis. I noted that, at one time, Janet's cell phone directory contained over 200 listings. Prior to cell phone access in Africa, most interaction had by necessity to occur at the face-to-face level because telephone land lines did not exist, were outdated, or in poor repair. Likewise, the national mail systems move through phases of corruption at the worst and poor efficiency at best.

Now, these women's operational spaces have extended out of their local villages across national borders and even into international spheres. Communications can now move quickly, efficiently, and privately within and across international borders. Youngs (2002) notes the role that such ease of communication plays in the exchange of ideas and increased realization of solidarity and action. I have noted women's knowledge of accessing Western Union, establishing bank accounts, and learning the intricacies of using air cargo for shipments.

The level of official organizational structure that provides a framework for these community activities varies. The women's group in Uganda is officially registered with the government, as is Alicia's church. Janet works with her church to acquire some resources through donations, but Annetta works alone in her endeavors, relying principally on her contacts with U.S. donors. These organizational structures may simply serve as the most readily available frameworks which the women can access as needed. The formalization of a registered non-governmental organization in each case is beyond the scope, energy, and political savvy needed to do the community work that the women currently perform.

Within their communities, these women's efforts have earned them the trust and respect of local authorities. While I cannot validate that their efforts have led to local, regional, or national policy changes, I do know that various governmental authorities with whom the women interact respect them and provide them with opportunities to move ahead with some of their initiatives. For example, Annetta's work on behalf of orphaned teenage girls keeps her highly visible with the headmasters and headmistresses with whom she visits on a regular basis. Annetta assumes the role of surrogate parent as she checks on students' academic progress, social development, and related needs. Alicia's work to forge ahead with her husband's dream of building a school has earned her the respect of members of the local town council with whom she worked closely to get land allotted, classrooms constructed, and teachers hired.

Janet's service to the incarcerated women in the national prison has been possible only through her efforts to build a good working relationship with the head warden and his assistants. Impressed by her regular visits to the women and commitment to improve their income-generating skills, the warden allows her to come unimpeded for visits to the prison and allows her to bring extra resources to improve the daily lives of the incarcerated women. Such visibility and earned respect counters the argument made by Moser (1993) that women's community efforts are largely invisible to the eyes and thinking of local government officials and others in authority. These women's efforts are indeed highly visible and their work is fully respected.

By stepping out into their communities and providing these alternative forms of assistance when the kinship network breaks down, these women are realizing a new level of self-assertion and empowerment (Bayles 2002). Two of these case studies show profound realizations of their roles as community activists. In email messages, Annetta frequently compares her present role in the village to that of five years ago when she was a respected hairdresser but nothing more. She mentions how her work in the community forces her to be a model citizen, especially for the young women, and to continually strive to maintain the respect of her neighbors.

The president of the women's group voices similar thoughts in email messages when she writes on behalf of the women in her group. She especially praises the women's creativity and skills with making the crafts and remarks that such skill has allowed them access to income, which in turn has been directed to the good of the community.

I cite these two because these are women whom I perceive to be least likely to become activists. Their rural roots, roles as homemakers, and limited educational backgrounds could have paralyzed them in their reproductive roles. Yet, they look beyond the day-to-day needs of their families and address the needs of AIDS orphans and other marginalized members of their communities. They recognize the helpless and nearly hopeless situations of the orphaned children and see far enough ahead to recognize the limited circumstances these children will face without schooling and basic care.

Now, with this strengthened "can do" capacity, the women are willing to voice expectations for the future. They express visions for their own homes, families, and their communities. All women want their own plots of land with their own dwellings so they can be freed from monthly rent and landlord whims. Annetta would like to start her own orphanage and wants her home to be a more embracing space that provides shelter and sustenance to many children in need. Janet's and Alicia's homes already provide housing and security for many people. Having homes of their own would allow them more freedom of action and ability to provide space for those in need.

Throughout these case studies, we have seen the common characteristics that have helped these women to be successful community activists. In return, as they perform their work to enhance the lives of members of their communities, we see their own skills grow, too.

CONCLUSION

This chapter is about a few women in East Africa doing a few activities to help their communities. They don't work under the auspices of large multi-donor structures. Some would say that, within the context of the AIDS pandemic's fierce grip on Africa, the work of these women is not profound. Yet, within their own communities, where poverty is too often the norm, their work and contributions are indeed significant in terms of impacts on individual lives, especially for AIDS orphans.

Contrary to the standard characterization of African women as victims, the women in these case studies are creative, assertive, and energetic local activists who work within the guidelines of their respective cultures to bring about change. As agents of change, they serve as sterling examples of responsible action in civil society. They use resources derived from productive roles and their innate nurturing reproductive roles to enact positive change.

By stepping out of the household and out of the shop, they shed the cloak of invisibility noted by Moser (1987, 1991, 1993). Their community actions serve the needs of the most marginalized in their communities. The women know their communities and are aware of those with greatest needs; they require little overhead to perform their work, and their administrative costs are minimal. They constantly monitor those whom they help. They are trustworthy and accountable with resources placed in their hands. The respect from local and government officials should serve in the future as a catalyst to encourage more grassroots efforts. The national and international development community would be wise to learn from these examples of women who, with minimal financial assistance but great energy and insight, are able to enact change within their neighborhoods and among the most marginalized.

REFERENCES AND FURTHER READING

Aspaas, Helen Ruth. 1992. "*Women's Small-Scale Enterprises in Rural Kenya: Coping with the Dynamics of Isolation.*" Ph.D. Thesis. University of Colorado, Boulder.

Aspaas, Helen Ruth. 1998. "Heading Households and Heading Businesses: Rural Kenyan Women in the Informal Sector." *Professional Geographer* 50: 192–203.

Aspaas, Helen Ruth. 1999. "AIDS and Orphans in Uganda: Geographical and Gender Interpretations of Household Resources." *Social Science Journal* 36: 201–226.

Bayles, Carolyn. 2002. "The Impact of AIDS on Rural Households in Africa: A Shock Like Any Other?" *Development and Change* 33: 611–632.

Bledsoe, Catherine. 1990. "The Policies of Children: Fosterage and the Social Management of Fertility Among the Mende of Sierra Leone." In *Births and Power: Social Change and the Politics of Reproduction*, edited by W. P. Handwerker. Boulder, CO: Westview Press.

Blondet, Cecilia. 1995. "Out of the Kitchens and Onto the Streets: Women's Activism in Peru." In *The Challenge of Local Feminisms: Women's Movements in Global Perspective*, edited by Amrita Basu. Boulder, CO: Westview Press.

Blumberg, Rae Lesser. 1988. "Income Under Female Versus Male Control: Hypotheses from a Theory of

Gender Stratification and Data from the Third World." *Journal of Family Issues* 9: 51–84.

Blumberg, Rae Lesser. 1991. *Gender, Family and Economy: The Triple Overlap*. Newbury Park: Sage Publications.

Brydon, Lynne and Sylvia Chant. 1989. *Women in the Third World: Gender Issues in Rural and Urban Areas*. New Brunswick: Rutgers University Press.

Castle, S. 1995. "Child Fostering and Children's Nutritional Outcomes in Rural Mali: The Role of Female Status in Directing Child Transfers." *Social Science and Medicine* 40: 679–693.

Castle, S. 1996. "The Current and Intergenerational Impact of Child Fostering on Children's Nutritional Status in Rural Mali." *Human Organization* 55: 193–205.

Fapohunda, Eleanor R. 1988. "The Non-Pooling Household: A Challenge to Theory," in *A Home Divided: Women and Incomes in the Third World*, edited by Daisy Dwyer and Judith Bruce. Stanford: University of Stanford Press.

Goody, E. 1982. *Parenthood and Social Reproduction: Fostering and Occupational Roles in West Africa*. Cambridge: Cambridge University Press.

Isaac, B.L. and S.R. Conrad. 1982. "Child Fosterage Among the Mende of Upper Bambara Chiefdoms, Sierra Leone: Rural–Urban Occupational Comparisons." *Ethnology* 21: 243–252.

Isiugo-Abanihe, C.U. 1985. "Child Fosterage in West Africa." *Population and Development Review I* 11: 53–73.

Kumar, Radha. 1995. "From Chipko to Sati: The Contemporary Women's Movement." In *The Challenge of Local Feminism*, edited by Amrita Basu. Boulder, CO: Westview Press.

Kusterer, Ken. 1993. "Women-Oriented NGOs in Latin America: Democratization's Decision Wage." In *Women at the Center: Development Issues and Practices for the 1990s*, edited by Gay Young, Vidyamali Samarasinghe, and Ken Kusterer. West Hartford, CT: Kumarian Press.

McFarren, Wendy. 1992. "The Politics of Bolivia's Economic Crises: Survival Strategies of Displaced Tin-Mining Households." In *Unequal Burden: Economic Crises, Persistent Poverty and Women's Work*, edited by Lourdes Beneria and Shelly Feldman. Boulder, CO: Westview Press.

Martin, Deborah. 2002. "Construction of the 'Neighborhood Sphere': Gender and Community Organizing." *Journal of Gender, Place and Culture* 9: 333–350.

Mehra, Rekha. 1993. "Gender in Community Development and Resource Development." In *Women at the Center: Development Issues and Practices for the 1990s*, edited by Gay Young, Vidyamali Samarasinghe, and Ken Kusterer. West Hartford, CT: Kumarian Press.

Moser, Caroline O.N. 1987. "Women, Human Settlements, and Housing: A Conceptual Framework for Analysis and Policy-Making." In *Women, Human Settlements and Housing: A Conceptual Framework for Analysis and Policy-Making*. London: Tavistock Publications.

Moser, Caroline O.N. 1991. "Gender Planning in the Third World: Meeting Practical and Strategic Gender Needs." In *Changing Perception: Writings on Gender and Development*, edited by Tina Wallace and Candida March. United Kingdom: Oxfam.

Moser, Caroline O.N. 1993. *Gender Planning and Development: Theory, Practice and Training*. London: Routledge.

Ndege, George Oduor. 2001. *Health, State and Society in Kenya*. Rochester: University of Rochester Press.

Page, H.J. 1989. "Childrearing Versus Childbearing: Co-Residence of Mother and Child in Sub-Saharan Africa." In *Reproduction and Social Organization in Sub-Saharan Africa*, edited by R.J. Lesthaeghe. Berkeley: University of California Press.

Reed, Maureen C. 2000. "Taking Stands: A Feminist Perspective on 'Other' Women's Activism in Forestry Communities of Northern Vancouver Island." *Gender, Place and Culture* 7: 363–387.

Sharma, K., B. Pandey, and K. Nantiyal. 1985. "The Chipko Movement in the Uttarkhand Region, Uttar Pradesh, India." In *Rural Development and Women: Lessons from the Field*, edited by S. Muntemba. Geneva: ILO/DANIDA.

Turner, Terisa. 1997. "Oil Workers and Oil Communities in Africa: Nigerian Women and Grassroots Environmentalists." *Labour, Capital and Society* 30: 66–89.

Youngs, Gillian. 2002. "Closing the Gap: Women, Communications and Technology." *Development* 45: 23–28.

Websites

https://www.cia.gov/library/publications/the-world-factbook/index.html Last retrieved February 18, 2008.

http://www.tasouganda.org Last retrieved February 18, 2008.

CHAPTER 32

Back to Nima

Jonathan D. Mayer

ABSTRACT

This chapter conveys one doctor's journey to Western Africa, where work in the field shifts from relationship building to health care to the emotional maintenance needed to be effective to patients. In Nima, the author establishes links, and later establishes a non-governmental organization, for some of the most marginalized people in Ghana. This chapter describes the various socio-environmental contexts, and personal connections, involved in working in a high-prevalence HIV area.

Today I saw a woman in Nima who will die in the next few months. In Seattle she would probably not die—at least there would be reasonable hope of preventing or delaying her death. In Nima, she'll certainly die, and soon. Though adequate health care facilities exist to treat her problem within three kilometers, she cannot afford the $10 a day for the hospital care that she needs, or the $25 a month that she needs for medication, and nobody will pay for her. So she, like thousands of other people in Nima, will die unpleasant deaths.

I first saw her after we visited Ahmad's aunt in her small room. His aunt had given birth to a 750g premature infant two months ago. Baby and mom are both doing fine, although baby was somewhat dehydrated; his fontanelles were OK, so the dehydration was not severe. Baby now weighs 1,700 g. Ahmad's aunt mentioned that two people in the family housing unit were currently sick. I asked if we could see them; both women were happy to talk to us.

Ahmad's grandmother is a woman of unknown age. Somewhat obese, she could barely walk because she was so short of breath, and I could hear her labored breathing and wheezing before I even saw her in the doorway. She had a pleasant face with expressive eyes, but her eyes expressed deep sadness and fatigue. I introduced myself and our team, and told her that we are working in Nima to try and improve health conditions. Ahmad translated this into Hausa, and she smiled. I sat down opposite her, and noticed her swollen ankles. Her jugular veins were distended above the angle of her jaw. These are all classic signs of congestive heart failure and, more specifically, right heart failure. Her heart was unable to pump sufficient blood to her lungs, and fluid was backing up in her cardiorespiratory system. Her degree of distress and degree of jugular vein distention indicated that her disease was very advanced. As we spoke, my attention focused totally on her, and I learned that she had had hypertension for as long as she could remember in her adulthood. She took appropriate medication for the hypertension, but had not been to the hospital or seen a doctor for the heart failure. I suggested that she should do that. In Hausa, she said, "There is no money for that." My heart finally broke; I had seen many others like her. A few dollars' worth of Lasix would make her feel better within a couple of hours, and in the U.S. this would be done immediately. She would be placed on oxygen and an ACE inhibitor. And I felt so impotent, so unable to do anything to help. I could have given her $10 or $100 and told her to go to the hospital. And it would have helped this one time. But what about the next time? And what about when her medication ran out? And what about her thousands of peers, and the false expectations that that would create that I would be able to solve their problems? Yes, her problem is medical, but her problem is also structural—there is no provision to get this woman to a hospital, to treat her disease, to treat her poverty, to prevent her hypertension. And I realized that tears were flowing down my cheeks after kilometers of deprivation, after seeing misery yet again on this visit to Nima, but I also knew then that our team is doing the right thing—working on community health assessment and intervention—trying to make a difference.

We also saw Jamaya. She lived in the same household. She came to see us, and I sat close to her, facing her, and looked into her eyes. They were sad eyes. She has fever—a generalized term usually taken to be malaria. She has not been to see a doctor, but has been to the pharmacy, and is taking chloroquine. She too has a history of hypertension, which is being treated with propanolol. As I question her more in English and Ahmad translates back and forth into Hausa, I learn that the fever comes regularly every two months, and has for years. This is not typical of malaria, and I wonder if it is one of the rarer periodic fevers, many of which have a hereditary basis. But I wonder too why she is so sad. I ask if she is lonely. Yes, she is very lonely. She does not go out of the house. She does not have any friends. Her illness makes her too tired to go out of the house, and nobody comes to visit her. I tell her that I hope that she can have some friends. She tells me that now she has a friend—that I am her friend, and that what Nima needs are people like us to help with the health conditions and the health of the people of Nima. And I feel deeply humbled and wonder if I am up to this task—that if I—if we—fail, we are not failing ourselves, but we are failing 150,000 people, and the thousands of people to come. Jamaya is so tired that I tell her that I think she needs to lie down. She smiles and says thank you for coming. And adds that next time we come, she hopes that she is alive. And I want to say something reassuring, but I cannot, so I say that I hope so too. When we talked about Jamaya's perception of the big health needs of Nima, her first answer—really, her only answer, was "Poverty. We need to banish poverty." She did not mention malaria, or diarrheal disease. This wise and lovely elderly woman pointed right to the crux of the matter—poverty, incredible poverty, poverty unknown in the United States, soul-sapping poverty, poverty that beats on the roof like the Accra sun in the dry season, 100-degree poverty on a day with 100 percent humidity, a day in a week in a month of nothing but hot days of poverty.

So we continue our circuit of Nima. Julia plays with the children. I think how unglorious it would be if I stumble into the feces-filled sewers. Sandy asks all the right questions and talks to the women. As a physician assistant with experience in Zaire and Mexico, she has done small-scale projects before. Courtney talks to the children and some adults. And our team is drawn closer by our commitment. This is going to be the hardest thing that I have ever done. But we have more smart and committed team members coming, people I have asked and urged to join us, capable people and compassionate people, people with technical skills and people with broad vision. Maybe if we join together, not so much with each other, but with the people of Nima, there will be a way. And somehow, knowing that, the many days ahead in Nima will be easier, and I feel a new sense of mission for myself, as though my years of study and work have all led up to this. May I be worthy of the trust and respect that those in Nima seem to accord me. False hopes are worse than no hopes at all.

Another day. We meet with an Islamic women's group. This group is one of our gateways into the community. We talk. They want some health education sessions. Sandy asks, "On what topics?" "Diabetes." So Sandy gives a couple of education sessions on diabetes a few days later. I can't go. I would have liked to have gone, but I had to go to some meetings, endless meetings, government officials and NGOs (non-governmental organizations), to set the stage for our projects. I hear that the sessions worked. I hear that the women danced. I hear that they were contemptuous of exercise, saying that impoverished people have no time for exercise. I hear that Sandy showed them that standing and dancing is exercise. I hear that people smiled and laughed. Dancing and laughing is a good way to exercise. I hear that an 84-year-old woman who had trouble standing stood up and danced and smiled and laughed. If Sandy can explain diabetes with her simple diagrams and get a few people to stand up and dance and laugh, and they can teach a few more people, and those other people stand and dance and laugh, then more people will exercise, and more people will laugh, and more will dance.

And another day. I learned that one of our cats, Mason, was murdered in Seattle. Murdered by one of the coyotes that has been plaguing our street. Murdered in the night and eaten, his hide discovered by Rachel, our daughter, the next day.

Another day, sunny. The day begins north of Accra as our minibus hits a goat, a baby goat, crippling him at least. The driver won't stop. He says he is afraid of being killed. So we go on. I am in the front seat, paralyzed by the suddenness of this. And why does the sudden death of a goat in front of me, or our pet cat, strike me as hard as the deaths of trauma victims in the operating room, or an elderly woman whose hand I held last year who died from a ruptured aortic aneurysm on the operating table? I have lost track of the days. I don't know which is which. We are taking a couple of days off from Nima to visit the area where the Krobos live—the people in Ghana who are hardest hit by HIV/AIDS. This is a different research project. We are in the area near the Akosombo Dam. We are going to a school and day care center for HIV orphans. First we go to the opening of a local voluntary counseling and testing center. Then a drive through a mountainous landscape, to the orphan center. Five hundred orphans in front of me. I look at them. I'm in front of all of them, and the Queen Mother who runs the school introduces me. She is one of the royal family of the Krobos. Five hundred. We talk to a couple of them. "My mother died. My father died. My uncle and aunt are dead. My sisters are gone. My brothers died. My grandparents died. I want to be a lawyer." This was after the Queen Mother told us that she is tired of researchers coming and taking from them and giving nothing back. She preaches to us. I feel the resentment building up and building further. Not a blind resentment or a fury, but an understanding and empathetic anger. I look her in the eyes, while understanding what she is saying and even agreeing. I tell her, "You've been frank with us. Now I will be frank with you. Don't presume to know what is in here [hand over my heart] or what motivates me or know how I will behave. Don't do that, because my heart is with you." She looks startled by both what I say and by my intensity. She smiles. She comes and hugs me. "Jonathan, now we are friends. Come, let's talk." So by being honest, by opening up, I have made a friend for life, an ally. The Queen Mother wants help for her orphans. I will help by trying to find foundations and funding sources with her. She wants to meet others, elsewhere, who are running similar schools.

And another day. Maybe to Nima again? But I am called by Joseph, who had set up a meeting with a big multinational NGO based in the U.S.A. He sounded desperate for me to come to the meeting, which was already going. He said we needed a show of force. So I grab a tie and jacket, round up a couple of people on our team. We go. What it boils down to is that this American NGO is also working in Nima. For the first time in Ghana I get a strong message that "This is our territory. Stay off our territory." I think about how to handle this. I decide to be honest. "The territory is neither yours nor mine. It is the people of Nima's and we are here to help them and to learn from them and to facilitate social change. That is what our team is about. Now why can't we try and cooperate rather than worry about territory?" And again I get a stunned look. But these two people get the message—and agree that this makes the most sense. And we agree to share and agree to start it there and then and shake hands and trade stories about books that we have read. Crisis averted. The next night I see one of these people at dinner. She is fun and kind and interesting.

Another day in Nima. Another day of going house to house. We split up into three teams of two people. We do a household survey. About eighty people live there, but nobody knows how many. Four generations. We say "Dagudi"—"Thank you" in Hausa. We trudge maybe a hundred meters when my mobile phone rings. It's Joseph. He is in another household. He doesn't know where, but he asks if I can come and see a young woman who has acute belly pain. He'll send Ahmad to meet me at a nearby mosque, and from there we'll go to the household. We need to meet with the eighteen tribal chiefs in Nima in less than half an hour, but I guess they will understand, and if they don't I'll send everybody else to the meeting. And so the days go. After a particularly stressful day, we got to "Trivia Night" at "Champ's Sport's Bar." A way to relax, to meet some expats and diplomats who might be able to help us. Our team comes in about halfway down the list of teams in the end. Of all things, we blew the questions on rock music and movies. Of all things.

Back to Nima, back to Nima, that's where I want to go now. On the streets and in the alleys, in the households, talking to people, being on the ground. There are so many details to take care of, too. This group that I've assembled, nurtured, brought together, look to me for leadership and wisdom. I'm learning that it's a heavy responsibility but it's not a team for the team's sake but for the sake of the people we work with, and if we believe what we say, then we work *for* them too, because the residents of Nima are the people we are here to help and here to help facilitate the changes that they themselves want. So the tasks and visions of leadership must get done. And I share the leadership because everybody in the group is a leader. And everybody has strengths. And some are good at one thing and others at another. Yet we are this amazing organic group of passion and commitment and talent that is almost as amazing to see as it is bringing up a child.

Yesterday at the orphanage, one of our members looked like he might break down. He was stunned. Overwhelmed by the sight of 500 orphans, this person who has worked with AIDS data for way over a decade had a crisis, could have crashed and burned. I always believe that most people have the inner psychological resources to deal with these overwhelming phenomena, even if they are overcome for the moment. The emotional crisis brought on by seeing these orphans is one that is not a bad crisis. It is one that people working with data need to have—to see the human side. And this person is fine today, if transformed by the experience. Two days later we go to a clinic in this general area that distributes antiretrovirals, and he observes his first patients. He sees his first clinical encounters, and gains a sense that a clinical encounter is a special social relationship built on trust. And even more special than that is when the nurse hands over a prescription for another month's supply of what will hopefully be life-saving medication. This is a husband and wife. They come a long distance to this rural clinic to assure anonymity, because the stigma of AIDS is strong. We give them a ride back toward their hometown in our van. In clinic we are free with our questions about their lives, their medical conditions, their coping. In the van, they are friends. It's been nice getting away from the pollution of the city to the open air of the country.

And tomorrow? Back to Nima. And back again. I see somebody with infectious endocarditis. A high fever and a worsening heart murmur, and another potential death. Same story, no money. This person needs to be hospitalized, urgently. Even in the U.S., the prognosis would not necessarily be good. I tell her she needs to be hospitalized, I tell her family, I tell her friends. They nod. I know it will be the same story, though. I say goodbye.

I begin to think of home. I'll be glad to return to Seattle. Familiar ground, loved ones, friends. But already I'm thinking of the proposals that we are working on, not only research for its own sake, but proposals with the community, with the chiefs, with the citizens, with the Noguchi Memorial Medical

Research Institute in Ghana. And already we're identifying people on our team who can live in Accra. My own home is not in Accra, but maybe home is also with those whom I serve. I have found a new sense of dedication, and one that is steeped in urgency. We've just got to deliver. These are the poorest of the poor in Ghana. They are Muslim in a very Christian city. They feel neglected and discarded by the society. One of our informants from outside Nima tells us, "All bad comes from Nima." But we have found good, and have been welcomed into people's homes, and their meetings, and have heard their life stories and their worries and their hopes. A haunting image of sounds still is with me: a discussion with the Islamic Women's Association on a Saturday morning in a schoolyard. That day was Koran school for the kids, and the women opened up about their lives and the structural problems of Nima to the beautiful sounds of children of all ages chanting the Koran, over and over. I don't know what they were saying. I am embarrassed that I have never read the Koran, and most of the women are speaking in Hausa, which must be translated. But I am reminded of another moment two decades ago when I stepped into an old cathedral in the U.K. for the aesthetic experience of experiencing Evensong, and it became a spiritual experience, not because of the words, but because of the music and the setting, both of which I had never experienced before.

My last day in Ghana. I want to say goodbye to Nima, but there isn't time. People are dropping by the hotel to discuss parts of our projects, to have lunch and to say goodbye for a few months until I return. I have mixed feelings. I'm happy about going home, but sad about leaving. Our team has become another family, and a very functional one. It's like leaving brothers and sisters. But the time comes to make it through the chaos of Kotoka Airport. It goes smoothly. I'm on the plane to Lagos and Frankfurt, looking down on Togo and Benin and feeling a bit empty.

I stay in Frankfurt for a day, overwhelmed as always by the return to mass Western culture, with people running about, tendering credit cards, and loudspeakers announcing flight departures to all over the world. There is some solace in my room in the airport hotel. I sleep. I exercise, and as I leave the exercise room I feel my foot rolling outwards on an uneven surface and I start falling. I hear a snap. An inversion sprain of my ankle. I let myself recover for a few minutes and hobble to my room. So much for going into Frankfurt. I have more time to think about Ghana as I ice my ankle. The one thing that I really look forward to at lunch is a big salad. And as I eat that wonderful salad, looking out at the Autobahn and the trees beyond, it strikes me again that, whereas pathogens cause infection and plaque causes atherosclerosis, those are the simple causes of ill-health. Causes not to be neglected, since they are so important. With the right antibiotics, many of the people I've seen over the past month would be fine. The conditions of poverty, prejudice, ignorance (I don't know how else to put it), and neglect—and, ultimately, social inequality—are key. With HIV/AIDS, the biggest task is to continue to communicate the message that it is an infectious disease like any other, and that how it is contracted is not really any different than how a respiratory infection is contracted. Get tested, get treated, save your life.

CHAPTER 33

Resilience and Meaning in Caregiving for Children Living with HIV/AIDS in Togo

Ami Moore

ABSTRACT

This study examines the experiences of caregiving to children with HIV/AIDS in the low-income country of Togo, West Africa. This study is important because HIV/AIDS is more prevalent in low resource areas, and the impacts are more devastating. Since allocation of resources to help people infected and affected by HIV/AIDS is not accessible to all, knowing how people affected by the disease—caregivers, especially—positively cope with it will lead to more immediate and practical ways in which others can effectively manage their challenges. Specifically, the chapter examines resilience and the ascribed meanings seropositive parents and seronegative caregivers gave to their experiences as ways of effectively coping with the challenges of caregiving.

Studies have documented the significant burden of informal caregiving to children living with HIV/AIDS (Bettoli-Vaughan, Brown, Brown, and Baldwin 1998; Lesar and Maldonato 1997; Lesar, Gerber, and Semmel 1995). Especially in resource-deprived areas where formal care for people with HIV/AIDS is generally rudimentary, family and friends face daily challenges of caregiving. Additionally, antiretroviral drugs are not readily available and affordable. Furthermore, there are insufficient resources in terms of health professionals such as physicians and nurses. Family and friends generally face a shortage of palliative care for their loved ones (Sepulveda, Habiyambere, Amandua, Borok et al. 2006) as well as hospices for terminally ill patients (Grant, Murray, Grant, and Brown 2003).

Caregivers of HIV/AIDS-infected and -affected children are also faced with a substantial burden because of the stigma that is often attached to the epidemic and are discriminated against along with their families (UNICEF 2002; Family Health International 2001). In some cases, the advanced age of the caregivers, in addition to their lack of resources and their own disabilities, compounds the demands of caring for children with HIV/AIDS (Johanson, Norman, and Staugård 1996; Moore, 2007–2008; Nyambedha, Wandibba, and Aagaard-Hansen 2003).

In cases where parents are themselves seropositive and are giving care to children who have HIV/AIDS, the issues become more complicated. In general, children who are HIV-infected were transmitted the disease by their mothers. Therefore, parents usually feel some guilt for infecting their children (Nagler, Adnopoz, and Forsyth 1995). They also face challenges over disclosing to the infected child her or his serostatus (Havens, Mellins, and Ryan 2005). Some mothers fear that the child will be angry at them for the contamination (Flanagan-Klygis, Ross, Lantos, Frader, and Yogev 2001; Wiener, Battles, Heilman, Sigelman, and Pizzo 1996; Waugh 2003).

All of these reports focused on the plights

of caregivers. However, it is important to know how caregivers manage these challenges because, as shown in the literature, people have different ways to cope with challenges that come into their lives (Rutter 2006a, 2006b). These differences in coping explain the differentials in the effects the challenges have on them (Pearlin 1991). Some efficient ways people react to difficulties is through the subjective meanings they attach to the event (Mead 1934; Blumer 1969; Simon 1997; Mirowsky and Ross 1989; Fife 2005) and/or the use of resilient traits they have (Evans 2005; DuMont, Wisdom, and Czaja 2007).

This study examines the experiences of caregiving to children with HIV/AIDS in the low-income country of Togo, West Africa. This study is important because HIV/AIDS is more prevalent in low resource areas, and the impacts are more devastating. Since allocation of resources to help people infected and affected by HIV/AIDS is not accessible to all, knowing how people affected by the disease—caregivers especially—positively cope with it will lead to more immediate and practical ways that others can effectively manage their challenges. Specifically, the chapter examines resilience and the ascribed meanings seropositive parents and seronegative caregivers gave to their experiences as ways of effectively coping with the challenges of caregiving.

BACKGROUND

Ascribed Meaning

Ascribing a meaning to an action or event is a framework that is found in both sociology and psychology. In sociology, ascribing a meaning to an act or event is an interpretative way of understanding the event. Thus, it's believed to be subjective. In fact, Max Weber is associated with this concept of subjective meaning. According to Weber, human beings always think, reason, and attach meaning and significance to most of what they do. Weber believed that understanding sociology is a matter of grasping the subjective meaning people attach to their individual social actions (Runciman 1978). Since human beings are part of a society, the subjective meaning they derive from their social action will be a function of their social, political, historical, and cultural environment, which ultimately forms them and gives them the necessary tools to interpret the actions or events.

The concept of meaning is also used in psychology. For psychologists, meaning is something that we experience and feel. As stated by Gendlin (1962:44), "meaning is experienced." We constantly construct meaning through life, although this meaning may change with life circumstances. The meaning ascribed to an event determines how this event is felt. For instance, when we ascribe meaning to suffering, we are able to have a certain significance of it. Thus, certain ascribed meanings of suffering may be liberating, therefore making the experience of suffering more bearable. This concept is well described by Frankl (1992:117) when he states: "In some way, suffering ceases to be suffering at the moment it finds a meaning, such as the meaning of sacrifice." In fact, putting a different perspective on events makes one accept difficult situations and experience them with grace and endurance. In a way, one shows resilience instead of retreat.

Resilience

Resilience is defined as a "successful adaptation under adverse conditions" (Luthar 2006). This is a special trait that is found among most humans (Taylor 1983). In the 1980s, the concept of resilience was mainly used in psychiatric risk research. However, today it is also used by researchers in child development, childhood, and family research and policy studies (Evans 2005). Basically, resilient people are those who are able to function under major life stressors. These people do not let their condition prevent them from living; they manage to find a way to function regardless of the gravity of the event. Although there are studies that warn that resilient people may have some emotional issues to contend with (Moskowitz 1983; Luthar 1991), resilience is a protective factor that helps people positively adjust to adversity in general.

Resilient people tend to possess some common traits. These characteristics are generally divided into two groups: personality and interpersonally related factors. While "personality factors encompass having a sense of self-efficacy, direction or mission, social problem-solving skills, empathy, humor, adaptive distancing, androgynous sex role behavior and realistic appraisal of the environment, interpersonally related factors include positive, caring relationships, positive environment, and high enough expectation" (Norman 2000:4). According to Wolin and Wolin (1993), having a sense of self-efficacy is having a sense of initiative. This most important trait of resilient people allows them to have confidence in themselves and believe that they can influence their internal and external environments (Norman 2000).

Another characteristic found in resilient people is a sense of direction or mission, which means having a sense of meaning, purpose, or responsibility. Having social problem-solving skills is also important, as well as empathy and a sense of humor. People with social problem-solving skills tend to have a good sense of self-esteem, sense of competence, and sense of mastery (Norman 2000). People with empathy usually understand and positively respond to others' problems and needs, a trait found to be common among resilient people (Werner 1986; Schwartz, Jacobson, Hauser, and Dornbush 1989). Additionally, humor also has helped resilient people maintain social relations and get through the challenges of life (Kumpfer 1993 cited in Norman 2000).

Other characteristics that are generally found in resilient people are their ability to adaptively distance themselves from problematic situations or persons that are the sources of adversity and their ability to realistically appraise their environment. They adaptively distance themselves by not blaming themselves for the cause or reason for the issues or troubles at hand (Beardslee 1989). They realistically appraise their environment by knowing their abilities and limits regarding how to act and affect the circumstance (Werner 1986; Garmezy and Masten 1986). They recognize the situations that they can influence and the ones that they cannot. The least commonly found characteristic of resilience is having androgynous sex role behavior (Norman 2000). This trait refers to people having traditionally both female and male sex-typed values and behaviors.

The interpersonal characteristics such as positive, caring relationships, as well as positive environments, help develop resiliency and sustain it. Positive, caring relationships seem to be an important protective factor in resilient people because through these relationships people learn to value themselves and become competent (Norman, Turner, and Zunz 1994). And having a positive environment centered on nurturing and caring relationships not only teaches people that life can be predicted (Walsh 1998), but also gives a sense of safety and support. Finally, having high enough but reachable expectations is a resiliency factor that motivates people and encourages them to excel in life regardless of their life circumstances (Norman 2000).

It is important to note that all these factors can be enhanced in people. Some experts (Rutter 1990; Luthar 1993) argue that resilience is not a universal or fixed trait that a person possesses. Rather, it is found in some specific areas in the life of a person due to her or his life circumstances. In order to understand the informal caregiving experiences of adults caring for children with HIV/AIDS in Togo, especially what motivated them not to give up in times of extreme difficulty, I examine the meanings that caregivers construe of these experiences. I also explore resilient factors that these caregivers possess. Knowing the meanings that caregivers construct will be beneficial for others who may be having difficulty coping with the challenges of caregiving, since the meanings they construct of the caregiving demands and challenges shape their positive responses to this difficult task of caregiving. Furthermore, their resilient attributes are protective factors that help them sustain caregiving. Others can be taught these traits as well. It will help HIV/AIDS service providers know how to teach caregivers to effectively cope with the challenges of caring for children with HIV/AIDS. Policymakers will better understand ways to efficiently allocate scarce resources.

SETTING

Togo is a low-income French-speaking country in West Africa. With an estimated 97,000 children aged 0 to 14 living with HIV/AIDS (UNICEF 2002), the number of Togolese families affected by the HIV/AIDS epidemic is significant. The estimated population is about 6.1 million inhabitants (UK Foreign Office 2007). The estimated average annual income is about $380 (World Bank 2005), and life expectancy is about 56 years for males and 60 years for females (CIA World Fact Book 2007). Although the prevalence rate of HIV/AIDS has declined from 6–7 percent in 2000 to 3.2 percent in 2007 (UNESCO 2007), the burden of HIV/AIDS is still important, especially among the poor, who seem to be the most affected (Moore and Williamson 2003; Moore and Henry 2005).

METHODS

The investigation is an in-depth qualitative study that explores resilience and ascribed meanings of the caregiving experiences of seronegative caregivers and seropositive parents in Togo. Following Taylor and Bogdan's (1998) suggestion, a qualitative method was used for the study because I was interested in collecting data on the lived experiences of caregivers of children with HIV/AIDS. Specifically, I was interested in learning about how these caregivers coped with the burdens and challenges that they encountered in their daily activities of caregiving. I wanted to know what motivated them to continue caring for the children.

Recruitment Procedure, Data Collection, and Sample

The data come from 6 seropositive parents of and 34 seronegative caregivers to children with HIV/AIDS in Togo. First, I contacted three HIV/AIDS centers that I have established research relationships with and discussed the research protocol with the directors. Six of the employees (two from each center) with at least a bachelor's degree were selected to help with the study. The employees were trained in a two-day workshop by the author. They watched the author conduct the first ten interviews as a part of their training. With the help of these centers, participants were recruited in Lomé and its surrounding areas for this study. The study was conducted from July to September 2006 in Lomé, Togo. Interviews were conducted in both English and Ewe, one of the native languages in Togo and lasted one hour on average.

To be included in the study, participants had to be the primary caregiver of a child with HIV/AIDS and have prior contact with the HIV/AIDS agencies before the study. The study was conducted in all three of the HIV/AIDS centers. Participants chose to come there because they were familiar and comfortable with the service providers at these centers. The purpose of the study was explained to each participant and oral permission to perform the study was obtained from each one of them. The study participants were asked to describe their experiences of caring for a child who has HIV or AIDS. Specifically, we wanted to know all the things caregivers did from dawn to dusk for the children, how they managed the caregiving demands, if family members helped with caregiving and ways that they helped, and how the caregiving has changed them, if at all. This study uses the subjective meaning and resilience framework to report mainly on what motivated caregivers to continue caring for children with HIV/AIDS. It is important to note that these concepts were derived from the data analysis.

Eighty-four percent of the sample was female. The average age of caregivers was about 42 years (range = 19 to 77). They had on average about 9 years of education (range = 2 to 19). They had been caring for 2 years, 7 months on average.

Analysis

Transcripts were read several times in order to be immersed with the data. Through inductive approach, data were condensed and key categories emerged. An inductive analysis allows emic analytical patterns to emerge from the data (Patton 1990). Ascribed meanings and resilience emerged as the central categories. The ways these two categories manifested in the data were analyzed by describing their key characteristics. The categories and the key characteristics were taken back to participants for feedback. They agreed that these reflected their caregiving experiences, especially motivation to endure the demands and challenges.

FINDINGS

Although all of the participants stated that caring for a child with HIV/AIDS was a difficult task that made them exhausted, they all reported that they could not give up on the children even when things became extremely tough. They gave different interpretations to caregiving in order to effectively cope with the demands and challenges. For instance, a 28-year-old woman who had a master's degree and was caring for a cousin replied as follows when asked how was she able to care for her 8-year-old cousin when things became unbearable:

> First of all, I love this child. Also, she is the only girl among her siblings. However, I have to always remind myself that she is innocent. She doesn't know what has happened to her. I am the adult person here who understands what has happened to her. Both of her parents are dead . . . She is not like other children. She will die one of these days. She will not grow old and have children. Thus, one must make her happy for the time that she is here. She has to be provided a lot. She is an innocent kid.

Several conclusions can be made from the above comment. Ascribing the meaning "innocent" to the child helped the caregiver meet the challenges. Also, this caregiver interpreted the condition of the child as imminent death. Thus, she had to be showered with all the necessary care. With these interpretations, she was able to overcome her caregiving challenges regardless of how difficult they were. She also stated later that, even though she did not get help and support from her family members, she could never abandon the child.

Other caregivers looked at all the little things that the children could do for them and held onto them as very meaningful. They also gave religious interpretations to their caregiving challenges, as commented by a 75-year-old grandmother who was caring for four seronegative and one seropositive grandchildren. She made the comments below when asked what motivated her in times of difficulties:

> The fact is when one has children one cannot give them up like that. One has to care for them. And these children are mine. When I am mad at the situation (caregiving), God always comforts me. The Lord gives us according to our capability. Thus, I cannot refuse what He has given me. See, when I come back from the market and fall asleep, the children wake me up . . . Whenever the children are happy, I am happy too. When they are old, they will say someday that grandma has suffered for us, and this will make me happy for them to grow up and recognize my efforts. This is what keeps me going.

Again, the interpretations that caregivers gave to the care they were providing made them continue regardless of the efforts they had to make. As shown in the excerpt above, this caregiver saw what she was doing as not only a natural responsibility, but also as something noble that will be later acknowledged by the grandchildren. Furthermore, her religious interpretation of her caregiving sustained her in times of difficulty. A grandmother of a 10-year-old seropositive boy commented as follows:

> In my difficult moments I always tell myself that one can hurt a foot and die. Thus, having HIV/AIDS is not the end of the world. He is still alive and well. This is what matters.

This grandmother had to banalize the condition of her grandson and her caregiving. In Togo, as in other low-income countries, it is not unusual that people may get a cut on their feet and later get infection and unfortunately die from it. Thus, to her, HIV/AIDS was not the "end of the world." One has to continue living despite HIV/AIDS.

The meanings that seropositive parents constructed were more holistic. They created meanings for their positive serostatus as well as their children's. However, they were more focused on their children's health. A seropositive, widowed father of an 11-year-old seropositive girl explained:

> No one in my family knows that my daughter is seropositive. I don't tell people that we are positive. I myself, I don't have it in my head that we are seropositive. It is an illness just like any illness and I'm dealing with it as I can . . . You see, even the fact that we are both seropositive doesn't worry me anymore. Even, if I worry, I cannot do anything to change that. Thus, I have abandoned everything in God's hands. All depends on God, that's why I am living without worrying . . . I give myself and my daughter to God. Whether I find something to eat or not is in God's hands. I know He will provide, even when things are hard. Sometimes, leaving the house is very difficult. I get really tired. However, she is my daughter. I can't abandon her and take a break. I'm obligated to do what I have to do regardless of my condition because there is no one to care for her.

This father like other seropositive parents strives to overcome the daily challenges of living with HIV/AIDS. Instead of equating HIV/AIDS to a death sentence, like most people, he constructed a different meaning to it: "just like any illness." Furthermore, he had a religious interpretation to his situation. All of these helped keep him going.

A seropositive mother replied as follows (choking in tears) when asked how she kept going despite all the challenges she faced with her seropositive 10-year-old boy and three other stepchildren. She also had a religious justification to her situation:

> I have to do whatever I need to care for her. Children don't know anything. When I able to care for them today, they will help me out later. I can't abandon them. No one helps us. . . . Since they are with me, I get to help them. I have to fight and help them regardless of my health. If you are suffering, you get to suffer with them. You can't say that since I'm suffering I must abandon them. If you do that then you sin against God.

A 49-year-old seropositive father of a 5-year-old seropositive girl described what kept him going even when he was exhausted by caregiving demands:

> This girl is my only hope in life. If she wasn't seropositive, I would say that God has really blessed me. But unfortunately, she is seropositive like myself. Oftentimes, I think about this . . . With God's help I'm feeling stronger and stronger everyday. I tell myself that if we don't die soon, a medication will be found to cure us. All my thoughts are about my daughter since I learned that she is positive like me. We have no one to care for us. Thus, I fight day in, day out for her. If I don't her future will be much more difficult. Her fate will be sealed. Thus, I told myself that whatever it is God will help us find a solution. Caring for her is a joy for me. She is my own. She didn't ask for this illness. It is our fault. It wasn't her that brought this illness into the family but me.

This parent had a sense of guilt for having a seropositive daughter. Also, he felt that he had to fight to keep both of them alive. He believed that if he did not provide for his daughter regardless of the challenges that they faced, then she would have more difficulty later on. His daughter was all he had and his hope was her. He considered it a "joy" caring for his daughter even though he admitted that caregiving wasn't an easy activity. These meanings that he had constructed in addition to a religious understanding of his experiences helped him meet his daily difficulties.

Similarly, a seropositive mother of two seronegative children and a 10-year-old seropositive son explained what motivated her to continue caring for her children when things became unbearable:

> I have to refocus myself because thinking and worrying will hasten my illness. But looking at my son's situation, I come to my senses. I tell myself that if I keep at it (worrying and thinking) I may get sick and he will not have anyone to care for him. Right now, I'm well but it's already difficult to care for him. So if I'm no more, who will care for him? With that, I return to my senses and give myself to God.

These caregivers had different meanings that sustained them even when things became extremely difficult. They all drew from the environment that they lived in. For instance, one had to compare the situation of her grandson to people who have a cut on a foot and get it infected and eventually die of infection. Others had to construct meanings from their religious beliefs. Still others had to ascribe meanings based on their social environment such as the father who did not share the seropositive status of both his daughter and himself, even to his family members, because of stigma and discrimination.

Furthermore, several protective attributes were found among the respondents. Both seropositive parents and seronegative caregivers showed a sense of self-efficacy or sense of meaning. For instance, when asked about how he was supporting his 11-year-old daughter, this father replied:

> Nowadays, things are very difficult. I wanted to be a security guard. I had a physical and was ready to start. However, the salary was really low (20,000CFA per month).[1] I would have to pay for transportation to and from work. By the end, I would not have anything left. Thus, I decided to sell gasoline. I went to a friend who delivers gasoline and explained my financial situation to him. He then decided to give me 20 liters of gas for sale and I pay him afterward. This is the only way I make money and I make sure I pay him when I sell the gas so that I will not lose that favor. I'm originally a mechanic. I used to repair Vespa,[2] but nowadays, people don't drive Vespa anymore.

A 46-year-old seropositive mother who had lost her husband nine years prior to the study and was caring for a 10-year-old seropositive son stated:

> Yes, at times, I'm very exhausted, but every day I have to go fetch water for the masons to earn money. In the evenings, my ribs hurt. I feel like I have wounds in my organs. However, this cannot prevent me from raising my children. I'm the only one who can help them. When I'm tired and sick, I buy medicines and take them.

It is important to note that, like this woman, most of the participants had a relatively steady income-generating activity prior to their seropositive status. However, because of health issues along with caregiving demands, they had to either stop the activity or spent all the money they used to have for the activity. Thus, they had to find something else that would help them earn a living. In fact the participants had a belief that they could influence their lot. They did not want to just retreat because there was no way out.

They also evidenced some of the other traits found among resilient people. They realistically appraised their environment, showed social problem-solving skills, and empathy. For instance, as shown in the earlier comments, the study participants recognized their limits. Some relied on their faith and abandoned themselves and their children in God's hands. In addition, they were not living in denial, but recognized that they would not be able to go through the challenges alone. They went to the HIV/AIDS centers for help and were grateful for all the support they received there. The following excerpt from a lady who was HIV positive, with one of her eight children, explains the points:

> When things get really heated at home, I wash the children and bring them over here [center]. The staff generally gives me and the children advice to help us handle our problem. They also tell us things to eat in order to stay healthy . . . I can honestly say that the center has saved my life.

It is worthwhile to note that these centers gave them some of the interpersonally related traits. Participants had caring, positive relationships with the staff at the centers. Also, these centers gave them an intimate, positive environment where they shared whatever might be troubling them and in return received valuable support.

Surprisingly, most of the caregivers were very empathetic. They willingly decided to care for the children with HIV/AIDS and, at times, along with a parent. When asked why they decided to care for the children, most of them stated that if they did not there would be no one to care for the children. This fact shows their sense of mission, as well. The following comments from a 75-year-old seronegative aunt of a seropositive mother and child illustrates the point:

> First my niece was abandoned by her husband. She was ill and did not have any means to buy medicines. There was no one to care for her . . . I'm retired and on a fixed income so at times it's really difficult.

All of the study participants showed this empathetic character in different ways. A seropositive father who was caring for his seropositive daughter reported the following:

> Prior to my having HIV/AIDS, I was caring for my nieces and nephews. They lived with me because I was the only one who succeeded in the family. I'm the only one who has a house. Now, my brothers and sisters took their children from me because they are afraid of me (HIV/AIDS). I now have only my younger sister's children with me. She would also have come for them had she had the means.

It is important to report that earlier this participant reported how difficult it has become for him to make ends meet because his health has been at times weak and has affected his business. However, he was still caring for his sister's children in addition to his seropositive daughter.

These were some of the resilient traits that transpired from the data. Since the goal of the study was not primarily to find resilient traits that participants possessed, there could have been more than the ones that have been discussed.

CONCLUSION

This study examined the experiences of caregiving to children with HIV/AIDS in Togo. It used resilience and ascribed meaning frameworks to analyze how seropositive parents and seronegative caregivers effectively coped with the challenges of caregiving. It was found that caregivers showed some resilient attributes. Most of them were very empathetic. They realistically appraised their environment and showed social problem-solving skills. They had a sense of mission as well as sense of efficacy or meaning. Additionally, the HIV/AIDS centers gave caregivers an intimate, positive environment where they shared whatever might be troubling them, and in return received valuable support. To overcome caregiving demands and challenges, caregivers constructed diverse meanings. For instance, some constructed meanings from their religious beliefs. Others ascribed meanings based on their social environment.

Several recommendations can be made from these findings. First, HIV/AIDS service providers can help caregivers who are having difficulty with caregiving challenges find a positive meaning to their experiences. Also, they can teach caregivers who are having problems some of the resilient characteristics and create more intimate environments where caregivers have positive, caring relationships with service providers. Finally, policymakers should actively support HIV/AIDS centers, since service providers at these centers basically become surrogate family to some of the caregivers.

ACKNOWLEDGMENTS

This study was funded by a Fulbright HIV/AIDS grant and would not have been possible without the help of the HIV/AIDS providers at the centers in Lomé, Togo, and the brave caregivers who participated in the project.

NOTES

1. $40 per month.
2. Vespa is a certain type of motorcycle.

REFERENCES AND FURTHER READING

Beardslee, W. R. 1989. The role of self-understanding in resilient individuals: The development of a perspective. *American Journal of Orthopsychiatry*, 59:266–278.

Bettoli-Vaughan, E., Brown, R. T., Brown, J. V., and Baldwin, K. 1998. Psychological adjustment and adaptation of siblings and mothers of children with HIV/AIDS. *Families, Systems and Health*, 16:249–266.

Blumer, H. 1969. *Symbolic interaction: Perspective and method*. Englewood Cliffs, NJ: Prentice-Hall.

CIA World Fact Book—Togo (2007). http://www.cia.gov/cia/publications/factbook/geos/to.html. Retrieved August 16, 2007.

DuMont, K. A., Widom, S. C., and Czaja, S. J. 2007. Predictors of resilience in abused and neglected children grown-up: The role of individual and neighborhood characteristics. *Child Abuse and Neglect*, 31:255–274.

Evans, R. M. C. 2005. Social networks, migration, and care in Tanzania: caregivers' and children's resilience to coping with HIV/AIDS. *Journal of Children and Poverty*, 11:111–129.

Family Health International (FHI). 2001. Care for orphans, children affected by HIV/AIDS and other vulnerable children: A strategic framework. http://www.fhi.org/en/HIVAIDS/pub/fact/carorphans.htm. Retrieved May 24, 2007.

Fife, B. 2005. The role of constructed meaning in adaptation to the onset of life-threatening illness. *Social Science and Medicine*, 61: 2132–2143.

Flanagan-Klygis, E., Ross, L. F., Lantos, J., Frader, J., and Yogev, R. 2001. Disclosing the diagnosis of HIV in pediatrics. *Journal of Clinical Ethics*, 12:150–157.

Frankl, V. E. 1992. *Man's search for meaning: An introduction to logotherapy*, 4th edition. Boston: Beacon Press.

Garmezy, N. and Masten, A. S. 1986. Stress, competence and resilience: Common frontiers for therapist and psychopathologist. *Behavior Therapy*, 57:159–174.

Gendlin, E. T. 1962. *Experiencing and the creation of meaning: A philosophical and psychological approach to the subjective*. New York: The Free Press of Glencoe.

Grant, E., Murray, S. A., Grant, A., and Brown, J. 2003. A good death in rural Kenya? Listening to Meru patients and their families talk about care needs at the end of life. *Journal of Palliative Care*, 19:159–167.

Havens, J. F., Mellins, C. A., and Ryan, S. 2005. Child psychiatry: Psychiatric sequelae of HIV and AIDS. In B. Sadock and V. Sadock (eds.), *Comprehensive textbook of psychiatry*, 8th edition. Baltimore, MD: Williams and Wilkins, pp. 3434–3440.

Johanson, M., Norman, C., and Staugård, A. 1996. Three anthropological perspectives addressing the influences of HIV/AIDS on the Bukoba urban and rural societies of Tanzania. In C. Cabrera, D. Pitt, and F. Staugård (eds.), *AIDS and grassroots: Problems, challenges and opportunities*. Gaborone: Ipelegeng Publishers, pp. 145–174.

Lesar, S., Gerber, M. M., and Semmel, M. I. 1995. HIV infection in children: Family stress, social support, and adaptation. *Exceptional Children*, 62:224–236.

Lesar, S. and Maldonato, Y. A. 1997. The impact of children with HIV infection on the family system. *Families in Society*, 78:272–279.

Luthar, S. S. 1991. Vulnerability and resilience: A study of high risk adolescence. *Child Development* 62(3):600–616.

Luthar, S. S. 1993. Annotation: Methodological and conceptual issues in research on childhood resilience. *Journal of Child Psychology and Psychiatry*, 34:441–454.

Luthar, S. S. 2006. Resilience in development: A synthesis of research across five decades. In D. Ciccheti and D. J. Cohen (eds.), *Developmental psychopathology: Risk, disorder, and adaptation*. New York: Wiley, pp. 740–795.

Mead, G. H. 1934. *Mind, self, and society*. Chicago: University of Chicago.

Mirowsky, J. and Ross, C. E. 1989. *Social causes of psychological distress*. New York: Aldine de Gruyter.

Moore, A. 2007–2008. Older poor parents who lost an adult child to AIDS in Togo, West Africa: A qualitative study. *Omega: Journal for Death and Dying*, 56:289–304.

Moore, A. R. and Henry, D. 2005. Experiences of older informal caregivers to people with HIV/AIDS in Lomé, Togo. *Ageing International*, 30:147–166.

Moore, A. R. and Williamson, D. A. 2003. Problems with HIV/AIDS prevention, care, and treatment in Togo, West Africa: Professional caregivers' perspectives. *AIDS Care*, 15:615–627.

Moskowitz, S. 1983. *Love despite hate*. New York: Schocken Books.

Nagler, S. F., Adnopoz, J., and Forsyth, B. W. C. 1995. Uncertainty, stigma and secrecy: Psychological aspects of AIDS for children and adolescents. In S. Geballe, J. Gruendel, and W. Andiman (eds.), In *Forgotten children of the AIDS epidemic*. New Haven, CT: Yale University Press, pp. 71–82.

Norman, E. 2000. Introduction: The strengths and perspective and resiliency enhancement—A natural partnership. In Elaine Norman (ed.), *Resiliency Enhancement: putting the strengths perspective into social work practice*. New York: Columbia University Press, pp. 1–16.

Norman, E., Turner, S., and Zunz, S. 1994. *Substance abuse prevention: A Review of the literature*. New York: New York State Office of Alcohol and Substance Abuse Services.

Nyambedha, E. O., Wandibba, S., and Aagaard-Hansen, J. 2003. "Retirement lost"—the new role of the elderly as caretakers for orphans in western Kenya. *Journal of Cross-Cultural Gerontology*, 18:33–52.

Patton, M. 1990. *Qualitative evaluation and research methods*. Newbury Park: Sage.

Pearlin, L. I. 1991. The study of coping: An overview of problems and directions. In J. Eckenrode (ed.), *The social context of coping*. New York: Plenum Press, pp. 2–21.

Runciman, W. G. 1978. *Max Weber: Selections in translation*. New York: Cambridge University Press.

Rutter, M. 1990. Psychosocial resilience and protective mechanisms. In J. Rolf, A. Masten, D. Chisshetti, K. Neuchterlein and S. Weintraub (eds.), *Risk and protective factors in the development of psychopathology*. New York: Cambridge University Press.

Rutter, M. 2006a. Implications of resilience concepts for scientific understanding. *Annals of the New York Academy of Sciences*, 1094:1–12.

Rutter, M. 2006b. The promotion of resilience in the face of adversity. In A. Clarke-Stewart and J. Dunn (eds.), *Families count: Effects on child and adolescent development*. New York and Cambridge: Cambridge University Press, pp. 26–52.

Schwartz, J., Jacobson, A. Hauser, S., and Dornbush, B. 1989. Explorations of vulnerability and resilience:

Case studies of diabetic adolescents and their families. In Degan and Coles (eds.), *The child in our times: Studies in the development of resiliency*. New York: Bruner/Mazel, pp. 134–144.

Sepulveda, C., Habiyambere, V., Amandua, J., Borok, M., Kikule, E., Mudanga, B., Ngoma, T., and Solomon, B. 2006. Quality care at the end of life in Africa. *British Medical Journal*, 327:209–213.

Simon, R.W. 1997. The meanings individuals attach to role identities and their implications for mental health. *Journal of Health and Social Behavior*, 38:256–274.

Taylor, S. 1983. Adjustment to threatening events: A theory of cognitive adaptation. *American Psychologist*, 38:1161–1173.

Taylor, S. J. and Bogdan, R. 1998. *Introduction to qualitative research methods: A guidebook and resource*, 3rd edition. New York: John Wiley and Sons Inc.

UK Foreign Office. 2007. Country profile: Togo. http://dmoz.org/Regional/Africa/Togo?Guides_and_Directories/. Retrieved on July 18, 2007.

UNESCO. 2007. HIV impact on education clearinghouse. HIV/AIDS in Togo. http://hivaidsclearinghouse.unesco.org/ev.php?ID=2840_201andID2=DO_TOPIC. Retrieved on March 3, 2007.

UNICEF. 2002. Orphans and other children affected by HIV/AIDS. http://www.unicef.org/publications/pub_factsheet_orphan_en_pdf Retrieved May 24, 2007.

Walsh, F. 1998. *Strengthening family resilience*. New York: Guilford Press.

Waugh, S. 2003. Parental views on disclosure of diagnosis to their HIV-positive children. *AIDS Care*, 15:169–176.

Werner, E. E. 1986. Resilient offspring of alcoholics: A longitudinal study from birth to age 18. *American Journal of Orthopsychiatry*, 59:72–81.

Wiener, L. S., Battles, H. B., Heilman, N., Sigelman, C. K., and Pizzo, P. A. 1996. Factors associated with disclosure of diagnosis to children with HIV/AIDS. *Pediatric AIDS HIV Infections*, 7:310–324.

Wolin, S. J. and Wolin, S. 1993. *The resilient self: How survivors of troubled families rise above adversity*. New York: Villard.

World Bank. 2005. World development indicators database. http://www.worldbank.org/data/databytopic/GNIPC.pdf. Retrieved September 9, 2006.

SECTION 9

Globalizing Theory on HIV/AIDS: Frameworks for the Future

FRAMING ESSAY

Globalization and Interacting Large-Scale Processes and How They May Affect the HIV/AIDS Epidemic

Samuel R. Friedman, Diana Rossi, and Nancy Phaswana-Mafuya

Social and economic change at the large-scale level has many impacts on people's lives and on their social interactions (Myer et al. 2003, 2004; Mann et al. 1994). These, in turn, affect how HIV/AIDS and other disease agents do or do not spread. The pathways through which all of this happens help us to understand how to reduce the damage that HIV/AIDS and other diseases do—and, likewise, the history of the HIV epidemic helps us understand these large-scale social and economic processes and how we might reduce the damage that they do.

In this chapter, we focus on globalization and other large-scale social and economic processes (such as wars, falling profit rates, sociopolitical transitions, global warming, migration, slummification, and social movements); what some of the pathways might be through which they come to affect different groups of human beings in distinct ways; and what this tells us about what should be done. This chapter is necessarily incomplete and, to a degree, speculative in that it makes some claims on the basis of logical extrapolation from the existing scholarship. Some of the pathways we point to have received little research attention as yet. Indeed, a few years ago (Friedman et al. 2006a), we helped write a relatively high-visibility article that drew attention to some (but by no means all) of the pathways, precisely in order to encourage research on these neglected areas.

The chapter is also somewhat eclectic rather than comprehensive. The sheer need to write it as a paper rather than as a multi-volume book forces us to pick and choose which pathways to gloss over and which to spend some (but too little even there) time on.

TWO SCHEMATIC DIAGRAMS AND THE PROCESSES THAT SHAPE HIV EPIDEMICS

One way to present a lot of material in a way that encourages taking an overview is to present a diagram of what you are discussing. This can also make it easy for readers to see what they disagree with in what you are presenting—and thus encourages both debate over what is being presented and research to clarify disagreements or areas of doubt. It may also make it easier to plan appropriate action.

Of course, diagrams also can be seductive. The unexamined presuppositions of the writers can be hidden from view by the sheer majesty of the diagram. This is less likely to happen to the degree that the various concepts and categories in the diagram come from a theoretically unified perspective that is known by the readers—particularly if the readers (and authors) are familiar with other theories that have different perspectives on the same scholarly domains. Unfortunately, the study of global epidemiology and prevention of HIV and other disease agents is not yet well theorized—so we, as authors, want to point to this as a weakness of what we are presenting.

Exhibit FE9.1 presents the logic of HIV transmission in a multidisciplinary context. It is useful because it illustrates some of the pathways by which the other categories in the diagram

Exhibit FE9.1 Risk is a socially conditioned probability. (Ovals are people; lines to and from ovals represent sexual or injection partnerships.)

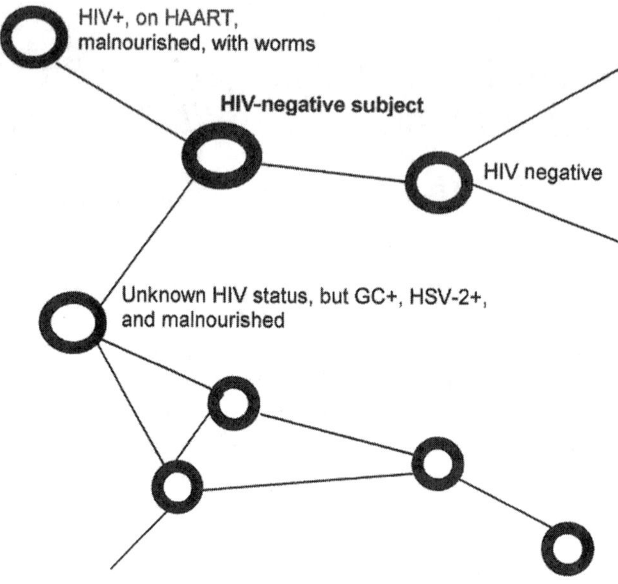

can affect HIV transmission. Specifically, it shows that the causes of viral transmission rates and events cannot be explained only in terms of individual risk-taking behavior. Networks of injection or sexual behaviors in a community are also very important (as is discussed further in Costenbader et al. 2006; Doherty et al. 2005; Friedman et al. 1997, 1999, 2002, 2004, 2005, 2007; Kottiri et al. 2002; Kretzschmar and Morris 1996; Latkin et al. 1995, 2003; Neaigus et al. 1994, 2006; Potterat et al. 2002; Rothenberg et al. 1998). This is because the community-wide network structuring of sexual (and injection) partnerships affects the probability that a given sexual or drug-injection event will involve discordant couples (that is, couples of whom one is infected and the other is not). It also affects the probability that one or both of them is infected with a sexually transmitted or blood-borne disease that increases HIV susceptibility or infectivity. Furthermore, social and economic dynamics, including the nature and extent of medical and mental health services, as well as the extent and distribution of severe malnutrition (Stillwaggon 2006), affect the probability that infected partners are on therapy that reduces the probability of HIV (or general herpes) transmission.

One implication of this, of course, is that interventions that address structural conditions of society rather than those that focus exclusively on individual behaviors are likely to have a substantial population-level impact (Friedman et al. 1994, 1995, 2006a; Mann 1993; Mann et al. 1994; Parker 1996; Teixera, 2002). Another is that the disruption of non-HIV-focused medical services (STI treatment, drug abuse treatment) during complex emergencies may create or heighten HIV epidemics (Hankins et al. 2002). A third is that structural approaches to social intervention are themselves insufficient to prevent HIV epidemics; we need to understand and intervene in processes of social change as well as in social structures.

Exhibit FE9.2 presents a table of some of large-scale social and economic processes that the authors think are particularly important for the arguments in this chapter. This chapter is eclectic, so we are knowingly not including some very important structures and processes in this table, even though we know that they condition everything being discussed. As one very important example, very little in Exhibit FE9.2 refers directly to gender. As we know, however, the power relations and cultural expressions of male–female interaction greatly affect every human institution and every social and economic process; and, as well, directly affect risk behaviors in both male–female and male–male sex and injection behaviors. Thus, gender conditions every box in this table and all of the causal patterns that connect these boxes with each other.

Two prefatory remarks are needed before explaining and discussing Exhibit FE9.2. First is an important caveat. Our efforts here to assign causal priority are tentative in many cases; and many of the processes presented here feed back on one another back and forth across columns and rows. Second, in some cases, an entry in a given row may be followed in the next column by an entry that is particularly related to it; but this is by no means always the case and, furthermore, as mentioned in the prior sentence, there is probably a great deal of mutual causation between every pair of boxes in the table. As we said, the research to support this table is only beginning.

The first column presents a number of social, economic, and other large-scale processes that have characterized the last several decades of human history. Most of these have been discussed in Friedman et al. 2006a (referred to above), Friedman and colleagues' paper on "Big Events" (2006b), or earlier papers (Friedman 1998a, 1998b; Friedman and Reid 2002). Mike Davis (2006) and Paul Farmer (2001) have written invaluable books on the growth of mass slums around the world and the implications of this for necessary action. Weiss and McMichael (2004) showed how these have been accompanied not only by HIV/AIDS but by other emerging infections.

The second column presents a number of what we are calling "second-order" processes. These are processes and conditions that seem to us to result to an important degree from the processes in the first column. Similarly, the third column follows from the first two (although reverse causal pathways no doubt exist, as well). Thus, for example, social processes like the transition in Russia disrupted the economy very severely; and this disrupted the authority of the parental generation over their children (and thus made "normative regulation" of the kind described by Heckathorn (1990) and Heckathorn et al. (1999) ineffective). The result of dashed economic hopes and weakened normative regulation meant that many teenagers took up sex work to earn money and casual sex and perhaps opiate use for enjoyment or to self-medicate against despair. This, in turn, led to a massive HIV epidemic (Aral et al. 2005; Friedman and Reid 2002; Rhodes et al. 2002; Rhodes and Simic 2005). Another example is that of the political and economic changes that South Africa experienced in the past two decades (building on the socioeconomic structures of the colonial and apartheid eras which created a number of structural vulnerabilities). These led to HIV/AIDS being the principal health threat in the country (Friedman and Reid 2002; Myer et al. 2003).

Wars or the economic changes precipitated by falling profit rates and the "race to the bottom" belt-tightening policies and programs that characterize globalization can similarly disrupt sexual and other networks, normative regulation, and economies, and furthermore lead to massive trauma and malnutrition and reduce the ability of governments or civil society to respond effectively to local epidemics—all of which can lead to increased HIV-related and STI-related risk behavior and, in the case of malnutrition, to increased susceptibility to sexual transmission and, among those infected, to increased HIV infectivity (Barnett et al. 2000; Friedman et al. 2006b; Hankins et al. 2002; Stillwaggon 2006; Wallace and Wallace 1998; Westerhaus et al. 2007). Furthermore, wars, transitions, globalization, and ecological-crisis-induced natural disasters also can devastate pre-existing programs to reduce HIV risk behaviors, cure sexually transmitted diseases, help those with problems with heroin, cocaine, or other drugs (Bastos et al. 2007), or provide therapy to the HIV-infected. Nevertheless, it is by no means foreordained that wars or other changes will have these effects. Gisselquist (2005) and Spiegel (2004), for example, have hypothesized that many African wars may have limited the extent of HIV spread by reducing the extent of sexual networks.

Finally, all of the first four columns, as discussed above, can influence the various constituent factors that affect the probability that any given sexual or injection event will result in HIV transmission.

Exhibit FE9.2 Large-scale processes and how they may affect HIV and other epidemics

Large scale processes: ALL of these interact with and condition the others	*Second-order processes (which may feed back and affect the large-scale processes as well as other second-order processes)*	*Third-order pathways (which may feed back and affect the higher-level processes)*	*Local processes*	*Behavioral and network interaction: The transmission event (see Exhibit FE9.1)*
Falling profit rates as a general condition of the capitalist economy in recent decades	Changes in the nature and quantity of work due to "race to the bottom" and related processes: Lower pay Longer hours Multiple job-holding Loss of career ladders Mass unemployment and underemployment—including an increase of numbers structurally excluded from any serious possibility of work Mass casualization of employment	Loss of hope in economic and/or social future among youth	Epidemiologic variables in cities, specific neighborhoods, and specific risk networks Population densities of high-risk groups (sex workers, IDUs, MSM, etc.) HIV prevalence among various groups STI prevalence among various groups AIDS among IDUs AIDS mortality among various groups	
Economic globalization	Destruction, shaking up and/or reforming of local community normative regulation due to social, economic, military, environmental, or other disruption	Shaking up and reforming of sexual and injection networks due to social, economic, military, environmental, or other disruption	Population prevalences of, distributions of, and mixing patterns of high-risk groups and high-risk events (such as group sex parties)	
Wars and imperial politics	Policy variables: Acceptance or rejection of neoliberal "belt-tightening" policies Budgets for: Health and mental health and drug-related problems Police and other security Education HIV-related programs and policies	Reduced (or increased) capability of intervening to reduce HIV and other transmission; progression; and infectivity. NB These interact with each other	Effectiveness of public health programs in reaching high-risk and other population groups	
Revolutions and transitions	Scapegoating (Friedman et al. 2006c) to counter the probability that these changes will lead to rebellion or revolution	Support for and opposition to HIV-related prevention, care, research, and other programs	Local peer norms towards sex, drugs, and partnership-formation programs	

	Drug war policies and campaigns Racial and ethnic scapegoating, cleansing, etc. Campaigns to "re-traditionalize" women's place Increased and intensified policing		
Ecological crisis, including global warming Floods Destruction of agriculture Industrial accidents, including nuclear ones that render large areas uninhabitable	Development of large-scale HIV, tuberculosis, or other, epidemics that themselves reshape national (or local) economies, military balances, normative regulation, or other key variables	Reduced (or increased) capability of intervening to reduce high-risk drug use or sex work behaviors, events, or settings. NB These interact with each other	Peer norms
Global and regional social movements such as World Social Forums and related activities, transnational activism by labor or by regional movements like Aboriginal groups	Extent and distribution of trauma, including that induced by large-scale or interpersonal violence, neighborhood disruption (Fullilove 2004), environmental or other catastrophes More scapegoating (immigrants bring the trouble)		Growth of travel to international meetings such as World Social Forums, religious conclaves, global programs Extent of anti-HIV transmission programs at these events
Growth of urban slums to incorporate a large proportion (25%?) of humanity—including considerable violence of poor against poor and also of police and vigilantes against the poor	Extent of serious malnutrition with its effects on (Stillwaggon 2006): a. susceptibility to infection by HIV b. infectivity among the infected c. mortality among the infected		
	Sociopolitical struggles against the symptoms and sequelae of the emerging global crisis (that have not led to transitions or revolutions—at least not yet) Some of these struggles may have impacts on risk environments, networks, or behaviors that may affect drug use or HIV risk behaviors.		
	International movement of people, including enormous rates of migration within and between countries		

Implications for Research and Action

What we have presented here may seem very distant from much of what is discussed in papers and programs to prevent HIV transmission. Nonetheless, we would maintain that these are the processes and causal relationships that will shape the future of the HIV epidemic. Educational and related programs that have been reasonably successful in preventing HIV transmission in the U.S.A. and Europe have been far less successful in much of Africa and the former Soviet Union. This seems to be due to the kinds of processes discussed in this chapter.

Furthermore, the extreme impacts of globalization and the other processes presented in the first column of Exhibit FE9.2 are not necessarily limited to poor or underdeveloped countries. During the first decade of the HIV epidemic, the Soviet Union seemed to be highly protected against HIV. Then, however, these large-scale processes led it to undergo a major social, political, and economic transition—which was followed by a massive HIV epidemic as discussed above. Similar economic and social processes are at work in every country today as a result of heightened global economic competition, the falling rate of profit, ecological disruption and uncertainty, and the apparent re-militarization of international relations. Putting it bluntly, given the near certainty that global warming will cause economic and agricultural disruption, coastal flooding, and massive population movements in the coming decades, and the high possibility that even developed countries may find themselves embroiled in internal or external wars as a result, it is only prudent to plan on the basis that, wherever the reader lives, it may happen "here" (Rischard 2002).

What are the implications of this worrisome outlook? Since there has been much less research than is needed into how these social and economic processes affect the magnitude and impact of the HIV epidemic, into how these impacts may be mediated by the general social and economic patterns of society and by social movements in reaction to these processes, and into how these processes affect HIV prevention efforts, such research is clearly needed (Barnett et al. 2000; Campbell 2003; Friedman 1998a, 1998b; Friedman and Reid 2002; Williams and Campbell 1999). As we have previously discussed (Friedman et al. 2006a, 2006b, 2007), not all wars, transitions, or other "Big Events" result in HIV epidemics. Some do, some do not. This provides the opportunity for research to discover what are the causal pathways that link the large-scale processes of the first column of Exhibit FE9.2 to the subsequent columns—and thus to discover what policies and programs on the part of governments, community-based organizations, social movements, or outside agencies are likely to make things better or worse. What we are likely to discover is three different types of situations:

1. Some of these processes may be impossible to control in some situations. Thus, it is possible that we might discover that, given the pre-existing economic relationships, social and risk networks, norms, traditions, and institutions of a given country, if it gets embroiled in a war or if global warming proceeds as anticipated, a massive HIV epidemic is a near certainty. In such cases, only action on the largest scale—the prevention of war, or a mammoth universal effort to reverse global warming—will prevent an HIV epidemic there.
2. In other cases, however, we might find that much more modest medical and social interventions during and after the war or ecological disruption might be all that is needed.
3. In a third set of cases, we might find that social intervention to maintain normative regulation of the upcoming generation in spite of economic disruption or widespread prevalence of disabling trauma among adults has a possibility of reducing the HIV-related impact of the Big Events.

The first and last categories of eventualities have very important implications for research and for public health. In most countries, perhaps in all countries, and in many ways, globally, we do not have the know-how nor the existing organizations or institutions to intervene successfully in these circumstances. Both for HIV-related reasons and for a host of other humanly vital reasons, since we are dealing with mass misery as well as with epidemic disease, we need to develop effective methods to intervene. We need to learn how to prevent wars and ecological disasters (situation 1). We also need to learn how to mitigate their impacts when and where they do occur.

This, along with identifying macro-social intervention approaches for the developing world, is the global agenda of public health for the coming decades and, we would suggest, for humanity as a whole.

ACKNOWLEDGMENTS

The authors would like to acknowledge support from a number of sources. Dr. Friedman was supported by National Institute on Drug Abuse projects R01 DA13336 (Community Vulnerability and Response to IDU-Related HIV), and P30 DA11041 (Center for Drug Use and HIV Research). Dr. Nancy Phaswana-Mafuya was supported by the Human Sciences Research Council, Social Aspects of HIV/AIDS and Health. Dr. Rossi was supported by Buenos Aires University UBACyT S118. Additional support was provided by Fogarty International Training and Research project D43 TW001037-06 (Mount Sinai New York State Argentina HIV Prevention).

REFERENCES AND FURTHER READING

Aral, S.O., St. Lawrence, J.S., Dyatlov, R., Kozlov, A. Commercial sex work, drug use, and sexually transmitted infections in St. Petersburg, Russia. *Social Science and Medicine* 2005;60(10):2181–2190.

Barnett, T. *HIV/AIDS and globalization: what is the epidemic telling us about economics, morality and pragnatism?* Overseas Development Group, East Anglia University (UEA) School of Development Studies, 2002.

Barnett, T., Whiteside, A., Decosas, J. The Jaipur paradigm—a conceptual framework for understanding social susceptibility and vulnerability to HIV. *South African Medical Journal* 2000;90:1098–1101.

Bastos, F.I., Caiaffa, W., Rossi, D., Vila, M., Malta, M. The children of Mama Coca: coca, cocaine and the fate of harm reduction in South America. *International Journal of Drug Policy* 2007;18(2): 99–106.

Campbell, C. *Letting them die: how HIV/AIDS prevention programmes often fail.* Cape Town, South Africa: Doublestorey Press, 2003.

Davis, M. *Planet of slums*. London: Verso, 2006.

Costenbader, E.C., Latkin, C. and Astone, N. The dynamics of injection drug users' personal networks and HIV risk behaviors. *Addiction* 2006;101:1003–1013.

Doherty, I.A., Padian, N.S., Marlow, C., Aral, S.O. Determinants and consequences of sexual networks as they affect the spread of sexually transmitted infections. *Journal of Infectious Diseases* 2005;191(Suppl. 1): S42–S54.

Farmer, P. *Infections and inequality: The modern plaques*. Berkeley: University of California Press, 2001.

Friedman, S.R. HIV-related politics in long-term perspective. *AIDS Care* 1998a:10 (Suppl. 2):S93–S103.

Friedman, S.R. The political economy of drug-user scapegoating—and the philosophy and politics of resistance. *Drugs: Education, Prevention, and Policy* 1998b:5(1):15–32.

Friedman, Samuel R., Bolyard, Melissa, Maslow, Carey, Mateu-Gelabert, Pedro, Sandoval, Milagros. Networks, risk-reduction communication, and norms. *Focus* 2005;20(1) (January):5–6.

Friedman, S.R., Bolyard, M., Mateu-Gelabert, P., Goltzman, P., Pawlowicz, M.P., Zunino Singh, D., Touze, G., Rossi, D., Maslow, C., Sandoval, M., Flom, P.L. Some data-driven reflections on priorities in AIDS network research. *AIDS and Behavior*, 2007.

Friedman, S.R., Cooper, H.L.F., Tempalski, B., Keem, M., Friedman, R., Flom, P.L., Des Jarlais, D.C. Relationships of deterrence and law enforcement to drug-related harms among drug injectors in U.S.A. metropolitan areas. *AIDS* 2006;20(1):93–99, January 2.

Friedman, S.R., Curtis, R., Neaigus, A., Jose, B., Des Jarlais D.C. *Social networks, drug injectors' lives, and HIV/AIDS*. New York: Kluwer/Plenum, 1999.

Friedman, S.R., Des Jarlais, D.C., Ward, T.P. Social models for changing health-relevant behavior. In R. DiClemente and J. Peterson (eds.), *Preventing AIDS: Theories and methods of behavioral interventions* (pp. 95–116). New York: Plenum Press. 1994.

Friedman, S.R., Flom, P.L., Kottiri, B.J., Sandoval, M., Neaigus, A., Maslow, C., et al. Networks, norms and HIV risk in New York City. *The Network Paradigm in Research on Drug Abuse, HIV, and Other Blood-borne and Sexually Transmitted Infections: New Perspectives, Approaches, and Applications, Meeting Proceedings.* 2002:41–49.

Friedman, S.R., Kippax, S.C., Phaswana-Mafuya, N., Rossi, D., Newman, C.E. Emerging future issues in HIV/AIDS social research. *AIDS* 2006a;20:959–960.

Friedman, Samuel R., Maslow, Carey, Bolyard, Melissa, Sandoval, Milagros, Mateu-Gelabert, Pedro, Neaigus, Alan. Urging others to be healthy: "Intravention" by injection drug users as a community prevention goal. *AIDS Education and Prevention* 2004;16:250–263.

Friedman, S.R., Neaigus, A., Jose, B., Curtis, R., Goldstein, M., Ildefonso, G., Rothenberg, R.B., Des Jarlais, D.C. Sociometric risk networks and HIV risk. *American Journal of Public Health* 1997;87(8):1289–1296.

Friedman, S.R., Neaigus, A., Jose, B., Curtis, R., Ward, T.P., Des Jarlais, D.C. Social models for altering health-relevant behavior. *Publicacion Oficial de la Sociedad Española Interdisciplinaria de S.I.D.A.* 1995(6)3:153–158.

Friedman, S.R., Reid, G. The need for dialectical models as shown in the response to the HIV/AIDS epidemic. *Int J Sociol Soc Policy* 2002;22:177–200.

Friedman, Samuel R., Rossi, Diana, Flom, Peter L. (2006b). "Big events" and networks: Thoughts on what could be going on. *Connections* 2006b 27(1):9–14.

Fullilove, Mindy Thompson. *Root shock: How tearing up city neighborhoods hurts America, and what we can do about it.* New York: Ballantine Books, 2004.

Gisselquist, D. Impact of long-term civil disorders and wars on the trajectory of HIV epidemics in sub-Saharan Africa. *Journal of Social Aspects of HIV/AIDS Research Alliance* 2005;1.

Hankins, C.A., Friedman, S.R., Zafar, T., Strathdee, S.A. Transmission and prevention of HIV and sexually transmitted infections in war settings: Implications for current and future armed conflicts. *AIDS* 2002;16(17), 2245–2252.

Heckathorn, Douglas D. Collective sanctions and compliance norms: A formal theory of group-mediated social control. *Amer Sociological Rev* 1990;55:366–384.

Heckathorn, Douglas D., Broadhead, Robert S., Anthony, Denise L., Weakliem, David L. AIDS and social networks: HIV prevention through network mobilization. *Sociological Focus* 1999;32:159–179.

Kottiri, B.J., Friedman, S.R., Neaigus, A., Curtis, R., and Des Jarlais, D.C. Risk networks and racial/ethnic differences in the prevalence of HIV infection among injection drug users. *Journal of Acquired Immune Deficiency Syndromes*, 2002;30(1): 95–104.

Kretzschmar, M., Morris, M. (1996). Measures of concurrency in networks and the spread of infectious disease. *Math Biosci.* 1996 (April 15) 133(2):165–195.

Latkin, C.A., Forman, V., Knowlton, A., Sherman, S. (2003). Norms, social networks, and HIV-related risk behaviors among urban disadvantaged drug users. *Social Science and Medicine* 56(3), 465–476.

Latkin, C.A., Mandell, W., Vlahov, D., Knowlton, A.R., Oziemkowska, M., Celentano, D.D. (1995). Personal network characteristics as antecedents to needle-sharing and shooting gallery attendance. *Social Networks*, 1995;17 (3–4):219–228.

Mann, J.M. Heterosexual transmission of HIV: a global view a decade later. *Int J STD AIDS* 1993;4:353–356.

Mann, J., Tarantola, D. The global AIDS pandemic. Toward a new vision of health. *Infect Dis Clin North Am* 1995;9:275–285.

Mann, J., Tarantola, D., O'Malley, J. Toward a new health strategy to control the HIV/AIDS pandemic. Global AIDS Policy Coalition. *J Law Med Ethics* 1994;22:41–52.

Myer, L., Morroni,C., Susser, E.S. Commentary: The social pathology of HIV/AIDS pandemic. *International Journal of Epidemiology*, 2003;32:189–192.

Neaigus, A., Friedman, S.R., Curtis, R., Des Jarlais, D.C., Furst, R.T., Jose, B., Mota, P., Stepherson, B., Sufian, M., Ward, T., Wright, J.W. The relevance of drug injectors' social networks and risk networks for understanding and preventing HIV infection. *Social Science and Medicine* 1994;38(1): 67–78.

Neaigus, A., Gyarmathy, V.A., Miller, M., Frajzyngier, V.M., Friedman, S.R., Des Jarlais, D.C. Transitions to injecting drug use among noninjecting heroin users: social network influence and individual susceptibility. *Journal of Acquired Immune Deficiency Syndromes* 2006;41(4):493–503.

Parker, R.G. 1996. Empowerment, community mobilization and social change in the face of HIV/AIDS. *AIDS* 10 (Suppl. 3)S27–S31.

Potterat, J.J., Muth, S.Q., Rothenberg, R.B., Zimmerman-Rogers, H., Green, D.L., Taylor, J.E., Bonney, M.S., White, H.A. Sexual network structure as an indicator of epidemic phase. *Sex Transm Infect* 2002; 78:152i–158.

Rhodes, T., Lowndes, C., Judd, A., Mikhailova, L.A., Sarang, A., Rylkov, A., Tichonov, M., Lewis, K., Ulyanova, N., Alpatova, T., Karavashkin, V., Khutorskoy, M., Hickman, M., Parry, J.V., Renton, A. Explosive spread and high prevalence of HIV infection among injecting drug users in Togliatti City, Russia. *AIDS* 2002;16(13):F25–F31.

Rhodes, T., Simic, M. Transition and the HIV risk environment. *BMJ* 2005;331:220–223.

Rischard, J.-F. *High noon: 20 global problems, 20 years to solve them.* New York: Basic Books, 2002.

Rothenberg, R.B., Potterat, J.J., Woodhouse, D.E., Muth, S.Q., Darrow, W.W., Klovdahl, A.S. Social network dynamics and HIV transmission. *AIDS* 1998:1529–1536.

Spiegel, P.B. HIV/AIDS among conflict-affected and displaced populations: Dispelling myths and taking action. *Disasters* 2004;28:322–339.

Stillwaggon, E. *AIDS and the ecology of poverty.* New York: Oxford University Press, 2006.

Teixeira, P.M. Program implementation and scaling up: Barriers and successes. 14th International AIDS Conference, Barcelona, Spain, 2002.

Wallace, D., Wallace, R. (1998). *A plague on your houses*. New York: Verso, 1998.
Weiss, R.A., McMichael, A.J. Social and environmental risk factors in the emergence of infectious diseases. *Nature Medicine*, 2004;10(12 Suppl.):S70–S76.
Westerhaus, Michael J., Finnegan, Amy C., Zabulon, Yoti, Mukherjee, Joia S. Framing HIV prevention discourse to encompass the complexities of war in northern Uganda. *Am J Public Health* 2007;97:1184–1186.
Williams, B., Campbell, C. Mines, migrancy and HIV in South Africa—managing the epidemic. *South African Medical Journal* 1996; 86:1249–1251.

CHAPTER 34

Feelings, Bodies, Places

New Directions for Geographies of HIV/AIDS

Jason Myers and Robin Kearns

ABSTRACT

The authors reflect on the shift towards alternative constructions of location and movement born of new developments in human geography: concerns with embodiment and emotions. Our concern is with how HIV/AIDS might more firmly be incorporated into the palpable world of everyday life in which literal place as well as place-in-the-world (e.g., status, identity) is irrevocably linked to one's appearance, demeanor, and feelings. We contend that the body can make a difference in the ways in which place is experienced, and that this concern informs an interest in the mobility of people living with HIV/AIDS (rather than movement of the virus itself). We explore the potential for the acquisition of HIV/AIDS to be constructed as a "moving experience," both in terms of the re/dislocations experienced in managing change, and the emotional transitions embedded in such moves.

OVERVIEW

Two recent items within the New Zealand print media speak to different geographies of HIV/AIDS that are distinctive for their interweaving of feelings, bodies and places. First, the *Christchurch Press* reports Hugh Board, a 42-year-old heterosexual, as dying of AIDS after having acquired HIV eighteen years ago. Board is reported to be starting a national peer support group for other straight men infected with HIV. His prompt is years of having been called a "faggot" and enduring "crude innuendo about his sex life." In his words, reflecting the spatial correlates of stigma, "people have literally backed away" when told of his HIV-positive status (*The Press* 2005). Second, the *Auckland City Harbour News* reports an "emotional farewell," not to an AIDS victim, but rather to Herne Bay House, New Zealand's only hospice for AIDS sufferers. The hospice's chief executive Dianne Robertson is quoted as saying "It's great that fewer people are dying of the disease." However, "a large number of the gay community, the main users of the facility, opposed the closure because of a strong emotional connection to it. Many have come here to tend to dying friends and partners. They have planted trees in the garden in memory of loved ones" (see Exhibit 34.1).

The foregoing stories speak to the importance of, and connection between, embodiment and emotion in geographical experience of HIV/AIDS. In the first example, the biomedical notion of someone being a "carrier" of a disease is transformed through recognising the way that disease as an experience is as much attributed through stigma as acquired through infection. In the second example, illness is revealed as embodied not only in the infected person, but also as more broadly memorialised in place. Thus, to those who have lost loved ones in a particular dwelling

Exhibit 34.1 Dianne Robertson mourns the closure of Herne Bay House

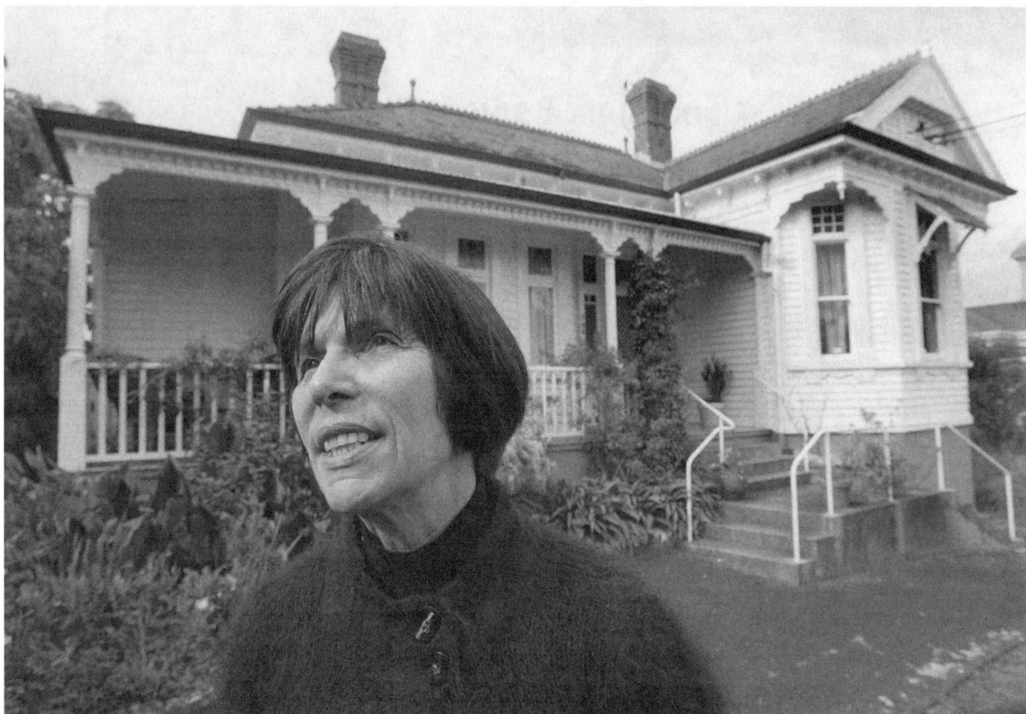

Source: Auckland City Harbour News, 16/9/2005

and site of care, its closure is "emotional" for the sense of loss and bereavement-of-place.

In this chapter, we acknowledge the valuable contribution that geographers have made in mapping aspects of location and movement in the early spread of HIV/AIDS. We argue, however, that a focus on these aspects of the disease has inevitably elided encounters with persons and places. Further, we follow earlier writers such as Michael Brown (1995a) in suggesting that such work risks a preoccupation with the geometric properties of space and a distancing from embodied human experience. We recognise that wider shifts in health geographies involving the so-called "qualitative turn" and acknowledgment of difference have resulted in some of the lived experiences of HIV/AIDS being heard (Gesler and Kearns 2002). However, we contend that there is scope for embracing everyday geographies to a greater extent. We pursue this contention by reflecting upon the move towards alternative constructions of location and movement born of new developments in human geography: concerns with embodiment and emotions.

Our primary concern is with how HIV/AIDS might more firmly be incorporated into the palpable world of everyday life in which literal place as well as place-in-the-world (e.g., status, identity) is linked to one's appearance, demeanor, and feelings. We address this concern by surveying the emerging field of "emotional geographies." Here, we follow recent calls to consider more deeply the ways that social life is constructed and lived through the emotions by suggesting the value in injecting "feeling" into geographies of HIV/AIDS. We draw on ideas of the body as a space marking the boundary between self and other, and as a site of struggle and contestation. We contend that the body can make a difference in the ways in which space is experienced, and that this concern informs an interest in the mobility of people living with HIV/AIDS (rather than the virus itself). Essentially, we explore the potential for the acquisition of HIV/AIDS to be constructed as a "moving experience," both in terms of the re/dislocations experienced in managing change, and the emotional transitions embedded in such moves.

HIV/AIDS AND GEOGRAPHY: CHARTING AN EPIDEMIC

The early and valuable contributions by geographers towards understanding spatial dimensions of HIV/AIDS have primarily centred on the *location* and *movement* of the disease (e.g., Dutt et al. 1987; Gardner et al. 1989; Shannon and Pyle 1989; Wood 1988). However, the application of these spatial-analytic approaches to examining HIV/AIDS involved a "preoccupation with the geometric properties of space" and took three main forms (Kearns 1996: 124). *First*, geographers mapped evidence of the disease, attempting to trace its origins. Among the earliest work, Wood (1988) examined the international patterns and paths of HIV/AIDS across a range of countries. A year later, Shannon and Pile (1989) suggested that, while a specific geography of the origin and diffusion of HIV remained incomplete, a partial reconstruction of the spatial pathways was a possibility. Using information reported to the World Health Organization, the authors developed a map proposing diffusion of AIDS during the 1970s and 1980s. In a *second* form of spatial-analytic work, geographers employed predictive modeling techniques to map the future spatial diffusion of HIV/AIDS. These models provided estimates of disease diffusion for actual regions and countries as well as predicting future infection paths within "high-risk" groups. Loyotonnen (1991), for example, employed statistics from 1982 to 1987 to predict future infection rates in Finland while Shannon et al. (1991) forecasted future infection rates among homosexuals, prostitutes, and intravenous drug users in the U.S. *Third*, and arguably most substantially, geographers have mapped the progression of HIV/AIDS across national and regional spaces. Dutt et al. (1987), for instance, analyzed data on the incidence of AIDS between 1981 and 1986 as reported to the United States Centers for Disease Control. This study emphasized national and regional patterns by sex, race, age cohorts, and survival rates. In a second example, Gardner et al. (1989) analyzed data from the first twenty-two months of the Department of Defense's HIV screening program for military applicants. While movement of the disease was linked to possible interventions, it disconnected from an understanding of on-the-ground experience.

An understanding of both the patterns or origin of HIV/AIDS and the mechanisms for infection and diffusion has undoubtedly been fundamental in the development of intervention strategies to try and control its spread. In this way, geographers added invaluable insight in the early years of the epidemic (Kearns 2003). However, notwithstanding the strength and quality of these studies, they have been critiqued for what they fail to represent. Most centrally, the spatial-science approach employed in the early years of geography's contribution to an understanding of HIV/AIDS, is said to have contributed to a silencing of the voices and experiences of those with the embodied experience of the disease. Indeed, Wilton asserts that, while the mapping of the virus has been important, it has provided "only a single, and necessarily partial, geography of AIDS" (1996: 70). Brown goes further in suggesting that the "pain, suffering and struggles that have certainly altered places where AIDS has struck" has not been captured (1995a: 174). These commentaries by geographers steeped in political and social traditions in the discipline align with a more general critique of medical geography that arose in the 1990s. This view held that, through its models and methods, the subdiscipline risked implicitly reducing the body to little more than a container of disease (Kearns 1993). It was claimed that medical geography distanced itself from gay men and their spaces in these early years and that the knowledge amassed about HIV/AIDS was produced at the expense of understanding its social dimensions. Writers such as Brown (1995a) contended that the uncritical adoption of an epidemiological model by medical geographers legitimated the focus for early studies of the virus and its travel across space. Essentially, occurrences of illness were commonly reduced to dots on a map, an abstraction seen by Dyck and Kearns (1995) to be culturally unsafe. As a consequence, gay men were "closeted by this spatial-scientific geography of AIDS" (Brown 1995a: 161).

EXPERIENCES OF ILLNESS: A SIGN OF THE TIMES

With the increasing use of the sub-disciplinary term "health geography" since the mid-1990s, geographers interested in disease and human wellbeing have embraced a shift in both the theories and concepts guiding their research as well as the methods employed (Gesler and Kearns 2002). Conventionally, quantitative methods have guided inquiry in medical geography. The emergence of humanistic geography, offering an explicit critique of the prevailing spatial paradigm in the 1970s, involved a modest but growing challenge to the prevailing mechanistic and purportedly "objective" research approaches in the discipline (Entrikin 1976). As the philosophical base of this critique differentiated and deepened over thirty years, the importance of meanings, values, and the human significance of life events has become deeply entrenched throughout much social and cultural geography. Alongside this shift, qualitative methodologies have become increasingly central in the practice of human geography (Dwyer and Limb 2001; Hay 2005). The maturity of this change is reflected in the observation that we have moved from seeing papers prefaced with legitimations of qualitative methods to observing debates among geographical methodologists over establishing orthodox approaches and standards in qualitative work (Crang 2002).

While the geographical pattern of any distribution of disease incidence or care services can be discerned, mapped, and explained, it is only relatively recently that "maps of meaning," or commonly understood ways of seeing the world (Jackson 1989) have become legitimate context for social inquiry within health geography. In seeking to acknowledge and interpret *experience*, we are in a position to discover more about the social determinants of health status, the plurality of health care modalities, and the multiple ways in which people, place, and health recursively constitute each other (Dyck and Kearns 1995). Fundamentally, geographers have embraced a shift towards a focus on "wellbeing" as opposed to a concern with essentially negative aspects of physical and mental health (i.e., illness, injury, impairment) (Kearns and Moon 2002). To this extent, connections with the more life-giving aspects of even severely challenging medical conditions becomes possible, especially given the breadth and depth of recent theoretical formulations like "therapeutic landscapes" (Gesler 1991).

Reflecting shifts in the wider discipline, alternative geographies of HIV/AIDS were crafted through the 1990s (see, e.g., Brown 1994, 1995a, 1995b, 1997; Geltmaker 1992; Wilton 1996, 1998, 1999). Brown's (1995b) work on AIDS politics in Vancouver, for example, provides a good example of a geography of AIDS distanced from the spatial science which characterized studies in the early years of the epidemic. The work of Geltmaker (1992), who considers AIDS activism in Los Angeles, is another. In this research, the author considers the ways in which struggles against the stigmatization of AIDS force gay men to reject the relative pleasures of the "closet." An insistence from within the gay community on the right to be "queer" comes out of such struggles (Geltmaker 1992). In a study surveying experiences of living with HIV/AIDS, Wilton (1996) suggests that the appearance of HIV, its development into AIDS, and the myriad of complications that accompany these events profoundly affects the geography of people's daily lives. He asserts that studies of the experience(s) of HIV/AIDS can serve to augment an overall understanding of the illness by illustrating the nature and extent of its impact. This wider understanding of the ways in which people live their lives post-HIV/AIDS diagnoses recognizes that there exists a variety of dimensions that combine to influence individual experience. Within this diversity, there are some important similarities which make it possible to conceptualize common life paths and trajectories. From diagnoses onwards, he suggests that a series of stages termed "shock," "cocoon," "emergence," "relapse" and "recovery" can be used to characterize the embodied experience of HIV post-diagnosis (Gesler and Kearns 2002). Words like "shock" and "cocoon," however, are charged with emotion and implications of embodied experience, challenging us to seek deeper understandings of the links between feeling, bodies, and place.

EMBODYING GEOGRAPHIES OF HIV/AIDS

A key recognition for appreciating the centrality of place in the experience of illness and disease is the contestation of the Cartesian mind/body dualism that has permeated much Western scholarship. As feminist geographers contend (e.g., Longhurst 1997), the body must be regarded as more than a mere container for consciousness. Rather, an understanding of bodily experience is crucial knowledge of people's relationships with physical and social environments. If this view is accepted, then the mind cannot be implicitly privileged over the body.

Upon acceptance of these contentions, we can begin to see the inherent interdependence of bodily experience and cognitive worldview. Indeed, the very idea of sense of place becomes transformed from a mental construct (as in "mental maps") to a recursive relation between actual experienced place and a Heideggerian notion of place-in-the-world (with implications of identity and status) (Eyles 1985). Thus, the notion of embodied human experience can be seen as incorporating mental, spiritual, and physical functions at an individual level, and by its very nature (i.e., being rooted in ideas of identity and perceived and attributed status) is social in character.

The writing of French theorist Henri Lefebvre can also assist in forging a place for the body as both experienced through place and in actively producing geographies of HIV/AIDS. In Lefebvre's (1991) discussion of the construction of social space, he gives a central place to the body, arguing that social practice presupposes the use of the body and that the body is inherent to the lived experience. As others have since contended, it is axiomatic that the world, including society, is perceived through the body via the senses (Rodaway 1994). In this way social practice is inherently a bodily experience that is involved in the process of constituting social spaces. Each living body both *is* space and *produces* space (Simonsen 2005). Extending these assertions to the theme of this chapter and book, it is paradoxical, perhaps, that the acquisition of a life-altering disease can lead to someone both "needing space" (to adjust to a changed identity) and being spatially isolated (through the experience of stigma). These deployments of space involve and invoke different emotions, a dimension of geographical experience to which we now turn.

EMOTIONAL GEOGRAPHIES: FEELINGS, BODIES, PLACES

In an often-cited editorial, Anderson and Smith (2001) consider the extent to which the human world is constructed and lived through the emotions and contend that emotions have been largely silenced in both social research and public life. The consequences of this silence have been noted (e.g., Williams 2001; Neu 2000; Pugmire 1998). In human geography, talk of emotion has conventionally been reserved for the cultural, and often feminist, domains of the discipline (see Koskela 2000; Nash 1998; Smith 2000 and Widdowfield 2000, for example). The "gendered nature of knowledge production is probably a key reason why the emotions have been banished from social science and most other critical commentary for so long" (Anderson and Smith 2001: 7). Indeed, it is claimed that the marginalization of emotion has been part of a "gender politics of research" (Anderson and Smith 2001: 7). Detachment, objectivity, and rationality have been valued and implicitly masculinized, while engagement, subjectivity, passion, and desire have been devalued and frequently feminized. The net result has been a discipline that Davidson, Bondi, and Smith (2005: 1) call "an emotionally barren terrain, a world devoid of passion, spaces ordered solely by rational principles." One reason for this situation is that emotions have often been considered as subjective and few attempts have been made to understand their connections to wider and often extremely crucial social processes. However, Koskela (2000) suggests that it remains crucial for us to interrogate the broader structures in which emotions are embedded. Whereas emotions themselves may be subjective, "emotional space" is social (Koskela 2000: 258). Anderson and Smith (2001) claim that a complete understanding of the world cannot be reached without a consideration of the place of emotions, a key set of relations through which lives are lived and societies made.

Wood and Smith (2004) argue that when considering aspects of everyday life, an understanding of emotions is crucial if we want to fully appreciate how the world of human interaction works. Agreeing that emotional experiences and relationships have been marginalized in human geography for too long, Wood and Smith (2004) claim that we need to understand emotions if we are to properly appreciate how lives are lived, histories experienced, geographies made, and futures shaped. Similarly, Davidson and Milligan argue that emotions:

> have tangible effects on our surroundings and can shape the very nature and experience of our being-in-the-world. Emotions can clearly alter the way the world *is* for us, affecting our sense of time as well as space. Our sense of who and what we are is continually (re)shaped by how we *feel*. (2004: 524)

Davidson and Bondi claim, emphatically, that "our emotions matter," for:

> whether we crave emotional equilibrium, or adrenaline thrills, the dynamic nature of our being-in-the-world entails a degree of instability for all of us. Whether joyful or heartbreaking, emotion has the power to transform the shape of our life-worlds, expanding or contracting, creating new fissures or fixtures we never expected to find. (2004: 373)

Following these calls for greater recognition of the place of feelings in everyday geographies, new lines of inquiry have emerged with emotion interrogated at a range of spatial scales. For example, while Twigg (2000) and Milligan (2003) have examined the place of emotion in the home, Blackman (1998) and Fielding (2000) survey "feelings" within institutional settings and Panelli et al. (2004) interrogate the place of emotion in communities. Arguably, however, the most popular site for discussions of emotion to date has been the body. Indeed, Davidson and Milligan (2004) suggest that much of the recent work on emotion has gained benefit from previous inquiry into geographies of the body. The body, after all, is the primary site of emotional experience and expression for even the most mundane of day-to-day tactics, such as eating, working, talking, and walking, cannot be carried out without some level of "feeling" (Davidson and Milligan 2004).

Geographers of health and illness have arguably been at the forefront in acknowledging emotions in conceptualizing the subjective experience of "feelings" and their links with place (Davidson and Milligan 2004). Moreover, they have often done so through examining the feelings of people experiencing illness or disabling conditions. Empirical investigations, for example, have highlighted the links between experiences of place, individual conceptions of health, and the provision of health care (Moss and Dyck 1996). Charmaz (1983) discusses the loss of self which accompanies the chronically ill and Wilton et al. (1997) assert that this loss of self can come from the construction of difference. The latter writers suggest that the production of difference is a "social and spatial process which allows the self to be partitioned from the other" (1997: 455). The end result of such processes is the stigmatization of entire classes of people and the production of rules for boundary maintenance between different groups.

The treatment of the chronically ill female body that Moss and Dyck (1996, 2003) offer is one example of how, for some time, health geographers have been considering the links between feelings, bodies, and places. The authors argue that in the reconceptualizing of health and illness that has accompanied a "new" medical geography, it is important not to take individual experiences of environment, health, and illness out of context (Moss and Dyck 1996). Women with chronic illnesses "negotiate meanings of health, illness, and body and forge their identities, both individual and collective, within a circumscription of multiple sets of social and structural relations" (Moss and Dyck 1996: 741). At home, for example, space is restructured in order to reassert control over sites originally designed for an able-bodied person. Elsewhere, a range of performances are mastered in the workplace so that the person appears as able-bodied as possible. These efforts are made in an attempt to adjust the process of "disablement" (Moss and Dyck 1996). We know that the ways in which people present themselves and "perform" in particular places is a result of both their awareness of what they know or believe themselves to be and how they believe others view them—and hence what they believe to be expected of them (Goffman 1963). To avoid social stigma, people who experience disabling conditions frequently attempt to "pass" as being as healthy as possible (Dyck 1999). These observations are readily transferable to concerns with HIV/AIDS.

The threat or actual experience of stigma, as well as concerns for managing one's performance of everyday life, can lead to movement in the lives of those experiencing HIV. Ellis (1996), for example, examined the movement of people living with AIDS in Florida. The study concluded that HIV diagnosis does have an effect on the spatial distribution of those people living with the virus and the most common move was one toward care facilities. Perhaps unsurprisingly, Ellis (1996) found that the stage of the illness determined the extent of movement. Those recently diagnosed with HIV were more likely to move to urban centers where care facilities and social networks were readily available. Those in the later stages of HIV and AIDS were more likely to move away to rural areas where, for example, they could be with families as they experienced the demise of their health (Ellis 1996). Thus, from Ellis's work, we can read the urban as a context of opportunity for care, if not cure, whereas the rural can be seen as a site of retreat and "therapeutic landscape" (Gesler 1991; Williams 1999).

RESEARCHING NEW SPACES OF, AND PLACES FOR, POSITIVE PEOPLE

Geographical research in the directions outlined by this chapter might begin with observation, and interpretation of the "ordinary" landscapes of everyday life. How, for example, is HIV/AIDS discussed in the media? Where are facilities targeting the needs of people who have acquired the virus? How are such facilities as Herne Bay House, discussed at the opening of this chapter, or Casey House in Toronto (see Chiotti and Joseph 1995), embodied in the landscape? How do users, providers, and members of the general public feel about their presence? Given their contribution to the landscape, how is emotion and embodiment deployed in billboard-based HIV prevention campaigns? Informal landscapes such as graffiti also speak to our themes of feelings, bodies and places as well as opening possibilities of observing sites of resistance (see Exhibit 34.2).

Closer engagement with these directions requires a deepening of understanding and a fostering of empathy. We are led to engage with ethics and experience, two domains less commonly encountered on a sustained basis by geographers working on patterns of HIV/AIDS. While the negotiations required by institutional committees to gain ethical approval to contact and interview those experiencing HIV/AIDS may stretch our patience as researchers, the gains may be a greater commitment to two-way flows of knowledge. Such efforts offer the possibility of offering some modest counterbalance to the way ill bodies—especially in the gay community—have been subjected to examination and inquiry. Further, creative and ethically sound methodologies offer possibilities that geographers might follow other social scientists and recognize what Butler (1999) calls the complexities involved in people's embodied experiences. These "complexities" risk remaining unheard in societies which are dominated by ableist and heteropatriarchal perspectives and power struc-

Exhibit 34.2 Graffiti suggesting sites of resistance, Downtown East Side, Vancouver, 1994

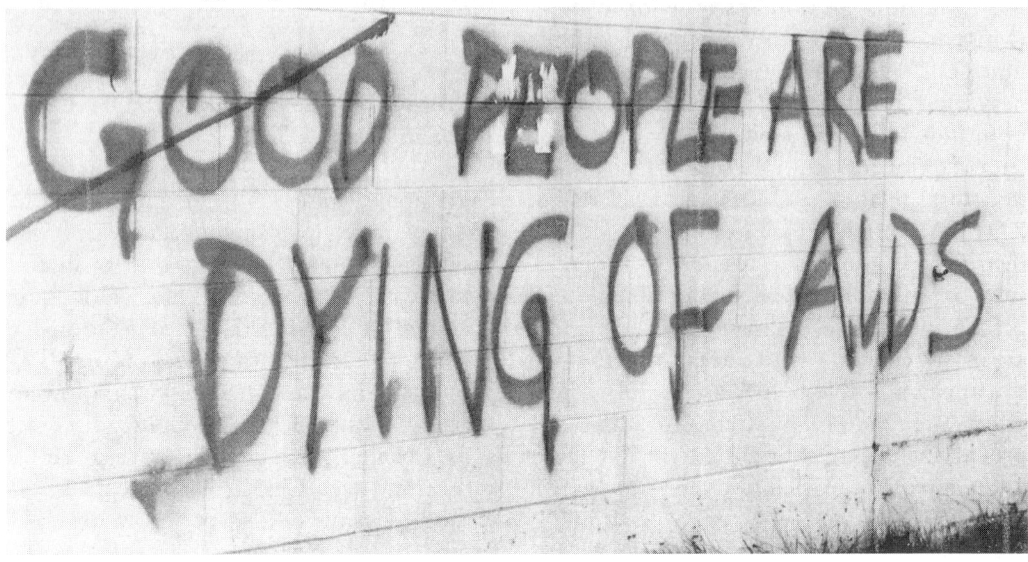

Source: Robin Kearns

tures. A knowledge of the powerful role of place in constructing and recreating the experience of illness also risks remaining unheard by society at large. Constructing and conveying this knowledge of connections between bodies, places, and feelings offers a niche for the geographic imagination two decades on from the emergence of HIV/AIDS.

ACKNOWLEDGMENT

We acknowledge the helpful conversations with Professor Peter Davis and Bonnie-May Shantz during the writing of this chapter.

REFERENCES AND FURTHER READING

Anderson, K. and Smith, S. 2001 Editorial: emotional geographies, *Transactions of the Institute of British Geographers*, 26: 7–10.

Auckland City Harbour News 2005 Herne Bay House closes: emotional farewell, Friday, September 16, p. 1.

Blackman, S. 1998 "Poxy cupid!" An ethnographic account of a resistant female youth culture: the new wave of girls, in Skelton, T. and Valentine, G. (eds.) *Cool places: geographies of youth cultures*, Routledge, London.

Brown, M. 1994 The work of city politics: citizenship through employment in the local response to AIDS, *Environment and Planning A*, 26: 873–894.

Brown, M. 1995a Ironies of distance: an ongoing critique of the geographies of AIDS, *Environment and Planning D: Society and Space*, 13: 159–183.

Brown, M. 1995b Sex, scale and the "new urban politics": HIV-prevention strategies from Yaletown, Vancouver, in Bell, D. and Valentine, G. (eds.) *Mapping desire: geographies of sexualities*, London: Routledge, 246–263.

Brown, M. 1997 *Replacing citizenship: AIDS activism and radical democracy*, London: Guilford Press.

Butler, R. 1999 Double the trouble or twice the fun? Disabled bodies in the gay community, in Butler, R. and Parr, H. (eds.) *Mind and body spaces: geographies of illness, impairment and disability*, New York: Routledge, 203–220.

Charmaz, K. 1983 Loss of self: a fundamental form of suffering in the chronically ill, *Sociology of Health and Illness*, 5(2): 168–195.

Chiotti, Q. and Joseph, A. 1995 Casey House: interpreting the location of a Toronto AIDS hospice, *Social Science and Medicine*, 41(1): 131–140.

Crang, M. 2002 Qualitative methods: the new orthodoxy? *Progress in Human Geography*, 26(5): 647–655.

Davidson, J. and Bondi, L. 2004 Spatialising affect; affecting space: an introduction, *Gender, Place and Culture*, 11(3): 373–374.

Davidson, J. and Milligan, C. 2004 Editorial: embodying emotion sensing space: introducing emotional geographies, *Social and Cultural Geography*, 5(4): 523–532.

Davidson, J., Bondi, L., and Smith, M. 2005 *Emotional Geographies*. Aldershot: Ashgate Press.

Dutt, A., Monroe, C., Dutta, H., and Prince, B. 1987 Geographical patterns of AIDS in the United States, *Geographical Review*, 77(1): 456–471.

Dwyer, C. and Limb, M. 2001 Introduction: doing qualitative research in human geography, in Limb, M. and Dwyer, C. (eds.) *Qualitative methodologies for geographers: issues and debates*, London: Arnold, 1–20.

Dyck, I. 1999 Body troubles: women, the workplace and negotiations of a disabled identity, in Butler, R. and Parr, H. (eds.) *Mind and body spaces: geographies of illness, impairment and disability*, London: Routledge, 119–137.

Dyck, I. and Kearns, R. 1995 Transforming the relations of research: towards culturally safe geographies of health and healing, *Health and Place*, 1(3): 137–147.

Ellis, M. 1996 The postdiagnosis mobility of people with AIDS, *Environment and Planning A*, 28: 999–1017.

Entrikin, N. 1976 Contemporary humanism in geography, *Annals of the Association of American Geographers*, 66(4): 615–632.

Eyles, J. 1985 *Senses of place*, Cheshire: Silverbrook Press.

Fielding, S. 2000 Walk on the left! Children's geographies and the primary school, in Holloway, S. and Valentine, G. (eds.) *Children's geographies: playing, living, learning*, London: Routledge, 230–244.

Gardner, L., Brundage, J., Burke, D., McNeil, J., Visintine, R., and Miller, R. 1989 Spatial diffusion of the Human Immunodeficiency Virus infection epidemic in the United States: 1985–87, *Annals of the Association of American Geographers*, 79: 25–43.

Geltmaker, T. 1992 The queer nation acts up: health care, politics, and sexual diversity in the County of Angels, *Environment and Planning D: Society and Space*, 10: 609–650.

Gesler, W. 1991 *The cultural geography of healthcare*, Pittsburgh: University of Pittsburgh Press.

Gesler, W. and Kearns, R. 2002 *Culture/place/health*, London: Routledge.

Goffman, E. 1963 *Stigma: notes on the management of spoiled identity*, New Jersey: Prentice Hall.

Hay, I. (ed.) 2005 *Qualitative research methods in human geography*, 2nd edition, Melbourne: Oxford University Press.

Jackson, P. 1989 *Maps of meaning*. London: Unwin Hyman.

Kearns, R. 1993 Place and health: towards a reformed medical geography, *Professional Geographer*, 45(2): 139–147.

Kearns, R. 1996 AIDS and medical geography: embracing the other? *Progress in Human Geography*, 20(1): 123–131.

Kearns, R. 2003 New geographies of disease: HIV/AIDS, in Rogers, A. and Viles, H. (eds.) *The student's companion to geography*, Oxford: Blackwell, 138–142.

Kearns, R. and Moon, G. 2002 From medical to health geography: novelty, place and theory after a decade of change, *Progress in Human Geography*, 26(5): 605–625.

Koskela, H. 2000 The gaze without eyes: video-surveillance and the changing nature of urban space, *Progress in Human Geography*, 24: 243–265.

Lefebvre, H. 1991. *The production of space*, trans. D. Nicholson-Smith. Oxford: Blackwell.

Longhurst, R. 1997 (Dis)embodied geographies, *Progress in Human Geography*, 21: 486–501.

Loyotonnen, M. 1991 The spatial diffusion of the human immunodeficiency virus type 1 in Finland, 1982–1987, *Annals of the Association of American Geographers*, 81: 127–151.

Milligan, C. 2003 Location or dis-location: from community care to long term care—the caring experience, *Social and Cultural Geography*, 4: 455–470.

Moss, P. and Dyck, I. 1996 Inquiry into environment and body: women, work and chronic illness, *Environment and Planning D: Society and Space*, 14: 737–753.

Moss, P. and Dyck, I. 2003 *Women, body, illness: space and identity in the everyday lives of women with chronic illness*, Maryland: Rowman and Littlefield.

Nash, C. 1998 Mapping emotion, *Environment and planning D: Society and Space*, 16(1): 1–10.

Neu, J. 2000 *A tear is an intellectual thing: the meanings of emotion*, New York: Oxford University Press.

Panelli, R., Little, J., and Kraack, A. 2004 A community issue? rural women's feelings of safety and fear in New Zealand, *Gender, Place and Culture*, 11(3): 445–467.

Pugmire, D. 1998 *Rediscovering emotion*, Edinburgh: Edinburgh University Press.

Rodaway, P. 1994 *Sensuous geographies, body, sense, place*, London: Routledge.

Shannon, G. and Pyle, G. 1989 The origin and diffusion of AIDS: a view from medical geography, *Annals of the Association of American Geographers*, 79: 1–24.

Shannon, G., Pyle, G., and Bashshur, R. 1991 *The geography of AIDS: origins and course of an epidemic*, New York: The Guilford Press.

Simonsen, K. 2005 Bodies, sensations, space and time: the contribution from Henri Lefebvre. *Geografiska Anneler Series B: Human Geography* 87: 1–14.

Smith, S. 2000 Performing the (sound)world, *Society and Space*, 18: 615–637.

The Press. 2005 Dying victim plans AIDS group, Wednesday, October 5, p. A9.

Twigg, J. 2000 *Bathing—the body and community care*, London: Routledge.

Widdowfield, R. 2000 The place of emotions in academic research, *Area*, 32: 199–208.

Williams, A. (ed.) 1999 *Therapeutic landscapes: the dynamic between wellness and place*, Lanham: University of Press of America.

Williams, S. 2001 *Emotion and social theory: corporeal reflections on the (ir)rational*, London: Sage.

Wilton, R. 1996 Diminished worlds? the geography of everyday life with HIV/AIDS, *Health and Place*, 2(2): 69–83.

Wilton, R. 1998 The constitution of difference: space and psyche in landscapes of exclusion, *Geoforum*, 29: 173–185.

Wilton, R. 1999 Qualitative health research: negotiating

life with HIV/AIDS, *Professional Geographer*, 51(2): 254–264.

Wilton, R., Gaber, S., and Takahashi, L. 1997 Seeing people differently: the sociospatial construction of disability, *Environment and Planning D: Society and Space*, 15: 455–480.

Wood, N. and Smith, S. 2004 Instrumental routes to emotional geographies, *Social and Cultural Geography*, 5(4): 533–548.

Wood, W. 1988 AIDS north and south: diffusion patterns of a global epidemic and a research agenda, *Professional Geographer*, 40: 266–279.

CHAPTER 35

A Global Clinic?

Prevention, Treatment, and the Problem of Scale in the World Health Organization's 3X5 Antiretroviral Treatment Program

Cindy Patton

ABSTRACT

The twenty-first century may come to be known as the century of scales. The coexistence of the massive and tiny creates huge problems in trying to articulate the experience of disease, and in defining policy that will work for the many peoples and countries affected by the epidemic. In this speculative chapter, the author reviews some of the history of representing the "experience" of HIV, summarizing the two principal modes of "understanding the global" that arose in the first decade of the AIDS epidemic. The bulk of the chapter suggests how these framings continue to inhabit the conceptual framework of global AIDS policy and, specifically, how this plays out in debates about the ethical implementation of worldwide distribution of antiretrovirals.

> The benefits of ARV treatment for patients are well documented. There is also evidence that ARV treatment generates benefits for households and society . . . Progress has been made towards developing a **public health approach to ARV treatment**. This aims to provide treatment for as many people as possible, while working towards universal access to ARV treatment. More specifically, the public health approach is based on standardized first- and second-line treatment regimens with simplified laboratory monitoring. The public health approach for scaling up ARV treatment also calls for early involvement of a range of stakeholders, including people with HIV and other community members . . . Community members and people with HIV must be involved in the design, implementation and monitoring as well as patient care, especially for supporting adherence to treatment and prevention . . . By maintaining a rights-based approach towards increasing the participation of people with HIV in a meaningful and appropriate way, ARV treatment programmes will ensure better outcomes for treatment and prevention . . . Healthcare workers, people with HIV, family members, and the community all have an important role to play in supporting patient adherence and protective behaviour, as well as in minimizing stigma and discrimination. (Dhaliwal et al. 2003, 7–8)

* * *

> A key element of the public health approach is to provide potent and effective ARV therapies that maximize the benefit for individual participants in programmes and preserve the treatment prospect for future participants, taking into account the special circumstances in the developing world . . . This can only be achieved if the selected treatments suppress viral replication in a high proportion of individuals. Only maximal suppression of viral replication can prevent the emergence of resistant strains.
> (Hammer et al. 2002, 23)

In 2003, the World Health Organization (WHO) announced a bold program to deliver HIV antiretrovirals (HIV-ARV) to three million people by 2005. Soon dubbed "3X5," the program was destined to fall under heavy criticism from all quarters. I do not wish to condemn the program, but rather to place its rationale in the context of failed AIDS initiatives. As the two documents cited above reveal, an importantly different spin was required to sell 3X5 to different groups: document 1 (the toolkit) was aimed at local program managers; document 2 (the treatment guidelines) was for government officials and policymakers. Responding to the likelihood that localities might remain skeptical about what looks for the world like a pharmaco-imperialist scheme, the toolkit takes pains to emphasize family and community participation (albeit, primarily, as monitors of adherence). The public health position paper guidelines, meanwhile, emphasize the importance of not screwing around with drug calibration and fancy experimental regimens. Constructing a "public health" approach from the shattered remains of advice that doctors gave individual patients of the developed world in the halcyon first years of "AIDS cocktails"—to hit early, hit hard[1]—the world, as represented by the World Health Organization, having vacillated far too long, masks its lateness with largesse: the explicit logic of 3X5 is hit hard, and hit as many as possible. The humanitarian platitudes about rights-based approaches barely disguise the very late arrival of treatment to low-resource settings, and the marketing of 3X5 on the local level seems ignorant of the very problem global planners pointed to—possibly correctly—as the rationale for not jumping in "too early" with the high-tech, experimental medicine used in the West: the very, very scary question of triggering drug-resistant HIV strains is underplayed in all the WHO's 3X5 materials. Despite the widespread and rampant problem of tuberculosis (TB) variants that are resistant to nearly every drug—a problem that both fuels and is fueled by the poor success rates in HIV containment[2]—the WHO seems to have made peace with the likelihood that particular mutations will occur, and appears confident that the so-called "four Ss" (when to start, substitute for toxicity, switch for failure, or stop and move to end-of-life care) (Kim and Gilks 2005[3]) are up to their clinical task in the low-resource context. With phrases like "preserve the treatment for future participants," the WHO documents only gloss what are, to many critics, substantial clinical issues in the particular drug combinations on the WHO formulary. As many critics have noted, for example, the use of an especially effective but highly mutagenic combination for pregnant and potentially pregnant women (among the most mediagenic "faces of AIDS" in "Africa") may well decrease perinatal transmission, but at the cost of throwing these mothers into the category of people who, once they fail on the first line treatments, will not be able to "switch"—an unfortunate personal outcome in the short and medium term, a potentially disastrous epidemiologic one in the long term, as these young women, with impossible-to-suppress viral load, will then be perfectly able to pass on the viral mutation to subsequent foetuses, as well as sexual and drug injection partners.

In fact, until recently, there was little attempt to deal with HIV in "resource-poor settings" (as we have now learned to call the Third World/developing world) using antiretrovirals as a means of decreasing total load in a population. This is especially the case in African locales.[4] Many letters and articles from doctors and public health officials in-country—and frequently *of* country—challenge the whole idea that their (or their colleagues') clinical experiments in delivery of drug trials should be swept upward via a uniform WHO program of standards and practices, and then distributed to locales in the downdraft. It becomes clear that "scaling up" feels much more like imposing down than the high-flown WHO rhetoric of community design and control suggests. "Cloning" might have been a better approach, constituting lateral relationships in which proximate and comparable programs could essentially share notes, as occurred in the NGO/ASO movement heavily supported by Global Program on AIDS in the 1980s, when prevention was the word of the hour. But there are impediments to a cloning approach: as Brown and Brown (2005) argue in a brief analysis of the theoretical problems of the 3X5 scheme that was published as a letter to the editors in response to an editorial praising the program in the journal *Lancet*, the "local" proof of principle projects were set up not *like* but *as* clinical trials (let's call them Phase V trials), to test applicability and uptake of outmoded formularies in the Third World context.[5]

I remain agnostic about the successes and failures of the 3X5 program to date: if wealthy America had bothered to take the African situation seriously in 1985, we would not even be in this situation today. Indeed, every undertaking in this epidemic has entailed a kind of complicated tango of steps forward, backward, and sideways—usually, followed by stumbling and yet more steps which might be part of a different dance altogether! The 3X5 program is no different. This does not mean stalling 3X5, but rather making it work to moral standards higher than those conceived by the hydra-headed beast of Big Pharma, the World Bank, and the World Health Organization—each a many-headed beast in its own right. Thus, I temper my skepticism with the observation that 3X5's success is likely to remain impossible to adjudicate because the "performance standards" derive from divergent medical thoughtstyles which conceive epidemic, its location(s), and solution(s) in fundamentally irreconcilable ways. I have no advice about what steps should come next, but I can consider what possibilities might open up if we resituate the debates—human rights versus public health, access versus continuity of care, national economic stabilization versus reduction in suffering, and so on (themselves an extension of the history that led to and informed 3X5)—in the context of a long-standing contest over the "right" way to understand disease on the global scale. The facts that are said to demonstrate success or failure for a given strategy change meaning and use as they are placed on one side, then another, of the contest. In this case, most of the facts in the global construction of AIDS are established in one scientific thoughtstyle (mostly in epidemiology, with its superior counting and visualization techniques), but applied using another (tropical medicine, which, however envious of the statistical skills of its larger, better-funded brother, is nevertheless more intimately involved in the lives of the actual bodies that possess the disease). After a quick summary of the current criticisms of 3X5, I will focus on the seemingly transparent concept of "scaling up," teasing out what goes on in the name of science by focusing on the different meaning that "scale" has within epidemiology and tropical medicine as they try to understand and implement "treatment" and "prevention," a kind of "two-by-two box" (Exhibit 35.1) that provides opportunities to slip morality into the pocket of science and vice versa.

In the case of epidemiology's hope to end a disease (hence the convergence of treatment and prevention), morality rears its head in the disdain for the very public health (or rather, for the public) it is in service of. Paradoxically, given its much-criticized role in the imperial projects that laid the groundwork

Exhibit 35.1 2X2

	Treatment	*Prevention*
Epidemiology	ARVs	Condoms and ARVs
Tropical Medicine	ARVs	Education + vaccine

for the current state of infrastructural disrepair and high rate of bodily need, tropical medicine imagines carrying on in the face of disease. But because in this case the first-line solution—education—involves discussion of sexuality and drug use, it wears its morality on its sleeve: either "liberal Western" or "traditionalist" (both explicitly Muslim and crypto-Christian).

In this context, "scaling up" leads to either of two problems—or to both: 1) it feeds epidemiology's desire to accumulate more and more data by raising a question it can never answer, that is, the relative contribution of prevention versus treatment in reducing overall viral load in a population; and 2) it engenders a struggle to conquer the developing world through "non-judgmental" approaches to the social engineering required to stop HIV transmission, or at least channel it into the apparently more manageable forms seen in the West.

For complex reasons—none admirable—we lived for two decades with the belief that, as one WHO publication put it, "education is our only vaccine." After hard-working clinician-researchers proved to the world that low-resource settings could consistently deliver ARVs in a compassionate, equitable (in the most local sense), and continuous treatment, one of the major pretenses for not making drugs available outside the West dropped with a resounding thud. The human rights rhetoric of access for all, already fairly successful in the West, was established as feasible and available to be applied to the low-resource world. But as I will show below, the rights position, despite being a vital tool, runs headlong into the complexities of managing a "right" and a resource in contexts that have a scarcity of both, and at the same time provides a cover for a project that is fundamentally more interested in reducing total viral load than in ensuring the care of people with HIV and the continuation of the cultures in which these myriad individuals exist. This set of refracting mirrors of competing interests is housed, I want to suggest, in the divergent meanings that "scale" embodies in the 3X5 debates, depending on whether we situate ourselves within epidemiology or tropical medicine.

TWO THOUGHTSTYLES OF LONG DURATION . . .

In earlier work (Patton 1995, 1996), I floated and then elaborated (Patton 2002) the position that 1980s AIDS policy and media discourse inherited its "truths" from two different and in most ways incompatible medical "thoughtstyles."[6] Broadly speaking, one was derived from tropical medicine and one from epidemiology. I was able to synthesize the differences in the chart reproduced here (Exhibit 35.2), and then demonstrate how policymakers and media writers tacked between the two, employing one, then the other, as the local, cultural elements of a story refused to line up with the global scientific logic. In particular I argued that an ongoing problem in the implementation of prevention and, later, treatment programs in the countries most reliant on the WHO (those in the then-deemed "developing world") was that HIV is predominantly conceptualized, monitored, and treated through the logic of epidemiology, while programs are implemented through a model of local care that emerged at the WHO as it took its place on the transnational stage in the late colonial/early post-colonial era (largely, that is to say, after the perplexing remapping of the globe following World War II), an approach I link to tropical medicine. I argued that these two ways of seeing disease and its translocation were at odds, but that the tension between them was manageable as long as the many possible locales/tropicals could be imagined as essentially *the same* in the "proof of principle" ideology of the initial distribution programs[7]—no matter that the settings were acutely different at the cultural level, nor that they were collaborating with the drug-supplying transnational agencies for a host of different reasons (to get resources, to look democratic, and so on). Even the rationale for launching the demonstration projects, however lifesaving and humanitarian these were in the individual locales, was shot through with racist ideas[8] about the people who were meant to be served; to wit, the epidemiological worry that it would be impossible to get "Third World people" to be compliant with drug

Exhibit 35.2 Competing medical thought styles

Tropical thinking	*Epidemiological thinking*
Argues through homology	Argues through metonymic production of statistical correlation
Is obsessed with proximity	Is obsessed with transfer, between bodies or disease pools
Always visualizes bodies in the colonial map	Abstracts bodies in data
Uses melodramatic narrative	Uses detective narrative
Sees disease "there"	Sees disease everywhere
Spatializes	Temporalizes
Is diasporal	Is vectorial
Defines bodies in advance and in relation to their original space	Defines and redefines bodies through categories related to disease
Considers all bodies	Acknowledges no meaning for bodies beyond their relation to a succession of diseases
Maps	Simulates
Presents immunity as the solution	Presents cure, breaking vectorial links as solution
Is confounded when bodies "go native"—may allow for vectoriality	Is confounded by employing fragmentary descriptions of previous diseases—may resort to tropical maps

Source: Patton, *Globalizing AIDS* (2002)

regimens, and the tropical medicine worry that developing countries were too backward (infrastructurally or scientifically) to deliver Western medical schemes (meaning, high-tech medicine). I want to extend that analysis here, updating our understanding of what underlies a key piece of the contemporary AIDS puzzle: *the ongoing failure to implement prevention as an emancipatory social project rather than a responsibilizing behavioral project.*

In an unintentional echo of the earlier (failed) hopes of the 1978 Alma Ata conference proclamation of "Health for All by the Year 2000," much of the 3X5 literature lauds what are constructed as two scientific breakthroughs that now enable the world to imagine providing ARVs *for all.* In the 3X5 narrative, biomedical science found a treatment for HIV (the "cocktails" of the 1990s), and then clinicians, with social science as their handmaidens, found the means to distribute ARVs to hard-to-serve populations in the developing world and the poorer quarters of the rest. But I would roll the beast over and look at the belly: between the important scientific break in the "early years" of HIV (in the deployment of AZT, roughly 1981–88), when it first became possible to imagine a cure (understood as the elimination of HIV from all bodies, individual and corporate), and the present moment of pharmaco-distributional justice (in which the hope of ridding the body of HIV is gone, but the hope of eliminating HIV from the whole lingers on), something important happened. A new category of disease appeared (or so it seemed, if we recall that syphilis in between the disease-defining Wasserman test and the disease eradicating penicillin looked awful darn similar), one that was communicable through discrete and socially frowned upon acts, but which once acquired took a chronic infectious, progressive, and, in the West, manageable form. The reconceptualization of differences between the modeling of infectious *and* chronic dimensions of this and other diseases is in its infancy, and the significance of the reality that HIV is *both* is still not well recognized. In my view, this oversight fatally hampers HIV social epidemiology. Behind the media fanfare about saving individual lives, the corridors of epidemiology echoed with a message about population health: ARVs could effectively reduce to nil the ability of the seropositive person to transmit virus; ARVs saved the individual patients, but also—and perhaps, to some, more importantly—reduced the total amount of virus the uninfected population might be exposed to. But ARVs did not fulfill the Final Solution fantasy of eradicating HIV altogether; because ARV treatment was not a cure, there was always the possibility that the population effect could be reversed if enough patients failed on or stopped taking their drugs. This realization ushered in the current moment, starting in 2001 and up to today, in which the important scientific and social scientific developments that I will now describe became entwined.

First, in the West, concern arose about prevention among those on ARVs. This was a new kind of stigmatizing placement of responsibility on those who contracted HIV since, in the early years, the silent belief lodged in epidemiology's mind had been that the epidemic would be semi-self-limiting because the infected were, by dint of their deviance, isolated, and would in any event die relatively quickly. Despite the massive efforts to situate "safe sex" in the context of emancipation for sexually marginalized groups (reduced now in the WHO documents to those who are "discriminated against"), prevention had been about containing HIV in pockets and preventing entry of new individuals into those pockets.

Second, several clinical research teams "proved" that people in resource-poor settings could actually adhere to ARV regimens and achieve treatment results quite similar to those in the West. This opened the door both to human rights arguments for access to ARVs and to the drug companies, who were quite happy to have a secondary market for proven products at a time when rapidly evolving trial drugs and highly tailored regimens for those with access to high-tech monitoring were threatening the stability of the established markets.

These shifts became entwined through a discourse that always puts the blame for HIV back on those who have it. Like the vigilance exercised over the responsibilized, seropositive safe sex practitioner—always at risk of "relapse" and, via acts, returning her or his infectivity into the disease pool—the compliant ARV taker is also always at risk of becoming a viral hazard through failure to adhere to drug regimens. However, the difference between reducing viral transmission through blocking viral replication (ARVs) and reducing transmission through blocking exchange of infected fluids (condoms or always and already-safe acts) is far more than just a matter of convenience to those who would rather pursue sex in a condom-free world.[9] If the fluid-blocking logic was made explicit in that early admonition that "education is our only vaccine," in the new scientific context that has blurred the functions of vaccine and treatment the slogan might need a makeover to reflect the faith in viral-blocking: "treatment is our only education."

And actually, that is more or less how the 3X5 program efforts manage the difference between epidemiology's emphasis on cure and tropical medicine's preference for education and vaccination. The availability of treatment dramatically increased the need for HIV testing if the plan was to transform the simulated "estimated seropositive population" into actual, treatable patients. For epidemiology, then, "scaling up" means going from the virtual to the real, from the statistical to the clinical. For tropical medicine, scaling up entails vertical linkages through homology; that is, a body is like the family is like the community is like the nation.

3X5 ON THE GROUND

I would like to turn now to an overview of the two principal debates over the implementation of 3X5.

HIV Testing: The Education Versus Access Argument Replayed in the Emerging Democracy Context

One of the issues that has vexed longtime activists and community-connected researchers is the role of HIV testing. As WHO plans note, in order to deliver ARVs to those in need, individuals and/or their care provider must recognize that the individual is HIV positive. The only way to do this, obviously enough, is to test people. Even in heavily impacted areas, the sero-prevalence rate is not that high, so you have to test *a lot* of people—between 100 and 100,000 to identify a single HIV-positive person. This problem is not new. As HIV treatment became available in the late 1980s, the U.S. and other governments proposed more aggressive programs for identifying those who were good candidates for treatment. Fair enough. But the price of submitting to HIV testing is the admission/recognition that one has engaged in risk-relevant behaviors that are, and remain, socially stigmatized and conflated with social categories that are subject to discrimination (thus, heterosexual sex is conflated with sex workers, promiscuity and anal sex with gay men, needle sharing with draconian images of "drug addicts"). I will not rehearse the complex history of confidentiality breaches. The WHO has recognized this problem—how could they not, when the world's activist community had spoken loudly and continuously about the necessity to provide confidentiality if not anonymity in testing? The organization appears to address this issue in their guidelines: "The provision of antiretroviral treatment can reinforce effective prevention campaigns, stimulate voluntary counseling and testing and help to destigmatize HIV infection" (Hammer 2002, 22). However, this position is of little comfort since it presumes that the stigma is the result of disease and not racism, homophobia, and misogyny.[10]

Local Knowledge Versus Central Planning: The Epistemological Fallacy

As various regional and local medical authorities argue, the scaling-up program, full as it is of rhetoric about the integration of the local into the national, nonetheless misunderstands the dynamic of knowledge production. There is an assumption that everything learned through "local experience" can be summarized and writ large as a national plan. Thus, while apparently respecting the local,[11] the scaling-up process intrinsically elides it, as Brown and Brown (2005) note in their letter to the *Lancet*: "The first consultants needed to design [nationwide AIDS] programmes are not ART experts from great university centers of the west. Rather, they are the lowly clinic nurses and doctors who tend to patients every day and thus have some genuine experience with which to advise national programs" (Brown and Brown 2005, 117–118). However, this cry for local voices to be heard still replicates a model of interplay between big and small scales, rather than arguing for lateral exchanges across, even without national borders. The loss of the local in the transposition to the national results from the use of outmoded social theories that see the macro as the sum of the micro; hence, any "macro" program contains the micro programs, and any macro program can be enacted in a local by making it small.[12]

It is not obvious in the rhetoric of scales that the implementation of local—and especially locally generated and controlled—initiatives to combat AIDS was a huge accomplishment, though it certainly was. The social and clinical knowledge that made local programs possible was assembled through organic but strategic networks of people working at various levels in organizations like the Red Cross, and by local activists (some united early on by the efforts of the late Jonathan Mann, initial director of the WHO's Global Program on AIDS, or GPA) who came from AIDS activism, gay liberation, and the prostitutes' rights movement. Indeed, a now obscured (or lost) document from 1989 enumerated extant NGOs (nongovernmental organizations) that were ready to take up the challenge of grappling with AIDS in various locales. The document (as much as the sentiment that resulted in the effort to involve NGOs) was remarkable for proposing who should be invested with authority to respond to the epidemic, groups dizzyingly collected, side by side, and functioning at wildly different scales. I was involved in a small way in the identification of the groups, and was also somewhat critical[13] of the effort's lack of comprehensiveness; indeed, I was not yet able to realize the impossibility of calibrating different kinds of groups' contributions at different scales. Thus the problem of scale that hounds

3X5 was already embedded in the uneasy coalition of the range of NGOs/CBOs (community-based organizations) that came to be recognized as the "experts" in cultural and social aspects of HIV in the late 1980s. This is in part why there are a host of mostly good people and groups who appear as the "community" that can affect the "scale-up" from local to national to regional.

INTERMINGLING PREVENTION AND TREATMENT: WHAT "SCALING UP" PREVENTION FINALLY MEANS

As the debates about a global treatment program grew complex,[14] with a wide variety of objections coming from human rights groups, the place of best retreat for promoters of global solutions was to reframe the challenges as an issue of balancing treatment and prevention. Hot on the heels of arguments to scale up treatment came a push to "intensify" or scale up prevention, even though this had already failed in most cases. Indeed, the UNAIDS document on scaling up education (UNAIDS 2005) contains proposals that sound virtually identical to those of the late 1980s, when all WHO constituent governments were urged to come up with a national AIDS plan centered on prevention, decreasing stigma, and outlawing discrimination. (Curiously, in current planning documents where discrimination is frequently mentioned and frowned upon, the possibility for legal recourse in such cases has been dropped, or possibly sublated in terms like finding the "political will.") But while WHO advocacy for "scaling up prevention" looks superficially like a retread, their context and relationship to 3X5 makes the old concepts quite different:

> Universal access to antiretroviral therapy for everyone who is deemed as needful of it through medical criteria opens up ways to accelerate prevention in communities in which more people will know their HIV status—and, critically, will *want* to know their status. As HIV/AIDS becomes a disease that can be both prevented and treated, attitudes will change, and denial, stigma, and discrimination will rapidly be reduced. Rolling out effective HIV/AIDS treatment is the single activity that can most effectively energize and accelerate the uptake and impact of prevention. Under 3X5, this will occur as part of a comprehensive strategy linking treatment, prevention, care, and full social support for people affected by HIV/AIDS. Such support is critical—both to ensure adherence to ARV therapy, and to reinforce prevention (WHO 2003, 6).

But the interlinking of prevention and treatment, including the subordination of the former to the latter, requires renewed vigor from social epidemiology. The accelerating interest in using classical statistical procedures to conduct joint analysis of something measurable (the amount of virus in individuals added together to estimate the amount of virus in a grouping of people, some of whom already have the virus and some of whom don't) with something that is not measurable (the net effect over time—measured in terms of amount of virus available to leap from body to body—of various pressures to cease practices that enable the virus to move at all) enables epidemiology, that is, *social epidemiology*, to pass off bad policy—i.e., giving up emancipatory prevention—as good science.

The Risk of Breaking Frame

> Tropical medicine is changing. At last week's launch of the spectacular third edition of *Principles of Medicine in Africa* (Cambridge University Press), Professor Eldryd Parry, the book's chief editor, spoke movingly and passionately about Africa's new landscape of danger. Human displacement, an emerging epidemic of non-communicable disease, collapsing health systems, the desperate need for palliative care as the tidal wave of HIV-AIDS continues, and a callous denial of access to vital medicines . . . First, there must be a commitment to creating in-country capacity, notably a human capacity that can determine for itself problems to be addressed instead of having a westernised impression of those problems imposed from outside . . . Second, there must be a commitment to listen to local voices . . . And finally, research must be put at the heart of policy development. While we accept experimental approaches to determine the effectiveness of clinical practices . . . we too

> often allow ideology to govern matters of political practice . . . Tropical medicine's future remains rooted in the lives, communities, conditions, and diseases of the tropics (*Lancet* 2004, 1087).

If it is possible to atone for complicity in the colonialist enterprise, then the bastard twins of the imperialist bitch[15]—tropical medicine and area studies—should start talking fast. While still marred by an overreliance on inherited definitions of region, the areas of cultural studies, feminism, and post-colonial theory have made serious inroads into the interdisciplinary study of places in the world. Apparently, the hand-wringing of the *Lancet* editorial's title—"*Tropical Medicine: a brittle tool of the new imperialism*"—notwithstanding, tropical medicine is still unable to loosen its ties to its imperialist past. It is a profound irony that in the African context two countries have been at the forefront of establishing the feasibility of local ARV programs: Uganda and South Africa. Uganda's unsavory political history is now partially redeemed by its early (and apparently accurate) perception that it should play along with the WHO/GPA desire for the transplantation of Western self-help models to non-Western contexts, and then the laundering of the history of those programmes to make them look "authentic." The AIDS Support Organization (TASO), which emerged from the interaction of Western activists and local service providers, and with the inexplicable blessing of the dictatorship, is now the model for an "empowered community" invoked in 3X5 and elsewhere. South Africa, meanwhile, emerged from apartheid rule during the first decade of the AIDS crisis and has been at the center of one of the most important contestations of Western hegemony in medical research. Unfortunately, the story of President Mbeki dismissing the findings of the country's Medical Research Council, preferring instead to discredit scientific dissidents of dubious politics (Duseburg's explanations for the patterning of AIDS—absent a virus like HIV—relies on racist and homophobic truisms) over the more mainstream advice of once-jailed political dissidents, itself reinforces racist and imperialist ideas about the superiority of Western science over other scientific systems.

The Mbeki episode shows that we are way past any assessment that the "inside" of Africa is anything but perfectly able to "determine for itself problems to be addressed" and that it is naive to imagine there is any "outside" to Western medicine such that there is much hope of anything but "westernised impressions" to be embraced or contested. But for me, it is the insistence on "research" that finally reveals the new tropical medicine's complicity with the latest form of medical imperialism, the assertion of evidence-based policy-making paralleled to (and modeled on) the evidentiary notions of the clinical trial. This is epidemiology envy of a very frightening sort. In the way that my earlier work suggested the collapse of epidemiology in tropical medicine, I here note the transmogrification of a central practice of epidemiology into a "brittle tool." Although the author of the editorial reasserts tropical medicine through the domestic tropes—"rooted in the lives, communities, conditions, and diseases of the tropics"—the assertion of research against ideology in a context in which research can only draw on its alter ego's practices finally informs us of what "[global] public health" must mean in the context of "scaling up ARVs": a plea to accept science over human rights or, better, to accept human rights only when there is a scientific basis for claims to their utility.

NOTES

1. In fact, virtually every new drug to hit the market also hit consumers early and hard—activists have long charged that AZT dosing in the late 1980s killed as many as it saved. Again in the 1990s, when protease inhibitors were added to the mix, so great was the enthusiasm for the "cocktail" that most North American clinicians went, for a time, to "universal" application to anyone who tested positive for HIV, regardless of the state of their immune system (usually measured in CD-4 count). As the realities of viral resistance and metabolic side effects became clear, treatment protocols moved toward lower and lower CD-4 count triggers. Today, with the complex range of treatments available, and with genotyping of virus making "boutique" combinations and sequences of therapies possible, clinicians differ on criteria for

deciding when to start antiretrovirals in "treatment naïve" patients, but in general, will have started ARVs by a CD-4 of 200 (the point at which the body is unable to manage its own endemic infections). Those who were the unfortunate recipients of "hit early, hit hard" may now be on "salvage therapies" as a result of both long-term infection and the resistances they engendered as a result of the (we now know) uncertainties about the effects of "hit early, hit hard." Déjà vu.

2. HIV treatment is made more complicated by co-treatment for TB, an infectious disease virtually endemic in developing countries and in poor neighborhoods of the developed world. Those with untreated HIV do not respond well to TB medications, and there are known drug interactions between current TB medications and the ARVs slated for use in the 3X5 protocol. This means that the morbidity and mortality of both TB and HIV are higher in low-resource contexts. In addition, since TB is an infectious airborne disease especially dangerous to people with poor health, the presence of co-infected people increases the total pool of TB, endangering those who do not have HIV. For a lay explanation of this problem and the solutions currently undertaken in various contexts, see *Scaling up prevention and treatment for TB and HIV* (Getahun and Reid 2005), which also makes a compelling case for applying to HIV-ARV programmes the directly observed therapy (DOT) now standard around the world for TB treatment. Halfway between public health surveillance and responsibilizing techne, DOT already has a major place in 3X5: both community health workers and family members are tasked with making sure the index patient has taken their drugs. (I want to note that the rise of DOT in the African context was in part necessitated by the lack of pediatric ARV formulations: adults pretended to take drugs, but took them home to their HIV+ children.)
3. Drs. Kim and Gilks are officials with the HIV/AIDS Department of the World Health Organization.
4. Despite the many projects in other low-resource contexts, it is always Africa that lies in the HIV imaginary as the "place" of Third World AIDS.
5. "PHASE I TRIALS: Initial studies to determine the metabolism and pharmacologic actions of drugs in humans, the side effects associated with increasing doses, and to gain early evidence of effectiveness; may include healthy participants and/or patients.

   PHASE II TRIALS: Controlled clinical studies conducted to evaluate the effectiveness of the drug for a particular indication or indications in patients with the disease or condition under study and to determine the common short-term side effects and risks.

   PHASE III TRIALS: Expanded controlled and uncontrolled trials after preliminary evidence suggesting effectiveness of the drug has been obtained, and are intended to gather additional information to evaluate the overall benefit-risk relationship of the drug and provide and adequate basis for physician labeling.

   PHASE IV TRIALS: Post-marketing studies to delineate additional information including the drug's risks, benefits, and optimal use" (US National Institutes of Health, available from www.clinicaltrials.gov).

   I proffer that a "Phase V Trial" would be one designed to determine how to maximize profit and utility of drugs that are no longer on the primary formularies of the original market; that is, how to successfully "dump" drugs in low-resource settings.
6. Throughout this chapter, I draw on Ludwig Fleck's (1979) concept of thoughtstyle. Fleck himself likely developed his idea from encounters with Karl Mannheim's early work in the sociology of knowledge. In a careful argument that derives from his clinical research in the field of syphilis and his historical research on syphilis treatment, Fleck demonstrates that a complex of factors—clinical training of researchers and physicians, social concepts of disease and of particular diseases, the state of scientific research and of treatment modalities—all serve to establish the facticity of a "scientific fact." Along with other thinkers of the late nineteenth and early twentieth century, he is very interested in the interplay between "esoteric" and "exoteric" knowledge and, like Mannheim, insists there is a way of thinking that is social as much as it is procedural. But the domains of the expert and "public" are not exclusive, since the expert also occupies the space of the public and *is* the public in relation to many other expert domains. Foucault's understanding of discourse/knowledge formations (elaborated in his *The Archaeology of Knowledge* 1969, *The Order of Things* 1970, and *Birth of the Clinic* 1973) combines nicely with Fleck's detailed account of the interplay of knowledge in the case of syphilis after the advent of the Wasserman test and salvarsan treatment, to provide a very nuanced and open model for understanding how broad "thoughtstyles" are inflected in the practices of medical subdisciplines, and how the argumentation of these subdisciplines can be invoked (often in a way that scientists recognize as commonsense) as citation of science in the media. (Also see Patton 2002.)
7. A range of funders were involved in these projects for noble, ignoble, and obscure reasons: Médecins Sans Frontières, The World Bank, the International Monetary Fund, the World Health Organization, universities from the North in partnership with regional universities (themselves largely the dividends of colonial-era education schemes), and many local AIDS service groups (most funded directly or indirectly by the WHO, the World Bank, Médecins Sans Frontières, and so on).
8. For further discussion on the bald racism in the construction of, especially, people in African

countries who are living with HIV, see my *Inventing African AIDS*, 1990a, and *Inventing AIDS*, 1990b.

9. I conflate safe sex with condoms here only for dramatic effect. From the early 1980s, I have been among those who promoted the widespread support for "already safe" practices, and have contested—in my critical writings and in various community organizing projects—the conflation of safe sex with condoms, especially as it stands in for the overall need for safe sex in eliminating HIV. Feminists have never spoken loudly enough in pointing out that there are more reasons than HIV to moderate the flow of semen. Negative consequences of pregnancy continue to rival or exceed HIV in causing misery and death for women.
10. For an excellent review of the problems of testing, see *Testing, Trials, and Re-thinking Human Rights* (Stephenson et al. 2005).
11. For example, the toolkit lists three assumptions underlying its approach, including that scaling up will "learn from and build on the existing experiences of providing ARV treatment at local, national or regional levels" (Dhaliwal et al. 2003, 3).
12. My team is currently engaged in a longer treatment of this problem, with a possible analytic solution based in Bourdieu's meso-analytic framework. We, along with a host of others, indict social epidemiology as resting on a faulty understanding of the social world, especially in its view of the relationship between systems and people—what we call the macro–micro problem.
13. My considerations have taken different forms. For two years, I chaired the ad hoc International Working Group on Women and AIDS, where my only real accomplishment was to create a list of groups and the work they were conducting in their locales. I parlayed some of that knowledge, as well as contacts I made as a consultant to GPA on an assessment of women's needs in the epidemic, into some comments on types and forms of activism in my *Last Served? Gendering the HIV Pandemic* (1994). My experience of these forays in and with GPA was the impetus for *Globalizing AIDS* (2002) which—perhaps belatedly—identified the "levels" at which connections around HIV were made, or better, how the complex relations between global and local were crafted through use of the two thoughtstyles I theorized.
14. Another important issue at the local level and in the ethics literature, but which is totally ignored in the WHO documents, is the question of criteria for choosing who gets ARVs first. Ethicists and epidemiologists have entered the fray, trying to split the difference between propositions based in a conviction that everyone should have an equal opportunity to go on ARVs and the proposition that those most likely to be compliant patients should be first. I want to toy—though only that—with the idea that neoliberalism, applied in the context of new democracies, offers rather different prospects than its cousin in the established democracies. I extend the suggestion by a number of writers in queer theory and other domains that "rights" mean, function, and constitute subjectivities differently in contexts in which there is rapid state transformation to "democracy." Paradoxically, although discriminated against for their transgression of having contracted HIV, those who undergo the responsibilizing transformation that the current enactment of 3X5 requires might produce the person living with HIV as the model citizen of the neo-neo-liberalized, post-dictatorship democracy.
15. I'm playing with a mixed metaphor here. I have always been fascinated by the small reality in the canine world that a female—bitch—can have puppies from more than one male—sire. Hence, I imagine here a promiscuous Imperialism being impregnated by, variously, modern medicine and the emergent (and perhaps, it is worth considering, first, interdisciplinary interdiscipline) international studies focused on specific regions, viewed through history, culture, and aesthetics.

REFERENCES AND FURTHER READING

Brown, R. C., and J. E. Brown. 2005. "Predicting the Failure of 3X5." Letter to the editors. *Lancet* 366(9480): 117–118.

Dhaliwal, M., A. Okero, I. Schillevoort, C. Green, S. Conway, and A. Jain. 2003. *A Public Health Approach for Scaling up Antiretroviral (ARV) Treatment: A Toolkit for Programme Managers*. Geneva: World Health Organization.

Fleck, L. 1979. *The Genesis and Development of a Scientific Fact*. Trans. F. Bradley and T. J. Trenn. Chicago: University of Chicago Press.

Foucault, M. 1970. *The Order of Things: An Archaeology of the Human Sciences*. New York: Vintage.

Foucault, M. 1972. *The Archaeology of Knowledge*. New York: Pantheon.

Foucault, M. 1973. *The Birth of the Clininc: An Archaeology of Medical Perception*. New York: Pantheon.

Getahun, H., and A. Reid. 2005. *Scaling Up Prevention and Treatment for TB and HIV*. Geneva: World Health Organization.

Hammer, S. (ed.) (with D. Havlir, E. Klement, F. Scano, J.-E. Malkin, J.-F. Delgraissy, J. Lange, L. Mungherera, L. Mofenson, M. Harrington, N. Kumarasamy, N. Durier, P. Salif Sow, S. Banoo, and T. Macharia). 2002. *Scaling up Antiretroviral Therapy in Resource-Limited Settings: Treatment Guidelines for a Public Health Approach*. Geneva: World Health Organization.

Kim, J. Y., and C. Gilks. 2005. "Scaling Up Treatment—Why we Can't Wait." *New England Journal of Medicine* 353(22): 2392–2394.

Lancet. 2004. "Tropical Medicine: a Brittle Tool of the New Imperialism." Editorial. *Lancet* 363(9415): 1087.

Patton, C. 1990a. "Inventing African AIDS." *New Formations* 10 (Spring).

Patton, C. 1990b. *Inventing AIDS*. New York: Routledge.

Patton, C. 1994. *Last Served? Gendering the HIV Pandemic*. Philadelphia: Taylor and Francis.

Patton, C. 1995. "Performativity and Spatial Distinction: AIDS Education and the End of AIDS Epidemiology." In A. Parker and E. K. Sedgwick (eds.), *Performance and Performativity (Essays from the English Institute)*, 173–196. New York: Routledge.

Patton, C. 1996. "Queer Peregrinations." In M. J. Shapiro and H. R. Alker (eds.), *Challenging Boundaries*, 363–382. Minneapolis: Minnesota University Press.

Patton, C. 2002. *Globalizing AIDS*. Minneapolis: University of Minnesota Press.

Stephenson, N., C. Webb, and M. Carman. 2005. *Testing, Trials, and Re-Thinking Human Rights*. Sydney: Australian Society for HIV Medicine.

UNAIDS (Joint United Nations Programme on HIV/AIDS). 2005. *Intensifying HIV Prevention: A UNAIDS Policy Position Paper*. Geneva: UNAIDS.

U.S. National Institutes of Health. *Glossary of Clinical Trial Terms*. http://www.clinicaltrials.gov/ct/info/glossary. Accessed February 21, 2008.

WHO (World Health Organization). 2003. *Treating 3 Million by 2005: Making it Happen: The WHO Strategy*. Geneva: World Health Organization.

CHAPTER 36

Towards an Interdisciplinary Research Agenda on HIV/AIDS in the Middle East and North Africa

New Directions for the Age of Globalization

Sandra Sufian

ABSTRACT

This chapter calls for strengthening and amplifying interdisciplinary research on HIV/AIDS issues in the Middle East and North Africa (MENA), a region where little research has been done and where there is a dire need for more. The MENA region is therefore a prime area to initiate an innovative, robust research strategy in a cohesive, organized way. The responsibility for averting disaster lies not only with national governments and citizens throughout the region but also with international agencies, civil society organizations, and the international AIDS community. In an age of globalization, national and international boundaries are no longer stable but rather fluid and "supernational" and therefore the global community must mobilize to keep HIV/AIDS under control in MENA, like it has in Africa and now India, Russia, and China.

OVERVIEW

This chapter calls for strengthening and amplifying interdisciplinary research on HIV/AIDS issues in the Middle East. It begins with an international news story that powerfully illustrates some of the forces and impact of globalization in the region. The Middle East and North Africa (MENA) is a region where little research has been done and where there is a dire need for more. The MENA region is therefore a prime area to initiate an innovative, robust research strategy in a cohesive, organized way. As we will see, just as the causes, routes of transmission and environmental conditions surrounding HIV/AIDS, its spread and solution, are interconnected in this region and others, research must reflect and interrogate these intersections.

A DIPLOMATIC SHOWDOWN: THE DILEMMA OF GLOBALIZATION AND HIV/AIDS

In May 2004, a Libyan court sentenced five Bulgarian nurses and one Palestinian doctor to death by firing squad. The crime for this sentence was the alleged deliberate HIV infection through contaminated blood products to 426 children in Fateh Children's Hospital in the city of Benghazi. Since that time, at least 53 of the infected children have died.

According to the Qaddafi government, these health providers infected the children and babies with HIV with the cooperation of the CIA, who purportedly supplied the virus.[1] The health workers claimed they were innocent; that they were forced to confess to intentional infection and that they, according to Amnesty International, were severely tortured while in prison.[2] The Bulgarian government believed that the Libyan government was using these medical professionals as scapegoats to divert attention away from internal problems in the Libyan health sector.[3]

In December 2005, after pressure from the Bulgarian Government, the U.S. government, and the European Union, the Libyan Supreme Court decided to overturn the conviction and retry the case in a lower court. The retrial was postponed several times. Judge Mahmoud Haouissa, the presiding judge of the three-person tribunal, denied the defense's request to release the workers on bail for fear that they would leave the country. They had been imprisoned since 1999.

The Libyan government was willing to set the health workers free if Bulgaria paid the children's families compensation in the amount of €4.4 billion. Bulgaria refused to pay the monies or forgive some of Libya's debt because it felt that would be an admission of guilt. However, it joined the U.S., the EU, and the Libyan government in setting up an aid fund for the families.[4]

Due to inaccurate testimony of Libyan experts about how the infection occurred, defense lawyers wanted international HIV/AIDS experts to testify about how HIV is transmitted and how the children's infection actually occurred. Thus, even before the death sentence, in July 2003, Luc Montagnier, the co-discoverer of HIV, testified that HIV was already present in the hospital *before* the arrival of the foreign medical workers. Its presence was likely due to a lack of upholding universal precautions.[5] Garrett wrote that sophisticated "molecular epidemiology techniques" should have been used early on to identify the origins of the particular HIV strain that the children contracted. Using such techniques, Garrett argued, would have confirmed Montagnier's claim about the chronology of contamination. Garrett added that it is likely that extreme shortages of needles and medical equipment in the hospital facilitated the spread of the virus throughout the facility.[6]

In response to the French and Bulgarian defense lawyers' request to provide more evidence, the judge postponed the retrial for a third time to July 4, 2006. On July 17, 2007, a year later and after much pressure, the Libyan government commuted the death sentences of the said medical workers. One week after that, after eight years of imprisonment and torture, the medical workers were released and flown from Libya to Bulgaria, thus putting an end to claims that they had deliberately infected more than 400 Libyan children with HIV. An undisclosed agreement of compensation to the children's families was settled on July 10, 2007.

This international news story, which the Associated Press termed a "diplomatic showdown,"[7] points not only to the dilemmas of dealing with HIV/AIDS infection in a Middle Eastern country, but also illustrates some of the forces of globalization and transnationalism in the Middle East region.

Boufford has identified certain factors that reflect the direct impact of globalization upon health and health care provision within societies. These include: 1) the flow of information, including popular culture as well as health and scientific education; 2) the movement of people through migration and travel; 3) new technologies that more easily link people together, including sophisticated communication and biomedical technologies; 4) emerging commercial markets and expanded modes of global commerce; 5) the effects of global debt; 6) religion and culture; 7) political conflicts; and 8) diseases and changes in the environment.[8] Many aspects of the Libyan case more or less recapitulate Boufford's broad categorization about the influence of globalization upon health: the migration of health workers, the involvement of political players (governmental, medical, and legal) other than Libyan in the case's adjudication, the call to use complex medical technologies to determine chronology and causality, the varying opinions (and therefore flow of information) of scientists, Libyan vs. non-Libyan, about the route of HIV infection of the children, the invocation of foreign debt in resolving the case, and the international media's reporting of the various aspects of the case. These dynamics, in turn, embody central, structural characteristics of globalization and current global exchanges: the transversal of national boundaries in conjunction with links between technology (medical and otherwise), disease, migrant work, domestic/foreign economies, and international law.

At the 2006 High Level Meeting on AIDS, the UN General Assembly recently recognized that AIDS itself is a global emergency that "poses one of the most formidable challenges to development, progress and stability of our respective societies and the world at large and requires an exceptional and comprehensive global response."[9] A global response to AIDS which utilizes "enhanced international cooperation and partnership" draws upon the same international media and flow of knowledge involved in the Libyan case. As an example of the connection between disease and globalization, AIDS goes beyond national boundaries in its spread and its response.

The processes of adjudication and postponements in the Libyan AIDS legal case plainly exhibit the country's past, present, and future negotiation with globalizing forces. Just as the Libyan legal case can be deconstructed in this way, so too the intricate and sometimes unpredictable relationships between the broad phenomenon of globalization, its country-wide economic effects, and its localized consequences upon people's health, need to be untangled in order to find the required, appropriate, and flexible responses to the AIDS epidemic.

How do we, as scholars, study such complex interactions and exchanges? In its description of the dynamics of globalization in the Middle East and its interface with HIV and AIDS, this chapter takes the theme of linkages inherent in the phenomenon of globalization and extends it to research. I argue that the sensibility of intersections and exchanges created and perpetuated in globalization—indeed forms that make up the essence of the phenomenon itself—should be practiced by scholars. As Ali Mirsepassi notes, an "epistemic shift" has occurred in a globalizing context where one can no longer find a singular subject or territory but rather a simultaneous multiplicity of experiences in multiple domains, geographic or otherwise.[10] In this way, I argue that the necessity of interdisciplinary research is a function of globalization itself—that research agendas must respond to this epistemological shift and incorporate into their own methods the thread of connectivity that exists today in our globalizing world. Research needs to capture the complex connectivity inherent in and between processes of globalization and the AIDS epidemic; at base, scholarship needs to catch up with the actual processes of global health. As globalizing forces cross the boundaries of nation-states, going beyond the borders of disciplines can only help us find more efficient programs and comprehensive interventions.

HIV/AIDS IN THE MIDDLE EAST: A GENERAL OVERVIEW

The Middle East and North Africa (MENA) region has managed, in relative terms, to maintain a low incidence and prevalence of HIV and AIDS as compared to other regions, such as sub-Saharan Africa (25.8 million) or Asia (8.3 million). Most definitions of the region include 22 Arab countries in addition to Israel, Turkey, and Iran. Out of the approximate 280 million Arabs living in the region, 65 million of them are illiterate, and two-thirds of those are women. One out of every five Arabs in the region lives on less than $2 a day. Of note as well, the GDP of the Arab states combined is still less than that of Spain.[11] The region as a whole, therefore, is not in a great economic, social, or political condition. Just as globalization is, according to contemporary Arab Muslim writers, "infecting the people," the region is also vulnerable to the infection of HIV/AIDS.[12]

UNAIDS estimates that the total number of people living with HIV in the MENA region has risen from 210,000 in 1998 and 380,000 in 2003 to 510,000 in 2007. Approximately 67,000 people became infected in 2005, and 58,000 adults and children died of AIDS-related illnesses in the same year.[13] According to the 2006 update on the AIDS epidemic, close to 350,000 of the 510,000 cases in MENA are in Sudan.[14] Although available data suggests low prevalence rates (2 percent at the end of 2005), such rates may mask small, vulnerable populations with high HIV/AIDS prevalence. In fact, UNAIDS has noted that the region has the third fastest rate of increase in new infections in the world.[15]

The problem with extant statistics about HIV/AIDS in MENA is that the quality and availability of surveillance data for the region is extremely scant. What statistics do exist are likely underestimations. The UNAIDS estimation of past and current regional prevalence lies within a very broad range of possible cases.[16] Most governments in the region are only now starting to establish systematic reporting systems. Fortunately, mobilization for HIV/AIDS prevention, care, and support is growing, but these efforts and the funds needed to continue or expand them are regularly eclipsed by international concerns about Africa, Russia, India, and China.[17]

Adding to the confusion about data is the fact that the composition of countries for the Middle East and North Africa region varies for each international agency working on HIV/AIDS.[18] Such variable definitions make clean comparisons on aggregate, regional MENA data between agencies complicated and sometimes cumbersome. Furthermore, several countries do not or cannot provide sufficient and updated information to these international agencies. The most recent data for Afghanistan, for instance, is from October 1999. The most recent epidemiological update on HIV/AIDS and STIs (Sexually Transmitted Infections) for Afghanistan (2006) and Iraq (2006) are almost entirely blank.[19] Sentinel surveillance numbers are not available for Iraq and detailed statistics on HIV/AIDS are given only up to 1999.

VULNERABLE POPULATIONS

The MENA region faces many socio-economic and political challenges in the context of globalization, which in turn affect HIV/AIDS.[20] These include a predominance of young populations, political conflicts, slow-growing economies, gender inequalities, population movement/migration, geographical proximity to high-prevalence regions (Central Asia and sub-Saharan Africa), foreign debt, armed conflict, issues with governance, a history of colonialism and post-colonial nationalism, as well as stressed or crumbling health infrastructures. A myriad of other social problems intensified by globalization like a drug trade, high unemployment rates, low educational levels, and migration also strongly influence the transmission of HIV/AIDS. At least half of HIV cases reported in Tunisia, for instance, are thought to be Libyans who crossed the border to undergo drug rehabilitation or receive antiretroviral treatment.[21] This type of migration has not been thoroughly studied and introduces a new type of global movement brought on by the pursuit of AIDS treatment. In fact, migration and the phenomenon of foreign work and its effect upon the spread of AIDS, in general, needs to be studied more thoroughly in the region.

Like other regions of the world, MENA possesses particularly vulnerable groups to HIV: men who have sex with men, female sex workers and their clients, injecting drug users, and prisoners. Other groups at risk likely include tourists, displaced persons, migrant workers, transport drivers, and women and young people. More research on all of these groups and their practices is desperately needed.[22]

MENA has not averted the consequences of a strong global drug trade. Being an injecting drug user in the Middle East is one of the primary risk factors for contracting HIV in the region. Based on evidence of increasing HIV infection among injecting drug users (IDU), the epidemic is focused upon IDUs in Iran and Libya and seems to be spreading among the general population in Djibouti and Sudan. HIV prevalence among IDUs in Tripoli, Libya is reportedly at 18 percent, in Sudan (2002) at 2 percent, and in Morocco at 1 percent in 2003.[23] HIV infection in Bahrain and Oman is also allegedly concentrated among injecting drug users.[24] It is probable that a concentrated epidemic among this risk group could develop soon in the region.

Sharing syringes among drug injectors appears to be quite prevalent. According to studies in Algeria, Egypt, and Lebanon, 41 percent, 55 percent, and 65 percent of IDUs in each respective country shared injecting equipment, putting them at high risk for HIV transmission.[25] Access to services, including provision and encouragement of condom use, for this population is strikingly low.

Sex work is another high-risk behavior that propels the spread of HIV/AIDS in some countries. Commercial sex workers (mostly of non-Turkish origin) are recognized as the "major driver of the epidemic" in Turkey. Turkey has an estimated 3,700 adult AIDS patients (ages 15–49, as of 2001 and 2004) and it should be noted that half of Turkey's total population is under the age of 25.[26] Yemen and Algeria have also reported that the sex work industry plays an important role in their country's modes of transmission. Out of its 9,100 HIV/AIDS total reported cases, Algeria's statistics from 2000 show a median prevalence of 1.7 percent of seropositivity (out of 117 sex workers tested) in the capital of Tamanrasett. An epidemiological map in the same report, however, shows a seropositive prevalence of 20 percent among commercial sex workers in Oran and Tamanrasett, respectively. For its part, Yemen had an approximate 12,000 HIV/AIDS cases in 2003 but surveillance is very poor. Statistics of sex workers points to an infection rate of 7 percent in 2001, up from 2.7 percent in 1999.[27] Domestic violence, rape, an inability to negotiate safe sex with their husbands, low levels of health education, and decreased social and economic power, put MENA women at high risk for HIV infection. The connections between political conflict, gender relations, education, and stigma are crucial and need in-depth study to understand how and why AIDS is spread in each country and then design programs to effectively intervene in these processes.

In addition to women, young people also constitute a vulnerable group in the Middle East. The region has a very young population overall. In Palestine, for instance, 66 percent of the total population is under the age of 24; Gaza has a younger population than the West Bank. Except for health fields, school and university curricula do not include information about HIV/AIDS in Palestine.[28] Extant research on university students in Palestine shows that, although most students have a basic knowledge about AIDS, there are some gaps in specific knowledge, especially about the life of the HIV virus, the incubation period of the virus, and routes of transmission. Most students want more information about the disease and on reproductive health. The report recommends that such education be integrated into secondary and university school curricula.[29]

DeJong notes that data on young people and HIV/AIDS is not widely available, but information from a high-prevalence country, Djibouti, provides one case example of the potential state of HIV/AIDS amongst young people in the region: of people living with HIV (AIDS) (PLWHA) in this country, 3.8 percent are young people between the ages of 15–19 and 43.6 percent are between the ages of 20–29 years old. Data from WHO EMRO, she writes, show that women acquire HIV at a younger age in the MENA region (25–29) than men (35–39).[30] The exact reasons for this difference are not given and likely vary from country to country. Investigating the various reasons and variability between Middle Eastern states could provide information about the particular directions the epidemic is heading and could provide clues as to how to educate young women and men more efficiently to stem those directions.

Overall, behavioral surveillance and research is highly inadequate, leaving governments, international agencies, and scientific researchers with the inability to securely identify trends in health behavior.[31] Multilayered studies by scholars about young people, drug users, women, mobile populations, and uniformed services are crucial. Needs assessment studies are vital for all countries. The information produced will be essential to adapt, inform, and design fitting interventions. These programs are particularly necessary in a perceived low prevalence context such as MENA, where the ability to reach those most in need with prevention information and services remains patchy and sporadic.

UNBOUNDED GOVERNANCE: INTERNATIONAL AND NATIONAL STEPS TOWARDS PREVENTION, MANAGEMENT AND TREATMENT

If governance is at issue, then past records of MENA governments on the whole have fallen short of due diligence. Until recently, the region has suffered from a lack of leadership in this regard and "widespread public policy denial."[32] In recent years, the region's governments have shown a variable response and success record with regard to the AIDS pandemic.

A slow but growing awareness is gradually manifesting itself among Middle Eastern governments about the great potential for a wide-scale epidemic in the region, especially in Iran, Djibouti, Algeria, Sudan, and Tunisia. Just as we saw in the Libyan court case, international players are playing an important role in efforts to deal with HIV/AIDS in MENA. UNAIDS and its affiliated agencies (UNICEF, UNFPA, UNDP, WHO, and the World Bank) have become more engaged with Middle Eastern governments to curtail the rise of its AIDS cases.[33]

The World Health Organization, the one UNAIDS agency that has worked in the region since the 1980s, developed a Regional Strategic Plan for the Eastern Mediterranean for the years 2002–2005. This Strategic Plan also outlines appropriate response elements and targets. Target goals include political commitment and advocacy (including budget guarantees and media advocacy), human resource development and capacity building, as well as applied research and the generation of knowledge. All of these elements mutually enforce one another. Researchers still need to interrogate how that dynamic has played out.

National AIDS programs and national steering committees in each country were set up to implement the strategic plans.[34] Actions by some National AIDS Committees and UN Theme Groups in the region—albeit incomplete—have included implementing universal health precautions, addressing the care of opportunistic infections, securing a safe blood supply, and providing antiretroviral therapy and counseling for AIDS patients.[35] Morocco, Algeria, and Lebanon, for instance, have developed improved surveillance and prevention programs.[36] Morocco worked with the World Bank on an AIDS Action Plan in 2001. It has instituted extensive services for the prevention and treatment of sexually transmitted infections, as heterosexual sex seems to be its main mode of transmission.[37] Despite this Plan, however, Morocco experienced a threefold increase of new infections between the years 2001–2003.[38] Tunisia developed a program in 1997 for their young population that offers regional and provincial comprehensive services in prevention, counseling, testing, and condom distribution.[39] Algeria also finalized a multi-sectoral strategic plan for 2003–2006.

Recognizing the importance of cross-communication and partnership, Turkey set up a national HIV case reporting system, an HIV/AIDS Action Plan and a National AIDS committee (established in 1996) with input from several ministries—including education, tourism, culture, foreign affairs, and labor—and non-governmental organizations. Tunisia developed a program as early as 1997, for instance, for their young population that offers regional and provincial comprehensive services in prevention, counseling, testing, and condom distribution.[40] For its part, Syria has instituted community-based HIV/AIDS education programs for out-of-school youth, coupling with local organizations for its implementation.

Drawing upon international agencies involvement in the region, both Yemen and Djibouti have received funding from the World Bank to implement a Health Reform Support Project on HIV/AIDS prevention and harm reduction and to examine HIV/AIDS transmission within the trucking industry, respectively.[41]

Iran has made extensive strides in the MENA region in confronting their HIV/AIDS problem. The Iranian government developed a national sentinel surveillance system with seventy-five sites in juvenile detention centers, prisons, and university clinics. It has set up an extensive network of triangular clinics for injecting drug users (IDUs) that implements harm-reduction programs and address HIV/AIDS and drug abuse education, care, and treatment. Their patient-centric approach provides social support for patients and families as well as community outreach. In addition, Iran has highlighted the concept of partnership and connectivity by setting up several regional committees with university participation, while its National AIDS Committee includes members from several governmental ministries and organizations. A National Harm Reduction Committee has also been formed.[42] Along with Morocco, Algeria, and Jordan, Iran received funding from the Global Fund to fight HIV/AIDS.[43]

The implementation and effectiveness of these plans is not yet fully known. Studies that look at the difficulties of executing these Strategic Plans and succeeding in building bridges between ministries, for instance, could shed light unto the health of the government itself and its ability to deliver on promises with regard to pressing health issues. What caused delays? What worked? What did not and why? How was the epidemiology of the disease affected by these programs, changes, and challenges? What new social and political practices have resulted? Have international players' roles intensified or not in this regard and how?

TREATMENT

Despite these initial and concerted efforts, we must keep in mind that prevention and harm reduction programs are not enough to address the complexity of the HIV/AIDS epidemic. In addition to social support programs, treatment programs are also needed to help those already living with HIV/AIDS. Not unlike antiretroviral therapy issues in other regions, access to treatment in the region poses a dilemma.[44] Only 5 percent of the at least 75,000 people who need antiretroviral treatment in the region receive it.[45]

Some Middle Eastern countries have started to address this fact, including trying to negotiate lower prices for antiretroviral drugs. Lebanon, for instance, signed an agreement in 2003 with a pharmaceutical company to reduce the cost of AIDS drugs by 15 percent from the market price, saving the Ministry of Health approximately $1 million dollars a year in expenses.[46] Since 1999, Jordan has provided ART free of charge and the Saudi Arabian government reportedly spent a total of SR15 million on prevention and treatment of AIDS in 2004.[47] ART is provided to all infected in Qatar but stigma associated with HIV/AIDS and at-risk populations is still noted as a major problem and therefore barriers to access still exist.[48] In addition to treatment, the government of Qatar provides limited programs like screening of HIV patients' families and tuberculosis patients, school lectures, and provision of antiretroviral therapy (ART). The Qatar government prescreens foreign labor for the virus upon entry to the country as well as new army recruits, but no recent data exists for pregnant women. Supplying ART to prevent mother–child transmission is even less common.

Difficulties with human resources, population distribution, general infrastructure, and funding/foreign debt—issues tied to the forces of globalization as discussed previously—all affect the delivery and efficacy of ART.[49] International patent law also complicates the accessibility and distribution of ART. Yet continued attempts to distribute ART in MENA may replicate savings experienced by countries like Brazil, where half the amount invested in ART treatment was recouped simply from a decrease in hospital admissions and complex treatment for AIDS-related diseases.[50]

The relationships between patent law, accessibility to ARV treatment and national economic savings in MENA countries need exploration. Health policy researchers, infectious disease specialists, economists and international legal scholars could all contribute to this needed knowledge. Understanding these relationships might make it easier to find ways to decrease barriers to treatment, increase accompanying social programs, and help MENA governments provide adequate care while also saving money in various aspects of the health field.

SOCIAL AND CULTURAL ISSUES: THE QUESTION OF ISLAM AS PROTECTIVE AND THE PRESENCE OF STIGMA TOWARDS PEOPLE LIVING WITH AIDS (PLWHA)

Just as there is a synergy between ART treatment and the forces of globalization, so too is there one between the social and cultural dynamics of globalization and HIV/AIDS in MENA. One of the greatest fallacies that exists is that a supposed increasing Islamic conservatism in the region (a response in part to globalization itself)[51] will keep the region from experiencing an all-out AIDS epidemic. Claims that the presence of Islam will either prevent the spread of HIV/AIDS or that religious states will not address this problem adequately have been shown to be wrong.

The Islamic Republic of Iran (Shi'a Islam) has made extensive strides in confronting their HIV/AIDS problem. It has developed a national sentinel surveillance system with seventy-five sites in juvenile detention centers, prisons, and university clinics. It has set up an extensive network of clinics for IDUs that address HIV/AIDS and drug abuse education, care, and treatment. Needles and syringes, for instance, are now available over the counter in pharmacies. Iran also has set up several regional committees with university participation, while its National AIDS Committee includes members from several governmental ministries (i.e., public health, drug control, religious affairs, law enforcement) and civil society organizations.[52] A National Harm Reduction Committee has also been formed.[53] As of June 2004, the Iranian government also committed itself to an AIDS prevention education project in the country's schools.[54]

Another Islamic state (Sunni Islam), Saudi Arabia, has established an HIV/AIDS Health Education Committee that includes governmental and non-governmental agencies. It has engaged in HIV surveillance since 1984. One of the major modes of transmission in Saudi Arabia is said to be extramarital sexual relations. The Saudi government has instituted health programs for at-risk populations and reproductive and sex education programs in schools, established three treatment centers, and held an HIV/AIDS conference in 2004. It has distributed booklets on AIDS at airports, universities, and public spaces. Saudi Arabia also supplies antiretroviral therapy for infected pregnant women.[55] Among all of these activities, however, strategies sanctioned by Islam—like prevention of non-marital sex, safe sex through legal marriage, and prevention of injecting drug abuse—are regularly raised and encouraged.[56] Despite recognition of AIDS being a development issue by the health director of Jeddah, the Kingdom has so far failed to integrate the HIV/AIDS issue into their general development plans.[57]

As opposed to the work of these Islamic states, the Oman government does not promote sex education for young people due to "cultural and religious traditions," although condoms are provided free of charge at supermarkets, family planning clinics, and private pharmacies.[58]

Most significantly, in November of 2004, Arab religious leaders, both Christian and Muslim, came together from various states to publish a response to the HIV/AIDS epidemic. The declaration's general principles state the support of the clergy for patients with HIV/AIDS and improvement of their lives. The section on prevention states:

> We emphasize the need to break the silence . . . we need to address the ways to deal with the HIV/AIDS epidemic based upon our genuine spiritual principles . . . and armed with scientific knowledge, aiming at innovation of new approaches to deal with this dangerous challenge. We reiterate that abstinence and faithfulness are the two cornerstones of our preventive strategies but we understand the medical call for the use of different preventive means to reduce the harm to oneself and others . . . we advocate the rights of women to reduce their vulnerability to HIV/AIDS.

The declaration goes on to state that all people with HIV/AIDS and their families should receive treatment, education, psychological, and economic guidance. Finally it calls for the establishment of awareness-raising centers and the encouragement of charitable organizations to provide care and support for people living with HIV/AIDS.[59] This is a major step for the region because religious leaders are a key sector whose involvement can change public attitudes and pressure governments into action.

Still like most other countries, HIV/AIDS will continue to spread in the region because, at base, talking about HIV/AIDS forces people to recognize the behaviors that are associated with the virus's spread: men who have sex with men (MSM), injecting drug use, sex with multiple partners, sex work, premarital sex, and so on.[60] Jocelyn DeJong and her colleagues (2005) reported that in general, governments in the region are reluctant to educate citizens about sexual health, especially young people.[61] DeJong cited scant evidence that suggests that young people's knowledge about sexually transmitted infections and HIV is extremely low. In a representative study of 16- to 19-year-old teens in Egypt, for instance, 19.7 percent of boys and 30 percent of girls did not know about HIV or STIs.[62]

Social customs or conventions like injection practices, tattooing, barber services, and traditional health practices are potential modes of transmission that need to be addressed in HIV/AIDS research and programs. Social issues like stigma, drug use, unemployment, and illiteracy compound the problem of attaining epidemiologic data of HIV/AIDS and remain substantial barriers to the reduction of AIDS cases because they limit the ability of MENA governments, nongovernmental organizations, and UN agencies to effectively respond to the problem. These interconnections must be considered an *essential characteristic* of the HIV/AIDS issue and must be addressed synergistically in research, rather than separately.

Strong stigmatization surrounding HIV in the MENA region has significant effects. Stigma makes extensive voluntary testing and counseling difficult to achieve and therefore reporting is inaccurate. It also complicates medical diagnosis and treatment. Some medical professionals in the region are reportedly hesitant to treat PLWHA, while employment discrimination and societal alienation and family rejection of PLWHA occur in many MENA countries. One example of addressing this issue is Iran's innovative and *integrated* campaign against HIV/AIDS in the injecting drug user community. This program also makes HIV-positive drug users visible by including them in outreach programs. Their participation is intended to avert stigma by showing that PLWHA are constructive members of society who can help others. Understanding that the problems of high-risk groups like injecting drug users are complex, Iran's triangular clinics address other, yet related, social problems by providing food and shelter, recreation, primary health care, employment, and family counseling. The clinics' integrated, comprehensive care approach is meant to reduce the effects of stigma by allowing patients to seek help for associated problems, instead of solely and clearly attending the clinic for HIV/AIDS.[63] This program can be seen as a model for planning and implementing interdisciplinary and interconnected interventions.

Hotlines throughout the region offering confidential counseling on HIV/AIDS try to disperse information about the disease, while also acknowledging the extent of social stigma and taboo that the subject engenders. Hotlines now exist in Tunisia, Lebanon, Egypt, Oman, and the West Bank and Gaza. Egypt's hotline, for example, receives, on average, 1,000 calls a month, mostly from young singles.[64]

Despite these efforts, powerful exclusionary sentiments continue to exist in the region. In 2002, Peter Piot, executive director of the Joint United Nations Program of HIV/AIDS (UNAIDS), gave a speech to MENA leaders in Beirut where he pleaded to "break the silence on AIDS" in the region. He stated:

> Most of AIDS in the Middle East and North Africa is still invisible. Progress is not possible unless AIDS becomes visible, unless stigma is challenged, and unless people living with HIV are encouraged to play their part in a community-wide AIDS response. All this requires resolute and courageous leadership at various levels.[65]

Towards this end, the UNDP (United Nations Development Program) sponsored a gathering in March 2003 in Cairo to raise awareness about HIV/AIDS in the Arab world. Actors, singers, and other media personalities in the Arab world attended the gathering.[66] Increasingly, civil society organizations that promote AIDS advocacy and information are being formed, but their voices in constructing AIDS policies are still not integrated.[67]

TOWARDS AN INTERDISCIPLINARY AGENDA FOR THE MIDDLE EAST AND NORTH AFRICA

UNAIDS has recommended improvements in behavioral surveillance, sero-surveillance among high-risk groups, and sexually transmitted infection surveillance in order to attain a better epidemiological profile of HIV/AIDS in the region. In addition, international leaders suggested in a recent High Level Meeting in May 2006 that a comprehensive response to the AIDS pandemic be met with multisectoral partnerships (between the United Nations, intergovernmental organizations, PLWHA, NGOs, business sector, trade unions, faith-based organizations, and scientific/educational institutions, among others).[68] This call requires a cohesive response by academic professionals.

Given the intricate relationships revealed in this chapter between various aspects of the HIV/AIDS epidemic and the dynamics of globalization in the MENA region, it is crucial for researchers to capture those interconnections in their research. In order to achieve this goal, researchers should form interdisciplinary teams and engage in interdisciplinary projects that incorporate *both* quantitative and qualitative methodologies within one project. These research teams should be comprised of either scholars indigenous to the Middle East itself and/or a mixture of scholars from the region along with scholars from outside of the region but who possess great investment and background in the region's languages and understand its considerable heterogeneity. Interdisciplinary research is especially needed between social scientists, humanities scholars, and medical/public health specialists.

Unfortunately the problem of HIV/AIDS has not been a topic seriously considered by Middle Eastern specialists to pursue in the recent past, but their expertise, including their language skills and cultural training, are in dire need. HIV/AIDS is a gender issue, a bioethical issue, a political economy, international trade and development issue wanting deep analysis, a social and demographic issue, as well as a basic public health, health policy, and medical problem. Quick, comprehensive responses informed by interdisciplinary perspectives will likely stave off the rapid transmission of the virus and will hopefully guard the region from severe economic, political, and social disaster.

Only by engaging in an interdisciplinary agenda can we as scholars of the region and of the disease learn about the various and complicated aspects of the emerging HIV/AIDS epidemic in the Middle East region and reach a comprehensive response to this growing problem. Particularly since the Middle East is, we think, at the beginning stages of an HIV/AIDS epidemic, it is essential to set out a research agenda that captures the complicated relationships that have emerged in a globalizing age.

EXAMPLES OF INTERACTIONS THAT NEED TO BE STUDIED

The current UN website for the MENA region clearly states: "Across the region, there is a clear need for more, better and in-depth information about the patterns of HIV transmission, especially the roles of sex work and of sex between men."[69] Therefore, projects on sex work, for instance, that combine anthropological with epidemiological and economics research might be able to better discern what the general labor market trends are and how they combine with specific economic incentives that exist for sex workers, what the level of risk for sex workers is for contracting HIV in a particular area, along with their social circumstances like housing, educational level, family circumstances, clientele, and length of time in the sex industry. A research team composed of these three disciplinary perspectives, for example, might be then able to see new connections between these variables that they could not see without each other, and may therefore be able, with the help of health education specialists, to construct an effective and very precise, community-sensitive intervention. Adding a gender studies scholar might provide even further insight into the roles of women and men in a given sub-population and how this translates into sex work practices.

A project focusing on sex between men may include a team of Middle East historians, anthropologists, sociologists, and health promotion specialists, among others. This team could, for example, produce a multilayered analysis of experiences of men, their ways of dealing (covert or overt) with their sexual preferences, marital status, and knowledge and attitudes towards using condoms. One of the layers of exploration could include looking at the history and politics of sexual identity in a particular country in the Middle East. Ethnography and historical documentation could be used to attain such information. Such an analysis would include changing policies, cultural taboos and stigma, geographies of meeting, forms of resistance to historical discrimination, and/or strategies for dealing with marginalized sexual identities. This information could then help further explicate the sociologist's and health promotion's work on condom use, family structure, and expectations and knowledge about HIV transmission. With all this data, the team could then together create an educational campaign that would be informed by political (national, social, and familial) and spatial constraints.

In addition to studying these vulnerable populations sufficiently, researchers have failed to ask wide-ranging questions about the connections between the workings of globalization and the spread of AIDS in the region. It is possible, for instance, that MENA's reported low AIDS rates are due, in part, to the fact that the region is largely marginalized with regard to global trade integration and the global economy.[70] Levine has pointed out, however, that "while MENA states remain fairly marginalized vis-à-vis indicators of global economic integration, they retain the large governments that characterize the most trade-dependent—that is, the most 'globalized'—societies."[71] In addition, he argues that MENA residents directly and forcefully experience the cultural aspects of globalization and have formed unique responses to them.[72]

Globalization's promise of economic growth through neoliberal policies has shown in many cases to be false; globalization has not translated into an increase in the health and welfare of people in developing countries or, for that matter, of marginalized or minority groups in developed countries. In fact, capitalist globalization has resulted in intensified social and economic divisions, an acceleration of disparities between "extremes of wealth and poverty."[73] Globalization has, according to Levine, engendered globalized chaos.[74] Ironically, however, MENA's relative marginalization from the global economic market may account for its low, absolute poverty levels.[75] Given this backdrop, it could be that the attenuation of absolute poverty levels—in spite of widespread gaps between the wealthy and poor in the region and extant poverty—has helped stem the spread of the HIV virus. How can we as scholars further explore this question? Clearly an economic analysis only will not suffice, as questions about governance, HIV transmission, and social welfare are also imperative to finding answers. A cohesive team consisting of a Middle East political scientist, a Middle Eastern historian, an economist, and an epidemiologist in a joint research project on the origins, politics, and social welfare status in poverty and health could look at these interconnections. In addition to an analysis within a MENA country (or city or rural area), it would be necessary to look at global trends over a certain period of time, the engagement of a named country in those patterns, and the differential effects of those trends on a particular country's poverty levels and HIV rates.

Although these ideas may seem promising and innovative, realistic constraints must be raised. Problems with actually doing this research, or any, in the region include access to materials and adequate funding, accessibility to high-risk groups, hesitation by individuals to discuss the dilemmas they face, and the risky behaviors in which they engage due to taboos on publicly discussing sexual practices, political conflict and economic vulnerability, and crumbling health infrastructures with relatively weak reporting systems.

On a high note, however, global networks are being established to deal with these obstacles. One organization is the GNR-MENA, the Global Network of Researchers on HIV/AIDS in the Middle East and North Africa, which acts as a forum for scientific exchange, debate, and networking for researchers from diverse perspectives and disciplines. The organization's seventy-five members represent universities, agencies, and ministries of health both from within and outside of the region who are interested in better understanding and effectively responding to the HIV/AIDS epidemic in the MENA region.

So far the network has produced strong relationships and collaborations between many of its members and has a listserv and research exchange program. The network has sponsored and presented Satellite Meetings at the International AIDS conferences in Bangkok and Toronto (2004 and 2006, respectively) and has exposed the Middle Eastern Studies community to the problem of HIV/AIDS. In addition, members of the network have begun to form a research team to initiate a multi-site survey on youth, stigma, and AIDS in the region.

CONCLUSION

Due to the early state of the epidemic in the region, a prime opportunity exists to conduct such research and institute appropriate programs that could pre-empt a regional catastrophe in the Middle East. Despite—indeed because of—low prevalence data on HIV/AIDS in the region, the time to act and invest in research and public health interventions is now. Our reliance upon data that suggests comparatively low rates of HIV/AIDS does not mean that a widespread epidemic is impossible or improbable. The responsibility for averting disaster lies not only with national governments and citizens throughout the region but also with international agencies, civil society organizations, and the international AIDS community. In an age of globalization, national and international boundaries are no longer stable but rather fluid and "supernational"[76] and therefore the global community must mobilize to keep HIV/AIDS under control in MENA (Middle East and North Africa), like it has in Africa and now India, Russia, and China.

Researchers hold a special responsibility in addressing this serious issue. Although some excellent programs exist in the Middle East and are increasing in number, a general lack of solid knowledge/research about the status of HIV/AIDS in MENA demands, in particular, an increased creation and flow of information about the epidemic in the region. This information should be based in multifaceted, complex approaches. As globalization has forced governments and others to recognize and deal with the relationships between diverse issues such as food policy, environmental and housing issues, military spending and education, so too must the academy adopt a rigorous research agenda to study these linkages and utilize diverse methodologies to most effectively find answers to complex research questions.

NOTES

1. Laurie Garrett (2006), "America shouldn't befriend Libya just yet," *International Herald Tribune*, June 11, 2006, http://www.iht.com/articles/2006/06/11/opinion/edgarrett.php.
2. Kaiser Family Foundation (2006a), "Defense Lawyers for Medical Workers Accused of Infecting Libyan Children with HIV Request HIV/AIDS Experts' Testimony," June 21, 2006, http://www.kaisernetwork.org/daily_reports/rep_hiv.cfm#38033; Khaled El-Deeb, "Judge Speeds Up Nurses' Trial in Libya," *The State*. Associated Press. June 13, 2006, http://hosted.ap.org/dynamic/stories/L/LIBYA_BULGARIA_AIDS_TRIAL?SITE=SCCOL&SECTION=HOME&TEMPLATE=DEFAULT.
3. Salah Sarrar (2006), "Foreign Medics' trial in Libya postponed to July 4," *Reuters*, June 20, 2006, http://today.reuters.co.uk/news/newsArticle.aspx?type=worldNews&story ID=2006-06-20T100534Z_01_L20587534_RTRUKOC_0_UK-LIBYA-TRIALxml&archived=False.
4. Sarrar (2006).
5. Katka, Krosnar (2003), "Libyan government lets AIDS experts comment on hospital deaths," *BMJ*, 327.7411 (August 16, 2003): 360; Luc Montag-

nier and Vittorio Colizzi (2003), "Final Report of Prof. Luc Montagnier and Prof. Vittorio Colizzi to Libyan Arab Jamahiriya on the Nosocomial HIV infection at the Al-Fateh Hospital, Benghazi, Libya," Paris, April 7, 2003, http://www.webcitation.org/5Mempgl11, 20–21.

6. Garrett (2006); Kaiser Family Foundation (2006b), "Retrial of Medical Workers Accused of Infecting Libyan Children with HIV Adjourned until June 20," June 14, 2006, http://www.kaisernetwork.org/daily_reports/rep_index.cfm?hint=1&DR_ID=37890.
7. El-Deeb (2006).
8. Jo Ivey Boufford (2005), "Leadership Development for Global Health," in *Global Health Leadership and Management*, ed. William Foege (San Francisco: Jossey-Bass, 2005), 153–154.
9. UNAIDS (2006a) Draft Political Declaration, June 2, 2006, http://www.un.org/ga/aidsmeeting2006, 1.
10. Mirsepassi (2006a), "Introduction," 17.
11. Mark Levine (2005a) "Chaos and Globalization in the Middle East," *Asian Journal of Social Science* 33 (2005): 397.
12. Mark Levine (2005b), "Globalization in the MENA and Europe: Culture, Economy and the Public Sphere in a Transnational Context," *Journal of Muslim Minority Affairs* 25.2 (August 2005): 154.
13. UNAIDS (2007) http://www.unaids.org/en/Regions_Countries/Regions/MiddleEastAndNorthAfrica.asp.
14. Joint United Nations Programme on HIV/AIDS, 2006 Report on the Global AIDS epidemic, http://data.unaids.org/pub/GlobalReport/2006/2006_GR_CH02_en.pdf, 48.
15. "North Africa, Middle East: HIV/AIDS Groups Aim to Nip a Rising Threat," January 28, 2005, excerpted from Susanna Howard, *Wall Street Journal*, January 27, 2005, http://www.thebody.com/cdc/news_updates_archive/2005/jan28_05/arab_countries_hiv.html#.
16. UNAIDS/WHO (2005), Middle East and North Africa Region, "Regional HIV and AIDS estimates, end 2005," http://www.thebody.com/unaids/pdfs/Epi05_13_ en.pdf.
17. One example of MENA's minimization among the international AIDS scientific community is that only one booth was dedicated to Middle Eastern organizations dealing with HIV/AIDS (out of hundreds) at the International AIDS Conference in 2006.
18. The World Bank, for instance, excludes Sudan, Somalia, and Israel. UNAIDS includes Israel and the Sudan but excludes Djibouti and Somalia. The World Health Organization includes the countries of the Middle East and North Africa within an Eastern Mediterranean regional name. It includes Sudan, Somalia, and Djibouti but excludes Israel within the purview of EMRO (Eastern Mediterranean Regional Office).
19. UNAIDS/WHO (2006a), Epidemiological Fact Sheet on HIV/AIDS. 2006 Update: Afghanistan, http://www.who.int/GlobalAtlas/predefinedReports/EFS2004/EFS_PDFs/EFS2006_AF.pdf; UNAIDS/WHO (2006b), Epidemiological Fact Sheet on HIV/AIDS. 2006 Update: Iraq, http://globalatlas.who.int/globalatlas/predefinedReports/EFS2004/EFS_ PDFs/EFS2006_IQ.pdf, 2.
20. Carol Jenkins and David Robalino (2003), *HIV/AIDS in the Middle East and North Africa: The Costs of Inaction* (Washington DC: The World Bank, 2003), xiv.
21. UNAIDS (2003). Middle East and North Africa Region, "Regional HIV and AIDS Estimates, End 2003," http://www.unaids.org/en/geographical+area/by+region/north+africa+and+middle+east+new.asp.
22. Ideas for such research are given at the end of this chapter.
23. Sammud, 2005 as cited in Joint United Nations Programme on HIV/AIDS, 2006 Report on Global AIDS Epidemic, http://data.unaids.org/pub/GlobalReport/2006/2006_GR_CH00FM_en.pdf, 49.
24. UNAIDS. Middle East and North Africa Region, "AIDS epidemic in the Middle East and North Africa Fact Sheet," http://www.unaids.org/en/geographical+area/by+region/north+africa+and+middle+east+new.asp.
25. Joint United Nations Programme on HIV/AIDS, 2006 Report on Global AIDS Epidemic, 50.
26. UNGASS (2003d) Turkey: Follow-up to the Declaration of Commitment on HIV/AIDS (UNGASS) country report format, reporting period: January–December 2002. Annexes 1 and 2. Written April 15, 2003; received April 23, 2003; posted March 31, 2003, http://www.unaids.org/EN/other/functionalities; Also UNAIDS/WHO Epidemiological Fact Sheet. 2004 Update: Turkey, http://globalatlas.who.int/globalatlas/predefinedReports/EFS2004/EFS_ PDFs/EFS2004_TR.pdf, 2.
27. UNAIDS/WHO (2004b), Epidemiological Fact Sheet. 2004 Update: Yemen, http://globalatlas.who.int/globalatlas/predefinedReports/EFS2004/EFS_ PDFs/ EFS2004_YE.pdf, 2.
28. Etaf Maqboul and Wafa Abu Ayyash Ramahi (2005), "Assessment of Palestinian Students' Knowledge about the Acquired Immunodeficiency Syndrome and their Attitudes towards AIDS Patients" (Bethlehem: Center for Sustainable Development and Community Health, 2005), unpublished paper, 2, 3.
29. Maqboul and Ramahi 2005: 65.
30. Jocelyn DeJong, Rana Jawad, Iman Nortagy, and Bonnie Shepard, "The Sexual and Reproductive Health of Young people in the Arab Countries and Iran," *Reproductive Health Matters* 13.25 (2005): 55.
31. Jenkins provided a summary of ad hoc surveys conducted in several countries that give a glimpse at trends in risk behaviors and risk groups. Carol Jenkins (2004), "Vulnerability to HIV/AIDS in the Middle East and North Africa: A Socio-Epidemiology Overview," paper given at Satellite

Meeting of Global Researchers of HIV/AIDS in the Middle East and North Africa Region, 15th International AIDS Conference, Bangkok, Thailand, July 13, 2004; UNAIDS (2006b), "Fact Sheet: AIDS Epidemic in the Middle East and North Africa," December 2006, http://data.unaids.org/pub/EpiReport/2006/20061121_epi_fs_mena_en.pdf."; Jenkins and Robalino 2003: xv.

32. DeJong et al. 2005: 55.
33. UNICEF is the United Nations Children's Fund; UNDP is the United Nations Development Programme; UNDCP is the United Nations International Drug Control Programme; UNFPA is the United Nations Population Fund; WHO is the World Health Organization.
34. WHO (2002), 8–10; Jenkins and Robalino 2003: xx.
35. Jenkins and Robalino 2003: xx.
36. UNAIDS (2006b), "Fact Sheet: AIDS Epidemic in the Middle East and North Africa"; UNAIDS (2003), Middle East and North Africa Region, "Regional HIV and AIDS Estimates, End 2003," http://www.unaids.org/en/geographical+area/by+region/north+africa+and+middle+east+new.asp.
37. Piot 2002: 4.
38. UNAIDS (2004), "Middle East and North Africa," in *UNAIDS AIDS Epidemic Update*, December 2004, http://www.unaids.org/wad2004/report_pdf.html, 66.
39. Jenkins and Robalino 2003: xx.
40. Ibid.
41. World Bank (2004), AIDS Regional Update: Middle East and North Africa, "An Opportunity for Prevention: HIV/AIDS Situation in the Middle East and North Africa Region," web.worldbank.org/WBSITE/EXTERNAL/NEWS, June 2004.
42. WHO (2004), "Best Practice in HIV/AIDS Prevention and Care for Injecting Drug Abusers: The Triangular Clinic in Kermanshah, Islamic Republic of Iran," Document WHO-EM/STD/052/E/U/05.04/1000 (Cairo: World Health Organization Regional Office for the Eastern Mediterranean, 2004), 13, 15, 25.
43. The Global Fund manages and disburses resources to fight AIDS, tuberculosis, and malaria. It does not implement programs but works with multilateral and bilateral organizations dealing with health and development issues in order to coordinate new programs with existing programs.
44. WHO/UNAIDS press release, "Access to HIV Treatment Continues to Accelerate in Developing Countries, But Bottlenecks Persist, Says WHO/UNAIDS Report," June 29, 2005, http://www.who.int/3by5/progressreportJune2005/en/.
45. As of June 2004, 440,000 people in low to middle-income countries are being treated with ART. The number of people being treated with ART worldwide has doubled in the past two years. Robert Steinbrook, "After Bangkok—Expanding the Global Response to AIDS," *New England Journal of Medicine* 351.8 (August 19, 2004): 738–742.
46. CDC (2003b), "Lebanon: AIDS Drug Deal to Slash Treatment Costs," *CDC News Updates*, April 21, 2003.
47. Mohammed Rasooldeen (2004), "SR15 Million Spent on AIDS Fight," *Arab News*, December 8, 2004.
48. UNGASS (2003b), Qatar: Follow-up to the Declaration of Commitment on HIV/AIDS (UNGASS) country report format, reporting period: January–December 2002, Annexes 1 to 3, written April 15, 2003; received April 23, 2003; posted March 31, 2003.
49. Hany Ziady (2004), WHO, "The Meaning of the 3 by 5 Initiative for Global Health and the Middle East," paper given at the Satellite Meeting of Global Network of Researchers on HIV/AIDS in the Middle East and North Africa. 15th International AIDS Conference, Bangkok, Thailand, July 13, 2004.
50. Pisani 2000: 65.
51. For Islamic movements as examples of "cultures of resistance," see Levine 2005a: 400–402.
52. For example, Prison Organization, Red Crescent Society, State Welfare Organization, etc.
53. WHO (2004), "Best Practice in HIV/AIDS Prevention," 13, 15, 25.
54. CDC (2003a), "AIDS Prevention Education to Go into Iranian Schools," HIV/AIDS Newsroom. *The Body*, www.thebody.com/cdc/news_updates_archive/2004/jun9_04/iran_aids_schools.html, June 7, 2004.
55. UNGASS (2003c), Saudi Arabia: Follow-up to the Declaration of Commitment on HIV/AIDS (UNGASS) country report format, reporting period January–December 2002, Annexes 1 and 2, written April 28, 2003; received May 2, 2003; posted March 31, 2003, http://www.unaids.org/EN/other/functionalities.
56. Tariq Madani, Yagoub Al-Mazrou, Mohammad Al-Jeffri, and Naser Al Huzaim, "Epidemiology of the Human Immunodeficiency Virus in Saudi Arabia; 18 Year Surveillance Results and Prevention from an Islamic Perspective," *BMC Infectious Diseases* 4.25 (2004): 2, 7–8.
57. Abdul Ghafour. (2004).
58. UNGASS (2003a), Oman: Follow-up to the Declaration of Commitment on HIV/AIDS (UNGASS) country report format, reporting period: January–December 2002, Annexes 1 and 2, written May 5, 2003; received May 12, 2003; posted March 31, 2003.
59. UNDP (2004), "The Cairo Declaration of Religious Leaders in the Arab States in Response to the HIV/AIDS Epidemic," UNDP HIV/AIDS Regional Programme in the Arab States, November 12–13, 2004.
60. Pisani 2000: 66.
61. DeJong et al. 2005: 55.
62. Ibid.
63. WHO (2004), "Best Practice in HIV/AIDS Prevention and Care for Injecting Drug Abusers: The Triangular Clinic in Kermanshah, Islamic Repub-

lic of Iran" (Cairo: World Health Organization Regional Office for the Eastern Mediterranean, 2004) 25, 27, Document WHO-EM/STD/052/E/U/05.04/1000.

64. DeJong et al. 2005: 56.
65. Piot 2002: 5.
66. UNDP (2003), "Key arts and media personalities gather to break the silence on HIV/AIDS in the Arab world," Press Release. United Nations Development Programme. www.undp.org/dpa/pressrelease/releases/2--3/march/05mar03.html.
67. DeJong et al. 2005: 56.
68. UNAIDS (2006a), Draft Political Declaration, June 2, 2006, http://www.un.org/ga/aidsmeeting 2006, 2.
69. UNAIDS (2007), http://www.unaids.org/en/Regions_Countries/Regions/MiddleEastAndNorthAfrica.asp.
70. Levine 2005b: 146.
71. Ibid.
72. Levine 2005a: 397.
73. Ali Mirsepassi (2006b), "New Geographies of Modernity," *Comparative Studies of South Asia, Africa and the Middle East* 26.1 (2006): 2, 4.
74. Levine 2005a: 394.
75. Levine 2005a: 397.
76. Mirsepassi 2006b: 4.

REFERENCES AND FURTHER READING

Boufford, Jo Ivey. (2005). "Leadership Development for Global Health," in *Global Health Leadership and Management*, ed. William Foege (San Francisco: Jossey-Bass 2005) 153–154.

CDC. (2003a). "AIDS Prevention Education to Go into Iranian Schools," HIV/AIDS Newsroom. *The Body*, www.thebody.com/cdc/news_updates_archive/2004/jun9_04/iran_aids_schools.html, June 7, 2004.

CDC. (2003b). "Lebanon: AIDS Drug Deal to Slash Treatment Costs," *CDC News Updates*, April 21, 2003.

DeJong, Jocelyn, Jawad, Rana, Nortagy, Iman, and Shepard, Bonnie. (2005). "The Sexual and Reproductive Health of Young People in the Arab Countries and Iran." *Reproductive Health Matters* 13.25 (2005): 55.

El-Deeb, Khaled. (2006). "Judge Speeds Up Nurses' Trial in Libya." *The State*, Associated Press, June 13, 2006, http://hosted.ap.org/dynamic/stories/L/LIBYA_BULGARIA_AIDS_TRIAL?SITE=SCCOL&SECTION=HOME&TEMPLATE=DEFAULT.

Garrett, Laurie. (2006). "America shouldn't befriend Libya just yet." *International Herald Tribune*, June 11, 2006, http://www.iht.com/articles/2006/06/11/opinion/edgarrett.php.

Ghafour, P.K. Abdul. (2004a). "Conference Puts AIDS in the Spotlight." *Arab News*. December 1, 2004.

Ghafour, P.K. Abdul. (2004b). "84 Children among Kingdom's AIDS Patients." *Arab News*. August 7, 2004.

Howard, Susanna. (2005). "North Africa, Middle East: HIV/AIDS Groups Aim to Nip a Rising Threat," January 28, 2005. Excerpted from Susanna Howard, *Wall Street Journal*, January 27, 2005, http://www.thebody.com/cdc/news_updates_archive/2005/jan28_05/arab_countries_hiv.html#.

Jenkins, Carol (2004). "Vulnerability to HIV/AIDS in the Middle East and North Africa: A Socio-Epidemiology Overview," paper given at Satellite Meeting of Global Researchers of HIV/AIDS in the Middle East and North Africa Region, 15th International AIDS Conference, Bangkok, Thailand, July 13, 2004.

Jenkins, Carol and Robalino, David. (2003). *HIV/AIDS in the Middle East and North Africa: The Costs of Inaction* (Washington DC: The World Bank, 2003) xiv.

Joint United Nations Programme on HIV/AIDS (2006). 2006 Report on the Global AIDS epidemic: A UNAIDS 10th Anniversary Special Edition. http://data.unaids.org/pub/GlobalReport/2006/2006_GR_CH02_en.pdf, 48.

Kaiser Family Foundation. (2006a). "Defense Lawyers for Medical Workers Accused of Infecting Libyan Children with HIV Request HIV/AIDS Experts' Testimony," June 21, 2006, http://www.kaisernetwork.org/daily_reports/rep_hiv. cfm#38033

Kaiser Family Foundation. (2006b). "Retrial of Medical Workers Accused of Infecting Libyan Children with HIV Adjourned until June 20," June 14, 2006, http://www.kaisernetwork.org/daily_reports/rep_index.cfm?hint=1&DR_ID=37890.

Krosnar, Katka. (2003). "Libyan Government Lets AIDS Experts Comment on Hospital Deaths," *BMJ*, 327.7411 (August 16, 2003): 360.

Levine, Mark. (2005a). "Chaos and Globalization in the Middle East," *Asian Journal of Social Science* 33 (2005): 397.

Levine, Mark. (2005b). "Globalization in the MENA and Europe: Culture, Economy and the Public Sphere in a Transnational Context," *Journal of Muslim Minority Affairs* 25.2 (August 2005): 154.

Madani, Tariq, Al-Mazrou, Yagoub, Al-Jeffri, Mohammad, and Al Huzaim, Naser. (2004). "Epidemiology of the Human Immunodeficiency Virus in Saudi Arabia; 18 Year Surveillance Results and Prevention from an Islamic Perspective," *BMC Infectious Diseases* 4.25 (2004): 2, 7–8.

Maqboul, Etaf, and Ramahi, Wafa Abu Ayyash. (2005). "Assessment of Palestinian Students' Knowledge about the Acquired Immunodeficiency Syndrome and their Attitudes Towards AIDS Patients" (Bethlehem: Center for Sustainable Development and Community Health, 2005) unpublished paper, 2, 3.

Mirsepassi, Ali. (2006a). "Introduction: Globalization and Place." Special volume, Beyond the boundaries of the old geographies: Natives, citizens, exiles and cosmopolitans, *Comparative Studies and South Asia, Africa and the Middle East*, 26(1).

Mirsepassi, Ali. (2006b). "New Geographies of Modernity," *Comparative Studies of South Asia, Africa and the Middle East* 26.1 (2006): 2, 4.

Montagnier, Luc, and Colizzi, Vittorio. (2003). "Final Report of Prof. Luc Montagnier and Prof. Vittorio Colizzi to Libyan Arab Jamahiriya on the Nosocomial HIV infection at the Al-Fateh Hospital, Benghazi, Libya," Paris, April 7, 2003, http://www.webcitation.org/5Mempgl11, 20–21.

Piot, Peter. (2002). "HIV/AIDS in the MENA Region: Challenges and Future Prospects." Beirut, Lebanon, 17 June 2002, www.unaids.org/html.pub/medial/speeches01/piot_Beirut_010602_en_doc.htm 4.

Pisani, Elizabeth. (2000). "AIDS into the 21st Century: Some Critical Considerations," *Reproductive Health Matters* 8(15) (May 2000): 65.

Rasooldeen, Mohammed. (2004). "SR15 Million Spent on AIDS Fight," *Arab News*, December 8, 2004.

Sarrar, Salah. (2006). "Foreign Medics' Trial in Libya Postponed to July 4," *Reuters*, June 20, 2006, http://today.reuters.co.uk/news/newsArticle.aspx?type=worldNews&storyID=2006-06-20T100534Z_01_L20587534_RTRUKOC_0_UK-LIBYA-TRIAL.xml&archived=False.

Steinbrook, Robert. (2004). "After Bangkok—Expanding the Global Response to AIDS," *New England Journal of Medicine* 351.8 (August 19, 2004): 738–742.

UNAIDS. (2003). Middle East and North Africa Region, "Regional HIV and AIDS estimates, end 2003," http://www.unaids.org/en/geographical+area/by+region/north+africa+and+middle+east+new.asp.

UNAIDS. (2004). "Middle East and North Africa," in *UNAIDS AIDS Epidemic Update*, December 2004, http://www.unaids.org/wad2004/report_pdf.html, 66.

UNAIDS. (2006a). Draft Political Declaration, June 2, 2006, http://www.un.org/ga/aidsmeeting2006.

UNAIDS. (2006b). "Fact Sheet: AIDS Epidemic in the Middle East and North Africa," December 2006, http://data.unaids.org/pub/EpiReport/2006/20061121_epi_fs_mena_en.pdf.

UNAIDS. (2007). Middle East and North Africa. Retrieved from: http://www.unaids.org/en/Regions_Countries/Regions/MiddleEastAndNorthAfrica.asp.

UNAIDS and WHO. (2004a). Epidemiological Fact Sheet. 2004 Update: Turkey, http://globalatlas.who.int/globalatlas/predefinedReports/EFS2004/EFS_PDFs/EFS2004_TR.pdf, 2.

UNAIDS and WHO. (2004b). Epidemiological Fact Sheet. 2004 Update: Yemen. http://globalatlas.who.int/globalatlas/predefinedReports/EFS2004/EFS_PDFs/EFS2004_YE.pdf, 2.

UNAIDS and WHO. (2005). AIDS epidemic update. Middle East and North Africa Region, "Regional HIV and AIDS Estimates, End 2005," http://www.thebody.com/unaids/pdfs/Epi05_13_en.pdf.

UNAIDS and WHO. (2006a). Epidemiological Fact Sheet on HIV/AIDS. 2006 Update: Afghanistan, http://www.who.int/GlobalAtlas/predefinedReports/EFS2004/EFS_PDFs/EFS2006_AF.pdf.

UNAIDS and WHO. (2006b). Epidemiological Fact Sheet on HIV/AIDS. 2006 Update: Iraq, http://globalatlas.who.int/globalatlas/predefinedReports/EFS2004/EFS_PDFs/EFS2006_IQ.pdf, 2.

UNDP. (2003). "Key Arts and Media Personalities Gather to Break the Silence on HIV/AIDS in the Arab World," Press Release. United Nations Development Programme, www.undp.org/dpa/pressrelease/releases/2--3/march/05mar03.html.

UNDP. (2004). "The Cairo Declaration of Religious Leaders in the Arab States in Response to the HIV/AIDS Epidemic," UNDP HIV/AIDS Regional Programme in the Arab States, November 12–13, 2004.

UNGASS. (2003a). Oman: Follow-up to the Declaration of Commitment on HIV/AIDS (UNGASS) country report format, reporting period: January–December 2002, Annexes 1 and 2, written May 5, 2003, received May 12, 2003, posted March 31, 2003.

UNGASS. (2003b). Qatar: Follow-Up to the Declaration of Commitment on HIV/AIDS (UNGASS) country report format, reporting period January–December 2002, Annexes 1 to 3, written April 15, 2003, received April 23, 2003, posted March 31, 2003.

UNGASS. (2003c). Saudi Arabia: Follow-Up to the Declaration of Commitment on HIV/AIDS (UNGASS) country report format, reporting period January–December 2002, Annexes 1 and 2, written April 28, 2003, received May 2, 2003, posted March 31, 2003, http://www.unaids.org/EN/other/functionalities.

UNGASS. (2003d). Turkey: Follow-Up to the Declaration of Commitment on HIV/AIDS (UNGASS) country report format, reporting period January–December 2002. Annexes 1 and 2, written April 15, 2003, received April 23, 2003, posted March 31, 2003, http://www.unaids.org/EN/other/functionalities.

WHO. (2002). "Improving Health Sector Response to HIV/AIDS and Sexually Transmitted Diseases in the Countries of the Eastern Mediterranean Region of WHO: Regional Strategic Plan, 2002–2005." (Cairo: WHO, 200) 8–10.

WHO. (2004). "Best Practice in HIV/AIDS Prevention and Care for Injecting Drug Abusers: The Triangular Clinic in Kermanshah, Islamic Republic of Iran," Document WHO-EM/STD/052/E/U/05.04/1000 (Cairo: World Health Organization Regional Office for the Eastern Mediterranean, 2004) 13, 15, 25.

WHO and UNAIDS. (2005). "Access to HIV Treatment Continues to Accelerate in Developing Countries, But Bottlenecks Persist, Says WHO/UNAIDS Report," June 29, 2005, http://www.who.int/3by5/progressreportJune2005/en/.

World Bank. (2004). "AIDS Regional Update: Middle East and North Africa, An Opportunity for Prevention: HIV/AIDS Situation in the Middle East and North Africa Region," web.worldbank.org/WBSITE/EXTERNAL/NEWS, June 2004.

Ziady, Hany (2004). WHO, "The Meaning of the 3 by 5 Initiative for Global Health and the Middle East," Paper given at the Satellite Meeting of Global Network of Researchers on HIV/AIDS in the Middle East and North Africa. 15th International AIDS Conference, Bangkok, Thailand, July 13, 2004.

CHAPTER 37

Viropolitics

How HIV Produces Therapeutic Globalization

Vinh-Kim Nguyen

ABSTRACT

With new "hot zones" springing up in the wake of the Afghan war, economic liberalization in China, and social restructuring in the former socialist states of Eastern Europe, it becomes difficult not to view the HIV epidemic as emblematic of globalization: systemic in nature and planetary in scope. The HIV epidemic itself produces globalization in novel and specific ways. The epidemic—both in the terrible devastation it has wrought on individuals and communities and in the response to that devastation—has shaped the way we interact as a global community and perhaps what is at stake in global politics.

It has been argued that Louis Pasteur, the man credited for the germ theory of disease causation, gave microbial agents the power to reorganize society, what Latour called the "Pasteurization of France." Latour was not just referring to the Pasteurian idea that microbes could cause disease and made them intelligible as unseen agents of misfortune. He was also indicating that the material practices that made microbes visible in the laboratory (from putrescence to Petri dishes) made them actors in the messy social world outside the laboratory. And once microbes were granted a kind of non-human citizenship in that messy social world—as causes of disease and agents to be governed through a range of sanitary rules and regulations—they were given the power to regulate human behavior, too. This view has come to be called "actor network theory," and informs my argument that HIV has reordered the world we live in. It has done so by linking together social phenomena (all the things that we have come to know as "risk" for HIV, ranging from individuals' sexual practices to large-scale social processes) to a range of material practices and technologies (condoms, safer sex, microbicides, gender empowerment). It has also catalyzed a transnational industry that brings together pharmaceuticals firms, activists, NGOs, and therapeutic entrepreneurs of all sorts. Together, these assemblages of ideas and practices have transformed the way we make love, the regulatory regimes that govern the circulation of pharmaceuticals, and even what is at stake in international intervention.

Now in its third decade, the HIV epidemic is often seen as globalization's biological hubris. As the epidemic continues to unfold in the twenty-first century, with new "hot zones" springing up in the wake of the Afghan war, economic liberalization in China, and social restructuring in the former socialist states of Eastern Europe, it becomes difficult not to view the epidemic as emblematic of globalization: systemic in nature, it is also irresolutely planetary in scope. As we see in this volume, the HIV epidemic is clearly a product of globalization, a dark side of the movement of populations, desires, and microbes and the new transnational inequalities that drive them. However, in this chapter, I want to explore the flip side of this view; namely, that the HIV epidemic itself produces novel and specific forms of globalization—what I will describe in this chapter as therapeutic globalization. The epidemic has crystallized contestation of global regimes (particularly with regard to intellectual property law and access to pharmaceuticals but increasingly over debt and poverty relief) and led to the rise of massive international AIDS relief, deployed by the Global Fund, the U.S. President's Emergency Program for AIDS Relief (PEPFAR) or the Gates Foundation, amongst many others. As these developments attest, the epidemic has shaped the way we interact as a global community around health issues, signaling a move to a "post-Westphalian" governance of health. However, it also marks a shift in what is at stake in global politics. The conjugation of military and humanitarian interventions since the Balkan wars of the late 1990s heralds a geopolitics where the projection of power can maim or kill, but can also make live.

This becomes clear in an ethnographic consideration of the evolution of the response to the HIV epidemic, as I will show below. The term "viropolitics" is used here to draw attention to the broad range of political phenomena that have clustered around HIV, ranging from negotiations between states about HIV policy to the micropolitics in the lives of those who live with the virus or are affected by it in some way. The term borrows from Foucault's notion of biopower, understood as a form of power that emerges with the rise of the modern state. Biopower manifests in the government of populations and individuals through technologies aimed at their bodily welfare. HIV has provided an organizing framework for the dissemination of a range of standardized political and social technologies across the globe. These technologies have worked to reshape subjectivities, biologies, and social relations in those that have used them; in this sense they have produced a form of therapeutic globalization. This chapter presents an ethnographic and historical overview of the response to the epidemic based on my own engagement with community-based organizations responding to the epidemic in the West African countries of Burkina Faso and Côte d'Ivoire.

A HUMANITARIAN INTERNATIONAL

This global response to HIV has come to constitute a veritable industry. It employs thousands and has deployed a range of technologies that manufacture specific products (management templates, pharmaceuticals, vaccines, condoms, self-help strategies; many of which are further discussed in this volume). Central to its expansion has been the growing market for the goods it produces. This is a humanitarian market, one that links social suffering and the global circulation of its representations with the attempts to alleviate it. Although the global AIDS industry often seeks alternatives to the free market economy that has so clearly failed to produce the global public good of health, it is nonetheless embedded in a global regime of value and exchange, however humanitarian its goals. Its products, however, are not limited to antiretroviral drugs or condoms; they include discourses, subjectivities, institutions, and even physiologies.

The global humanitarian industry has come under increasing scrutiny since the new millennium. Alex de Waal's critical scholarship of the "Famine Industry" and the "Human Rights International" (de Waal 1997) suggests that we can today speak of a "humanitarian international." The everyday reality and political implications of this humanitarian international emerges from ethnographic scrutiny of a myriad of humanitarian sites, from refugee camps and NGOs to the military-humanitarian complex in the Balkans (Douzinas 2003; Duffield 2001; Fassin and Vasquez 2005; Fischer 1997; Malkki 1995, 1997, 2001; Pandolfi 2000). This research has largely focused on the globalized nature of these large-scale institutional responses to humanitarian catastrophes; less visible has been attention to how these responses in fact produce a particular kind of humanitarian globalization, one that tracks both forwards (to its intended recipients) and backwards (to its beneficent instigators), to embrace them in a moral economy.

The violence of the Biafran civil war in Nigeria in the late 1960s was the first time that the widespread suffering of civilian populations triggered a global reaction, and that moment is often credited with the birth of modern humanitarianism (Weber 2000). To this day, the "French doctors" who first denounced the atrocities are seen as emblematic of the humanitarian figure, who braves injustice to denounce the suffering of the powerless and voiceless. Modern humanitarianism is based on a politics of witnessing, ushering an era where mass-media representations of suffering are instrumentally linked with attempts to alleviate that suffering (Redfield 2006). We have all, at some point, been moved by representations of suffering while at times wondering whether we are not in some way being subject to manipulation. This concern informed Boltanski's sociology of distant suffering, which inquired as to how representations of abjection—such as the iconic starving African child—could trigger responses of concern for anonymous strangers that would not occur in everyday life, and the implications of this phenomenon for social relations (Boltanski 1993; Kleinman and Kleinman 1996). Globalization is commonly thought of as a form of bringing the world closer; Boltanski's argument suggests that it might also be a form of distancing, as suffering becomes only manageable in a distant stranger—rather than in an intimate figure who might share our everyday world. As though we might need the distant suffering of global others to better endure the immediacy of social suffering in our midst.

Anthropologists have sought to bring distant suffering closer empirically and theoretically. An engaged perspective was developed by scholars of "social suffering," who argued that suffering is caused by social relations that inflict violence on the powerless. This enormously influential school began with Farmer's seminal work that showed how AIDS in Haiti was the outcome of a centuries-old structure of persistent and continuing racism (Farmer 1993). As Farmer and many others have shown, globalization has exacerbated the inequalities that produce social suffering, whether this be epidemic diseases or others. Scholars working in this tradition have endeavored to unmask the structural violence these forms of inequality constitute by linking suffering to social and economic processes. Ethnographic research has sought to link suffering at home and abroad to common, global processes and provide vivid accounts of the devastation wrought by these processes, taking the politics of witnessing to the heart of ethnographic research. The call for a "militant" anthropology has not gone unheeded, and has had a significant impact on the response to the epidemic. It was instrumental in recasting the AIDS epidemic as a humanitarian emergency. Today, unprecedented resources are flowing into many developing countries to combat the AIDS epidemic, swelling the AIDS industry and staging a massive humanitarian intervention. In this chapter, I argue this massive humanitarian intervention paved the way for the globalization of a very specific form of biopolitics. The features of this biopolitics emerge from empirical consideration of the response to the epidemic, to which I now turn.

THE RESPONSE TO THE EPIDEMIC: A BRIEF HISTORY

While the global history of AIDS has yet to be written, it is already possible to distinguish three generations in the response to the epidemic. Each generation disseminated a different set of technologies that layered onto the previous set—to varying biological, social, and institutional effect. The pre-1994 classical public health strategy was sharpened by a focus on rights (1994–2000) which paved the way, after 2000, for an aggressive interventionist approach to testing and treatment, in many ways resurrecting a more orthodox public health approach. The ideal-type of the first generation of the response was incarnated in WHO's model medium-term plans, used by national Ministries of Health as blueprints for designing programs to respond to the epidemic. A mix of classical public health approaches to controlling infectious diseases as reflected in these plans, which stressed epidemiological surveillance (with a particular focus on high-risk groups and rapid "knowledges, attitudes, behaviours and practices" or KABP studies) and achieving behavior change. These programs deployed a range of social technologies: voluntary counseling and testing (particularly for pregnant women and high-risk groups), social marketing of condoms, and "IEC" (Information–Education–Communication) campaigns. These aimed to raise awareness of HIV and how to prevent it, as well as to gather data that would paint a more finely grained epidemiological picture. Considerable efforts were made to broaden the scope of this response beyond narrowly defined "affected and vulnerable" populations by reframing AIDS as a problem of development. The broadened response was to be multi-sectoral, concerned with addressing the social determinants of vulnerability by integrating AIDS programs within all branches of government and development assistance. This first generation of response was characterized by a managerial and epidemiological ethos concerned with mapping the epidemic and deploying standardized policy responses. Remarkably, in many parts of the world where the epidemic was already ravaging populations, this translated into little or no actual services to meet actual needs—HIV testing rates remained low and the epidemic coursed, largely invisible and silent, even in the hospital wards that filled with patients suffering from opportunistic infections (Mann and Tarantola 1996).

Even as this public health framework began to take hold across the globe, a coalition of AIDS and social activists (some of whom had become powerful AIDS bureaucrats) came together to contest what they feared was an "exclusion and control" approach, arguing that instead "rights and empowerment" should be stressed (Seidel 1993). This crystallized as a policy of "greater involvement of people with HIV and AIDS" or GIPA in 1994. This policy aimed to "give a face" to the epidemic through active empowerment of people with HIV and AIDS by involving them at the front lines of the response as prevention workers and lay counselors. GIPA helped shift the response to an emphasis on individual empowerment. People with HIV were trained to "come out" and affirm their rights in a workshop that used what have been called "confessional technologies" by myself and others to build the skills to testify about being HIV in public (for a fuller account, see Nguyen 2005a). These technologies had originated in small and large group awareness training groups pioneered in the civil rights, feminist and countercultural movements of the American 1960s (Lee 2002). They included open-ended questions, role plays, trust-building exercises, and many others. In the late 1970s they migrated to a host of other social change movements, including gay liberation, playing a central part in the gay community's response to the epidemic in America in the 1980s particularly through the "buddy" system that matched AIDS patients with caregivers who would support them through their illness. As I have argued elsewhere, they were powerful technologies for training, but also for producing new socialities and subjectivities (Nguyen 2005b). This second generation of the response was marked by an ideology of rights and empowerment and the practical deployment of a range of individualizing technologies that in effect addressed a transnational public of people living with HIV.

As a result, a small army of HIV-positive activists was trained across the world, which helped to shift the paradigm of the response by 2000. Access to effective treatment for the infection, which had been available in the north since 1995 but had been considered too expensive, too complex, and not cost-effective in the south, became a political issue (most notably in the context of the 2000 U.S. Presidential campaign). Health was forcefully argued to be a human right, and this came to be viewed through the lens of access to treatment—and the complex welter of institutional, policy, and even geopolitical issues that hindered that access. The stage was set for casting the epidemic as a humanitarian medical emergency. It was not long before a wave of "emergency" programs emerged to treat AIDS—most notably, WHO's "3×5" initiative inspired by Paul

Farmer's group at Harvard and President Bush's Emergency Program for AIDS Relief (PEPFAR). It is worth stressing that it was advances in biomedical research (that is, the discovery of life-saving highly active antiretroviral therapy in 1994) that were able to reframe a public health crisis deeply rooted in decades of neglect of global public health as a humanitarian emergency. Biomedical technologies—antiretrovirals, but also the technologies to diagnose HIV and monitor the medications—have become the driving force of the response. This is now increasingly concerned with scaling up access to treatment, and in the future will be called to attend to the complex logistical and policy challenges of managing millions of people in poor countries who depend on continual treatment for survival.

HIV-Testing Programs

Distinguishing three generations in the response provides a shorthand to historicizing the epidemic, although of course "in the field" the reality was, and continues to be, more complex. I started working with community-based organizations in Burkina Faso and Côte d'Ivoire in 1994. In those early years, HIV testing programs were relatively few and far between—in the Ivoirian metropolis of Abidjan, for example, there was only one site that provided free and anonymous testing in 1995. In Burkina Faso, there was little or no access to HIV screening—including for screening blood transfusions. As a result, only a handful number of people knew their HIV status. The few who were tested were often not told of their diagnosis. In the main hospital in Ouagadougou, Burkina Faso, for example, HIV testing was done sporadically for inpatients in 1994–1995, but the majority were not told; the few who were informed of their diagnosis had an "A" scrawled in red on their charts.

In the mid-1990s, two large clinical trials of AZT for the prevention of mother to child transmission of HIV (commonly abbreviated as "pMTCT") were conducted in West Africa; one sponsored by the French national AIDS research agency (ANRS) and the other by the rival American Centers for Disease Control (CDC). The French study tested 14,385 women in Bobo-Dioulasso (Burkina Faso) and Abidjan while the American study tested 12,668 women in Abidjan. All the women, of course, received state-of-the-art pre-test counseling for HIV. Of the total of over 27,000 women tested, 3,424 were found to be HIV positive. However, in the American study 618 HIV-positive women never returned for their results and the post-test counseling; in the French study the figure was 648—almost a third. Researchers told me that the rate of drop-out was lower in HIV-negative women, suggesting that women suspected their diagnosis and decided not to return for results. Of the HIV-positive women who did return for their results, only 711 were included in the actual trials, the remaining 2,713 women having either not returned for follow-up as just discussed, been excluded for various reasons, or simply not consented (Dabis et al. 1999; Wiktor et al. 1999).

The trials had an enormous impact in shaping the early response to the epidemic—simply through the sheer number tested. Based on my own fieldwork with HIV prevention and care programs in both countries in the mid-1990s, the majority of people who knew their HIV status had found out by having been recruited by the trials. Of course, only a small minority actually were enrolled in the trials, which had to screen a very large number to have a significant pool from which to enrol a necessarily smaller number of selected, eligible study subjects. There were numerous reasons which disqualified women—not arriving early enough in pregnancy to receive the AZT, or suffering from anemia (which could be dangerously worsened if they received AZT) were among the most common. Women who had tested positive but had not been eligible to enrol in the trials complained bitterly that they had been "discarded." They resented that they did not have access to what they perceived to be a panoply of services for the women who had been included in the trials and therefore had been randomized to the receive either placebo or AZT. Indeed, women who were included in the trial did receive medical care and social services that were not available to others. Many women found their way into community groups after having been tested in search of material and social support; some even set up organizations for their fellow would-be trial subjects. They made up the bulk of the membership of early groups of people living with HIV in both countries.

At the same time, international donors were stressing "empowerment" of people living with HIV and AIDS as a human-rights-based response to the epidemic. The first step of empowerment was disclosure: being able to be "out" and talk about being HIV positive. This was a difficult step for many of the women, for whom disclosure could lead to blame, violence, and even being disowned by husband and family. Women—most of whom had found out about being HIV positive through the clinical trials—were swept up in the wave of empowerment training workshops that coursed across Africa after 1995. The workshops trained Africans to give testimonials about being HIV positive (Nguyen 2005b). They did so using experiential and active listening techniques first developed by social psychologists after World War II that then disseminated into management schools and self-awareness movements in America. These confessional technologies were remarkable because they were so effective—participants reported to me putting them into practice immediately after they finished the workshops: mirroring the posture of their interlocutors, asking open-ended questions, practicing active listening. These social technologies were the foundation of what were to become therapeutic communities.

A Social Tissue of Disclosure

When they returned to their community associations, workshop participants set up discussion groups to encourage other people with HIV to talk about their affliction. I attended these groups regularly from when they first started, in 1998. In Côte d'Ivoire and Burkina Faso, however, in the first few years, the groups did not seem particularly successful. Very few men attended. Attempts to get participants talking were at first met by silence and, eventually, halting attempts at self-expression that more often than not were a litany of complaints that seemed devoid of affective content. But, over time the dynamic in the groups began to change. After awkward, embarrassed beginnings a more convivial atmosphere began to prevail. Previously laconic participants became voluble and animated. Gradually, the charismatic side of some of the participants emerged.

Their narratives were frequently couched in an evangelical idiom, describing the process of being diagnosed with HIV as the beginning of a conversion-like process, the first step on a road that led to greater enlightenment and the adoption of a more responsible, moral life. These declarations were inevitably followed by exhortations to the audience to get tested. These evangelical idioms disturbed many of the Western aid workers employed by the agencies that funded these efforts. Thee workers had come to international AIDS work through AIDS activism in the north, and many from the gay community. Needless to say, the moralizing tone of message conflicted with aid workers' personal values that stressed empowerment, sexual openness, and tolerance.

Initially, I suspected that that these evangelical forms were either historical residues of the colonial period or a reflection of the growing popularity of Pentecostal churches. I spent considerable time interviewing volunteers and adepts in religious organizations. Some of these organizations were responding directly to the epidemic in various ways—volunteering at the hospital, holding prayer services, providing emotional and material support—while others were not so directly involved with epidemic but concerned with affliction more broadly understood. Some spoke of volunteering to work with the ill and dying as a religious experience, while others expressed the desire to offer solace to those afflicted. Common to all was a powerful sense that what was at stake was the way in which HIV reframed moral dilemmas and required transformation in response.

In other words, faced with the prognosis of certain disease and death—and little in the way of resources to alter that prognosis—what was at stake was how the good life was to be defined and how it might be attained. In this way, the moral dilemmas surrounding the HIV diagnosis (framed by popular understandings of HIV as a disease of sexual immorality) were transformed into ethical predicaments. Sufferers had little to work with—in fact, they had only themselves. Ethics was about attaining the good life (no matter how damaged the prospects might seem) through self-transformation; ethics was about the care of the self and the relationship to others. These circulating, global discourses about AIDS were taken up in local ethical projects, in local economies of self-fashioning. What these ethical predicaments share, perhaps, with evangelical movements is the way in which they make available instruments and strategies which individuals may then take up to equip themselves to better navigate the moral economies in which they are enmeshed. In the era of globalization and NGO discourses about AIDS, these moral economies are starkly juxtaposed, making this task particularly acute for people living with HIV and AIDS in settings where the only source of solidarity is family. The market for testimonials, anchored in Western notions of self-help through confession, offered the best opportunity to gain resources that could help feed family and maintain one's position in the kinship networks that, in the absence of a viable state, are the only available forms of social solidarity.

Until recently, in the absence of any real political or economic engagement to address the structural issues driving the epidemic, it was possible to view these testimonials as only so much post-colonial theatre. But confessional technologies not only produced the desired testimonials; they also were instrumental in turning people living with HIV, many of whom first learned of their diagnosis through a clinical trial, into activists. More significantly, perhaps, they created a tissue of social relations organized around shared disclosure.

SOCIAL TRIAGE

As the supply of donated drugs increased from 1998, self-help groups of people living with HIV were increasingly faced with the gut-wrenching prospect of deciding who should get the drugs. No matter how many donations were received, demand always outstripped supply. In a setting where poverty is endemic, and where the state is a hollow shell providing little—if any—services, any organization offering even the most minimal services is quickly overrun. This was certainly the case of the HIV/AIDS groups where fear of stigma did not appear to be much of a barrier to a steadily increasing stream of would-be beneficiaries. Many were ill, or suspected themselves to be HIV positive because they had lost a spouse.

The concept of triage was developed on the battlefield, as a way to most rationally use scarce treatment resources: those most likely to live are prioritized to receive care, while those whose prognosis is poor are left to die. Many organizations of people with HIV were faced with the same kind of situation. They made the difficult decision of who should benefit from the limited source of drugs by adopting a form of social triage. Those whose continued health was most likely to translate into increased resources for the group were the first beneficiaries. Those who were most charismatic, most able to deliver effective testimonials, would be the best advocates for getting more drug donations. The discussion and self-help groups, which were ideally suited to cultivating and demonstrating testimonial skills, were sites where charisma and other social arts could emerge—and where they could be translated into access to medications. It was a subtle, implicit process, but it highlighted how the discussion groups were veritable social laboratories, where confessional technologies could be used to experiment new forms of disclosure and subtly constitute social triage.

Sometimes the decision as to who should get the drugs was more directly pragmatic. Prioritizing access to drugs for beneficiaries who could be counted upon to facilitate the group's work in virtue of their professional position, for instance as a customs officer, was an example of how groups used drugs to increase access to medications. These strategic forms of social triage contrasted with the rhetoric that framed international donors' aid, which was meant to target the most vulnerable members of society, not the most valuable.

Over time, those who were gifted communicators also became those with the most direct experience with the drugs. Echoing the experience of AIDS activism in the north, these patients were often the most knowledgeable people around when it came to their treatments. Now, as drug programs expand, they are ideal candidates for assuming leadership roles in treatment literacy and expanded access programs. Some, however, had already left as part of a therapeutic migration that brought them to Europe—and antiretrovirals. In some countries, those living with HIV and AIDS benefit from a "humanitarian exception" from deportation by virtue of their biomedical condition. This therapeutic migration was not without consequence for domestic and foreign policy in Europe (Fassin 2001, 2005; Ticktin 2006).

These stories are representative of many whose early experiences with the AIDS industry, its discourses of empowerment, and its confessional technologies trained them to become effective advocates. While South Africa's Treatment Action Campaign (several media profiles of its founder, Zackie Achmat, have made him the best-known African AIDS activist in the north; see Power 2003) is an example of an organization that explicitly harnessed this process to identify and train future activists from the ranks of patients, throughout Africa the inchoate strategies of other groups and activists amounted to the same (Robins 2005, 2006). While some individuals, particularly well versed in the social arts or endowed with charisma, were naturally well suited to draw on the repertoire of confessional techniques to mobilize others, even those less skilled were able to benefit from the drills, exercises, and training that proliferating workshops disseminated throughout the continent. But this "production of activists" was not exclusively driven by social forces.

The issue of access to ARV treatment in effect simultaneously provided both a therapeutic telos and the means to sustaining the therapeutic quest; it grafted seamlessly onto the ethical project that had been fashioned by sufferers through their involvement with HIV groups. Bluntly put, skill at telling the right stories got activists drugs, and kept them alive. The confessional technologies drawn upon on in this therapeutic quest were conjugated with the growing availability of antiretrovirals to fashion, biologically and socially, therapeutic citizens. The activist slogan of "drugs into bodies" tellingly illustrates how social forms are incorporated into individual biology.

FROM TRIAGE TO COMMUNITY

The early years of social triage were a conflicted time. While the discourse of empowerment imagined a community of solidarity and self-help, differential access to medications belied the message. In Abidjan, for instance, not all of the women who had met through the trials and gone on to form self-help groups were able to subsequently get access to the treatments. As time wore on, the women in the groups on treatment grew healthy and plump, while those who did not became thinner. In one group, three women died in one year. Not surprisingly, much rumor and suspicion surrounded the question of access to the medicines, at times poisoning group life.

In the context of generalized poverty, material issues also generated tensions. GIPA policies meant that donors funded organizations of people living with HIV to provide peer-counseling services for prevention and treatment programs. Micro-credit programs were also experimented with by the agencies, while some resorted to outright handouts of food. Taken together, these faltering attempts at something between empowerment and charity generated competition between group members. Eventually, it led to a paradoxical phenomenon: rather than promoting solidarity between group members, these attempts to help created a dynamic of fission as members split off to form their own groups. They reasoned that having one's own group would make it easier to compete for resources from the outside rather than from within the group.

As resources became more plentiful, and donors adjusted their policies to encourage teamwork amongst organizations, competition receded, and the tissue of social relations amongst those who had survived the early years thickened. The shared experience of social triage bound together the first generation of activists. Even between rivals, attendance at workshops and conferences fostered a hesitant and ambivalent comradeship that nonetheless, over time, smoothed over previous conflict. The divisive experience of triage was burnished into an ethic of care of the self—and a sense of obligation to others, who should no longer be allowed to die for lack of treatment. This bivalent ethic of transformation was reflected in the growth of treatment activism, as members of therapeutic communities, trained in the arts of public testimonies, became increasingly politicized and advocated for greater access to the medications. It is difficult not to see in this activism the reflection of the searing experience of the early years of the epidemic. Beyond overt activism, however, this ethic of care of the self and of others was further nurtured by the growth of ARV clubs and discussion groups aimed to support members' being adherent to their medications. Peer support and peer counseling in effect worked to bind people living with HIV and their families into communities marked by shared therapeutic work and the increasingly dense moral economy into which this work embedded them. This moral economy, initially built on an ethic of disclosure and positive living, became increasingly material as the flow of resources (drugs, food aid, micro-credit, credits for school fees for children and orphans, and peer-counseling jobs) from donor agencies increased.

With the drugs came better health and with better health the urge to plan for the future and, for many, start a family. Women, who make up the majority of those in the self-help groups and associations that make up this therapeutic community, were mainly tested in the early years in clinical trials or because their husbands had died. It was thus inevitable that, with improved health, people within the groups began to marry and have children. Ironically, many women had come to the groups through trials aimed at preventing mother-to-child transmission of HIV. They were now having more children, and safely—not so much because of pMTCT interventions, but because they themselves were now on treatment. While the core of these groups was formed around a first generation of activists largely drawn from the ranks of those tested through the pMTCT trials, the subsequent expansion of pMTCT and HIV treatment programs rapidly swelled the mass of the community and self-help groups, already densified by the earlier dynamic of fission. Today these groups offer a plethora of activities and services that in materially powerful ways transform the condition of being HIV positive into social identity and social relations. The glue that holds this all together, both synchronically and diachronically, is antiretroviral treatment—as a common goal, experience, and the chance to have a future together. Remarkably, in these groups it is possible to witness a flattening of hierarchies (for example, between patients and doctors) as the experience of being HIV positive—or of being on ARVs—confers legitimacy and authority. These characteristics —a shared social identity and social relations, a common moral economy, and a flattening of hierarchies—have been described before, in therapeutic communities pioneered in post-World War I psychiatry, and remind us of Goffman's "total institutions" (Mills and Harrison 2007; Goffman 1961). They certainly merit that we see HIV groups as therapeutic communities in the most robust sense.

While confessional technologies and discourses of empowerment provide the tools for building these therapeutic communities, being diagnosed with HIV focuses attention on what is at stake in this activism. Growing availability of ARV drugs, which dramatically restore health in those who are ill and keep them healthy, in effect sustains activism not only by keeping activists alive and healthy, but also by putting flesh on the biomedical discourse that preaches the very real biological efficacy of these drugs. Living through a diagnosis, with all the uncertainties and challenges it raises, is one thing; living through the "resurrection" one experiences after one has been ill and has recovered because of the drugs is a whole other magnitude of experience. No wonder that the medicines have only confirmed the evangelical aura that surrounds HIV and its treatments.

THERAPEUTIC CITIZENSHIP

Until now treatment activism has largely focused on the availability of the treatments for a number of reasons. Certainly the life-saving drugs, with their prohibitively high cost rooted in a complex web of intellectual property and pharmaceutical industry, were powerful symbols of global capital and a tangible rallying point for activism. In 1999–2000 this activism conjugated with the emergence on the global drug market of generic ARVs manufactured by Indian, Thai, and Brazilian pharmaceuticals firms, triggering a rapid collapse in drug prices, suddenly making the drugs far more accessible. However, mechanisms for procuring and supplying the drugs have not been able to keep up. The disintegration of the public health infrastructure in Africa means that, today, drugs can only be delivered through programs patched together from NGOs, community groups, public and mission hospitals, and workplace health centres. In some cases, health care systems are cannibalized in order to piece together ARV distribution mechanisms.

As a result, for many, antiretroviral programs will be one of the few—or maybe the only—interaction they have with the kind of modern institutions those who live in industrialized countries take for granted. In effect, the growing numbers who take part in antiretroviral programs—and the discourses and forms of discipline they embody—do so in an environment where they are otherwise largely disconnected from the cardinal features of global modernity. These features can be summed up as the ability to live in a world where the future has promise because large stable institutions manage the domains of the social world necessary to individual and collective thriving: health, education, public services, economy, etc. This management in effect insures against the vicissitudes of chance events (an illness, a drought, a conflict) that would otherwise always threaten to compromise the future.

Structural adjustment programs, enacted in the context of the contemporary neoliberal consensus, effectively dismantled what infrastructure was in place to provide social services throughout Africa. With the implementation of user fees for schools and health care, those less well off found themselves unable to pay. The growth of the informal economy in Africa from the 1980s testifies to the inability of the formal economy to integrate a new generation that increasingly found itself on the outside of modernity, looking in. In this context, where citizenship is limited and the state's ability to deliver on the promises of modernity is impaired, ARV programs offer partial access to a depleted modernity, an access mediated by the biological condition of its beneficiaries. This depleted modernity is a truncated version of the "full" modernity we enjoy in wealthier countries with functional health, social, and economic systems that do deliver on "promissory notes" of modernity.

Access to this depleted modernity is conditioned by an economy of deprivation. In effect, access is only granted through programs to palliate conditions that have themselves been generated by contemporary globalized processes of dispossession. These processes are driven by macro-economic policies and trade regimes that, for instance, impose tariffs on developing country exports while subsidizing exports from industrialized countries, or protect the intellectual property of corporations while putting indigenous knowledge in the public domain. These processes have compromised livelihoods, driven migration, and weakened the health of the poor, even as basic common goods (clean air and water) are fenced off and commodified. Programs to treat AIDS and other epidemics alleviate poverty, address the needs of "orphans and vulnerable children," and palliate epidemics fanned by many of these processes. In so doing, they produce specific populations that are made available for intervention, in effect paving the way for future relief efforts and justifying the programs that made these populations available in the first place.

BIOAVAILABILITY AND VIROPOLITICS

In his description of the patterns of resort of Indian women organ donors, medical anthropologist Lawrence Cohen (2005) shows how enrollment into family planning programs—often the only contact these poor women had with the state—initiated a "therapeutic" trajectory that continued on to selling one's organs. Cohen uses the term "bioavailability" to refer to this condition. The term plays on the concept of bioavailability in clinical medicine, where it is used to refer to the portion of a biologically active substance that can actually be used by the body once it is ingested (some drugs, for instance, are more "bioavailable" than others because they are more readily absorbed or are metabolized by the liver into more active forms). In the sense introduced by Cohen, bioavailability refers to how historical interconnections between biomedical knowledges and technologies (family planning and transplantation) drive programs that seek out and target specific populations for intervention. Etymologically, Cohen links this concept with Foucault's historical studies of the rise of the modern, governmental state. This, Foucault argued, was inextricably linked to the dissemination of practices designed to manage the population through the internalization of rules and procedures aimed at keeping bodies docile and productive. This "governmental" form of state power focuses on producing a healthy, lively population rather than on asserting territorial sovereignty through force—hence Foucault's term "biopower," where "bio" refers to the emphasis on "life." This is indistinct to classical notions where state power resided in the ability to enforce territorial boundaries and the law through the use of violence.

The global response to the epidemic can be seen as new variant of biopower. It is one that operates transnationally and largely independently of recipient states, and which focuses on a very narrow dimension of population life: the biological futures of those living with HIV. While it participates in the global shift in governance, where politics is displaced by policy and citizens are constituted as objects of management, it signals a marked intensification of processes of individualization, as people become subjects of their biomedical fate. In doing so they regain a partial and depleted citizenship, one that is based on lack and exclusion rather than on wholeness and inclusion. The diffusion of this biomedical subjectivity would not have occurred without the existence of humanitarian networks of concern and intervention. These made it possible to frame HIV in terms of human rights and lack of access to treatment, mobilize political support in wealthy countries, and frame both the problem and its solution in terms of an emergency. Paradoxically, as the response to the epidemic has been transformed into a global industry it has introduced a new aspect of globalization: the globalization of the therapeutic subject, defined in terms of bare, biological existence rather than full participation as a citizen of the modern world.

REFERENCES AND FURTHER READING

Boltanski, Luc. 1993. *La Souffrance à distance*. Paris: Metailié.

Cohen, Lawrence. 2005. "Operability, Bioavailability and Exception." In Aihwa Ong and Stephen Collier, eds. *Global Assemblages: Technology, Politics and Ethics as Anthropological Problems*. London: Blackwell.

Dabis, François, Philippe Msellati, Nicolas Meda, Christiane Wiffens-Ekra, Bruno You, Olivier Manigart, Valériane Leroy, Arlette Simonon, Michel Cartoux, Patrice Combe, Amadou Ouangré, Rosa Ramon, Odette Ky-Zerbo, Crépin Montcho, Roger Salamon, Christine Rouzioux, Philippe Van de Perre, Laurent Mandelbrot for the DITRAME Study Group. 1999. 6-month efficacy, tolerance, and acceptability of a short regimen of oral zidovudine to reduce vertical transmission of HIV in breastfed children in Côte-d'Ivoire and Burkina Faso: a double-blind placebo-controlled multicentre trial. *Lancet* 353:786–793.

De Waal, Alex. 1997. *Famine Crimes: Politics and the Disaster Relief Industry in Africa*. Bloomington: Indiana University Press.

Douzinas, Costas. 2003. "Humanity, Military Humanism and the New Moral Order." *Economy and Society*. 32:159–183.

Duffield, Mark. 2001. *Global Governance and the New Wars: The Merging of Development and Security*. London and New York: Zed Books.

Farmer, Paul. 1993. *AIDS and Accusation: Haïti and the Geography of Blame*. Berkeley: University of California Press.

Fassin, Didier. 2001. "Quand le corps fait loi. La raison humanitaire dans les procédures de régularisation des étrangers en France." *Sciences Sociales et Santé* 19:5–34.

Fassin, Didier. 2005. "Compassion and Repression: The Moral Economy of Immigration Policies in France." *Cutural Anthropology* 20:362–387.

Fassin, Didier and Paula Vasquez. 2005. "Humanitarian Exception as the Rule: The Political Theology of the 1999 Tragedia in Venezuela." *American Ethnologist* 32:389–405.

Ferguson, James. 2006. *Global Shadows: Africa in the Neoliberal World Order*. Durham: Duke University Press.

Fischer, William F. 1997. "Doing Good? The Politics and Antipolitics of NGO Practices." *Annual Review of Anthropology* 26:439–464.

Goffman, Erving. 1961. *Asylums: Essays on the Social Situation of Mental Patients and Other Inmates*. New York: Doubleday Anchor.

Kleinman, Arthur and Joan Kleinman. 1996. "The Appeal of Experience; The Dismay of Images: Cultural Appropriations of Suffering in Our Times." *Daedulus* 125: 1–24.

Lee, Laura Kim. 2002. "*Changing Selves, Changing Society: Human Relations Experts and the Invention of T Groups, Sensitivity Training and Encounter in the United States, 1938–1980*." Ph.D. dissertation, University of California, Los Angeles.

Malkki, Liisa. 1995. "Refugees and Exile: From 'Refugee Studies' to the National Order of Things." *Annual Review of Anthropology* 24:495–523.

Malkki, Liisa. 1997 "Speechless Emissaries. Refugees, Humanitarism and Dehistoricization." In Akhil Gupta and James Ferguson, eds. *Culture, Power, Place: Explorations in Critical Anthropology*. Durham: Duke University Press.

Malkki, Liisa. 2001. "Nongovernmental Organizations, Grassroots, and the Politics of Virtue." *Signs* 26: 1187–1211.

Mann, Jonathan and Daniel Tarantola. 1996. *Aids in the World II*. Oxford: Oxford University Press.

Mills, John A. and Tom Harrison. 2007. "John Rickman, Wilfred Ruprecht Bion, and the Origins of the Therapeutic Community." *History of Psychology* 10:22–43.

Nguyen, Vinh-Kim. 2005a. "Antiretroviral Globalism, Biopolitics, and Therapeutic Citizenship." In Aihwa Ong and Stephen J. Collier, eds. *Global Assemblages: Technology, Politics, and Ethics as Anthropological Problems*, London: Blackwell.

Nguyen, Vinh-Kim. 2005b. "Uses and Pleasures: Sexual Modernity, HIV/AIDS and Confessional Technologies in a West African Metropolis." In Vincanne Adams and Stacy Leigh Pigg, eds. *Sex in Development: Science, Sexuality, and Morality in Global Perspective*. Durham: Duke University Press.

Pandolfi, Mariella. 2000. "L'Industrie humanitaire: une souveraineté mouvante et supracoloniale. Réflexion sur l'expérience des Balkans." *Multitudes* 3:97–105.

Power, Samantha. 2003. "The AIDS Rebel." *The New Yorker*, May 19. Accessed June 2007 at http://www.pbs.org/pov/pov2003/stateofdenial/special_rebel.html.

Redfield, Peter. 2006. "A Less Modest Witness: Collective Advocacy and Motivated Truth in a Medical Humanitarian Movement." *American Ethnologist* 33:3–26.

Richey, Lisa Ann and Stefane Ponte. 2006. *Better (RED)™* than Dead: "Brand Aid," Celebrities and the New Frontier of Development Assistance. Copenhagen, Danish Institute for International Studies. Accessed June 2007 at http://www.diis.dk/sw27885.asp.

Robins, Steven L. 2005. "From 'Miraculous Cures' to 'Normal(ised)' Medicine: AIDS Treatment, Activism and Citizenship in the UK and South Africa," *IDS Working Paper 252*. Brighton, UK: Institute of Development Studies.

Robins, Steven L. 2006. "From Rights to 'Ritual': AIDS Activism and Treatment Testimonies in South Africa." *American Anthropologist* 108:312–323.

Seidel, Gill. 1993. "The Competing Discourses of HIV/AIDS in Sub-Saharan Africa: Discourses of Rights and Empowerment vs Discourses of Control and Exclusion." *Social Science and Medicine* 36:175–194.

Silla, Eric. 1998. *People are Not the Same: Leprosy and Identity in Twentieth-Century Mali*. London: Heinemann.

Ticktin, Miriam. 2006. "Where Ethics and Politics Meet: The Violence of Humanitarianism in France." *American Ethnologist* 33:33–49.

Weber, Olivier. 2000. *French Doctors*. Paris: Robert Laffont.

Wiktor, Stefan Z, Ehounou Ekpini, John M. Karon, John Nkengason, Chantal Maurice, Sibailly T. Severin, Thierry H. Roels, Moise K. Kouassi, Eve M. Lackritz, Issa-Malick Coulibaly, and Alan E. Greenberg. 1999. "Short-Course Oral Zidovudine for Prevention of Mother-to-Child Transmission of HIV-1 in Abidjan, Côte-d'Ivoire: A randomised Trial." *Lancet* 353:781–785.

THE GLOBAL HIV/AIDS EPIDEMIC

A timeline of key milestones

(Reproduced with permission from The Kaiser Family Foundation)

Introduction *On June 5, 1981, the United States Centers for Disease Control and Prevention (CDC) issued its first warning about a relatively rare form of pneumonia among a small group of young gay men in Los Angeles, which was later determined to be AIDS-related. Since that time, more than 65 million people have been infected with HIV worldwide, including 39.5 million estimated to be living with HIV/AIDS today. The Global HIV/AIDS Timeline is designed to serve as an ongoing reference tool for the many political, scientific, cultural, and community developments that have occurred over the history of the epidemic.*

Pre-1981 *While 1981 is generally referred to as the beginning of the HIV/AIDS epidemic, scientists believe that HIV was present years before the first case was brought to public attention.*

1981 *U.S. Centers for Disease Control and Prevention (CDC) reports first cases of rare pneumonia in young gay men in the June 5 Morbidity and Mortality Weekly Report (MMWR), later determined to be AIDS. This marks the official beginning of the HIV/AIDS epidemic. CDC also issues report on highly unusual occurrence of rare skin cancer, Kaposi's Sarcoma, among young gay men in the July 4 MMWR.*

First mainstream news coverage of the CDC's June 5 MMWR by the Associated Press and the LA Times on the same day it is issued. The San Francisco Chronicle reports on it the next day.

New York Times publishes its first news story on AIDS on July 3, 1981.

1982 *U.S. CDC formally establishes the term Acquired Immune Deficiency Syndrome (AIDS); refers to four "identified risk factors" of male homosexuality, intravenous drug abuse, Haitian origin and hemophilia A.*

ABC World News Tonight: October 18, 1982. Cause of AIDS epidemic still unknown, now present in many states.

First AIDS case reported in Africa.

First U.S. Congressional hearings held on HIV/AIDS.

"GRID" or "gay-related immune deficiency" increasingly used by the media and health care professionals, mistakenly suggesting inherent link between homosexuality and the syndrome.

Gay Men's Health Crisis, the first community-based AIDS service provider in the U.S., established in New York City.

City and County of San Francisco, working closely with San Francisco AIDS Foundation, Shanti Project and others, develops the "San Francisco Model of Care," which emphasizes home and community-based services.

1983 *The U.S. Public Health Service issues recommendations for preventing transmission of HIV through sexual contact and blood transfusions.*

U.S. CDC clarifies its use of term "high risk group" and urges that it not be used to justify discrimination or unwarranted fear of casual transmission.

U.S. CDC adds female sexual partners of men with AIDS as fifth risk group.

The Orphan Drug Act is signed into U.S. law, providing incentives to drug companies to develop therapies for rare diseases.

People living with AIDS (PWAs) take over plenary stage at U.S. conference and issue statement on the rights of PWAs referred to as The Denver Principles.

National Association of People with AIDS (NAPWA), National AIDS Network (NAN) and Federation of AIDS Related Organizations form.

AIDS Candlelight Memorial held for the first time.

1984 *HIV, the virus, isolated by Luc Montagnier of the Pasteur Institute and Robert Gallo of the National Cancer Institute; later named the Human Immunodeficiency Virus (HIV).*

ABC World News Tonight: November 23, 1984. San Francisco officials order bathhouses closed; major public controversy ensues and continues in Los Angeles, New York and other cities.

CDC states that abstention from intravenous drug use and reduction of needle-sharing "should also be effective in preventing transmission of the virus."

AIDS Action Council is formed by small group of AIDS service organizations from across the United States.

1985 *First International AIDS Conference held in Atlanta. Hosted by U.S. Department of Health and Human Services (DHHS) and the World Health Organization (WHO).*

At least one HIV/AIDS case has been reported from each region of the world.

First HIV case reported in China.

The U.S. Public Health Service issues first recommendations for preventing transmission of HIV from mother to child.

First HIV test licensed by the U.S. Food and Drug Administration (FDA), detects antibodies to HIV. Blood banks begin screening the U.S. blood supply.

Pentagon announces that it will begin testing all new recruits for HIV infection and will reject those who are positive.

ABC World News Tonight: October 2, 1985. Rock Hudson announces that he has AIDS and dies later this year.

Ryan White, an Indiana teenager with AIDS, is barred from school; goes on to speak out publicly against AIDS stigma and discrimination.

New York production of "The Normal Heart", by playwright Larry Kramer, opens; first major play about the early days of the AIDS epidemic.

American Foundation for AIDS Research (amfAR) is founded by Co-Chairs Mathilde Krim and Michael S. Gottlieb, and National Chair Elizabeth Taylor.

Project Inform founded to advocate for faster government approval of HIV drugs.

1986 *President Reagan first mentions the word AIDS in public.*

Informal distribution of clean syringes begins in Boston and New Haven.

ABC World News Tonight: September 19, 1986. AZT, the first drug used to treat AIDS, begins clinical trials.

2nd International AIDS Conference, Paris, France.

U.S. Surgeon General Koop issues "Surgeon General's Report on AIDS", calling for education and condom use.

International Steering Committee for People with HIV/AIDS (ISC) created; becomes Global Network of People Living with HIV/AIDS (GNP+) in 1992.

First HIV cases reported in Russia and India.

National Academy of Science issues report critical of the U.S. response to "national health crisis;" calls for a $2 billion investment.

First panel of the AIDS Memorial Quilt created.

Ricky Ray, a 9-year-old hemophiliac with HIV, is barred from a Florida school and his family's home is burned by arsonists in the following year.

Institute of Medicine report calls for a national education campaign and creation of National Commission on AIDS.

Robert Wood Johnson Foundation creates "AIDS Health Services Program", providing funding to hard hit U.S. cities; program is precursor to Ryan White CARE Act.

1987 *First antiretroviral drug – Zidovudine or AZT (a nucleoside analog) – approved by U.S. FDA.*

Global Programme on AIDS launched by the World Health Organization.

3rd International AIDS Conference, Washington DC.

The AIDS Support Organisation (TASO) formed in Uganda.

ABC World News Tonight: April 1, 1987. President Reagan makes first public speech about AIDS; establishes Presidential Commission on HIV (Watkins Commission).

U.S. FDA sanctions first human testing of candidate vaccine against HIV.

U.S. FDA creates new class of experimental drugs, Treatment Investigational New Drugs (INDs), which accelerates drug approval by two to three years.

U.S. Congress approves $30 million in emergency funding to states for AZT.

U.S. adds HIV as a "dangerous contagious disease" to its immigration exclusion list; mandates testing of all applicants.

U.S. Congress adopts Helms Amendment banning use of federal funds for AIDS education materials that "promote or encourage, directly or indirectly, homosexual activities," often referred to as the "no promo homo" policy.

U.S. FDA adds HIV prevention as a new indication for male condoms.

U.S. CDC launches first AIDS-related public service announcements, "America Responds to AIDS".

U.S. CDC holds its first National Conference on HIV and communities of color.

"And the Band Played On: Politics, People and the AIDS Epidemic", a history of the early years of the epidemic by Randy Shilts, is published.

Entertainer Liberace dies of AIDS.

AIDS Memorial Quilt displayed on National Mall in Washington DC for first time.

The National Black Leadership Commission on AIDS, the National Minority AIDS Council, and the National Task Force on AIDS Prevention form in the U.S.

AIDS Coalition to Unleash Power (ACT UP) established in New York in response to proposed cost of AZT; the price of AZT is subsequently lowered.

First issue of "AIDS Treatment News" published to provide HIV treatment information to community members.

1988 *World AIDS Day first declared by World Health Organization on December 1.*

UNAIDS reports that the number of women living with HIV/AIDS in sub-Saharan Africa exceeds that of men.

4th International AIDS Conference, Stockholm, Sweden.

International AIDS Society Forms.

U.S. Surgeon General and CDC mail brochure "Understanding AIDS" to all U.S. households; first and only national mailing of its kind.

The U.S. Health Omnibus Programs Extension (HOPE) Act of 1988 authorizes the use of federal funds for AIDS prevention, education, and testing.

U.S. National Institutes of Health (NIH) establishes Office of AIDS Research (OAR) and AIDS Clinical Trials Group (ACTG).

U.S. FDA allows the importation of unapproved drugs for persons with life-threatening illnesses, including HIV/AIDS.

ACT UP demonstrates at FDA headquarters in protest of slow pace of drug approval process.

First comprehensive needle exchange program (NEP) established in North America in Tacoma, WA. New York City creates first government-funded NEP and San Francisco establishes what becomes largest NEP in the nation.

ABC World News Tonight: January 8, 1988. WHO reports AIDS cases has jumped 56% worldwide.

ABC World News Tonight: June 17, 1988. A scientist injects himself with an experimental vaccine to help find a cure.

ABC World News Tonight: June 24, 1988. A special commission on AIDS presents a tough report to President Reagan.

ABC World News Tonight: August 29, 1988. A young girl with AIDS can only attend school if she is in a glass enclosure.

ABC World News Tonight: October 6, 1988. A reversal in Department of Justice policy: AIDS/HIV patients can no longer be discriminated against.

ABC World News Tonight: October 17, 1988. A TV commercial campaign about AIDS awareness is aimed at minorities.

1989 *First guidelines for the prevention of Pneumocystis carinii pneumonia (PCP), an AIDS-related opportunistic infection and major cause of morbidity and mortality for people with HIV, are issued by U.S. CDC.*

ABC World News Tonight: April 6, 1989. A foreigner with AIDS is not allowed into the U.S. because he has the virus.

5th International AIDS Conference ("The Scientific and Social Challenge of AIDS"), Montreal, Canada.

U.S. Congress creates the National Commission on AIDS.

Head of NIH's National Institute of Allergy and Infectious Diseases (NIAID), Dr. Anthony Fauci, endorses parallel track policy, giving those that do not qualify for clinical trials access to experimental treatments.

AIDS activists stage several major protests about AIDS drugs during the year, including at the Golden Gate Bridge, the New York Stock Exchange, and U.S. headquarters of Burroughs Wellcome.

ABC World News Tonight: December 1, 1989. First "Day Without Art" organized by Visual AIDS to acknowledge the impact of AIDS on the arts.

Dancer and choreographer Alvin Ailey dies of AIDS.

Photographer Robert Mapplethorpe dies of AIDS.

1990 *6th International AIDS Conference ("AIDS in the Nineties: From Science to Policy"), San Francisco, CA. To protest U.S. immigration policy, domestic and international non-governmental groups boycott the conference. (The 1992 conference, scheduled to take place in Boston, is moved to Amsterdam.)*

ABC World News Tonight: April 8, 1990. Ryan White dies at the age of 18.

ABC World News Tonight: April 9, 1990. The Ryan White Comprehensive AIDS Resources Emergency (CARE) Act of 1990 is enacted by the U.S. Congress, providing federal funds for community-based care and treatment services. In the first year, it is funded at $220.5 million.

U.S. FDA approves use of AZT for pediatric AIDS.

Americans with Disabilities Act of 1990 enacted by the U.S. Congress, prohibiting discrimination against individuals with disabilities, including people living with HIV/AIDS.

First National Conference on Women and AIDS held in Boston.

"Women, AIDS and Activism," developed by ACT UP's Women's Caucus, is published, becoming the first book of its kind.

Pop artist Keith Haring dies of AIDS.

Kimberly Bergalis, of Florida, is believed to have been infected with HIV by her dentist, causing major public debate.

1991 *NBA legend Earvin "Magic" Johnson announces that he is HIV-positive and retires from basketball.*

7th International AIDS Conference ("Science Challenging AIDS"), Florence, Italy.

Housing Opportunities for People with AIDS (HOPWA) Act of 1991 enacted by the U.S. Congress, to provide housing assistance to people living with AIDS through grants to U.S. states and local communities.

U.S. CDC recommends restrictions on the practice of HIV-positive health care workers and Congress enacts law requiring states to take similar action.

ICASO (International Council of AIDS Service Organizations) forms as global network of non-governmental and community-based organizations.

Red ribbon introduced as the international symbol of AIDS awareness at the Tony Awards by Broadway Cares/Equity Fights AIDS and Visual AIDS.

Freddie Mercury, lead singer of the rock band Queen, dies of AIDS.

1992 *8th International AIDS Conference ("A World United Against AIDS"), Amsterdam; would have taken place in Boston, but was moved due to U.S. immigration ban.*

ABC World News Tonight: December 18, 1992. Teenager Ricky Ray, whose home was torched because he and his siblings were HIV-positive, dies of AIDS.

International Community of Women Living with HIV/AIDS (ICW) is founded.

FDA licenses first rapid HIV test, which provides results in as little as ten minutes.

AIDS becomes number one cause of death for U.S. men ages 25 to 44.

Mary Fisher and Bob Hattoy, each HIV-positive, address the Republican and Democratic National Conventions, respectively.

Tennis star Arthur Ashe announces he has AIDS.

1993 *President Clinton establishes White House Office of National AIDS Policy (ONAP).*

9th International AIDS Conference, Berlin, Germany.

U.S. FDA approves female condom for sale in U.S.

Women's Interagency HIV Study (WIHS) and HIV Epidemiology Study (HERS) begin; both major U.S. federally-funded research studies on women and HIV/AIDS.

President Clinton signs HIV immigration exclusion policy into law.

U.S. Congress enacts the NIH Revitalization Act, giving the OAR primary oversight of all NIH AIDS research; requires NIH and other research agencies to expand involvement of women and minorities in all research.

U.S. CDC expands case definition of AIDS to reflect fuller spectrum of the disease, including adding a condition specific to women and those more prevalent among injection drug users.

U.S. CDC initiates HIV prevention community planning process for local distribution of federal prevention funding.

"Angels in America", Tony Kushner's play about AIDS, wins the Tony Award and Pulitzer Prize.

First annual "AIDSWatch" – hundreds of community members from across the U.S. converge in Washington DC to lobby Congress for increased AIDS funding.

World class ballet dancer Rudolf Nureyev dies of AIDS.

Katrina Haslip, leading advocate for women with AIDS in prison, dies of AIDS.

1994 *U.S. Public Health Service recommends use of AZT by pregnant women to reduce perinatal transmission of HIV, based on "076" study showing up to 70% reduction in transmission.*

10th International AIDS Conference ("The Global Challenge of AIDS: Together for the Future"), Yokohama, Japan.

AIDS becomes leading cause of death for all Americans aged 25 to 44; remains so through 1995.

U.S. FDA approves an oral HIV test, the first non-blood-based antibody test for HIV.

NIH issues guidelines requiring applicants for NIH grants to address "the appropriate inclusion of women and minorities in clinical research."

Elizabeth Glaser, co-founder of the Pediatric AIDS Foundation, dies of AIDS.

Pedro Zamora, a young gay man living with HIV, appears on the cast of MTVs popular show, The Real World; dies later this year at age 22.

ABC World News Tonight: February 22, 1994. Randy Shilts, author of "And the Band Played On," dies of AIDS at age 42.

1995 *First protease inhibitor, saquinavir, approved in record time by the U.S. FDA, ushering in new era of highly active antiretroviral therapy (HAART).*

President Clinton establishes Presidential Advisory Council on HIV/AIDS.

First guidelines for the prevention of opportunistic infections in persons infected with HIV issued by U.S. CDC.

First White House Conference on HIV/AIDS.

First National HIV Testing Day created by the National Association of People with AIDS.

ABC World News Tonight: February 23, 1995. Olympic Gold Medal diver Greg Louganis discloses that he is living with HIV, leading to public debate regarding disclosure of HIV status.

Rap artist Eric Wright (Eazy-E of NWA) dies of AIDS.

1996 *11th International AIDS Conference ("One World, One Hope"), Vancouver, Canada; highlights effectiveness of HAART, creating period of optimism.*

UNAIDS begins operations; established to advocate for global action on the epidemic, and to coordinate HIV/AIDS efforts across the UN system.

Brazil begins national ARV distribution, first developing country to do so.

U.S. FDA approves first non-nucleoside reverse transcriptase inhibitor (NNRTI), nevirapine.

U.S. FDA approves HIV urine test and first HIV home testing and collection kit.

U.S. FDA approves viral load test, a new test that measures the level of HIV in the body.

The number of new AIDS cases diagnosed in the U.S. declines for first time in history of epidemic, though experience varies by sex, race and ethnicity.

HIV no longer leading cause of death for all Americans ages 25–44; remains leading cause of death for African Americans in this age group.

U.S. Congress reauthorizes the Ryan White CARE Act.

The Levine Committee, a blue ribbon advisory panel, calls for overhaul of NIH AIDS research, including stronger role for OAR and increased support for vaccine-related and investigator-initiated research.

International AIDS Vaccine Initiative (IAVI), a nongovernmental organization (NGO), forms to speed the search for an effective HIV vaccine.

Time Magazine names AIDS researcher Dr. David Ho as its "Man of the Year."

Former heavyweight boxing champion Tommy Morrison announces he is HIV-positive.

ABC World News Tonight: February 1, 1996. Interview with AIDS researcher Dr. David Ho on a new AIDS drug.

ABC World News Tonight: February 1, 1996. ABC News poll on public attitudes towards AIDS.

ABC World News Tonight: July 8, 1996. A period of optimism begins – being HIV-positive is no longer a death sentence.

ABC World News Tonight: July 8, 1996. AIDS awareness ad campaigns target everyone, not only high-risk groups.

ABC World News Tonight: July 8, 1996. Images of what the AIDS virus looks like in the body.

1997 *AIDS-related deaths in the U.S. decline by more than 40 percent compared to the prior year, largely due to HAART.*

President Clinton announces goal of finding an effective vaccine in 10 years and the creation of Dale and Betty Bumpers Vaccine Research Center.

U.S. Congress enacts FDA Modernization Act of 1997, codifying accelerated approval process, and allowing dissemination of information about off-label uses of drugs.

1998 *Minority AIDS Initiative created in U.S., after African American leaders declare a "state of emergency" and Congressional Black Caucus (CBC) calls on the Department of Health and Human Services to do the same.*

12th International AIDS Conference ("Bridging the Gap"), Geneva, Switzerland.

U.S Department of Health and Human Services issues first national guidelines for the use of antiretroviral therapy in adults.

First large scale human trials (Phase III) for an HIV vaccine begin.

Despite earlier optimism, several reports indicate growing signs of treatment failure and side effects from HAART.

Ricky Ray Hemophilia Relief Fund Act of 1998 enacted by U.S. Congress, authorizing payments to hemophiliacs infected through unscreened blood-clotting agents between 1982 and 1987.

U.S. Department of Health and Human Services Secretary Shalala determines that needle exchange programs are effective and do not encourage the use of illegal drugs, but Clinton Administration does not lift the ban on use of federal funds for such purposes.

The U.S. Supreme Court in Bragdon v. Abbot rules that the Americans with Disabilities Act covers those in earlier stages of HIV disease, not just AIDS.

Treatment Action Campaign (TAC) forms in South Africa; grassroots movement pushes for access to treatment.

Global AIDS and human rights activists Jonathan Mann and Mary Lou Clements-Mann are killed in a plane crash en route to World Health Organization in Geneva.

1999 *President Clinton announces "Leadership and Investment in Fighting an Epidemic" (LIFE) Initiative to address the global epidemic; leads to increased funding.*

First human vaccine trial in a developing country begins in Thailand.

Congressional Hispanic Caucus, with the Congressional Hispanic Caucus Institute, convenes Congressional hearing on impact of HIV/AIDS on Latino community.

Reggie Williams, founder of the National Task Force on AIDS Prevention, dies of AIDS.

2000 *13th International AIDS Conference ("Breaking the Silence"), Durban, South Africa; first to be held in a developing nation, heightens awareness of the global pandemic.*

U.S. and UN Security Councils each declare HIV/AIDS a security threat.

G8 Leaders acknowledge need for additional HIV/AIDS resources during Okinawa Meeting.

President Clinton issues Executive Order to assist developing countries in importing and producing generic forms of HIV treatments.

UNAIDS, WHO and other global health groups announce joint initiative with five major pharmaceutical manufacturers to negotiate reduced prices for AIDS drugs in developing countries.

Global AIDS and Tuberculosis Relief Act of 2000 enacted by U.S. Congress, authorizing up to $600 million for U.S. global efforts.

Millennium Development Goals, announced as part of Millennium Declaration, include reversing the spread of HIV/AIDS, malaria and TB as one of eight key goals.

U.S. Congress reauthorizes the Ryan White CARE Act for the second time.

President Clinton announces Millennium Vaccine Initiative, creating incentives for development and distribution of vaccines against HIV, TB and malaria.

U.S. CDC reports that, among men who have sex with men in the U.S., African American and Latino cases exceed those among whites.

President Clinton creates first ever Presidential Envoy for AIDS Cooperation.

U.S. CDC forms Global AIDS Program (GAP).

U.S. Department of Health and Human Services approves first state 1115 Medicaid expansion waivers for low-income people with HIV in Maine, Massachusetts and District of Columbia; in 2001, Massachusetts becomes first state to enroll new clients.

2001 *United Nations General Assembly convenes first ever special session on AIDS, "UNGASS."*

ABC World News Tonight: June 25, 2001. The state of treatment for AIDS patients.

June 5 marks 20 years since first AIDS case reported.

First Annual National Black HIV/AIDS Awareness Day in the United States.

UN Secretary-General Kofi Annan calls for a global fund, a "war chest", to fight AIDS, during African Summit on HIV/AIDS in Abuja, Nigeria.

The World Trade Organization, meeting in Doha, Qatar, announces "DOHA Agreement", to allow developing countries to buy or manufacture generic medications to meet public health crises, such as HIV/AIDS.

Newly appointed U.S. Secretary of State, Colin Powell, reaffirms U.S. statement that HIV/AIDS is a national security threat.

Generic drug manufacturers offer to produce discounted, generic forms of HIV/AIDS drugs; several major pharmaceutical manufacturers agree to offer further reduced drugs prices in developing countries.

2002 *The Global Fund to Fight AIDS, Tuberculosis, and Malaria begins operations; approves first round of grants later this year.*

ABC World News Tonight: July 7, 2002 AIDS & African Americans

HIV is leading cause of death worldwide, among those aged 15–59.

UNAIDS reports that women comprise about half of all adults living with HIV/AIDS worldwide.

14th International AIDS Conference ("Knowledge and Commitment"), Barcelona, Spain.

U.S. National Intelligence Council releases report on "Next Wave" of the Epidemic, focused on India, China, Russia, Nigeria, and Ethiopia.

Approval of OraQuick Rapid HIV-1 Antibody Test, by U.S. FDA; first rapid test to use finger prick. OraQuick granted a Clinical Laboratory Improvement Amendments (CLIA) waiver in 2003, enabling the test to be performed outside of the laboratory, allowing more widespread use.

2003 *President Bush announces PEPFAR, the President's Emergency Plan for AIDS Relief, during the State of the Union Address; PEPFAR is a five-year, $15 billion initiative to address HIV/AIDS, tuberculosis, and malaria primarily in hard hit countries.*

"3 by 5" Initiative announced by World Health Organization, to bring treatment to 3 million people by 2005.

The William J. Clinton Presidential Foundation secures price reductions for HIV/AIDS drugs from generic manufacturers, to benefit developing nations.

First Annual National Latino AIDS Awareness Day in the United States.

The South African Government announces new antiretroviral treatment program.

G8 Evian Summit includes special focus on HIV/AIDS, new commitments to the Global Fund announced.

2004 *15th International AIDS Conference ("Access for All"), Bangkok, Thailand; first to be held in Southeast Asia.*

The Global Fund to Fight AIDS, Tuberculosis, and Malaria holds first ever "Partnership Forum," in Bangkok, Thailand; 400 delegates participate.

Leaders of the Group of Eight (G8) nations call for creation of "Global HIV Vaccine Enterprise," a consortium of government and private sector groups designed to coordinate and accelerate research efforts to find an effective HIV vaccine.

U.S. Department of Health and Human Services announces expedited review process by FDA for fixed dose combination and co-packaged products – to be used by U.S. in purchasing medications under PEPFAR.

PEPFAR, President Bush's Emergency Plan for AIDS Relief, begins first round of funding.

UNAIDS launches The Global Coalition on Women and AIDS to raise the visibility of the epidemic's impact on women and girls around the world.

OraQuick Rapid HIV-1 Antibody Test approved for use with oral fluid by U.S. FDA. Oral fluid rapid test is granted a CLIA waiver.

Keith Cylar, long time AIDS activist and founder and co-president of Housing Works, Inc. in the United States, dies at age 45.

ABC World News Tonight: July 12, 2004. AIDS in China

ABC World News Tonight: July 13, 2004. Kofi Annan compares the war on terror to the war on AIDS.

2005 *U.N. General Assembly High-Level Meeting on HIV/AIDS to review progress on targets set at 2001 U.N. General Assembly Special Session on HIV/AIDS (UNGASS).*

United Kingdom hosts G8 Summit at Gleneagles; focus on development in Africa, including HIV/AIDS.

At historic and unprecedented joint press conference, the World Health Organization, UNAIDS, the United States Government, and the Global Fund to Fight AIDS, Tuberculosis and Malaria announce results of joint efforts to increase the availability of antiretroviral drugs in developing countries. An estimated 700,000 people had been reached by the end of 2004.

At World Economic Forum's Annual Meeting in Davos, Switzerland, priorities include a focus on addressing HIV/AIDS in Africa and other hard hit regions of the world.

First Annual National Asian and Pacific Islander HIV/AIDS Awareness Day in the United States.

The U.S. Food and Drug Administration grants "Tentative Approval to Generic AIDS Drug Regimen for Potential Purchase Under the President's Emergency Plan for AIDS Relief", marking first ever approval of an HIV drug regimen manufactured by a non-U.S.-based generic pharmaceutical company, under FDA's new expedited review process.

Ranbaxy becomes first Indian drug manufacturer to gain U.S. Food and Drug Administration approval to produce generic antiretroviral for PEPFAR.

2006 *June 5 marks a quarter century since first AIDS case reported.*

United Nations convenes follow-up meeting and issues progress report on the implementation of the Declaration of Commitment on HIV/AIDS.

16th International AIDS Conference ("Time to Deliver"), Toronto, Canada.

U.S. Centers for Disease Control and Prevention releases revised HIV testing recommendations for health care settings, recommending routine HIV screening for all adults, aged 13–64, and yearly screening for those at high risk.

First Eastern European and Central Asian AIDS conference (EECAAC) held (Moscow).

Russia hosts G8 Summit for first time (St. Petersburg); HIV/AIDS is addressed.

U.S. Congress reauthorizes the Ryan White CARE Act for the third time.

First Annual National Women and Girls HIV/AIDS Awareness Day in the United States.

2007 *President Bush calls on Congress to reauthorize PEPFAR at $30 billion over 5 years (White House Press Release).*

International HIV/AIDS Implementers Meeting held in Kigali, Rwanda and hosted by the Rwandan Government. It draws over 1,500 delegates from around the world to share lessons on HIV prevention, treatment, and care from the field. Co-sponsors include PEPFAR, The Global Fund, UNAIDS, WHO, the United Nations Children's Fund (UNICEF), The World Bank, and GNP+.

The World Health Organization and UNAIDS issue new guidance recommending "provider-initiated" HIV testing in health care settings.

The World Health Organization and UNAIDS recommend that "male circumcision should always be considered as part of a comprehensive HIV prevention package."

CONTRIBUTORS

Peter Aggleton is a Professor at the Thomas Coram Research Unit of the Institute of Education at the University of London. He is editor of the "Social Aspects of AIDS" and the "Sexuality, Culture and Health" series of books and of the journal "Culture, Health and Sexuality."

K. Rivet Amico is a consultant for intervention design, research methods, adherence, and statistical analyses at the Center for Health, Intervention, and Prevention at the University of Connecticut.

Helen Ruth Aspaas is Associate Professor, Bachelor of Urban Studies and Geography Program in the Wilder School of Government and Public Affairs at Virginia Commonwealth University.

Laëtitia Atlani-Duault is Associate Professor of Cultural Anthropology at Paris X Nanterre University. She has authored the books *Au Bonheur des Autres. Anthropologie de l'Aide Humanitaire* (2005) and *Humanitarian Aid in Post-Soviet Countries: An Anthropological Perspective* (2007).

Kriss Barker is Vice President for International Programs at Population Media Center, an international organization that works with broadcast media to produce entertainment-education programs. She has trained numerous media and health communication professionals in the Sabido methodology for behavior change communication.

Francisco I. Bastos is a senior researcher at the Oswaldo Cruz Foundation (FIOCRUZ), Brazil, and a physician with extensive experience working on studies about populations at high-risk of HIV infection in Brazil.

Ronald Bayer is Professor at the Center for the History and Ethics of Public Health in the Department of Sociomedical Sciences at the Columbia University Mailman School of Public Health. He serves as Co-Director of the Ethics, Policy, and Human Rights Core in the HIV Center.

Anne Rygaard Bennedsen works at the University of Copenhagen.

Jannette Berkley-Patton is a Research Assistant Professor in the Psychology Department at the University of Missouri-Kansas City. She conducts research on strategies for translating components from a randomized clinical trial focused on adherence to HIV antiretroviral therapy (Project MOTIV8) to sustainable real world applications.

Neilane Bertoni joined the Oswaldo Cruz Foundation in Brazil in 2005. He joined the Oral HIV Testing project there, first as a research assistant and then as a supervisor of fieldwork.

James F. Blanchard is Associate Professor of Community Health Sciences at the University of Manitoba (Canada), Canada Research Chair in Epidemiology and Global Public Health, and Director of Canada's National Collaborating Centre for Infectious Diseases.

Kim Blankenship is Associate Director for the Center for Interdisciplinary Research on AIDS, Associate Director of the Law, Policy and Ethics Core there, and Associate Research Scientist in Epidemiology and Public Health at Yale University.

Andrea Bradley-Ewing is a Research Associate in the Department of Psychology at the University of Missouri-Kansas City where she serves as an enhanced motivational counselor on Project MOTIV8.

Deborah J. Brief is Acting Section Chief, Substance Abuse Services in the Veterans Affairs Boston Healthcare System and director of residential and outpatient treatment programs for veterans with substance use disorders in VA Boston system. Brief is an Assistant Professor of Psychiatry at Boston University School of Medicine and Psychology at Boston University.

Scott Burris is a Professor at Temple University's Beasley School of Law. He has written extensively in the areas of HIV and public health law.

Tara L. Carruth, a social worker, is the Project Coordinator for an NIH-funded randomized clinical trial focused on adherence to HIV antiretroviral therapy (Project MOTIV8) in the Department of Psychology at the University of Missouri-Kansas City.

Patricia Case is Senior Research Scientist at the Fenway Institute in Boston, Massachusetts. Case has been collaborating on research activities such as HIV/AIDS prevention, lesbian health, and injection drug use since 1986.

Siv Cheng is Media Advisor for Internews Cambodia, an international media development organization devoted to the employment of media in emerging democracies.

Scott Clair spent five years in a joint appointment with the Hispanic Health Council, and Yale University in their Center for Interdisciplinary Research on AIDS. Clair focuses on examining HIV risk behaviors of drug users, the effects of oral HIV testing on HIV transmission beliefs, the application of social network models to risk behavior, and the dissemination of effective interventions.

Megan Comfort is a sociologist at the Center for AIDS Prevention Studies at the University of California, San Francisco. She authored *Doing Time Together: Forging Love and Family in the Shadow of the Prison* (University of Chicago Press), an ethnographic study of the social and cultural impact of incarceration on wives, fiancées, and girlfriends of male state prisoners.

Aine Costigan is a medical microbiologist at the University of Manitoba Medical College and serves as Co-Director of the Strengthening Sexually Transmitted Diseases (STD)/HIV Control in Kenya Project.

Susan Craddock is Associate Professor in Global Studies and Women's Studies at the University of Minnesota. Recent publications include "Market Incentives, Human Lives, and AIDS Vaccines," *Social Science and Medicine* 2007 and "AIDS and Ethics: Clinical Trials, Pharmaceuticals, and Global Scientific Practice," in *HIV and AIDS in Africa: Beyond Epidemiology*, E. Kalipeni, S. Craddock, J. Oppong, and J. Ghosh, eds., 2004.

Colleen P. Crittenden is a National Institutes of Health-funded Postdoctoral Fellow in the Rollins School of Public Health, Department of Behavioral Sciences and Health Education at Emory University, where she is working on the evaluation of STI/HIV prevention programs for high-risk adolescents.

Marie-Marcelle Deschamps is Secretary General of GHESKIO (Haitian Study Group on Kaposi's Sarcoma and Opportunistic Infections) and a Senior Researcher at the *Institut National de Laboratoire et de Recherches* and Cornell Infectious Disease Unit.

Jessy G. Dévieux, a clinical psychologist, is Associate Professor of Public Health at Florida International University, and Co-Director of the Florida International University AIDS Prevention Program.

Ralph J. DiClemente is Charles Howard Candler Professor of Public Health and Associate Director for Prevention Science, Emory Center for AIDS Research. He is the author of more than 200 publications, including the recent books *Handbook of Adolescent Health Risk Behaviors, Handbook of HIV Prevention; Adolescents and AIDS: A Generation in Jeopardy*, among others.

Hansjörg Dilger is an Assistant Professor at the University of Florida, Department of Anthropology and Centre for African Studies (CAS). He is author of the monograph *Living with AIDS: Illness, Death and Social Relationships in Africa* (2005; in German) and co-editor of *Anthropologies of AIDS: The Morality of Illness, Treatment and Death in Africa* (forthcoming).

Martin C. Donoghoe is currently the Senior Adviser on HIV/AIDS, Injecting Drug Use and Harm Reduction for the World Health Organization Regional Office for Europe's HIV/AIDS program.

Michael Duke, a social anthropologist, is a Research Scientist with the Prevention Research Center of the Pacific Institute for Research and Evaluation in Berkeley, California.

Ramani Durvasula is Assistant Professor of Psychology at California State Los Angeles (CSLA). Her current area of focus is the neuropsychiatric effects of HIV, and she has been doing work with HIV-positive men and women for the past seven years.

Delia Easton is Senior Research Scientist at Battelle. In addition to various positions at Hispanic Health Council, Albert Einstein Medical Center, the Philadelphia Geriatric Center, Centers for Disease Control and Prevention, and Hunter College, she was the Deputy Director of the Office of Outcomes Evaluations in the HIV/AIDS Bureau at the New York City Department of Health and Mental Hygiene.

Ruth Edwards is Senior Research Scientist and former Director of the Tri-Ethnic Center for Prevention Research at Colorado State University. She is a member of the editorial board of *Substance Use and Misuse*.

Antonio L. Estrada is Professor of Public Health and Mexican American Studies and Director of the Mexican American Studies and Research Center (MASRC) at the University of Arizona.

He is currently the Co-Principal Investigator for an EXPORT Grant from the National Center for Minority Health and Health Disparities focused on Diabetes and Substance Abuse among Mexican Americans and the Navajo.

Barbara Estrada is the owner and president of Impact Consultants, Inc. a consulting firm specializing in research and program evaluation.

Todd Faubion is a doctoral student in the Department of Geography at the University of Washington. His specific interests include health, health care access, HIV/AIDS, globalization, critical development studies, and the emerging literature surrounding HIV care and responsibility.

Amy C. Finnegan was working with the Africa Division of World Education, Boston at the time of the study on which the chapter is based.

Mary Fisher is a globally recognized artist, author and AIDS advocate. Since being the keynote speaker at the Republican National Convention in 1992, Fisher has authored five books about HIV/AIDS. In May 2006, she was appointed by the UN General Secretary as Special Representative for the Joint United Nations Program on HIV/AIDS.

Tim Frasca currently directs an AIDS program involving seven southern U.S. states. In 1988 he joined five other volunteers to form the first AIDS prevention and advocacy organization in Chile and served as its executive director from 1993 to 2000.

Samuel R. Friedman is Senior Research Fellow and the Director of the Theoretical Synthesis Core in the Center for Drug Use and HIV Research at National Development and Research Institutes, Inc. He is Associate Editor for Social Science of the *International Journal of Drug Policy* and is a published poet.

Mary M. Gerkovich is a Research Associate Professor in the Psychology Department at the University of Missouri-Kansas City. She is a co-investigator and Project Director of a NIH-funded randomized clinical trial focused on adherence to HIV antiretroviral therapy (Project MOTIV8).

Dr. Jayati Ghosh is Professor in the school of Business and Leadership at the Dominican University of California in San Rafael, CA.

Kathy Goggin is Associate Professor in the Department of Psychology at the University of Missouri—Kansas City. Together with Drs. Wilson and Gqaleni, she is currently co-leading a National Center for Complimentary and Alternative Medicine funded clinical trial to explore the safety of a traditional medication frequently used by Traditional Health Practitioners who care for HIV-positive individuals.

Nceba Gqaleni is Professor in the Department of Science and Technology/National Research Foundation Research Chair on Indigenous Health Care Systems at the Nelson R. Mandela School of Medicine at University of KwaZulu-Natal. Gqaleni serves on the Presidential Task team on Traditional Medicines and the World Health Organization (African region) Expert Committee on Traditional Medicines.

Sande Gracia Jones is an Assistant Professor in the School of Nursing at Florida International University. Her experience includes being an HIV/AIDS Adult Nurse Practitioner, and her research includes symptom management in HIV/AIDS, medication adherence/side effect management of HIV/AIDS medications, and HIV prevention.

Geeta Rao Gupta is President of the International Center for Research on Women (ICRW), a leading global authority on women's role in development, women's empowerment and the protection and fulfillment of women's human rights.

Olena Hankivsky is Associate Professor in Political Science at Simon Frasier University and a research associate at the Canadian Centre for Policy Alternatives. She is the author of *Social Policy and the Ethic of Care* (2004) and co-author of *The Dome of Silence: Sexual Harassment and Abuse in Sport* (2000).

Peter Ibembe is a medical doctor with the Family Planning Association of Uganda.

Michèle M. Jean-Gilles, clinical pediatric psychologist, is a Research Assistant Professor of Public Health in the AIDS Prevention Program of Florida International University. She is also a Health Disparities Scholar for the National Center on Minority Health and Health Disparities.

Ezekiel Kalipeni is an Associate Professor of geography and African Studies at the University of Illinois at Urbana-Champaign. Kalipeni is a population/medical/environmental geographer interested in demographic, health, environmental, and resource issues in sub-Saharan Africa. He is currently working on HIV/AIDS in Africa and population and environmental issues in Malawi.

Clair Kaplan is a Women's Healthcare Nurse Practitioner and Assistant Professor at Yale University School of Nursing. She is jointly appointed as the Director of Women's Healthcare Services at two state psychiatric hospitals and practices per diem at Planned Parenthood.

Terence M. Keane is Director of the National Center for PTSD-Behavioral Sciences Division and Associate Chief of Staff for Research and Development at VA Boston Healthcare System. He is Professor and Vice Chairman in the Division of Psychiatry at Boston University School of Medicine and holds the rank of Professor of Clinical Psychology at BU.

Robin Kearns is Professor in the School of Geography at the University of Auckland. Kearns researches the links between culture, place and health. He edits three journals: the *New Zealand Geographer, Health and Place*, and *Health and Social Care in the Community*.

Alyx Kellington is a photojournalist who has worked for clientele, such as *Newsweek, The Los Angeles Times, The New York Times, The Washington Post* and *The Boston Globe*. Alyx covered events in Central America, the Caribbean and Mexico, including the political and economic changes in Haiti from August 1992 to December 1994.

Stephen Koester is a Professor of Anthropology and Health and Behavioral Sciences and former Director of the Ph.D Program in Health and Behavioral Sciences, University of Colorado—Denver.

Zita Lazzarini co-authored *Human Rights and Public Health in the AIDS Pandemic* as well as national surveys on health information privacy, syringe-related laws, and HIV testing and counseling provisions.

JiangHong Li is a Research Associate at the Institute for Community Research in Hartford, Connecticut, where she serves as a PI, Co-PI, and Data Analyst on numerous federal funded research studies. She has over 15 years of experience in public health and social behavioral research, as well as program evaluation in both the United States and China.

Monica Malta is a psychologist and Researcher in the Social Science Department of the Sergio Arouca School of Public Health, Oswaldo Cruz Foundation, Brazil. In 2005 she was a NIDA/NIH visiting researcher in the Mental Health department of the Johns Hopkins Bloomberg School of Public Health.

David Martinez is a McNair Scholar and currently a first year graduate student in the Clinical Health Psychology Program at the University of Missouri—Kansas City.

Jonathan Mayer is Professor in the Departments of Geography, Medicine (Division of Allergy and Infectious Diseases), Epidemiology, Family Medicine, and Health Services at the University of Washington.

Virginia McCoy is a Professor of Public Health and serves as Director, Office of Public Health Practice and Director, Center for Health Research and Policy Public Health at Florida International University.

Roger McLean is a professor in the Health Economics Unit, Department of Economics at the University of the West Indies, St. Augustine, Trinidad.

Lisa Metsch is Associate Professor of Epidemiology and Public Health at the University of Miami Miller School of Medicine. She directs the Miami-Dade County and Broward County sites of CDC's National HIV Behavioral Surveillance Study.

Ami Moore is Assistant Professor of Sociology at the University of North Texas, specializing in HIV risk and caregiver issues in Western Africa.

Donald Morisky is Professor in the UCLA School of Public Health, Director of the Pre-Doctoral Training Program in the Social and Behavioral Determinants of HIV/AIDS, and Program Director of the Executive Masters of Public Health Program for Health Professionals in the Department of Community Health Sciences.

Stephen Moses is Professor in the Departments of Community Health Sciences and Medical Microbiology, and Director of the Office of International Health in the Faculty of Medicine, University of Manitoba. He is the Project Director of a large HIV/AIDS prevention and control program funded by the Bill and Melinda Gates Foundation.

Joia Mukherjee works with Partners in Health, Boston.

Jason Myers is a doctoral candidate in the department of geography at The University of Auckland. His Ph.D. dissertation uses solicited photo-diaries to construct "emotional geographies" of HIV in the context of Auckland, New Zealand.

Vinh-Kim Nguyen is Adjunct Faculty in the Department of Anthropology at McGill University.

Seth M. Noar is Assistant Professor and Associate Member of the graduate faculty in the Department of Communication at the University of Kentucky.. Noar is co-editor of *Communication Perspectives on HIV/AIDS for the 21st Century* (2007).

Lisa Norman works in the Laboratory of Viral Immunology in the AIDS Research Program and Department of Microbiology at the Ponce School of Medicine in Ponce, Puerto Rico.

John O'Neil is the Dean of the Faculty of Health Sciences at Simon Fraser University. O'Neil was a CIHR Seniour Investigator and the Chair of the Advisory Board for the Institute for Aboriginal People's Health at the Canadian Institutes for Health Research from 2000 to 2005.

Gerald M. Oppenheimer is Professor of Health and Nutritional Sciences at Brooklyn College. His research includes analysis of health services in New York City, the costs of funding health services for those with HIV/AIDS, ethical issues raised by a private health insurance system in the U.S. and by the HIV/AIDS epidemic, and the history of the HIV/AIDS epidemic in the United States and South Africa.

Joseph Oppong is Associate Professor, University of North Texas Health Sciences Center in Forth Worth. He has published widely in the field of medical geography and HIV/AIDS in Africa. He is a co-editor of *Beyond Epidemiology: HIV/AIDS in Africa* (2004).

Treena Orchard is a medical anthropologist working from the British Columbia Centre for Excellence in HIV/AIDS as part of a community-based HIV prevention project with survival sex workers in Vancouver.

Tasleem J. Padamsee is a Visiting Research Scholar at Ohio State University. Her research focuses on HIV/AIDS policy; relationships between health policy and contemporary welfare states; the roles of discourses in shaping social policy in the industrialized world; and the influences of race, class, and gender on the policy-making process.

Jean William Pape, MD, is the founding and current Director of GHESKIO (The Haitian Group for the Study of Kaposi's Sarcoma and Opportunistic Infections) in Port-au-Prince and a Professor of Medicine at Cornell University. He has received France's Legion of Honor Award for his contribution to the improvement of health and was elected to the United States National Academy of Sciences Institute of Medicine in June 2003.

Richard Parker is chair of the Department of Sociomedical Science and Director of the Center for Gender, Sexuality, and Health in the Mailman School of Public Health at Columbia University. His research focuses on the social and cultural construction of gender and sexuality, the social aspects of HIV/AIDS, and the relationship between social inequality, health, and disease. He has conducted long-term research in Brazil since the early 1980s, as well as comparative studies in Asia, Africa, North America, and other parts of Latin America and the Caribbean.

Cindy Patton holds the Canada Research Chair in Community Culture and Health at Simon Fraser University in British Columbia, where she is Professor of Women's Studies and Sociology. Her major publications include *Inventing AIDS* (1990), *Last Served? Gendering the HIV Pandemic* (1994), *Fatal Advice* (1996), *Queer Diasporas* (w/Benigno Sanchez-Eppler 2000) and *Globalizing AIDS* (2002).

Cynthia Pearson is a Research Scientist at the University of Washington in the department of psychology and a doctoral candidate in the Health Services department. Her work investigates ARV access and adherence in Mozambique.

Nancy Phaswana-Mafuya is the youngest native woman appointed Research Director in the Social Aspects of HIV/AIDS and Health at Human Sciences Research Council. She recently received a National Institutes on Drug Abuse foreign scholar award and two young scientist finalist awards by the National Science and Technology Forum.

Megan Pinkston is a doctoral candidate in the Department of Psychology at the University of Missouri—Kansas City. She is currently completing a clinical internship at University of Maryland School of Medicine and Baltimore Veterans Hospital Consortium.

Thandi Puoane is an Associate Professor at the School of Public Health, University of the Western Cape. Dr. Puoane conducts participatory action research on obesity and cardio-vascular risk reduction among Africans in the Khayelitsha Township outside of Cape Town, South Africa.

Eve Rose is Director of Programs in the Rollins School of Public Health, Department of Behavioral Sciences and Health Education at Emory University, where she currently directs several randomized controlled HIV prevention interventions funded by National Institutes of Mental Health and the Centers for Disease Control and Prevention.

Rhonda Rosenberg is Research Assistant Professor with the AIDS Prevention Program at Florida International University's Stempel School of Public Health. She has published in screening and cost/benefit issues of alcoholism prevention in primary care, and in HIV/AIDS prevention and intervention design.

Diana Rossi is Professor at the Social Sciences School and in postgraduate courses at Buenos Aires University. She is also Research Coordinator at the Intercambios Civil Association, a non-governmental organization working with drug-related problems in Buenos Aires.

Gilbert Saint-Jean is Research Assistant Professor in the Department of Epidemiology and Public Health at the University of Miami. He coordinated HIV counseling and testing services for the Miami-Dade County Health Department and served as the Coordinator of the Micossukee Tribe of Indians Health Department. He is an NIH Health Disparities Scholar.

Jessica M. Sales is Research Assistant Professor in the Rollins School of Public Health, Department of Behavioral Sciences and Health Education at Emory University, where she is working on the development and evaluation of STI/HIV risk-reducing programs for adolescents. Her expertise pertains to adolescent coping ability and psychosocial factors contributing to emotion regulation and coping in youth.

Claudia Santelices is Associate Research Scientist, Center for Health Prevention and Intervention, University of Connecticut. She is currently the project director of PHRESH, a five-year CDC-funded study on sexual behaviors and condom negotiation among African American and Puerto Rican youth in Hartford.

Susan Sherman is Associate Professor in the Department of Epidemiology. She is the co-investigator on several network oriented interventions designed to prevent viral infections among drug users in Thailand and street children in Pakistan.

Jane Simoni is Professor in Psychology at the University of Washington. Her current research includes work in Seattle, Beijing China, and among Native Americans in the United States.

Merrill Singer is Senior Research Scientist at the Center for Health, Intervention and Prevention at the University of Connecticut. He is the recipient of the Rudolph Virchow Prize, the George Foster Memorial Award in Practicing Anthropology, and the Prize for Distinguished Achievement in the Critical Study of North America.

Paul Spiegel, a medical epidemiologist, is the Senior HIV Advisor at the United Nations High Commissioner for Refugees (UNHCR) in Geneva. He is responsible for global HIV policy and programs for refugees and internally displaced persons.

Sandra Sufian is Assistant Professor of Medical Humanities and History at University of Illinois-Chicago. Her first book, *Healing the Land and the Nation: Malaria and the Zionist project in Mandatory Palestine, 1920–1947*, was published in 2007.

Steve Sussman is Professor of preventive medicine and psychology at the University of Southern California. He received the honor of Research Laureate for the American Academy of Health Behavior in 2005, and is President there (2007–2008).

Laurie Novick Sylla was a co-founder of the AIDS Council of Northeastern New York and the Community Research Initiative of New England. She is presently Research Project Director at the Yale AIDS Program and is the Connecticut Site Coordinator for the Global Campaign for Microbicides.

Kylie Thomas is a post-doctoral fellow in the Department of Fine Arts and Visual Studies at Rhodes University. She has worked on two book projects *LongLife: Positive HIV Stories* (2003) and *Nobody Ever Said AIDS: Poems and Stories from Southern Africa* (2004).

Taigy Thomas is a Research Analyst for the Orange County Health Care Agency in the Office of Quality Management. She has conducted research nationally and internationally, addressing environmental risk perceptions, HIV/AIDS risk and prevention, and perinatal substance exposure.

Nikki Thomson is a Research Assistant at the University of Missouri-Kansas City in the Department of Psychology. Thomson counsels HIV+ patients to assist them in achieving optimal adherence to antiretroviral therapy (ART) with the Project MOTIV8 study.

Anne Thurland is the Director of the Bureau of Health Education and Project Director of the Diabetes Prevention and Control Program for the Virgin Islands Department of Health. In 2002 she was elected president of the national organization, the Directors of Health Promotion and Education, and became the first minority president in 56 years and the first to serve who came from a territory.

Ashley Toombs graduated from Fairfield University in 2007 and currently works as a Peace Corps volunteer in Peru.

Lianne Urada is a doctoral candidate in Social Welfare at the University of California, Los Angeles. She is a Pre-Doctoral Training Fellow in the Social and Behavioral Determinants of HIV/AIDS Prevention, UCLA School of Public Health/Department of Community Health Sciences.

Jon Vernick is Associate Professor and Co-director of The Johns Hopkins Center for Gun Policy and Research.

Melanie J. Vielhauer is the Acting Section Chief, General Mental Health Programs, in VA Boston Healthcare System and a Clinical Instructor in Psychiatry at Boston University School of Medicine. Her primary clinical and research interests are in the areas of trauma and posttraumatic stress disorder, mood disorders, and integrated mental health and primary care services.

Karla D. Wagner is a doctoral student at the University of Southern California Keck School of Medicine. She is the Principal Investigator on a study evaluating the effectiveness of an overdose prevention program for opiate users on Skid Row in downtown Los Angeles.

Ellen Weiss is the Senior Technical Advisor for Research Utilization at the International Center for Research on Women.

Michael J. Westerhaus works at Brigham and Women's Hospital, Boston. Massachusetts.

Douglas Wilson is currently leading a clinical trial funded by the National Center for Complimentary and Alternative Medicine to explore the safety of a traditional medication frequently used by Traditional Heath Practitioners who care for HIV+ individuals in South Africa.

Yoti Zabulon works with the Department of HIV/AIDS, Lacor Hospital, Gulu, Uganda.

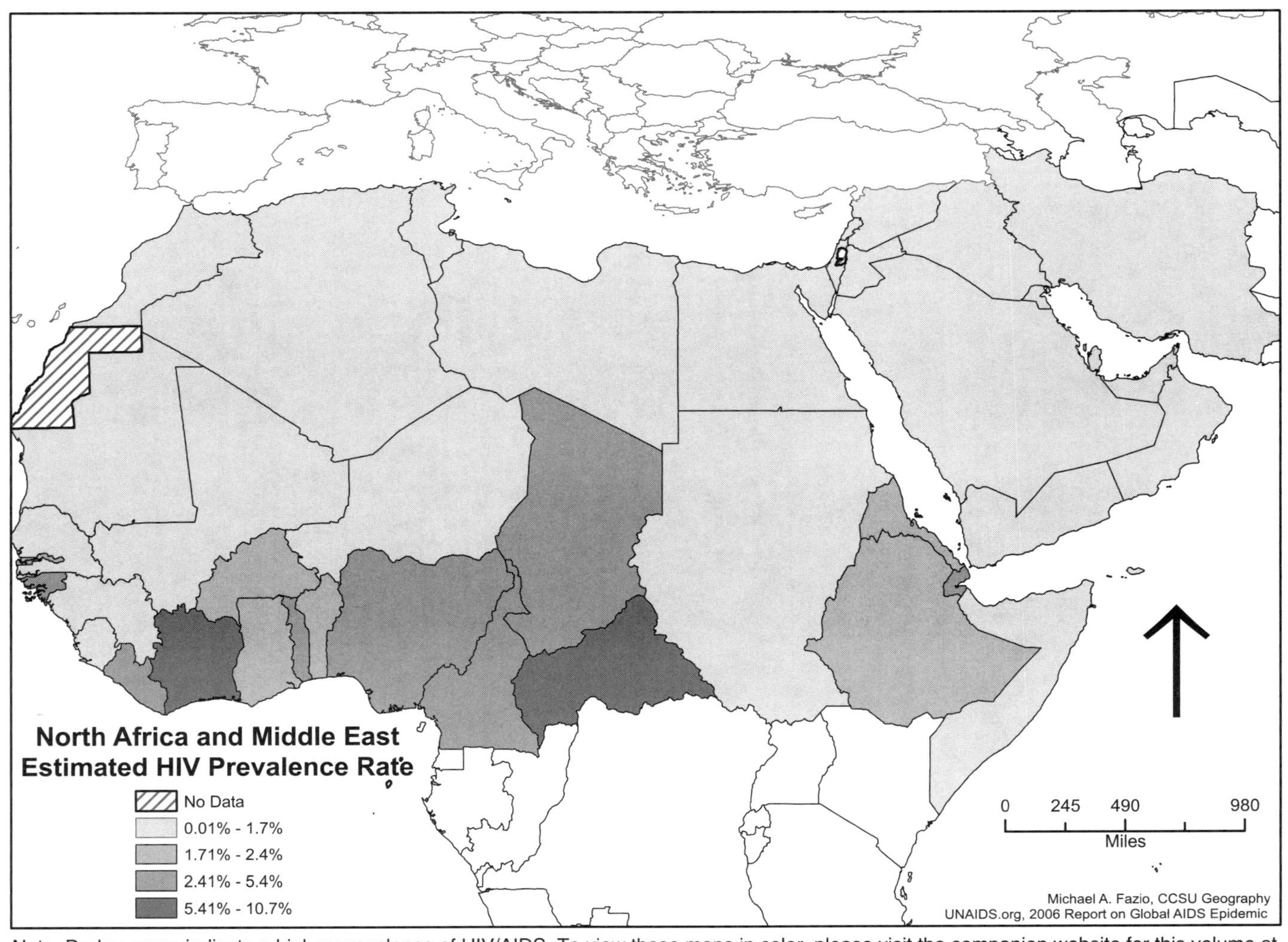

Note: Darker areas indicate a higher prevalence of HIV/AIDS. To view these maps in color, please visit the companion website for this volume at www.routledge.com/textbooks/9780415953832.

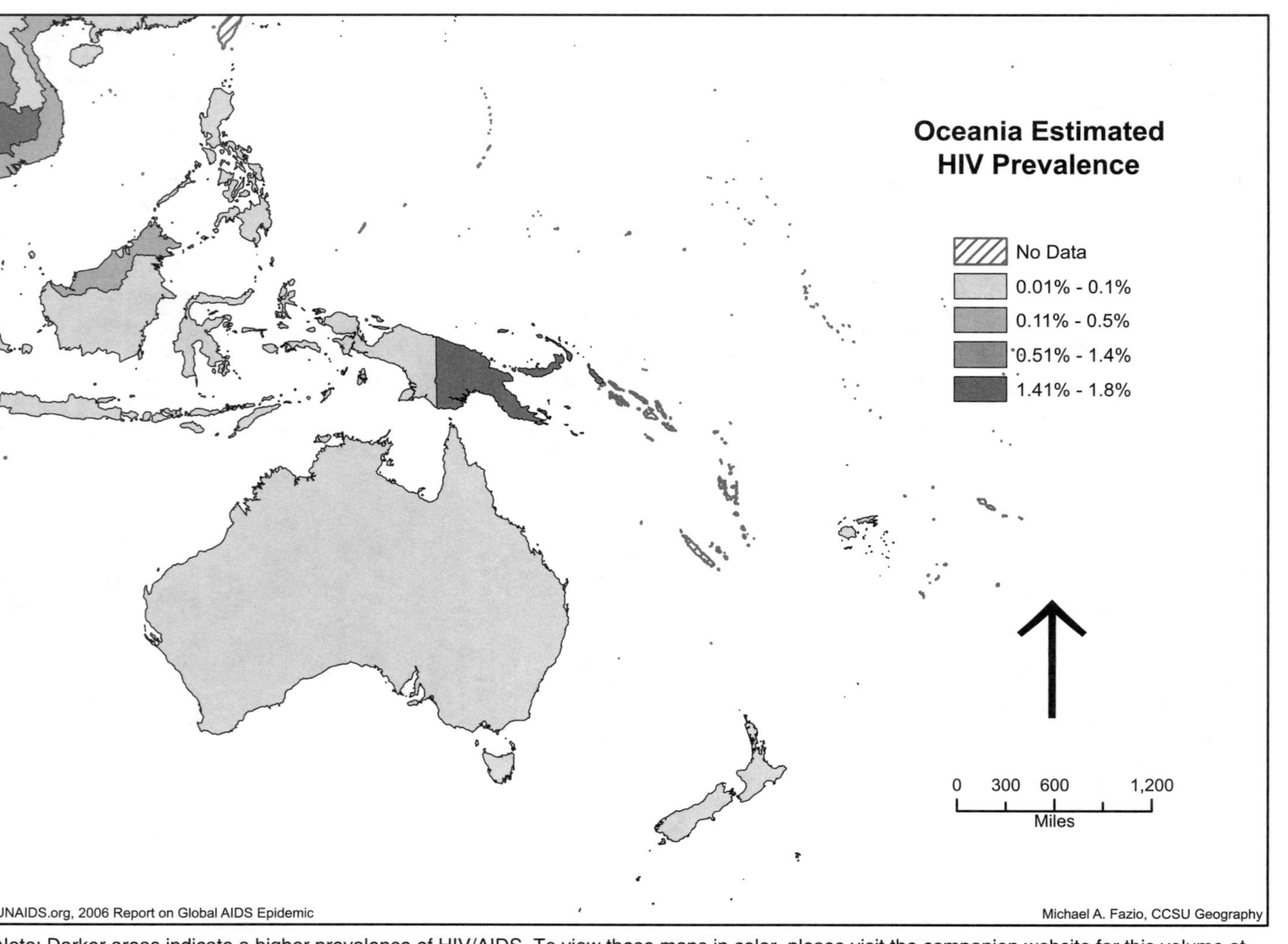

Note: Darker areas indicate a higher prevalence of HIV/AIDS. To view these maps in color, please visit the companion website for this volume at www.routledge.com/textbooks/9780415953832.

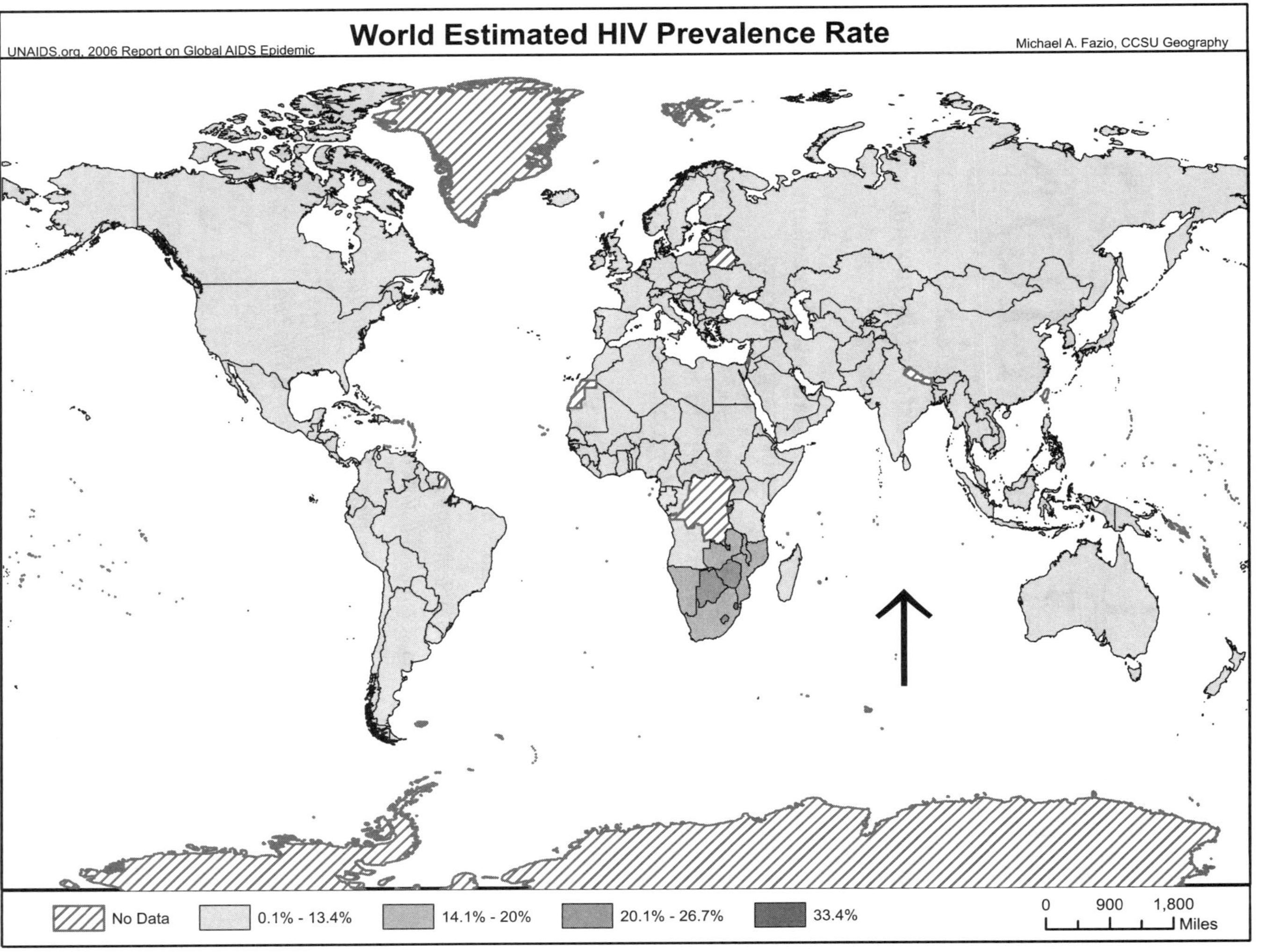

Note: Darker areas indicate a higher prevalence of HIV/AIDS. To view these maps in color, please visit the companion website for this volume at www.routledge.com/textbooks/9780415953832.